Abdominal Surgery: Clinical Perspectives

Abdominal Surgery: Clinical Perspectives

Edited by Idris Adams

hayle medical

New York

Hayle Medical,
750 Third Avenue, 9th Floor,
New York, NY 10017, USA

Visit us on the World Wide Web at:
www.haylemedical.com

ISBN: 978-1-63241-617-9

Printed in China.

Cataloging-in-Publication Data

Abdominal surgery : clinical perspectives / edited by Idris Adams.
p. cm.
Includes bibliographical references and index.
ISBN 978-1-63241-617-9
1. Abdomen--Surgery. 2. Abdomen--Diseases. 3. Gastrointestinal system--Surgery.
4. Clinical medicine. I. Adams, Idris.
RD540 .A23 2019
617.55--dc23

Table of Contents

Preface

This book has been a concerted effort by a group of academicians, researchers and scientists, who have contributed their research works for the realization of the book. This book has materialized in the wake of emerging advancements and innovations in this field. Therefore, the need of the hour was to compile all the required researches and disseminate the knowledge to a broad spectrum of people comprising of students, researchers and specialists of the field.

Abdominal surgery is a broad term encompassing a number of surgical procedures that involve the opening of the abdomen. These include appendectomy, inguinal hernia surgery, cesarean section, laparoscopy, exploratory laparoscopy, etc. There can arise complications during abdominal surgery, such as adhesions, shock, bleeding, paralytic ileus, infection, etc. Antibiotics, sterile technique, aseptic post-operative care and vigilant post-operative monitoring can reduce such complications. This book contains some path-breaking studies in the field of abdominal surgery. The various studies that are constantly contributing towards advancing practices and procedures of abdominal surgery are examined in detail in this book. It is a vital tool for all researching or studying this field as it gives incredible insights into emerging trends and concepts.

At the end of the preface, I would like to thank the authors for their brilliant chapters and the publisher for guiding us all-through the making of the book till its final stage. Also, I would like to thank my family for providing the support and encouragement throughout my academic career and research projects.

Editor

1

Methods of Patient Warming during Abdominal Surgery

Li Shao[1], Hong Zheng[3], Feng-Ju Jia[1], Hui-Qin Wang[1], Li Liu[1], Qi Sun[4], Meng-Ying An[1], Xiu-Hua Zhang[1], Hao Wen[2]*

1 Department of Operation Room, The First Teaching Hospital of Xinjiang Medical University, Urumqi, Xinjiang Uygur Autonomous Region, China, **2** Department of Surgery, The First Teaching Hospital of Xinjiang Medical University, Urumqi, Xinjiang Uygur Autonomous Region, China, **3** Department of Anesthesiology, The First Teaching Hospital of Xinjiang Medical University, Urumqi, Xinjiang Uygur Autonomous Region, China, **4** Department of Statistic Counseling, The First Teaching Hospital of Xinjiang Medical University, Urumqi, Xinjiang Uygur Autonomous Region, China

Abstract

Background: Keeping abdominal surgery patients warm is common and warming methods are needed in power outages during natural disasters. We aimed to evaluate the efficacy of low-cost, low-power warming methods for maintaining normothermia in abdominal surgery patients.

Methods: Patients (n = 160) scheduled for elective abdominal surgery were included in this prospective clinical study. Five warming methods were applied: heated blood transfusion/fluid infusion vs. unheated; wrapping patients vs. not wrapping; applying moist dressings, heated or not; surgical field rinse heated or not; and applying heating blankets or not. Patients' nasopharyngeal and rectal temperatures were recorded to evaluate warming efficacy. Significant differences were found in mean temperatures of warmed patients compared to those not warmed.

Results: When we compared temperatures of abdominal surgery patient groups receiving three specific warming methods with temperatures of control groups not receiving these methods, significant differences were revealed in temperatures maintained during the surgeries between the warmed groups and controls.

Discussion: The value of maintaining normothermia in patients undergoing abdominal surgery under general anesthesia is accepted. Three effective economical and practically applicable warming methods are combined body wrapping and heating blanket; combined body wrapping, heated moist dressings, and heating blanket; combined body wrapping, heated moist dressings, and warmed surgical rinse fluid, with or without heating blanket. These methods are practically applicable when low-cost method is indeed needed.

Editor: Sara Cheng, University of Colorado, United States of America

Funding: The authors have no support or funding to report.

Competing Interests: The authors have declared that no competing interests exist.

* E-mail: dr.wenhao@163.com

Introduction

In recent years, core body temperature has been considered one of the basic measurements in monitoring patients undergoing general anesthesia. As early as the mid-1990s, observers reported hypothermia in as many as 60% of patients during surgery, with 30% of patients having a core body temperature below 35°C [1]. As a result, complications such as ventricular tachycardia, hypertension, and increased risk of infection associated with intra- and perioperative hypothermia have come to the attention of surgeons and anesthesiologists [2], and various methods of patient warming have been promoted for clinical use to lower the risk of hypothermia associated with administering general anesthesia.

During natural disasters such as earthquakes, tsunami or major flooding, power is generally lost and alternative methods are available, including body wraps and the use of heated moist dressings as well as warmed fluids and blood transfusions and the use of heated blankets. Heating is an option with commonly used practices such as infusion of fluids, blood transfusion, and the application of body wraps, dressings, and blankets. Combinations of these warming methods may be feasible.

The purpose of the present research was to evaluate low-cost, low- or no-power, and readily available alternative warming methods for maintaining normothermia in abdominal surgery patients.

Methods

Patient Selection

The present study is a prospective study conducted in the surgical center of the First Hospital of Xinjiang Medical University, Xinjian, China. One hundred sixty patients who scheduled for elective abdominal surgery between October 2009 and May 2010 were selected. Inclusion criteria were as follows: patients between the ages of 18 and 60 with an ASA score of I or II [3]; three days of preoperative temperature within the normal range; procedure conducted under combined intravenous and inhalation anesthesia; patient in supine operative position; procedure not done *per anum*; patient able to tolerate placement of temperature sensor in nasopharynx and rectum; operation time limited to within 5 hours. Exclusion criteria were as follows: presence of systemic metabolic disease; presence of infection or abnormal body temperature three days before operation; hypothermia or shock induced by surgery; surgery interrupted by need to obtain frozen section; change in surgical method due to inconsistency between preoperative and intraoperative diagnoses; cessation or intensification of warming measures due to hyperthermia or hypothermia. Random sampling was applied to select patients for groups receiving various warming methods during surgery.

The study was approved by the ethics committee of the First Affiliated Hospital of Xinjiang Medical University. All patients who participated in the study signed informed consent forms indicating that they knew of the existence of the study, understood its purpose, and agreed to participate.

Data Collection

Data were collected for five factors (methods of warming) on two levels, one level involving heating or specific application and one without heating or specific application. Five factors were configured as follows: blood transfusions and fluid infusions were either heated or not; patients' bodies were either wrapped or not; moist dressings were heated or not; surgical field rinse was either heated or not; and heating blankets were either used or not. According to the permutations of the factors (2^5), a total of 32 combinations were set, and each group received specific combinations repeated 5 times for the total number of 160 patients (Table 1 and 2). The present study used random sampling of patients to determine groups receiving specific warming methods and a double-blind design. The double blind was carried out by having one researcher seal each envelope containing warming instructions and then having the envelope opened by a second researcher, with the operation and warming method conducted according to the instructions in the envelope.

The average normal environmental temperature of a patient in the supine position is 23°C. For this study, the core body temperature was measured by rectal temperature, which reflects the temperature of major internal organs such as the liver while the nasopharyngeal temperature reflects the temperature of the brain.

The five methods of warming were carried out as follows: 1) Blood and fluid warming: a MIR-162 electric incubator (Sanyo, Osaka, Japan) was used to warm fluid to 37°C before use; the 37°C fluid was then infused into the patient. Banked blood for transfusion was warmed to 37°C by means of a DK series water bath (Shanghai Jinghong Laboratory Instrument Co., Ltd., Shanghai, China) for half an hour. 2) Body wrap: the patient's limbs were wrapped from the lower third of the thighs to the feet; the neck and shoulders were also wrapped using lightweight pads that were not prewarmed. 3) Warmed moist dressing: the moist dressings were made of Xinjie brand surgical gauze (Kangqiang Medical Equipment Co., Urumqi, Xinjiang Uyghur Autonomous Region, China) soaked with normal saline warmed to 37°C and applied intraoperatively. 4) Warming of fluid for surgical field flush: the fluid was warmed to 37°C with an electric thermostat. 5) Heating blanket: An Astopad Plus electric blanket (Stihler Electronic, Stuttgart, Germany) was prewarmed and then set to 38.5°C and spread beneath the patient's body except for the head.

The temperature of the operating room was set at 23°C with humidity at 50%. The temperature sensors for the patient's nasopharynx and rectum were first connected to a BeneView T6 model vital signs monitor (Shenzhen Mindray Bio-Medical Electronics Co., Ltd., Shenzhen, China). Rectal and nasal probes were then inserted into awake patients. The nasopharyngeal temperature sensor was inserted into the nasopharynx as far as the distance between the inner side of the nasal ala and the earlobe. The rectal temperature sensor was inserted to a depth of more than 6 cm from the anus. The patient's age, height, and weight; preoperative temperature, heart rate, and blood pressure; fluid volume of the surgical field flush; intraoperative volumes of bleeding, blood transfusion, and fluid infusion; urine volume; and surgeon's name were recorded. Temperatures in the nasopharynx and rectum were monitored and recorded continuously from the time of patients' entrance into the operating room until completion of the surgery. Rectal and nasal probes were removed before patients leave the operating room. Nasophayngeal and rectal temperatures are those recorded at the end of surgery as described below.

Table 1. Array of the 32 groups of patients.

			D1		D2	
			E1	E2	E1	E2
A1	B1	C1	A1B1C1D1E1	A1B1C1D1E2	A1B1C1D2E1	A1B1C1D2E2
		C2	A1B1C2D1E1	A1B1C2D1E2	A1B1C2D2E1	A1B1C2D2E2
	B2	C1	A1B2C1D1E1	A1B2C1D1E2	A1B2C1D2E1	A1B2C1D2E2
		C2	A1B2C2D1E1	A1B2C2D1E2	A1B2C2D2E1	A1B2C2D2E2
A2	B1	C1	A2B1C1D1E1	A2B1C1D1E2	A2B1C1D2E1	A2B1C1D2E2
		C2	A2B1C2D1E1	A2B1C2D1E2	A2B1C2D2E1	A2B1C2D2E2
	B2	C1	A2B2C1D1E1	A2B2C1D1E2	A2B2C1D2E1	A2B2C1D2E2
		C2	A2B2C2D1E1	A2B2C2D1E2	A2B2C2D2E1	A2B2C2D2E2

Key: A1: Bood transfusion and fluid infusion not heated. A2: Blood transfusion and fluid infusion heated. B1: Patient's body not wrapped. B2: Patient's body wrapped. C1: Moist dressings not heated. C2: Moist dressings heated. D1: Surgical field rinse not heated. D2: Surgical field rinse heated. E1: Heating blanket not used. E2: Heating blanket used.

Statistical Analysis

Means and standard deviations with range or frequency and percentage were summarized for each variable unless otherwise stated. Rectal and nasopharyngeal temperatures were measured over the study period and analyzed at completion of surgery. Comparisons were performed with analysis of variance (ANOVA) with post hoc comparison adjusted by Tukey's test. Data were analyzed with SAS 9.0 software (SAS Institute Inc, Cary, NC, USA), and a *P* value <0.05 was considered statistically significant.

Results

The 160 patients selected for the study were between 18 and 60 years old; they included 82 males and 78 females. In terms of ethnicity, 116 patients were Han Chinese; 30 patients were Uyghurs; and ethnic minorities such as Kazaks included 14 patients. No complications or adverse effects were caused by the warming methods used in the study. Differences in patients' age, height, and weight; preoperative temperature, heart rate, and blood pressure; volume of fluid used to rinse the surgical field; intraoperative volumes of bleeding, blood transfusion, and fluid infusion; and patients' urine volume in each group were not considered statistically significant (Tables S1 and S2).

Postoperative Comparison of Nasopharyngeal Temperatures

The mean nasopharyngeal temperature of the group warmed by a combination of body wraps and a heating blanket was 37.3±0.51°C,- which was a statistically significantly difference compared to that of control groups A1B1C1D1E1 (Table 1), in which none of the

Table 2. Factors and levels.

Group	Factors and levels					Subject number				
1	A1,	B1,	C1,	D1	E1	27	37	87	97	139
2	A1,	B1,	C1,	D1	E2	15	36	79	100	152
3	A1,	B1,	C1,	D2	E1	13	63	95	123	136
4	A1,	B1,	C1,	D2	E2	7	40	88	121	154
5	A1,	B1,	C2,	D1	E1	32	51	67	119	135
6	A1,	B1,	C2,	D1	E2	4	53	75	128	146
7	A1,	B1,	C2,	D2	E1	18	39	85	106	159
8	A1,	B1,	C2,	D2	E2	12	35	82	105	153
9	A1,	B2,	C1,	D1	E1	30	52	92	122	157
10	A1,	B2,	C1,	D1	E2	3	50	73	126	143
11	A1,	B2,	C1,	D2	E1	5	57	86	116	158
12	A1,	B2,	C1,	D2	E2	11	45	66	127	142
13	A1,	B2,	C2,	D1	E1	23	44	90	107	129
14	A1,	B2,	C2,	D1	E2	26	55	81	120	138
15	A1,	B2,	C2,	D2	E1	2	38	74	110	160
16	A1,	B2,	C2,	D2	E2	16	60	76	98	155
17	A2,	B1,	C1,	D1	E1	22	48	68	111	130
18	A2,	B1,	C1,	D1	E2	24	43	80	113	151
19	A2,	B1,	C1,	D2	E1	8	62	70	112	131
20	A2,	B1,	C1,	D2	E2	28	46	84	114	144
21	A2,	B1,	C2,	D1	E1	21	58	91	103	149
22	A2,	B1,	C2,	D1	E2	1	54	69	108	150
23	A2,	B1,	C2,	D2	E1	29	33	94	118	148
24	A2,	B1,	C2,	D2	E2	19	61	93	104	132
25	A2,	B2,	C1,	D1	E1	9	41	78	99	147
26	A2,	B2,	C1,	D1	E2	20	59	83	102	145
27	A2,	B2,	C1,	D2	E1	17	49	77	125	140
28	A2,	B2,	C1,	D2	E2	10	47	89	117	133
29	A2,	B2,	C2,	D1	E1	25	64	72	101	141
30	A2,	B2,	C2,	D1	E2	31	42	96	109	134
31	A2,	B2,	C2,	D2	E1	14	34	71	115	156
32	A2,	B2,	C2,	D2	E2	6	56	65	124	137

warming methods were used (Table 3). $P<0.05$; this method was the most effective method of patient warming. The second most effective method of warming was a combination of body wraps, heated moist dressings, and a heating blanket. The mean nasopharyngeal temperature of patients in this group was 37.12±0.26°C, which was a statistically significant difference compared to that of control groups A1B1C1D1E1, $P<0.05$ (Figure 1). The third most effective method of warming was a combination of body wraps, heated moist dressings, warming of the surgical rinse fluid, and a heating blanket. The mean nasopharyngeal temperature of patients in this group was 37±0.33°C, which was a statistically significant difference compared to that of control groups A1B1C1D1E1, $P<0.05$ (Table 3). Figure 1 shows the measurement of temperature over time during surgery; the temperatures in the control groups A1B1C1D1E1 dropped slightly over time while temperatures were maintained in the selected groups receiving warming methods.

Postoperative Comparison of Rectal Temperatures

The mean rectal temperature of the patient group warmed by a combination of body wraps and a heating blanket was 37.44±0.5°C, which was a statistically significant difference compared to that of control groups A1B1C1D1E1, $P<0.05$. The rectal temperature of patients in the group warmed by a combination of body wraps, heated moist dressings, and a heating blanket was 37.42±0.15°C, which was a statistically significant difference compared to that of control groups A1B1C1D1E1, $P<0.05$. The rectal temperature of patients in the group warmed by a combination of body wraps, heated moist dressings, and warming of the surgical rinse fluid was 37.42±0.49°C, which was statistically significant difference compared to that of control groups A1B1C1D1E1, $P<0.05$. Similar to the record of nasopharyngeal temperatures in Figure 1, Figure 2 shows the rectal temperatures measured over time during surgery. The temperature in control group A1B1C1D1E1 dropped slightly over time

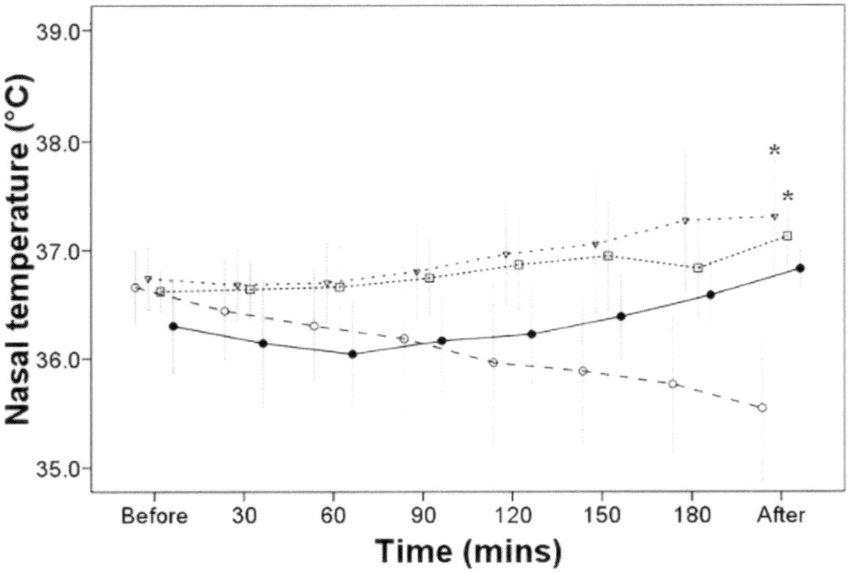

Figure 1. Selected groups of patients' nasopharyngeal temperatures during surgery. ○ Control group; ▽ Body wraps and heating blanket group; □ Body wraps, heated moist dressing, and heating blanket group; ● Heated blood transfusion and fluid infusion, body wraps, heated moist dressing, heated surgical field rinse, and heating blanket group. Mean ± SD, n = 5, *$P<0.05$ compared to control group at end of surgery after Tukey's test.

while temperatures were maintained in the selected groups receiving warming methods.

Discussion

In this study, we evaluated the use of low- or no-power, low-cost and readily available alternative warming methods to help maintain normothermia in abdominal surgery patients. When we compared temperatures of abdominal surgery patient groups receiving three specific warming methods with temperatures of control groups not receiving these methods, significant differences were revealed in temperatures maintained during the surgeries between the warmed groups and controls. The three most effective warming methods in order of levels of efficacy in maintaining normothermia were: 1) a combination of body wraps and a heating blanket, 2) a combination of body wraps, heated moist dressings, and a heating blanket, and 3) a combination of body wraps, heated moist dressings, warming of the surgical rinse fluid, and with or without a heating blanket. These methods all use less or no electric power and readily available supplies, and are inexpensive. As such they are practical and applicable for use in certain geographic areas or specific circumstances, including in power outages during natural disasters.

Core temperature can be measured in several ways based on the site of measurement. Oral sublingual temperature and rectal temperature measurements are the two most frequently used methods for measuring core temperature in thermoregulatory investigations [4]. A review of core measurement methods indicated that rectal measurement is considered the gold standard for core measurements, although it is slower to reach temperature [5]. Oral (sublingual) measures were sometimes found to be inaccurate but nasopharyngeal measurements were more reliable. Other measures such as tympanic temperature measurement, bladder and arterial measurements, and esophageal temperature measurement are not convenient and are reserved for specific clinical circumstances; esophageal temperature measurement is not advised for general core measurements because of the difficulty of inserting the thermistor and general patient discomfort. Therefore, for this study, we relied on measurements of nasopharyngeal and rectal temperatures, which are both easily measured and relatively stable.

The value of maintaining normothermia in patients undergoing abdominal surgery under general anesthesia is accepted. Mild hypothermia is recognized when the patient's core temperature is 35–36.4°C; the intraoperative incidence rate of mild hypothermia is reported to be 50%–70% [6]. Recent studies of patient safety during the perioperative period and the consequent development of relevant research have shown that there are several forms of serious impairment to the human organism when the core temperature of a patient falls below 36°C [7]. A higher incidence of cardiovascular complications is caused by hypothermia, including angina, myocardial infarction, and cardiac arrest [8]. Hypothermia inhibits blood coagulation, which may increase intraoperative blood loss. Blood loss in turn may lead to a higher rate of postoperative complications [9]. In addition, hypothermia has an impact on the immune system, which markedly increases the incidence of wound infections [10], extended hospitalization, and a worsening of the patient's prognosis [11]. A decrease in core body temperature slows the metabolism of anesthetic agents, which in turn delays the patient's recovery from general anesthesia [12]. Since hypothermia is known to increase susceptibility to complications [13], the higher risk of complications during the perioperative period, the higher rate of postoperative complications, and a prolonged stay in the hospital may lead to increases in the patient's financial burden [7]. However, extending the warming methods to the perioperative period can provide beneficial effects that may also be preventative in the sense of reducing risks, and at only minimal additional cost [13].

Hypothermia during abdominal surgery is the result of heat loss through radiation, convection, conduction, and evaporation. The operating room in our hospital is equipped with a clean laminar airflow, with room temperature set at 23°C and humidity at 50%. It is a cool environment for abdominal surgery patients, and this factor increases the loss of body heat that causes hypothermia. The use of a disinfectant fluid at low temperature prior to the operation

Table 3. Postsurgical nasopharyngeal and rectal temperatures (°C).

Group	Heated transfusion and fluid infusion	Body wraps	Heated moist dressing	Heated surgical filed rinse	Heating blanket	Nasopharyngeal temperature	Rectal temperature
1						35.54±0.65	36.02±0.65
2					Y	36.9±0.37*	37.26±0.26*
3				Y		36.32±0.91	36.62±0.71
4				Y	Y	36.1±0.96	36.5±0.97
5			Y			36.12±0.26	36.36±0.09
6			Y		Y	36.7±0.49	36.96±0.5
7			Y	Y		36.54±0.35	36.44±0.38
8			Y	Y	Y	36.74±0.52	37.06±0.49
9		Y				36.46±0.93	36.76±0.82
10		Y			Y	37.3±0.51*	37.44±0.5*
11		Y		Y		36.86±0.33	36.98±0.35
12		Y		Y	Y	36.92±0.26*	37.1±0.23
13		Y	Y			36.12±0.34	36.36±0.3
14		Y	Y		Y	37.12±0.26*	37.42±0.15*
15		Y	Y	Y		37±0.58*	37.42±0.49*
16		Y	Y	Y	Y	37±0.33*	37.38±0.49*
17	Y					36.44±0.8	36.64±0.77
18	Y				Y	36.78±0.13	37.14±0.09
19	Y			Y		36.02±0.83	36.36±0.74
20	Y			Y	Y	36.94±0.22*	37.32±0.13*
21	Y		Y			36.52±0.88	36.98±0.76
22	Y		Y		Y	36.46±0.39	36.74±0.47
23	Y		Y	Y		36.2±0.35	36.42±0.36
24	Y		Y	Y	Y	36.64±0.51	37.04±0.21
25	Y	Y				36.48±0.36	36.82±0.4
26	Y	Y			Y	36.16±0.58	36.5±0.51
27	Y	Y		Y		36.72±0.51	36.86±0.49
28	Y	Y		Y	Y	36.84±0.47	37.04±0.21
29	Y	Y	Y			36.38±0.38	36.96±0.29
30	Y	Y	Y		Y	36.92±0.42*	37.16±0.53
31	Y	Y	Y	Y		36.3±0.84	36.74±0.73
32	Y	Y	Y	Y	Y	36.82±0.18	37.04±0.21

*$P<0.05$ compared to control group after Tukey's test.

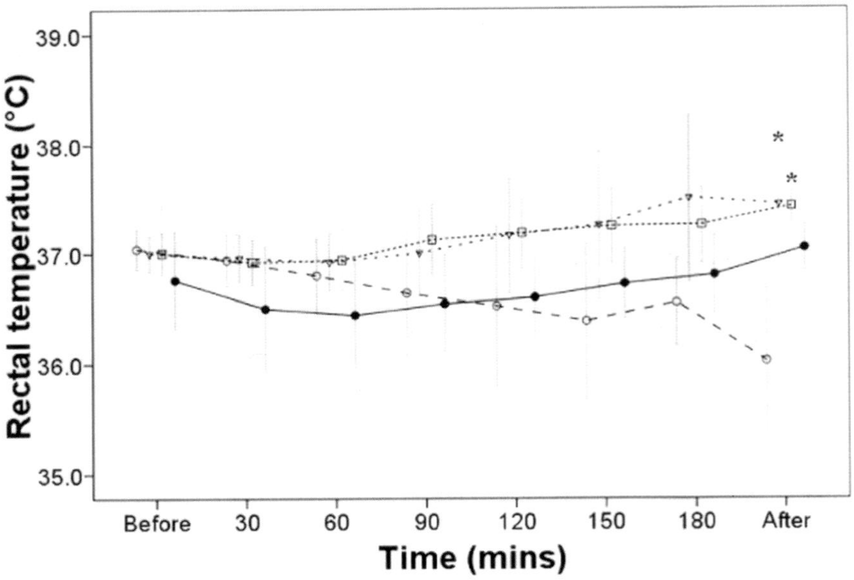

Figure 2. Selected groups of patients' rectal temperatures during surgery. ○ Control group; ▽ Body wraps and heating blanket group; □ Body wraps, heated moist dressing, and heating blanket group; ● Heated blood transfusion and fluid infusion, body wraps, heated moist dressing, heated surgical field rinse, and heating blanket group. Mean ± SD, n = 5, *$P<0.05$ compared to control group at end of surgery after Tukey's test.

leads to loss of body heat through conduction and evaporation. General anesthesia depresses the mechanisms of body thermoregulation; thus a lengthy abdominal surgical procedure that exposes the internal organs induces hypothermia. A study of the effects of intravenous fluid warming and skin surface warming for elderly patients undergoing abdominal surgery demonstrated that skin surface warming was more effective in preventing hypothermia and maintaining acid-base balance during administration of general anesthesia, although it didn't sustain normal body temperatures in these elderly patients [14].

Unintentional hypothermia occurs commonly during surgery and measures are introduced to prevent heat loss. To compensate for inadvertent hypothermia, operating rooms usually introduce some method of warming patients, including warming blankets with circulating water, air insulation blankets, or warmed fluid to maintain patients' body temperature. It is also possible, however, to work out the best methods for maintaining body temperature using traditional warming techniques instead of advanced equipment for general surgical patients in certain locations–such as the author's present hospital–that are under financial constraints. The low-cost method evaluated in this study are ideal for institutions with financial constraints; these methods use materials that are readily available in almost all operating rooms and that are easily applied, which makes them practical and applicable in circumstances in which technology-intensive methods are not available. The results of this research demonstrate that the combined use of warming measures contributes to the best outcome for patients. The loss of heat generated inside the body occurs primarily through exposure of the body surface to the surrounding environment. Since the greater portion of an abdominal surgery patient's body is exposed in a low-temperature operating room, the greatest the amount of heat lost is via the skin. Wrapping the body surface except for the sterile surgical field to reduce loss of body heat via radiation, and obstructing immediate contact between the skin and the cold environment is effective in minimizing intraoperative heat loss. The same rationale applies to the use of a heating blanket; however, a heating blanket is an active heat preserving measure that provides an environment with a relatively higher temperature than the patient's body. Heating blankets are effective in preventing loss of body heat and elevating body temperature by reducing heat loss through the skin via radiation and conduction. They even reverse the processes of radiation, conduction, and convection through the flow of heat from the blanket to the contacted skin surface. Recently, thermal suits constructed of special heat-preserving textiles were shown to be a good alternative to conventional warming measures in reducing heat loss in surgical procedures using regional anesthesia, although conventional methods such as heating blankets and

Table 4. The marginal effects of each factor is demonstrated for nasopharyngeal temperature and rectal temperature.

	Nasopharyngeal temperature, p value	Rectal temperature, p value
Heated transfusion and fluid infusion	0.445	0.814
Body wraps	0.003	0.003
Heated moist dressing	0.585	0.410
Heated surgical filed rinse	0.288	0.556
Heating blanket	<0.0001	<0.0001

warmed intravenous fluids were used simultaneously [15]. Although the thermal suits did not entirely prevent decreases in patients' body temperatures, they did so to a greater extent than in controls who received the conventional methods only. The low temperature of wet dressings is another leading contributor to intraoperative hyothermia, although moist dressings soaked with normal saline at a temperature of 37°C have the effect of a certain amount of thermal warming. Using surgical field rinse warmed to 37°C reduces the gap in temperature between the abdominal organs and the fluid, whose temperature may even be higher than that of the abdominal cavity and, as such, may help to maintain body temperature by minimizing the effects of radiation and convection between the exposed organs and the environment.

The limitation of this study is that we have compared all 32 individual groups and it wasn't powered for this approach. The proper analysis for factorial approach is to evaluate the marginal effects of each factor. From the analysis for the marginal effects of each factor (Table 4), body wraps and heating blanket are the two major factors having marginal effects. The analysis result is well fit in our conclusion.

Conclusion

We conclude that the use of a combination of body wrapping and a heating blanket is the most effective method of warming abdominal surgery patients to ensure successful anesthesia and surgery, and to reduce the risk of postoperative complications. The second most effective method is a combination of body wrapping, heated moist dressings, and a heating blanket. The third best method is a combination of body wrapping, heated moist dressings, and warmed surgical rinse fluid, with or without a heating blanket. These methods are practically applicable when low-cost methods are indeed needed.

Author Contributions

Conceived and designed the experiments: LS. Performed the experiments: F-JJ H-QW LL M-YA X-HZ. Analyzed the data: QS. Contributed reagents/materials/analysis tools: QS. Wrote the paper: LS F-JJ HW HZ.

References

1. Frank SM, Fleisher LA, Bresow MJ, Higgins MS, Olson KF, et al. (1997) Perioperative maintenance of normothermia reduces the incidence of morbid cardiac events. A randomized clinical trial. The Journal of the American Medical Association 277: 1127–1134.
2. Putzu M, Casati A, Berti M, Pagliarini G, Fanelli G (2007) Clinical complications, monitoring and management of perioperative mild hypothermia: anesthesiological features. Acta Bio Medica 78: 163–169.
3. Harling DW (1995) Consistency of ASA grading. Anaesthesia 50: 659.
4. Moran DS, Mendel L (2001) Methods for core temperature measurements. Harefuah 140: 1078–1083.
5. Sund-Levander M, Forsberg C, Wahren LK (2002) Normal oral, rectal, tympanic and axillary body temperature in adult men and women: a systematic literature review. Scand J Caring Sci 16: 122–128.
6. Liu XY, Wu XM (2003) Intraoperative hyperthermia. Chinese Journal of Anesthesiology 23: 712–714. (in Chinese).
7. Sessler DI (2001) Complications and treatment of mild hypothermia. Anesthesiology 95: 531–543.
8. Frank SM, Beattie C, Christopherson R, Norris EJ, Perler BA, et al. (1993) Unintentional hypothermia is associated with postoperative myocardial ischemia. The Perioperative Ischemia Randomized Anesthesia Trial Study Group. Anesthesiology 78: 468–476.
9. Sheng ZR (1996) Clinical Anesthesiology in Practice (3rd ed.). Shenyang: Liaoning Science and Technology Publishing House (in Chinese).
10. Kurz A, Sessler DI, Lenhardt R (1996) Perioperative normothermia to reduce the incidence of surgical-wound infection and shorten hospitalization. Study of Wound Infection and Temperature Group. New Eng J Med 334: 1209–1215.
11. Hervey GR (1988) Themoregulation. In Emslie-Smith D, Paterson C, Scratcherd T, Read N, eds. Textbook of Physiology (BDS) (11th ed) Edinburgh: Churchill-Livingstone pp510–533.
12. Sessler DI (1997) Perioperative thermoregulation and heat balance. Annals of the New York Academy of Sciences 813: 757–777.
13. Wong PF, Kumar S, Bohra A, Whetter D, Leaper DJ (2007) Randomized clinical trial of perioperative systemic warming in major elective abdominal surgery. Br J Surg 94: 421–426.
14. Park H, Yoon H (2007) A comparison of the effects of intravenous fluid warming and skin surface warming on perioperative body temperature and acid base balance of elderly patients with abdominal surgery. J Korean Acad Nurs 37: 1061–1072.
15. Hirvonen EA, Niskanen M (2011) Thermal suits as a way to keep patients warm perioperatively: a randomised trial. Eur J Anaesthesiol 28: 376–381.

2

Association between Duration of Carbon Dioxide Pneumoperitoneum during Laparoscopic Abdominal Surgery and Hepatic Injury

Hao Lai[1 ❡ ¶], **Xianwei Mo**[1 ❡ ¶], **Yang Yang**[1 ❡ ¶], **Jun Xiao**[1], **Ke He**[2], **Jiansi Chen**[1*], **Yuan Lin**[1*]

1 Department of Gastrointestinal Surgery, Affiliated Cancer Hospital of Guangxi Medical University, Nanning, Guangxi Autonomous Region, China, 2 Department of Neck and Head Surgery, Affiliated Cancer Hospital of Guangxi Medical University, Nanning, Guangxi Autonomous Region, China

Abstract

Background: The aim of this study is to accurately assess whether the duration of intraoperative carbon dioxide pneumoperitoneum (CDP) is associated with the induction of hepatic injury.

Methods: We conducted a systematic review of PubMed, Embase, and Cochrane Library databases (through February 2014) to identify case-match studies that compared high-pressure CDP with low-pressure CDP or varied the duration of CDP in patients who underwent abdominal surgery. The outcome of interest was postoperative liver function (ALT, AST, TB).

Results: Eleven comparative studies involving 2,235 participants were included. Overall, levels of ALT, AST, and TB (on postoperative days 1, 3, and 7) were significantly elevated in the study groups. However, the results of the subanalyses of those who underwent laparoscopic colorectal cancer resection (LCR) versus open colorectal cancer resection (OCR) and those who underwent laparoscopic gastric bypass (LGBP) versus open gastric bypass (OGBP) were inconsistent.

Conclusions: The current evidence suggests that the duration of CDP during laparoscopic abdominal surgery may be associated with hepatic injury. Additional large-scale, randomized, controlled trials are urgently needed to further confirm this.

Editor: Helge Bruns, University Hospital Heidelberg, Germany

Funding: These authors have no support or funding to report.

Competing Interests: The authors have declared that no competing interests exist.

* Email: Chenjiansi168@sina.cn (JSC); doctoryuanlin@sina.cn (YL)

❡ These authors contributed equally to this work.

¶ HL, XWM, and YY are co-first authors on this work.

Introduction

Laparoscopic surgery is one of the most significant surgical advances of the twentieth century. Its numerous advantages are well known: shorter hospital stays and convalescence, limited postoperative pain, more rapid recovery,, and a reduction in complications and lost working days [1,2,3,4]. However, these clinical advantages must be compared with the effects caused by the pressure and duration of carbon dioxide pneumoperitoneum (CDP) on liver function during laparoscopic abdominal surgery.

With the increasing use of laparoscopic surgery, new concerns have arisen regarding the effects of CDP on cardiovascular and respiratory systems. An important hemodynamic change is the transient reduction in hepatic blood flow caused by CDP. In 1994, Halevy et al. [5] were the first to report that the pressure created by CDP and its duration influence the degree of hepatic ischemia and can cause liver enzyme elevation.

To date, conflicting results have been reported regarding the effects of CDP on splanchnic and liver perfusion. Most reports have suggested that there is a direct correlation between duration of CDP and hepatic injury [6,7,8,9,10,11,12], but several other retrospective analyses have reported *no* effect [13,14,15,16]. These differences leave uncertainty in the surgical field regarding the effects of CDP on the induction of hepatic injury. Thus, it is important to assess all the available data and review controversial or inconclusive results.

We assumed that the duration of CDP would be associated with hepatic injury in those who underwent laparoscopic abdominal surgery. Then, we performed a systematic meta-analysis to evaluate this assumption.

Materials and Methods

Search strategy

The Pubmed, Embase, and Cochrane Library electronic databases were searched for comparative studies published up to February 2014. The following medical subject heading (MeSH) terms and words were used for the search in all possible combinations: "pneumoperitoneum," "insufflation," "aeroperitoneum," "liver function," and "hepatic function." A filter for identifying comparable studies recommended by the Cochrane Collaboration was used to filter out non-randomized studies in Pubmed and Embase [17]. A manual search of the reference lists of relevant articles was also performed. No language or time restriction was used. Data were extracted from each study by two independent reviewers (Hao Lai and Xianwei Mo). Disagreements were resolved by consensus.

Eligibility criteria

Studies were considered eligible if they met the following inclusion criteria: Study design—case-match design (random controlled trials or controlled clinical trials); population—patients undergoing laparoscopic abdominal surgery; intervention—some period of CDP in the intraoperative period; comparator—patients undergoing laparoscopic abdominal surgery with lower pressure CDP or patients undergoing open abdominal surgery; and all included studies had to report at least one of the following postoperative outcome measures: ALT, AST, TB, ALP, GGT, and Alb.

Studies were excluded if any of the following criteria were met: not a case-match design, animal experiment, primary outcome was not the one of interest, interventions other than duration of CDP, raw data could not be extracted in an appropriate format and could not be obtained from the authors or other published results.

Data extraction

Data were independently extracted from all eligible publications by two investigators (Hao Lai and Xianwei Mo) according to the aforementioned inclusion criteria. Disagreements were resolved by discussion during a consensus meeting with a third reviewer (Yuan Lin). Data extracted included first author's last name, year of publication, study design, country, type of surgery, patient population, type of CDP, and postoperative results of liver function (ALT, AST, TB, ALP, GGT, LDH, and Alb).

Outcome variables were considered suitable for analysis if they met the following criteria: continuous outcomes were reported as means and standard deviations, and the same variables were reported for a minimum of five comparison groups and a minimum of two days postoperatively. Three outcome variables were considered the most suitable for analysis: postoperative results for ALT (days 1, 3, 7), AST (days 1, 3, 7), and TB (days 1, 3, 7).

Risk of bias assessment

Risk of bias was evaluated by the reviewers using the Cochrane Handbook for Systematic Reviews of Interventions [17]. The assessment was based on sequence generation, allocation concealment, blinding, incomplete outcome data, selective outcome reporting, and other sources of bias. Agreement was achieved through discussion when necessary.

Statistical analysis

Statistical analysis for continuous variables was performed using the standard mean difference (SMD) and a random-effects or fixed-effects model was used depending on the presence or absence of heterogeneity. We used the Q-based chi-square test and the I^2 statistic to assess heterogeneity between studies, with a P-value of less than 0.10 representing statistical significance. Sensitivity and subgroup analyses were used to explore potential causes of heterogeneity. Subgroup analyses were performed to examine whether hepatic injury varied by duration of CDP and type of surgery. Publication bias was also evaluated by constructing a funnel plot with a visual assessment of asymmetry [18,19]. All analyses were performed using STATA software (ver. 9.0; Stata Corp, College Station, TX).

Results

Literature search

Figure 1 depicts a PRISMA flow chart for study inclusion and exclusion. A total of 1,132 records were retrieved from the database search and 13 were identified through manual searches of the reference lists of relevant articles. After omitting duplicate results, 1,030 records remained. Of these, 19 were selected for full-text examination. Eight of these were then excluded for the following reasons: raw data could not be extracted in an appropriate format ($n = 5$) [20,21,22,23,24], the comparator was not of interest ($n = 1$) [12], or no full text was available ($n = 2$) [25,26]. Eleven studies fulfilled the inclusion criteria and were included in the meta-analysis [6,7,8,9,10,11,13,14,15,16,27].

Study characteristics

The characteristics of the 11 studies included, which were published between 2003 and 2013, are presented in Table 1. Six studies used randomized controlled trials [6,7,9,10,14,27], and the other five used controlled clinical trials [8,11,13,15,16]. One study was conducted in China [6], one in India [7], three in Turkey [8,10,27], one in Bosnia and Herzegovina [9], two in Korea [13,16], two in Japan [11,15], and one in the United States [14]. There was a total of 1,539 patients were in the study group and 696 in the control group. The operations performed included cholecystectomy, colorectal cancer resection, distal gastrectomy, and gastric bypass. In three studies [7,9,10], laparoscopic techniques were performed with standard-pressure CDP (12–14 mmHg) in the study group and low-pressure CDP (7–10 mmHg) in the control group. In eight studies [6,8,11,13,14,15,16,27], the CDP pressure ranged from 8 to 15 mmHg in the study group, whereas it was zero (i.e., open surgery) in the control group. Among the eight studies that described the inclusion criteria for patients [6,7,8,9,10,11,13,14], seven of them presented preoperative normal serum liver enzyme values as the most common reason for inclusion [6,7,8,9,10,11,14]; the remaining studies included patients with any disease that might cause liver enzymes to be elevated preoperatively [13]. In the eight studies describing the exclusion criteria for patients, the most common reason for exclusion was the presence of any condition that might cause serum liver enzymes to be elevated in the preoperative period [6,7,8,10,14,15,16,21,27]. The outcome measures of these studies varied and included some index of postoperative liver function from days 1 to 7.

Quantitative synthesis of data

ALT. (Fig. 2. Table 2A) Ten studies described ALT results on postoperative day 1 [6,7,8,9,10,11,14,15,16,27]. ALT was not significantly elevated in the laparoscopic colorectal cancer resection (LCR) versus open colorectal cancer resection (OCR) ($SMD = -0.02$, 95% CI $= -0.23$–0.20, $P = 0.86$; $I^2 = 75.7\%$ and $P_Q = 0.02$ for heterogeneity) or the laparoscopic gastric bypass (LGBP) versus open gastric bypass (OGBP) ($SMD = -0.04$, 95% CI $= -0.70$–0.61, $P = 0.90$) subanalyses, but other subgroups showed inconsistent results. The overall pooled estimate results showed significant ALT elevations in the study groups ($SMD = 0.58$, 95% CI $= 0.48$–0.68, $P < 0.01$; $I^2 = 91.3\%$ and $P_Q < 0.01$ for heterogeneity).

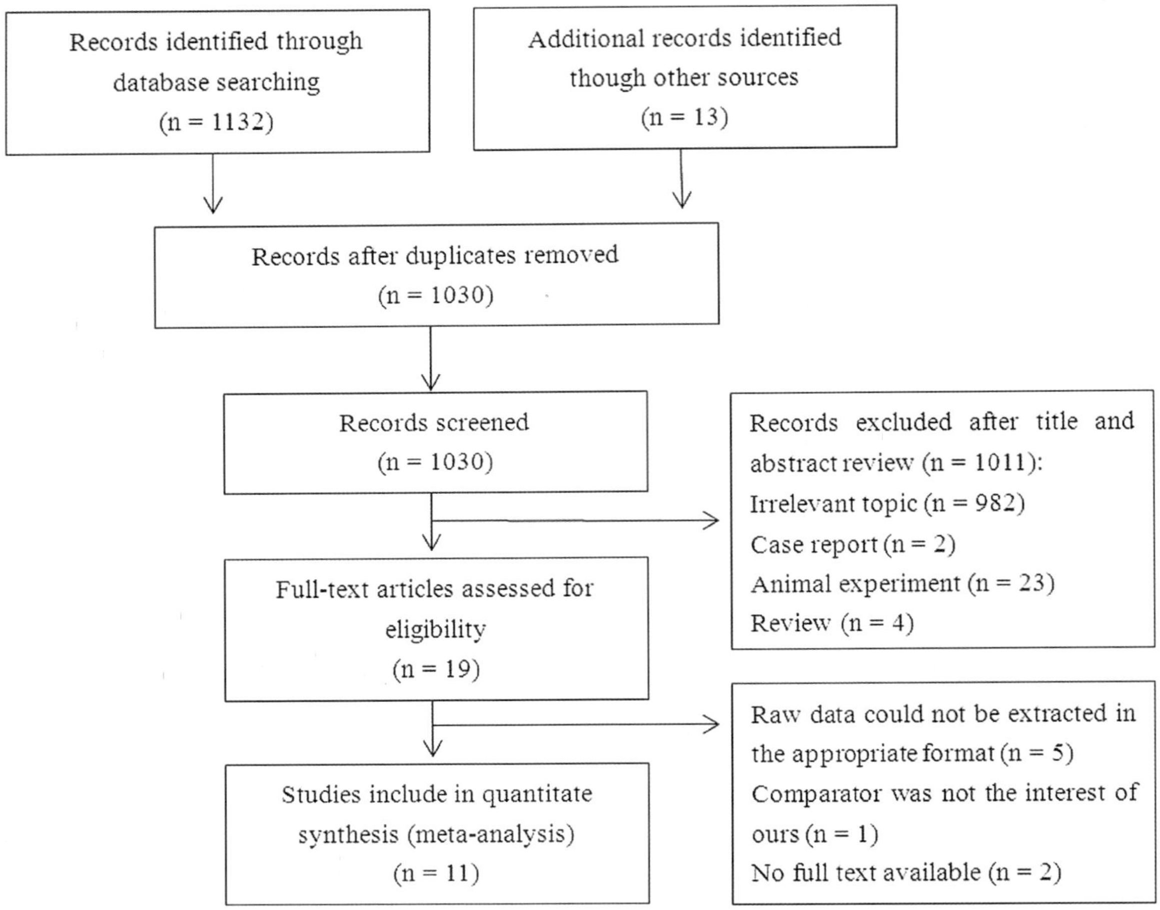

Figure 1. Flow chart for the systematic search and study selection strategy.

Four studies evaluated ALT results on postoperative day 3 [11,15,16,27] and seven studies evaluated them on postoperative day 7 [6,11,13,14,15,16,27]. Subgroup analyses showed significant elevations of ALT in all subgroups, and the overall estimated results supported this finding.

In the analyses above, there was a high degree of heterogeneity across trials. Publication bias was not evident in the results of postoperative day 1 ($P = 0.30$) or day 7 ($P = 0.36$), but it was observed in the results of postoperative day 3 ($P = 0.02$, Fig. 3B).

AST. (Fig. 4, Table 2B) Ten studies evaluated AST results on postoperative day 1 [6,7,8,9,10,11,14,15,16,27]. Subgroup analyses showed significant differences in all subgroup comparisons, except for LGBP versus OGBP ($SMD = -0.21$, 95% CI = −0.87–0.61, $P = 0.44$) and LCR versus OCR ($SMD = 0.05$, 95% CI = −0.16–0.26, $P = 0.64$; $I^2 = 0\%$ and $P_Q = 0.43$ for heterogeneity). The overall pooled estimates showed significant differences between the study and control groups ($SMD = 0.53$, 95% CI = 0.43–0.63, $P < 0.01$; $I^2 = 91.6\%$ and $P_Q < 0.01$ for heterogeneity).

Results on postoperative day 3 were reported in four studies [11,15,16,27]. Subgroup analysis continued to show significant elevations in AST in all treatment groups analyses the except LCR versus OCR comparison ($SMD = 0.09$, 95% CI = −0.14–0.32, $P = 0.44$; $I^2 = 0\%$ and $P_Q = 0.83$ for heterogeneity), and the overall estimates revealed significant differences between the study and control groups ($SMD = 0.39$, 95% CI = 0.27–0.52, $P < 0.01$; $I^2 = 96.5\%$ and $P_Q < 0.01$ for heterogeneity).

Eleven studies evaluated AST results on postoperative day 7 [6,7,8,9,10,11,13,14,15,16,27]. Most studies showed that AST was significantly elevated in the high-pressure CDP groups, and the overall estimates also supported this ($SMD = 0.53$, 95% CI = 0.43–0.63, $P < 0.01$; $I^2 = 85.9\%$ and $P_Q < 0.01$ for heterogeneity). However, no significant differences were found in the LC versus OC ($SMD = 0.35$, 95% CI = −0.04 subgroup 0.74, $P = 0.08$) and LCR versus OCR ($SMD = 0.12$, 95% CI = −0.10 subgroup 0.33, $P = 0.29$; $I^2 = 31.6\%$ and $P_Q = 0.23$ for heterogeneity) subgroup analyses.

In these analyses, there was evidence of significant heterogeneity across the trials. No publication bias was detected, with the exception of the results for postoperative day 3 (P = 0.04, Fig. 3C).

TB. (Fig. 5, Table 2C) On postoperative days 1, 3, and 7, only the LADG versus ODG subgroup analysis showed a significant TB elevation. However, the overall pooled estimates continued to show significant differences between study and control groups. In these analyses, lower heterogeneity was seen across all trials, except for the results on postoperative day 7. No publication bias was evident in the studies ($P > 0.05$).

Sensitivity analysis

The inclusion criteria for this meta-analysis were subjected to a sensitivity analysis to determine whether modification of the inclusion criteria of the meta-analysis affected the results (Fig. 3a). A single study involved in the meta-analysis was deleted each time to assess the influence of each individual data set on the pooled

Table 1. Characteristics of included studies.

First author	Study design	Country	Patients population	Type of surgery	Type of CDP	Inclusion criteria	Exclusion criteria
Tan2003	RCT	China	143 VS 40 143 VS 40 18 VS 23	LC VS OC (group 1) LC VS OC (group 2) LCR VS OCR	12–14 mmHg VS open 12–14 mmHg VS open 12–14 mmHg VS open	Patients had normal values of serum liver enzymes preoperative	Patients who underwent ERCP or EST within one week preoperative; Patients who developed complications which might cause serum liver enzymes elevated
Gupta2013	RCT	India	51 VS 50	LC VS LC	14 mmHg VS 8 mmHg	Patients with normal preoperative LFTs	Patients with a history of jaundice, with common bile duct stones, or with abnormal preoperative LFTs
Güven2007	CCT	Turkey	267 VS 54	LC VS OC	12–14 mmHg VS open	Patients with fully completed data on results of liver function test	Patients who with disease which might cause serum liver enzymes elevated preoperative
Hasukic2005	RCT	Tuzla	25 VS 25	LC VS LC	14 mmHg VS 7 mmHg	Patients without history of previous liver diseases and exhibited normal values on preoperative liver function tests.	Patients who with disease which might cause serum liver enzymes elevated preoperative; age ≤18 years, pregnancy and lactation, previous extensive abdominal surgery, and an ASA grade of 3 or more.
Eryılmaz2012	RCT	Turkey	23 VS 20	LC VS LC	14 mmHg VS 10 mmHg	ASA physical status I or II patients	Patients with liver failure, coagulopathy, and known allergy to medication drugs
Sakorafas2005	RCT	Turkey	72 VS 36	LC VS OC	14 mmHg VS open	NA	Patients who with disease or complication which might cause serum liver enzymes elevated in perioperative period
Jeong2011	CCT	Korea	91 VS 124 43 VS 78	LADG VS ODG LCR VS OCR	12 mmHg VS open 12 mmHg VS open	NA	Patients underwent any surgical technique which might affect their liver function during surgery.
Kinjo2011	CCT	Japan	199 VS/120 324 VS 56	LADG VS ODG LCR VS OCR	8 mmHg VS open 8 mmHg VS open	NA	Patients with liver tumor, hepatic disease or whose liver function were abnormal preoperative
Yoon2011	CCT	Korea	18 VS 32	LADG VS ODG	12 mmHg VS open	Liver cirrhosis patients; fatty liver patients, healthy hepatitis B virus carriers; and healthy hepatitis C virus carriers.	NA
Etoh2007	CCT	Japan	147 VS 58	LADG VS ODG	10 mmHg VS open	LADG was selected for tumors limited to the mucosal layer or superficial submucosal layer and ODG for those invading deep submucosal layer.	NA
Nguyen2003	RCT	USA	18 VS 18	LGBP VS OGBP	15 mmHg VS open	Patients being evaluated for surgical treatment of morbid obesity	Patients who had undergone previous obesity or gastric surgery, had a large abdominal ventral hernia, or a history of cirrhosis

Note: ASA: American Society of Anesthesiology; LC: laparoscopic cholecystectomy; OC: open cholecystectomy; LCR: laparoscopic colorectal cancer resection; OCR: open colorectal cancer resection; LADG: laparoscopic assisted distal gastrectomy; OADG: open assisted distal gastrectomy; LGBP: laparoscopic gastric bypass; OGBP: open gastric bypass; NA: not available;

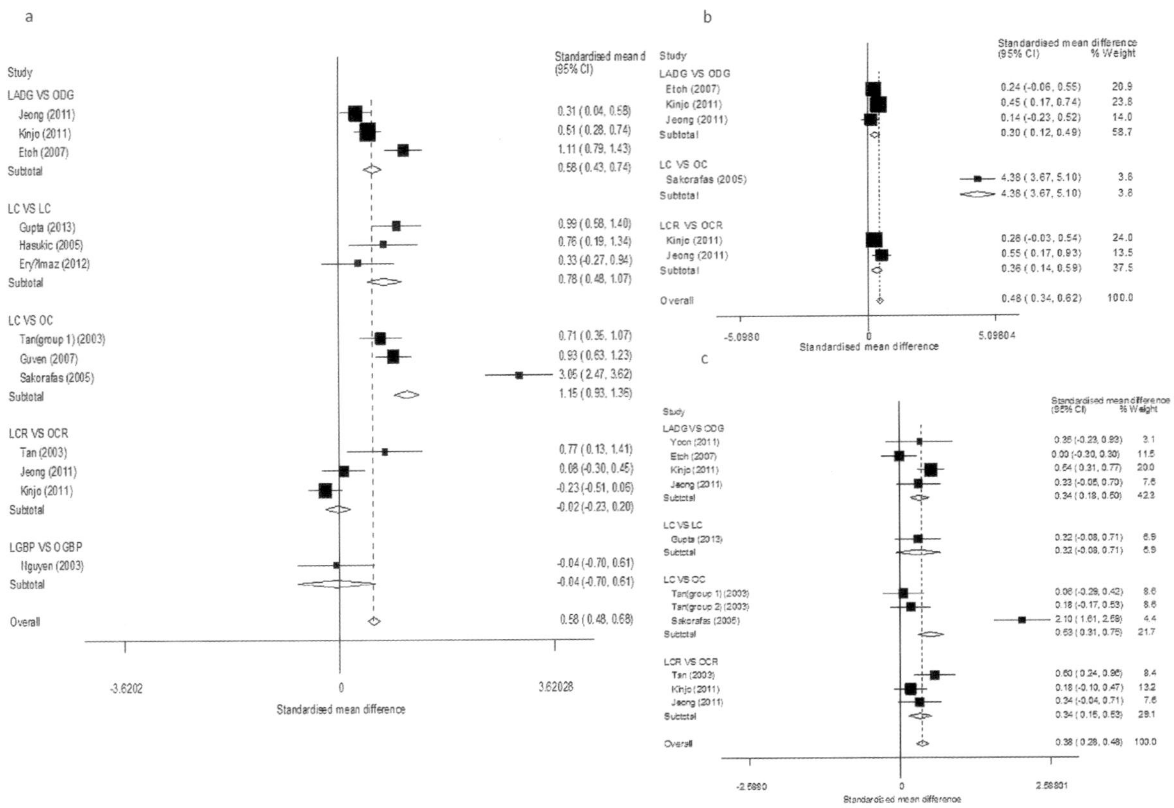

Figure 2. Forest plots of postoperative ALT results in subgroup analysis. (a: day 1; b: day 3; c: day 7).

SMDs. The corresponding pooled SMDs were essentially unaltered (data not shown), thereby indicating that our results were statistically sound.

Risk of publication bias

Funnel plots of the studies included in our outcome analysis of the postoperative results regarding ALT, AST, and TB were prepared to assess publication bias. The funnel plot showed the CI and effect estimate. The latter showed a symmetrical distribution around the effect estimate, thereby indicating that publication bias was likely minimal for the results evaluating postoperative liver function in patients who underwent laparoscopic abdominal surgery ($P>0.05$).

However, publication bias was evident in the ALT ($P=0.02$, Fig. 3b) and AST results ($P=0.04$, Fig. 3c) on postoperative day 3. This may have been because of the limited number of studies that evaluated these outcomes on postoperative day 3. The funnel plot should be interpreted with some caution. Linear regression analysis was not conducted to determine funnel plot asymmetry, because none of the dichotomous outcomes were included in a sufficient number of trials for this method.

Discussion

Presently, the association between the duration of CDP in laparoscopic abdominal surgery and hepatic injury is not fully understood. Increasing evidence suggests that the duration of CDP may be associated with reduced hepatic blood flow and induce hepatic injury. However, other studies have suggested that elevated liver enzyme values may be caused by direct liver manipulation or aberrant hepatic artery ligation rather than CDP [16]. Brundell *et al.* even suggested that duration of CDP had *no* effect on hepatic blood flow [28]. Our meta-analysis of 11 comparative studies provides evidence that the duration of CDP in laparoscopic abdominal surgery is associated with hepatic injury.

"The higher the pressure, the better the view" used to be the axiom of surgeons who needed adequate exposure for laparoscopic procedures. To provide good exposure of the surgical field, generally 10 to 15 mmHg pressure ranges are used during pneumoperitoneum [27,29,30]. However, when CDP is created, there may be some side effects [31,32]. The primary mechanism for elevation of liver enzymes after laparoscopic abdominal surgery is likely due to the increased intra-abdominal pressure and its effects on portal venous flow. The 11–15 mmHg of CO_2 that is used is higher than the normal portal blood pressure of 7–10 mmHg, which results in reduced portal blood flow [33,34,35,36]. On this occasion, free radicals are generated at the end of a laparoscopic procedure, possibly as a result of an ischaemia-reperfusion phenomenon induced by the inflation and deflation of the pneumoperitoneum [27]. Free radicals can damage tissues and organs, particularly the Kupffer and the endothelial cells of the hepatic sinusoids [37]. Therefore, the elevated intra-abdominal pressure due to pneumoperitoneum may be responsible for the increase in liver enzymes after laparoscopic abdominal surgery. However, other unmeasured confounding factors may also be responsible for elevation of liver enzymes, such as extended liver traction in large laparoscopy procedure that lead to hepatocyte damage [16], and the intraoperative "squeeze" pressure effect on the liver that free liver enzymes into the blood stream [6]. This mechanism remains to be further confirmed in animal models.

Table 2. Results of pools SMDs and test for heterogeneity.

a		Test for heterogeneity			b		Test for heterogeneity			c		Test for heterogeneity		
Subgroups	**Pools SMDs**	*P*	I^2	P_Q	**Subgroups**	**Pools SMDs**	*P*	I^2	P_Q	**Subgroups**	**Pools SMDs**	*P*	I^2	P_Q
Results for postoperative day 1					Results for postoperative day 1					Results for postoperative day 1				
LADG vs. ODG	0.58 (0.43, 0.74)	0.00	86.2%	0.00	LADG vs. ODG	0.51 (0.36, 0.66)	0.00	84.4%	0.00	LADG vs. ODG	0.34 (0.18, 0.51)	0.00	0%	0.50
LC vs. LC	0.78 (0.48, 1.07)	0.00	34.9%	0.22	LC vs. LC	0.82 (0.52, 1.11)	0.00	69.7%	0.04	LC vs. LC	0.28(−0.01, 0.56)	0.06	34.9%	0.22
LC vs. OC	1.15 (0.93, 1.36)	0.00	96%	0.00	LC vs. OC	0.97 (0.76, 1.19)	0.00	97.4%	0.00	LCR vs. OCR	0.11(−0.12, 0.33)	0.35	34.2%	0.22
LCR vs. OCR	−0.02 (−0.23, 0.20)	0.86	75.7%	0.02	LCR vs. OCR	0.05 (−0.16, 0.26)	0.64	0%	0.43	Overall	0.26 (0.15, 0.39)	0.00	12.6%	0.33
LGBP vs. OGBP	−0.04(−0.70, 0.61)	0.90	-	-	LGBP vs. OGBP	−0.21(−0.87,0.61)	0.44	-	-					
Overall	0.58 (0.48, 0.68)	0.00	91.3%	0.00	Overall	0.53 (0.43, 0.63)	0.00	91.6%	0.00					
Results for postoperative day 3					Results for postoperative day 3					Results for postoperative day 3				
LADG vs. ODG	0.31 (0.12, 0.49)	0.00	0%	0.39	LADG vs. ODG	0.35 (0.19, 0.50)	0.00	85.4%	0.00	LADG vs. ODG	0.38(0.22, 0.55)	0.00	0%	0.55
LC vs. OC	4.39 (3.67, 5.10)	0.00	-	-	LC vs. OC	4.43 (3.71, 5.14)	0.00	-	-	LCR vs. OCR	0.08(−0.15, 0.30)	0.50	0%	0.37
LCR vs. OCR	−0.36 (−0.14, 0.59)	0.00	33.1%	0.22	LCR vs. OCR	0.09 (−0.14, 0.32)	0.44	0%	0.83	Overall	0.39 (0.27, 0.52)	0.00	38.6%	0.16
Overall	0.48 (0.34, 0.62)	0.00	95.9%	0.00	Overall	0.39 (0.27, 0.52)	0.00	96.5%	0.00					
Results for postoperative day 7					Results for postoperative day 7					Results for postoperative day 7				
LADG vs. ODG	0.34 (0.18, 0.50)	0.00	61.2%	0.05	LADG vs. ODG	0.09(−0.06, 0.23)	0.00	0%	0.87	LADG vs. ODG	0.22(0.06, 0.38)	0.01	73%	0.01
LC vs. LC	0.32 (−0.08, 0.71)	0.11	-	-	LC vs. LC	0.35 (−0.04, 0.74)	0.08	-	-	LC vs. LC	−0.06(−0.45,0.34)	0.78	-	-
LC vs. OC	0.53 (0.31, 0.75)	0.00	96%	0.00	LC vs. OC	0.41 (0.19, 0.63)	0.00	96.7%	0.00	LCR vs. OCR	0.18(−0.05, 0.41)	0.12	76.8%	0.04
LCR vs. OCR	0.34 (0.15, 0.53)	0.00	38.3%	0.20	LCR vs. OCR	0.12 (−0.10, 0.33)	0.29	31.6%	0.23	Overall	0.18 (0.06, 0.30)	0.00	64.8%	0.01
Overall	0.38 (0.28, 0.48)	0.00	84.1%	0.00	Overall	0.53 (0.43, 0.63)	0.00	85.9%	0.00					

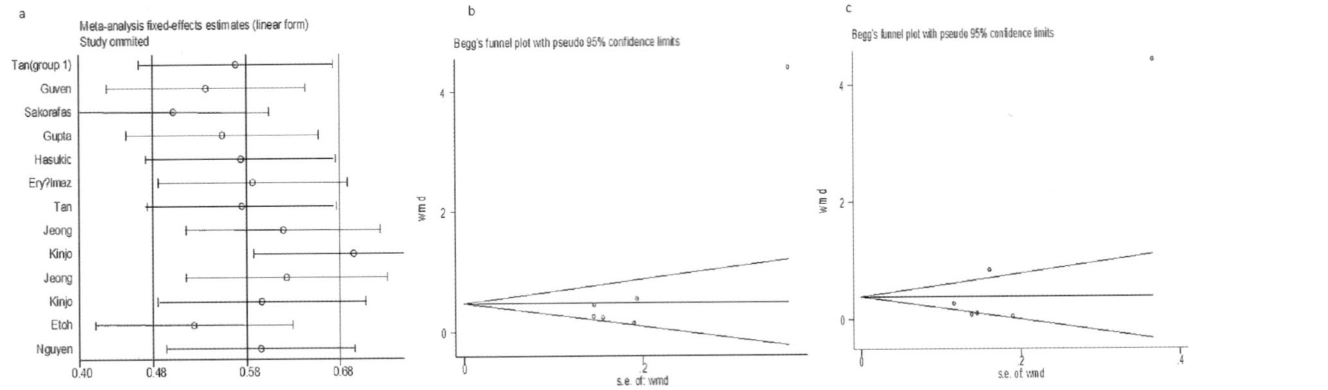

Figure 3. a. Sensitivity analysis. b. Funnel plot analysis to detect publication bias for ALT results on postoperative day 3; each point represents a separate study for the indicated association. c, Funnel plot analysis to detect publication bias for AST results on postoperative day 3; each point represents a separate study for the indicated association.

Generally, this effect might be positively correlated with the pressure of CDP and its duration [20]. For example, the higher elevation of hepatic transaminases after LGBP (six-fold) than LC (two-fold) may reflect the longer operative time for LGBP [14]. However, not all results demonstrated this trend. This heterogeneity is a problem in the interpretation of the results as the studies were very heterogeneous (Table 2).

We performed a sensitivity analysis on the subgroup analyses. The LCR versus OCR subgroup analysis always produced contrary results. The study conducted by Kinjo *et al.* examined a lower pressure of CDP (8 mmHg) in the subgroup analysis and included a larger population ($n = 324$) in the study group than other studies (Table 1) [15]. However, omitting this study did not yield discordant postoperative results, eliminate the statistical significance of the results ($P>0.05$), or reduce the degree of heterogeneity ($I^2 = 70.7\%$). Sensitivity analysis showed that the studies conducted by Guven *et al.*, Etoh *et al.*, and Sakorafas *et al.* exerted a major impact on our results [8,11,27]. Omitting these three studies from the analysis did not increase the trend seen with regard to the relationship between the duration of CDP and postoperative liver function nor did it eliminate the statistical significance of the results. The control groups in three studies included those who underwent laparoscopic surgery with low-pressure CDP (7–10 mmHg) [7,9,10], whereas the remaining studies included those who underwent open surgery. The results for the cohorts were analyzed separately in the subgroup analysis.

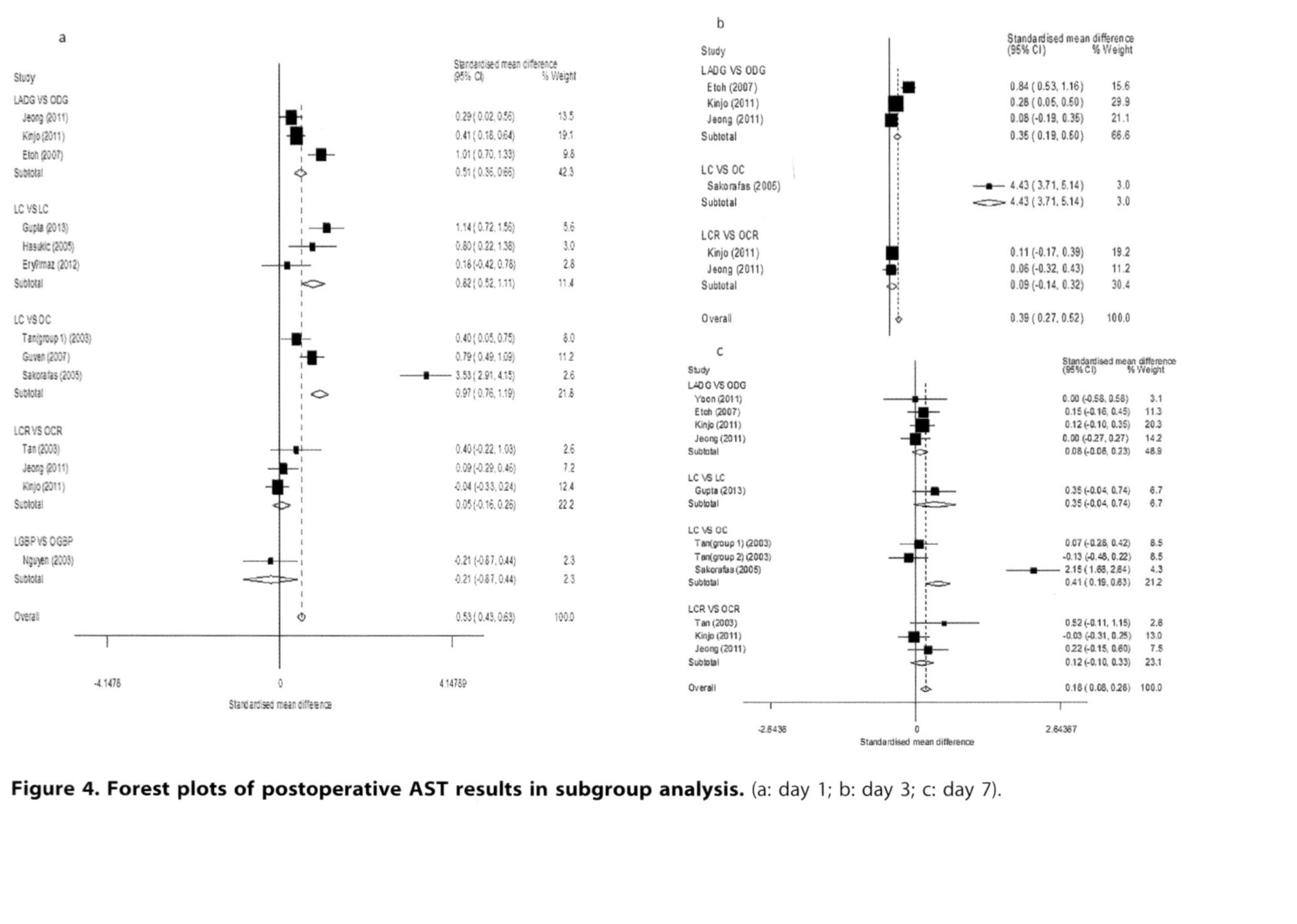

Figure 4. Forest plots of postoperative AST results in subgroup analysis. (a: day 1; b: day 3; c: day 7).

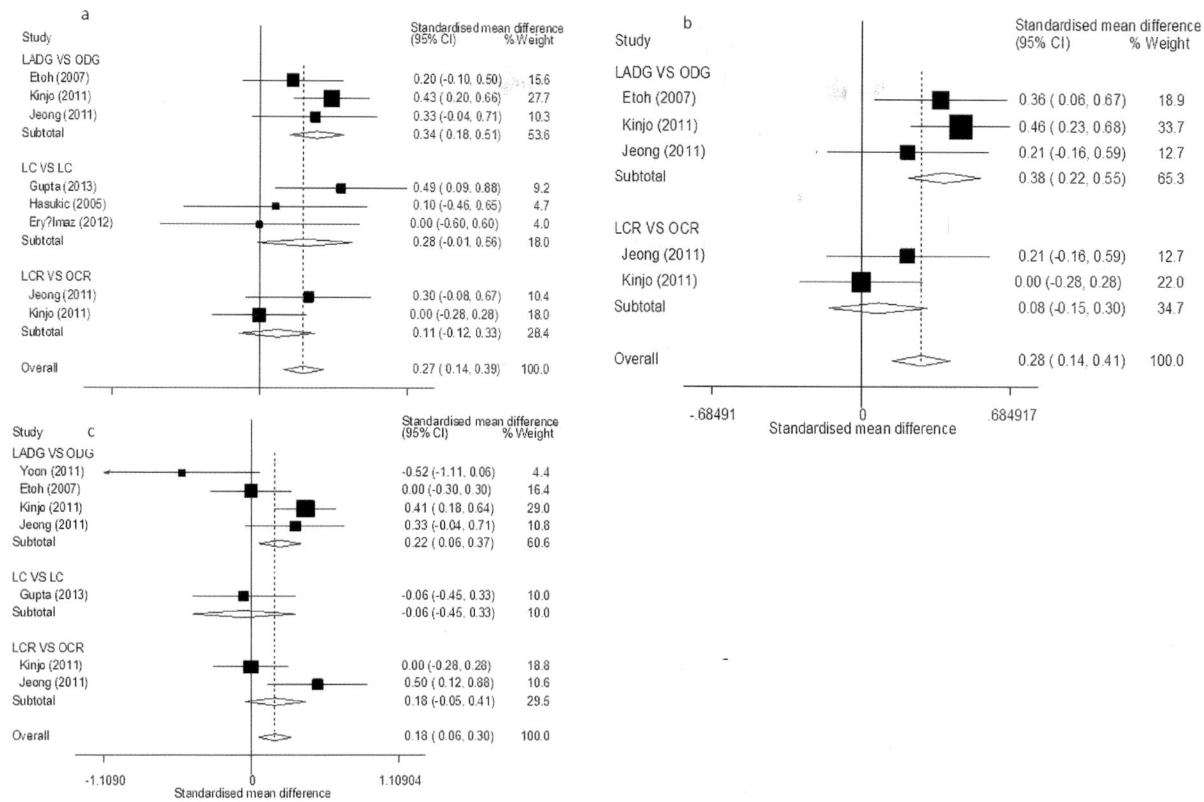

Figure 5. Forest plots of postoperative TB results in subgroup analysis. (a: day 1; b: day 3; c: day 7).

However, no trend toward higher statistical significance in the laparoscopic surgery group versus the open surgery group was found.

Explanations for these differing results of the subgroup analyses may include that the small numbers of cases in some studies and the limited number of trials in the subgroup analyses increased the possibility that chance alone accounted for the results. Additionally, the CDP used for patients in the study groups was not uniform. For example, three studies involved LCR versus OCR, and these showed inconsistent results [6,15,16]. However, the study conducted by Kinjo *et al.* involved 8 mmHg CDP for patients in the study group, which is approximately equal to the normal portal blood pressure (7–10 mmHg) [15]; thus, hepatic blood flow may not have always been reduced intraoperatively. In contrast, in the two other studies, the CDP pressure was 12–14 mmHg in the study groups [6,16], thereby leading to reduced hepatic blood flow. Our meta-analysis showed that the postoperative liver enzyme elevation was significant in "small" laparoscopic surgical procedures, but that a significant difference was rarely found in "larger" surgeries, such as LGBP versus OGBP. Thus, it is possible that the potential mechanisms for the postoperative elevation of liver enzymes after laparoscopic surgery in these procedures are not limited to reduced portal blood flow due to CDP; they may also include the effects of anesthetic drugs and/or local hepatic parenchymal injury from the mechanical retraction of the left lobe of the liver [14], especially given that the open control groups in these studies showed similar side effects. This was demonstrated by Clarke *et al.* [38], who found that liver enzymes increased two-fold after open gastric and biliary surgery, but that no change was seen after "small" surgical procedures, such as cystoscopy and a superficial biopsy.

We included several abdominal surgeries and then performed subgroup analyses regarding the duration of CDP according to type of surgery or control group. There is sufficient evidence in the 11 comparative studies to conclude that the duration of CDP is associated with the induction of hepatic injury in patients undergoing laparoscopic abdominal surgery.

To the best of our knowledge, this is the first reported meta-analysis to systematically evaluate the relationship between the duration of CDP and hepatic injury and to demonstrate a significant effect in this regard. Despite the variation in the results of individual studies, the accumulating evidence and large sample provided the statistical power to produce more precise and reliable efficiency estimates. Overall, the published evidence supports the assumption that the duration of CDP is associated with the induction of hepatic injury. Therefore, surgeons should pay attention to the following take home messages. First, surgeons should be cautious before planning to perform laparoscopic abdominal surgery in patients with known hepatic insufficiency. Second, we recommend using low pressure CDP (10 mmHg or lower), particularly for those undergoing prolonged laparoscopic surgery. This is because low-pressure CDP is not only feasible for decreasing hemodynamic variations but also add on to already existing benefits of endoscopic surgery [7]. Third, the potential occurrence of hepatic dysfunction should be carefully monitored after laparoscopic abdominal surgery in patients with chronic hepatic disease.

Our meta-analysis has several limitations. First, the interesting aspect of our study is the significance of this transient abnormality of liver enzymes and its clinical impact. Most studies reported that a transient increase in serum transaminase activities was most prominent on postoperative day 1, but returned to normal levels within several days after surgery [6,8,16,29,39]. Further, in some studies [8], elevated liver enzymes are not always consistently elevated; significant elevations after high-pressure CDP laparoscopic surgery compared with low-pressure CDP laparoscopic surgery or open surgery has been defined for only AST and ALT levels. Additionally, these liver enzyme alterations observed after laparoscopic abdominal surgery have not been reported to be clinically important in some studies [6,20,27,29]. Since most of the studies included in our meta-analysis [6,7,8,10,11,14] mentioned preoperative normal serum liver enzyme values as the most common reason for inclusion for patients, we cannot precisely conclude that these enzyme changes reflect a true hepatic injury in these patients, but this may be more relevant in patients with chronic liver disease like cirrhosis. This aspect needs to be investigated in future. Although the clinical importance of these enzyme elevations has not been fully clarified, surgeons should be cautious, as we suggested earlier. Second, the study design, type of CDP used for patients in the study groups, and inclusion and exclusion criteria were frequently not uniform (Table 2), thereby leading to the potential for bias. Third, several included studies had small sample sizes [7,9,10,13,14], and the types of surgery were limited. Thus, larger-scale, multi-center trials focusing on other types of surgery, such as laparoscopic appendectomies and hysterectomies, are required to provide evidence that the duration of CDP can be associated with the induction of hepatic injury. Fourth, substantial heterogeneity was present among the studies, and residual confounding is a concern. Uncontrolled or unmeasured confounding factors, such as the effects of anesthetic drugs and local hepatic parenchymal injury from mechanical retraction of the left lobe of the liver, can potentially produce biases. Unfortunately, several studies did not fully describe all their procedures. Furthermore, because currently available data on the effects of the duration of CDP in laparoscopic surgery are sparse, we were unable to assess this fully.

Conclusions

The current evidence suggests that the duration of CDP during laparoscopic abdominal surgery may be associated with hepatic injury. Additional large-scale, randomized, controlled trials are urgently needed to further confirm this.

Author Contributions

Conceived and designed the experiments: YL. Performed the experiments: HL XWM YY. Analyzed the data: HL XWM YY. Contributed reagents/materials/analysis tools: JX KH JSC. Contributed to the writing of the manuscript: HL XWM YY.

References

1. Li X, Zhang J, Sang L, Zhang W, Chu Z, et al. (2010) Laparoscopic versus conventional appendectomy–a meta-analysis of randomized controlled trials. BMC Gastroenterol 10: 129.
2. Markar SR, Blackburn S, Cobb R, Karthikesalingam A, Evans J, et al. (2012) Laparoscopic versus open appendectomy for complicated and uncomplicated appendicitis in children. J Gastrointest Surg 16: 1993–2004.
3. Liang Y, Li G, Chen P, Yu J, Zhang C (2011) Laparoscopic versus open gastrectomy for early distal gastric cancer: a meta-analysis. ANZ J Surg 81: 673–680.
4. Chen K, Xu XW, Zhang RC, Pan Y, Wu D, et al. (2013) Systematic review and meta-analysis of laparoscopy-assisted and open total gastrectomy for gastric cancer. World J Gastroenterol 19: 5365–5376.
5. Halevy A, Gold-Deutch R, Negri M, Lin G, Shlamkovich N, et al. (1994) Are elevated liver enzymes and bilirubin levels significant after laparoscopic cholecystectomy in the absence of bile duct injury? Ann Surg 219: 362–364.
6. Tan M, Xu FF, Peng JS, Li DM, Chen LH, et al. (2003) Changes in the level of serum liver enzymes after laparoscopic surgery. World J Gastroenterol 9: 364–367.
7. Gupta R, Kaman L, Dahiya D, Gupta N, Singh R (2013) Effects of varying intraperitoneal pressure on liver function tests during laparoscopic cholecystectomy. J Laparoendosc Adv Surg Tech A 23: 339–342.
8. Guven HE, Oral S (2007) Liver enzyme alterations after laparoscopic cholecystectomy. J Gastrointestin Liver Dis 16: 391–394.
9. Hasukic S (2005) Postoperative changes in liver function tests: randomized comparison of low- and high-pressure laparoscopic cholecystectomy. Surg Endosc 19: 1451–1455.
10. Eryilmaz HB, Memis D, Sezer A, Inal MT (2012) The effects of different insufflation pressures on liver functions assessed with LiMON on patients undergoing laparoscopic cholecystectomy. ScientificWorldJournal 2012: 172575.
11. Etoh T, Shiraishi N, Tajima M, Shiromizu A, Yasuda K, et al. (2007) Transient liver dysfunction after laparoscopic gastrectomy for gastric cancer patients. World J Surg 31: 1115–1120.
12. Atila K, Terzi C, Ozkardesler S, Unek T, Guler S, et al. (2009) What is the role of the abdominal perfusion pressure for subclinical hepatic dysfunction in laparoscopic cholecystectomy? J Laparoendosc Adv Surg Tech A 19: 39–44.
13. Yoon HM, Yang HK, Lee HJ, Park DJ, Kim HH, et al. (2011) Comparison of liver function after laparoscopically assisted and open distal gastrectomies for patients with liver disease. Surg Endosc 25: 1761–1765.
14. Nguyen NT, Braley S, Fleming NW, Lambourne L, Rivers R, et al. (2003) Comparison of postoperative hepatic function after laparoscopic versus open gastric bypass. Am J Surg 186: 40–44.
15. Kinjo Y, Okabe H, Obama K, Tsunoda S, Tanaka E, et al. (2011) Elevation of liver function tests after laparoscopic gastrectomy using a Nathanson liver retractor. World J Surg 35: 2730–2738.
16. Jeong GA, Cho GS, Shin EJ, Lee MS, Kim HC, et al. (2011) Liver function alterations after laparoscopy-assisted gastrectomy for gastric cancer and its clinical significance. World J Gastroenterol 17: 372–378.
17. Higgins JPT, Green S (eds) (2011) Cochrane handbook for systematic reviews of interventions, version 5.1.0. Available at: http://www.cochrane-handbook.org. Accessed January 1, 2012.
18. Egger M, Davey SG, Schneider M, Minder C (1997) Bias in meta-analysis detected by a simple, graphical test. BMJ 315: 629–634.
19. Begg CB, Mazumdar M (1994) Operating characteristics of a rank correlation test for publication bias. Biometrics 50: 1088–1101.
20. Morino M, Giraudo G, Festa V (1998) Alterations in hepatic function during laparoscopic surgery. An experimental clinical study. Surg Endosc 12: 968–972.
21. Hasukic S, Kosuta D, Muminhodzic K (2005) Comparison of postoperative hepatic function between laparoscopic and open cholecystectomy. Med Princ Pract 14: 147–150.
22. Omari A, Bani-Hani KE (2007) Effect of carbon dioxide pneumoperitoneum on liver function following laparoscopic cholecystectomy. J Laparoendosc Adv Surg Tech A 17: 419–424.
23. Bickel A, Weiar A, Eitan A (2008) Evaluation of liver enzymes following elective laparoscopic cholecystectomy: are they really elevated? J Gastrointest Surg 12: 1418–1421.
24. Andrei VE, Schein M, Margolis M, Rucinski JC, Wise L (1998) Liver enzymes are commonly elevated following laparoscopic cholecystectomy: is elevated intra-abdominal pressure the cause? Dig Surg 15: 256–259.
25. Said-Ahmed HAEF (2004) Effect of laparoscopy on hepatic function. Acta Anaesthesiologica Italica/Anaesthesia and Intensive Care in Italy 55: 120–131.
26. Bohm B, Junghans T, Neudecker J, Schwenk W (1999) Hepatic and renal function following laparoscopic and conventionell resection of colorectal cancer - Results from a prospective randomized trial. Viszeralchirurgie 34: 20–24.
27. Sakorafas G, Anagnostopoulos G, Stafyla V, Koletis T, Kotsifopoulos N, et al. (2005) Elevation of serum liver enzymes after laparoscopic cholecystectomy. N Z Med J 118: U1317.
28. Brundell SM, Tsopelas C, Chatterton B, Touloumtzoglou J, Hewett PJ (2002) Experimental study of peritoneal blood flow and insufflation pressure during laparoscopy. Br J Surg 89: 617–622.
29. Saber AA, Laraja RD, Nalbandian HI, Pablos-Mendez A, Hanna K (2000) Changes in liver function tests after laparoscopic cholecystectomy: not so rare, not always ominous. Am Surg 66: 699–702.
30. Dexter SP, Vucevic M, Gibson J, McMahon MJ (1999) Hemodynamic consequences of high- and low-pressure capnoperitoneum during laparoscopic cholecystectomy. Surg Endosc 13: 376–381.
31. Gutt CN, Oniu T, Mehrabi A, Schemmer P, Kashfi A, et al. (2004) Circulatory and respiratory complications of carbon dioxide insufflation. Dig Surg 21: 95–105.

32. Osman Y, Fusun A, Serpil A, Umit T, Ebru M, et al. (2009) The comparison of pulmonary functions in open versus laparoscopic cholecystectomy. J Pak Med Assoc 59: 201–204.
33. Takagi S (1998) Hepatic and portal vein blood flow during carbon dioxide pneumoperitoneum for laparoscopic hepatectomy. Surg Endosc 12: 427–431.
34. Sato K, Kawamura T, Wakusawa R (2000) Hepatic blood flow and function in elderly patients undergoing laparoscopic cholecystectomy. Anesth Analg 90: 1198–1202.
35. Tunon MJ, Gonzalez P, Jorquera F, Llorente A, Gonzalo-Orden M, et al. (1999) Liver blood flow changes during laparoscopic surgery in pigs. A study of hepatic indocyanine green removal. Surg Endosc 13: 668–672.
36. Richter S, Olinger A, Hildebrandt U, Menger MD, Vollmar B (2001) Loss of physiologic hepatic blood flow control ("hepatic arterial buffer response") during CO2-pneumoperitoneum in the rat. Anesth Analg 93: 872–877.
37. Glantzounis GK, Tselepis AD, Tambaki AP, Trikalinos TA, Manataki AD, et al. (2001) Laparoscopic surgery-induced changes in oxidative stress markers in human plasma. Surg Endosc 15: 1315–1319.
38. Clarke RS, Doggart JR, Lavery T (1976) Changes in liver function after different types of surgery. Br J Anaesth 48: 119–128.
39. Saber AA (2007) Non ominous changes in liver function tests after laparoscopic cholecystectomy. J Gastrointestin Liver Dis 16: 427–428.

Myocardial Injury after Surgery Is a Risk Factor for Weaning Failure from Mechanical Ventilation in Critical Patients Undergoing Major Abdominal Surgery

Shu Li[1], You-zhong An[1], Jing-yi Ren[2], Feng-xue Zhu[1], Hong Chen[2]*

1 Department of Critical Care Medicine, Peking University People's Hospital, Beijing, China, 2 Department of Cardiology, Peking University People's Hospital, Beijing, China

Abstract

Background: Myocardial injury after noncardiac surgery (MINS) is a newly proposed concept that is common among adults undergoing noncardiac surgery and associated with substantial mortality. We analyzed whether MINS was a risk factor for weaning failure in critical patients who underwent major abdominal surgery.

Methods: This retrospective study was conducted in the Department of Critical Care Medicine of Peking University People's Hospital. The subjects were all critically ill patients who underwent major abdominal surgery between January 2011 and December 2013. Clinical and laboratory parameters during the perioperative period were investigated. Backward stepwise regression analysis was performed to evaluate MINS relative to the rate of weaning failure. Age, hypertension, chronic renal disease, left ventricular ejection fraction before surgery, Acute Physiologic and Chronic Health Evaluation II score, pleural effusion, pneumonia, acute kidney injury, duration of mechanical ventilation before weaning and the level of albumin after surgery were treated as independent variables.

Results: This study included 381 patients, of whom 274 were successfully weaned. MINS was observed in 42.0% of the patients. The MINS incidence was significantly higher in patients who failed to be weaned compared to patients who were successfully weaned (56.1% versus 36.5%; $P<0.001$). Independent predictive factors of weaning failure were MINS, age, lower left ventricular ejection fraction before surgery and lower serum albumin level after surgery. The MINS odds ratio was 4.098 (95% confidence interval, 1.07 to 15.6; $P=0.04$). The patients who were successfully weaned had shorter hospital stay lengths and a higher survival rate than those who failed to be weaned.

Conclusion: MINS is a risk factor for weaning failure from mechanical ventilation in critical patients who have undergone major abdominal surgery, independent of age, lower left ventricular ejection fraction before surgery and lower serum albumin levels after surgery.

Editor: Yiru Guo, University of Louisville, United States of America

Funding: The authors have no funding or support to report.

Competing Interests: The authors have declared that no competing interests exist.

* Email: chenhong0418@aliyun.com

Introduction

Prolonged mechanical ventilation has been associated with significant morbidity and mortality. Therefore, weaning should be considered as early as possible during the course of ventilation [1]. Postoperative patients are generally able to resume spontaneous ventilation as soon as they have recovered from anesthesia; therefore, the mode of ventilation should have little impact on the decision to extubate these patients. However, approximately 3 to 6% of patients admitted to the adult intensive care unit (ICU) require prolonged mechanical ventilation (cumulative duration of 24 hours) [2–3]. The rate of weaning failure is 5 to 8% in all surgical patients [4–5]. However, in patients who require prolonged mechanical ventilation, the rate of weaning failure is greater than 10%, and mortality and complication rates are also increased compared with other patients [6–8]. Unfortunately, the criteria and strategies for their successful weaning have been unclear [2]. Parameters of respiratory mechanics and oxygenation have commonly been used to wean patients with chronic obstructive pulmonary disease and other pulmonary disorders from long-term mechanical ventilation. However, these parameters are not sufficient for patients undergoing abdominal surgery whose pulmonary function is relatively normal.

Acute heart dysfunction or failure is another primary cause of weaning failure, largely due to acute myocardial ischemia during the perioperative period [9]. However, emerging evidence has suggested that many patients sustain myocardial injury during the perioperative period that does not satisfy the diagnostic criteria for myocardial infarction [10]. There have been only a limited number of studies that have reliably evaluated the incidence of myocardial injury after surgery, not to mention the effects of myocardial injury on weaning. Myocardial injury after noncardiac surgery (MINS) was recently proposed as a new concept [11]. The definition of MINS is broader than that of myocardial infarction because it includes not only the latter but also other prognostically relevant perioperative myocardial injuries due to ischemia. Evaluating patients for the presence of MINS, rather than myocardial infarction alone, could help physicians to avoid missing the majority of patients who develop prognostically relevant perioperative myocardial injury.

Therefore, we investigated the relationships of MINS and other perioperative parameters with the incidence of weaning failure in a cohort of critical patients who underwent major abdominal surgery. The aim of this study was to determine whether MINS and these parameters serve as risk factors of weaning failure.

Materials and Methods

Study design and patients

This study retrospectively analyzed patients who underwent abdominal surgery in the Department of Critical Care Medicine of Peking University People's Hospital between January 2011 and December 2013. All of the participants provided written informed consent. This study was approved by the Institution of Human Subjects Committee at Peking University People's Hospital. Critically ill patients were selected as the study subjects, according to the following inclusion and exclusion criteria.

Inclusion criteria. Patients meeting all of the following criteria were included in this study: (1) age >18 years old; (2) Acute Physiological and Chronic Health Evaluation II (APACHE II) score >8; (3) underwent endotracheal intubation and mechanical ventilation for abdominal surgery under general anesthesia; and (4) cumulative duration of postoperative mechanical ventilation >24 h. These criteria imply that patients who were not extubated within 24 hours as well as those who had one or more unsuccessful extubation attempts that resulted in an accumulated duration of at least 24 hours of mechanical ventilation were included.

Exclusion criteria. Patients who met the following criteria were excluded from this study: (1) patients who died or discontinued mechanical ventilation due to other reasons before weaning, (2) pregnant or nursing women, (3) patients who would underwent sequential noninvasive mechanical ventilation after weaning as planned, (4) patients who underwent tracheotomy, and (5) patients whose etiologies of elevated TnT were both ischemic and non-ischemic or could not be confirmed.

Study procedures

Mechanical ventilation modes. According to the patient's condition, the treatment team responsible for the patient made decisions together regarding any adjustments of the mode and parameters of mechanical ventilation. The modes used for all of the patients included volume controlled ventilation, pressure controlled ventilation, and synchronized intermittent mandatory ventilation (pressure/volume), plus pressure support ventilation and pressure support ventilation.

Weaning procedure. The treatment team responsible for the patient evaluated daily whether the patient met the indications for weaning. If the patient met the indications, a spontaneous breathing trial (SBT) was conducted. For patients who succeeded in the trial, the tracheal cannula was immediately removed. Continuous electrocardiographic monitoring provided dynamic monitoring of arterial blood pressure, heart rate and finger oxygen saturation. Blood gas analysis was performed every 12 h. The patients were continuously observed for 48 h to determine whether weaning was successful.

Indications for weaning. When the patient essentially met the following indications for weaning [8], the treatment team responsible for the patient decided to initiate SBT.

Clinical evaluation criteria: forceful cough; no excessive airway secretion; the patient's underlying disease improved or began to improve.

Objective evaluation criteria: stable clinical condition; stable hemodynamic status; heart rate ≤140 beats/min; systolic blood pressure between 90 to 160 mm Hg; no or low-dose vasoactive drugs; stable metabolic status; modified oxygenation index ≥ 150 mm Hg; and positive end-expiratory pressure (PEEP) ≤8 cm H_2O.

Respiratory function measurements: respiratory rate ≤35 times/min; pH >7.3; and arterial carbon dioxide pressure ($PaCO_2$) of 35–50 mmHg.

SBT implementation methods. Every patient underwent one of the following methods. According to previous studies, there were no significant differences in sensitivity or specificity between the two SBT implementation methods in determining whether patients could be weaned from a breathing machine.

1) The tracheal cannula was connected to the breathing machine in pressure support mode. Inspiratory pressure ranged from 6 to 8 cm H_2O, PEEP was 3 to 4 cm H_2O, and the fraction of inspired O_2 (FiO_2) was 40%, lasting for 60–120 min.
2) The tracheal cannula was connected to an artificial nose. The oxygen flow was 3 to 5 l/min, lasting for 60–120 min.

SBT failure criteria. Patients who showed changes in mental status, including anxiety, restlessness, delirium, and somnolence, and/or who demonstrated the following criteria [8]:

Arterial oxygen pressure (PaO_2) ≤50–60 mm Hg, $PaCO_2$ ≥ 50 mmHg or increase >8 mm Hg; respiratory rate ≥35/min or increase ≥50%, heart rate ≥140 beats/min or ≥20% increase, systolic blood pressure ≥180 mm Hg or ≥20% increase, systolic blood pressure <90 mm Hg, or arrhythmia.

Weaning failure criteria. If the patients met any of the following criteria and required reintubation or if they died within 48 h after weaning, it was judged to be weaning failure [8]:

1) Respiratory rate ≥25 times/min for more than 2 h;
2) Heart rate ≥140 beats/min or persistent increase/decrease of ≥20%;
3) Patients developed evidence of respiratory muscle weakness or significant increase in breathing work, with oxygen saturation (SO_2) <90%;
4) PaO_2 <80 mm Hg, when FiO_2 ≥50; or
5) Hypercapnia ($PaCO_2$ >45 mm Hg or ≥20% increase compared with that before weaning) and pH <7.33.

Grouping

The patients were divided into successful weaning and weaning failure groups according to whether they were successfully weaned or not.

Observation indicators

Basic demographic characteristics of the patients included age, sex and body mass index (BMI).

The indicators for outcome evaluation included 28-day survival rate and the length of ICU stay.

Preoperative conditions included hypertension, diabetes, chronic renal disease, old myocardial infarction, chronic obstructive pulmonary disease, history of smoking, APACHE II score and preoperative left ventricular ejection fraction (LVEF).

Surgical data included intraoperative blood loss, duration of surgery and whether reoperation was performed within 24 h or not.

Postoperative data included pleural effusions, pneumonia, MINS, sepsis, acute kidney injury (AKI), duration of mechanical ventilation before weaning and Simplified Acute Physiology Score II (SAPS II) at the time of weaning.

Postoperative laboratory parameters included blood cardiac troponin I (cTnI), cTnT, N-terminal pro-brain natriuretic peptide (NT pro-BNP), calcium, magnesium, serum creatinine (SCr), hemoglobin (Hb) and albumin (Alb) levels.

Laboratory tests were routinely performed for all patients as indicated below. TnT and TnI were measured every 6 hours during the first 12 hours, every 24 hours during the following 3 days, and twice weekly until the patients were discharged from the ICU. These measurements were also obtained at the time of weaning and assessed more frequently if necessitated by additional conditions. NT pro-BNP, calcium, magnesium, SCr, Hb and Alb levels were measured daily, whereas urine volume was record by a nurse every 2 hours until the patient was discharged from the ICU.

Definition of MINS

The definition used was prognostically relevant myocardial injury due to ischemia that occurred during or within 30 days after noncardiac surgery [11]. The diagnostic criterion for MINS was any peak TnT of 0.03 ng/ml or greater that was judged as resulting from myocardial ischemia. Each elevated TnT was evaluated to ensure an ischemic etiology.

Definition of AKI

AKI was defined as a ≥0.3 mg/dl (≥26.5 mol/l) increase in SCr within 48 hours; or an increase in SCr of ≥1.5 times baseline, which is known or presumed to have occurred within the prior 7 days; or urine volume <0.5 ml/kg/h for 6 hours [12].

Statistical analysis

SAS statistical software (SAS Institute Inc., Cary, NC, USA), version 9.1, was used for the statistical analyses. Measurement data are expressed as the means ± standard deviations or the medians (25th to 75th percentile). Enumeration data are expressed as absolute frequencies and percentages. For inter-group comparisons of basic demographic characteristics and clinical indicators, Student's t test was used for normally distributed measurement data, and the rank sum test was used for non-normally distributed measurement data. The χ^2 test was used for comparisons of rates. Binary logistic regression was used for multivariate analysis. All of the tests were conducted at a level of significance of $\alpha = 0.05$.

Results

Baseline clinical and demographic characteristics

Between January 2011 and December 2013, 4,205 patients were treated in the Department of Critical Care Medicine of Peking University People's Hospital. Among these patients, 381 were selected and included in this study. A flowchart of patient inclusion is shown in Figure 1. General patient information is shown in Table 1.

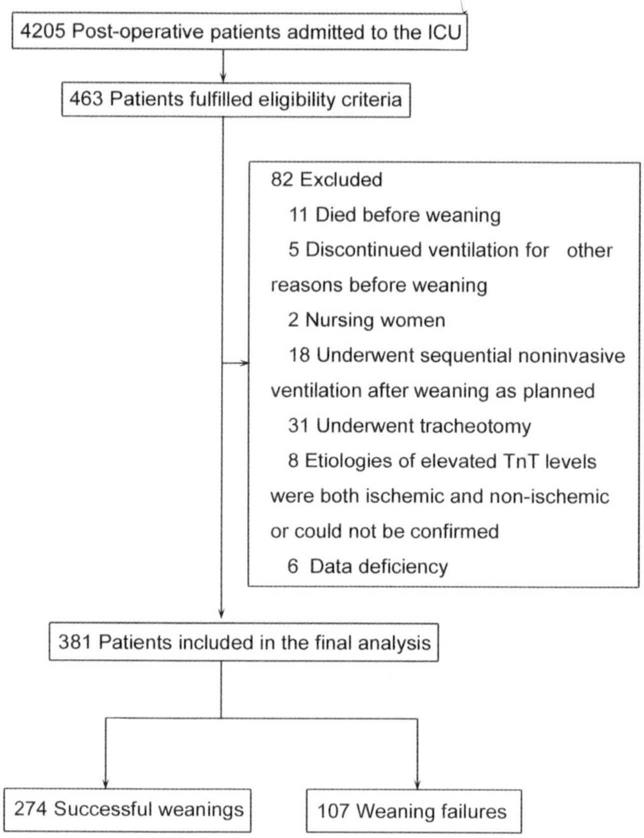

Figure 1. Patient flow chart.

Comparison of clinical characteristics at admission to the ICU

According to whether they were successfully weaned or not, the patients were divided into successful weaning and weaning failure groups. The statistical results showed that patients in the successful weaning group were younger with a lower rate of hypertension, fewer chronic renal diseases, higher preoperative LVEF and lower APACHE II score on admission to the ICU than patients in the weaning failure group. These differences were statistically significant ($P<0.05$). Detailed results are shown in Table 2.

Comparison of intraoperative and postoperative situations

The statistical results showed that the patients in the successful weaning group had lower incidences of postoperative pneumonia, pleural effusion, MINS and AKI and a shorter duration of mechanical ventilation before weaning than the patients in the weaning failure group. These differences were statistically significant ($P<0.05$). Detailed results are shown in Table 3.

Comparison of laboratory indicators and disease condition scores at the time of weaning

The statistical results showed that patients in the successful weaning group had higher blood albumin and lower SAPS II scores than patients in the weaning failure group. These differences were statistically significant ($P<0.05$). Detailed results are shown in Table 4.

Table 1. Patient Demographic and Clinical Characteristics.

Characteristic	Value
Male sex, n (%)	212 (55.6)
Mean age (years)	63.8±16.5
Mean BMI (kg/m^2)	23.4±4.4
Mean length of stay in ICU (days)	6 (4 to 12)
Duration of mechanical ventilation before weaning (hours)	66 (39 to 144)

Data are presented as medians (25th to 75th percentile) or numbers (% of patients). BMI, body mass index; ICU, intensive care unit.

Outcome comparison between the successful weaning and weaning failure groups

In the successful weaning group, 5 patients died with 28-day mortality of 1.82%; in the weaning failure group, 41 patients died with 28-day mortality of 38.32%. This difference was statistically significant ($\chi^2 = 91.85$, $P<0.001$). The median length of ICU stay was 6 days in the successful weaning group and 9 days in the weaning failure group. This difference was statistically significant ($t = -4.179$, $P<0.001$).

Risk factors for weaning failure

In accordance with the above results, binary nonconditional logistic regression analysis was performed using the backward LR method, with parameters that showed statistically significant differences between the two groups in the previous analysis as the independent variables and weaning success as the dependent variable. Age, LVEF and blood albumin were the continuous variables, while postoperative occurrence of MINS was a categorical variable (with MINS = 1, without MINS = 0). The results showed that advanced age, low preoperative LVEF, postoperative occurrence of MINS and low blood albumin at the time of weaning were independent risk factors influencing the weaning success rate. Of all the MINS patients, 79.4% (127/160) were diagnosed within 24 hours after surgery, 97.5% (156/160) were diagnosed within 72 hours after surgery, and 98.6% (158/160) were diagnosed within the first week. Regarding the 2 cases who were not diagnosed within the first week, one was diagnosed on the 8th day, whereas the other patient was diagnosed on the 9th day after surgery. Detailed results are shown in Table 5.

Discussion

Postoperative occurrence of MINS is an important factor influencing cardiovascular function. In our study, regression analysis showed that MINS was an independent risk factor for weaning failure with a greater than 4-fold increased risk of failure. Acute myocardial ischemia during the perioperative period is not always due to local stenosis or spasm of the coronary artery. After surgery, patients are in a state of stress because of the pain after recovery from anesthesia, the stress of the surgery itself and intolerance to the tracheal cannula, all of which contribute to a significant increase in blood catecholamines. This increase leads to an increased cardiac load and a significant increase in the risk of myocardial ischemia [11]. In addition, intraoperative and postoperative hemodynamic instability is the main cause of myocardial hypoperfusion, ischemia, hypoxia and particularly myocardial injury. If patients have concurrent coronary heart disease and chronic heart disease, perioperative hemodynamic instability and systemic ischemia and hypoxia are more likely to cause cardiac dysfunction during weaning, ultimately resulting in extubation failure [13–14]. Following abdominal surgery, factors such as postoperative abdominal pain, the use of abdominal bandages, long-term immobilization, intra-abdominal infections

Table 2. In-ICU Variables.

Variables	Success (n = 274)	Failure (n = 107)	*P* value
Mean age (years)	60.95±16.84	70.3±13.76	<0.001
Male sex, n (%)	154 (56.2)	58 (54.2)	0.732
Mean BMI (kg/m^2)	23.22±4.20	23.72±4.96	0.487
Complications, n (%)			
Hypertension	80 (29.2)	64 (59.8)	<0.001
Diabetes mellitus	28 (10.2)	18 (16.8)	0.082
Chronic renal disease	6 (2.19)	14 (13.1)	<0.001
Previous myocardial infarction	8 (2.92)	6 (5.61)	0.230
Chronic obstructive pulmonary disease	12 (4.38)	5 (4.67)	0.545
Smoking	30 (10.9)	8 (7.48)	0.348
LVEF (%)	68.9 (65 to 72)	65.6(59.3 to 70.7)	0.039
APACHE II	18 (14 to 21)	25 (20 to 29)	0.027

Data are presented as medians (25th to 75th percentile) or numbers (% of patients). BMI, body mass index; LVEF, left ventricular ejection fraction; APACHE II, Acute Physiology and Chronic Health Evaluation II.

Table 3. Intraoperative and Postoperative Variables.

Variables	Success (n = 274)	Failure (n = 107)	*P* value
Operative blood loss (ml)	650 (200 to 1950)	500 (150 to 1450)	0.200
Duration of surgery (hours)	4.5 (3 to 6.5)	3.5 (2.5 to 5)	0.079
Reoperation in 24 hours, n (%)	10 (3.65)	4 (3.74)	0.587
Pleural effusion, n (%)	86 (31.4)	46 (43.0)	0.041
Pneumonia, n (%)	70 (25.5)	48 (44.9)	<0.001
MINS, n (%)	100 (36.5)	60 (56.1)	<0.001
Sepsis, n (%)	88 (32.1)	46 (43.0)	0.056
Acute kidney injury, n (%)	70 (25.5)	50 (46.7)	<0.001
Duration of mechanical ventilation before weaning (hours)	46.5 (42.5 to 37.5)	75.5 (14 to 184)	0.048

Data are presented as medians (25th to 75th percentile) or numbers (% of patients). MINS, myocardial injury after noncardiac surgery.

and diaphragmatic dysfunction often influence intrathoracic pressure and lung volume. The effects of these factors on respiratory function and hemodynamics cannot be ignored.

Potential insufficient cardiovascular reserve and compensatory capacity before surgery are important factors that influence postoperative weaning failure. In our study, multivariate regression analysis showed that advanced age and low preoperative LVEF were independent risk factors for weaning failure. In addition, patients in the weaning failure group had a higher proportion of concomitant underlying high-risk cardiovascular diseases, with higher rates of hypertension and chronic renal disease than the patients in the successful weaning group. These are all important factors that can lead to cardiovascular dysfunction and decreased compensation.

It has been estimated that the global population will show a trend of accelerated aging over the next 20 years, and the elderly population requiring surgery will be more than 4 times larger than the population in other age groups [15]. Increased age leads to a higher rate of perioperative complications [16]. Among the various perioperative complications in elderly patients, cardiovascular diseases have the highest incidence. In a study of patients between 75 and 84 years old, 19% of men and 12% of women had one or more cardiovascular diseases of varying severity [17]. Thus, these patients were more likely to have insufficient cardiac reserves before surgery. In our study, echocardiography also showed that, although patients in both groups had LVEF values within the normal range, patients in the successful weaning group had higher LVEF values than those in the weaning failure group.

In this study, patients with definite diagnoses of underlying cardiovascular diseases were few in number. The patients in the successful weaning group had a slightly higher rate of cardiovascular diseases than patients in the weaning failure group. However, perhaps due to the small sample size, the difference was not statistically significant. This finding does suggest, however, that it is not sufficient to focus only on the presence of documented underlying cardiovascular diseases during preoperative evaluations. The evaluation and improvement of potentially insufficient cardiovascular reserve and compensation are of great importance for improving the postoperative weaning success rate.

Poor nutritional status has consistently been recognized as one of the factors influencing weaning difficulty. Theoretically, patients with poor nutritional status are in negative nitrogen balance after surgery, which can induce disorders and dysfunctions of respiratory muscle strength and can even result in pulmonary interstitial edema. Patients with a low body mass index can develop respiratory drive suppression, decreased muscle volume and weaning difficulty [18]. The results of our study also showed that after abdominal surgery, critically ill patients who were successfully weaned had significantly higher blood albumin levels at the time of weaning than patients who failed weaning. Hypoalbuminemia was an independent risk factor for weaning failure. Despite this observation, few studies have investigated the associations between low albumin levels and weaning failure. While low albumin levels

Table 4. Variables before Weaning.

Variables	Success (n = 274)	Failure (n = 107)	*P* value
cTnI (ng/ml)	0.020 (0.007 to 0.035)	0.034 (0.009 to 0.067)	0.319
NT pro-BNP (pg/ml)	217 (73 to 405)	247 (108 to 424)	0.908
Ca^{2+} (mmol/l)	1.15 (1.11 to 1.19)	1.135 (1.09 to 1.18)	0.222
Mg^{2+} (mmol/l)	0.55 (0.49 to 0.63)	0.55 (0.48 to 0.64)	0.613
SCr (μmol/l)	61.5 (49 to 85.5)	69 (57.5 to 118)	0.116
Hb (g/l)	97.44±14.11	96.32±13.58	0.617
Alb (g/l)	33.94±4.17	30.36±5.01	<0.001
SAPS II	24 (18 to 31)	37 (23 to 52)	0.016

Data are presented as medians (25th to 75th percentile) or numbers (% of patients). cTnI, cardiac troponin I; NT pro-BNP, N-terminal pro-brain natriuretic peptide; SCr, serum creatinine; Hb, hemoglobin; Alb, albumin; SAPS II, Simplified Acute Physiology Score II.

Table 5. Multiple Regression.

Variables	*P* value	Odds ratio (95% CI)
Age	0.006	1.100 (1.028–1.176)
LVEF before surgery	0.008	0.861 (0.772–0.962)
MINS	0.040	4.098 (1.070–15.63)
Serum albumin level	0.043	0.812 (0.664–0.993)

LVEF, left ventricular ejection fraction; MINS, myocardial injury after noncardiac surgery.

might suggest poor nutritional status, they can also be related to the surgical procedure. Further, patients usually cannot eat a normal diet after abdominal surgery. Low albumin itself can be corrected through treatment in a relatively short time. However, further studies are required to investigate in greater detail whether hypoalbuminemia is a reflection of poor nutritional status, of a metabolic disorder or of other issues.

Our study analyzed the outcomes of critically ill patients after abdominal surgery. The results showed that patients who were successfully weaned had shorter ICU stays and overall durations of mechanical ventilation than patients who failed weaning. Furthermore, there was a significant difference in 28-day mortality between the two groups. There are many factors that influence the outcomes of critically ill patients after abdominal surgery. Because this study was a retrospective case analysis, it was impossible to determine whether weaning was a risk factor for poor outcomes due to the limited case data. Our available results were similar to the results from other domestic and overseas studies. Other studies have indicated that after statistical adjustment for disease conditions, underlying diseases and age, weaning failure remains an independent risk factor for predicting in-hospital mortality [19]. Additionally, weaning failure exacerbates the deterioration of underlying diseases and complications, such as aspiration, atelectasis and even pneumonia [20]. These complications, combined with the direct complications caused by reintubation and the instability of the disease condition between extubation and reintubation, contribute to the increased mortality of patients who fail weaning. Prolonged mechanical ventilation also causes side effects that can contribute to a poor outcome. For example, the incidence of nosocomial pneumonia increases after prolonged mechanical ventilation. The development of these complications is also an independent risk factor for inpatient mortality [21–22]. Thus, exploring the methods and means needed to improve the postoperative weaning success rate is extremely important for improving patient outcomes and reducing perioperative mortality.

The present study has its strengths and limitations. This is the first study demonstrating that MINS is an independent risk factor for weaning failure in critical patients who have undergone major abdominal surgery. Our results also indicate that potentially insufficient cardiovascular reserve and compensatory capacity before surgery and poor nutritional status are important factors that potentially influence postoperative weaning failure. Our study also has several limitations. First, it is a single center study. Although numerous confounding factors could influence weaning from ventilation, we only included a limited number of factors given the small sample size. Second, this study is retrospective, and medical history and diagnosis data could alter the accuracy of our results.

In conclusion, MINS, as diagnosed based on any peak TnT of 0.03 ng/ml or greater, was a risk factor for weaning failure in critical patients who underwent major abdominal surgery, independent of age, lower LVEF before surgery and lower serum albumin level after surgery. For patients with underlying heart disease and MINS, it is therefore necessary to further evaluate whether their heart function can tolerate the load that results from weaning, as well as the current indications for weaning. Advanced age and low blood albumin at the time of weaning were also risk factors influencing the weaning success rate. For these patients, the indications and the timing of weaning should be strictly monitored to improve the weaning success rate and patient outcomes.

Author Contributions

Conceived and designed the experiments: SL YZA FXZ HC. Performed the experiments: SL YZA. Analyzed the data: SL JYR FXZ HC. Contributed reagents/materials/analysis tools: JYR HC. Wrote the paper: SL JYR HC.

References

1. Thille AW, Richard JC, Brochard L (2013) The decision to extubate in the intensive care unit. Am J Respir Crit Care Med 187: 1294–1302.
2. Siddiqui MM, Paras I, Jalal A (2012) Risk factors of prolonged mechanical ventilation following open heart surgery: What has changed over the last decade. Cardiovasc Diagn Ther 2: 192–199.
3. Dunning J, Au J, Kalkat M, Levine A (2003) A validated rule for predicting patients who require prolonged ventilation post cardiac surgery. Eur J Cardiothorac Surg 24: 270–276.
4. Epstein SK (2009) Noninvasive ventilation to shorten the duration of mechanical ventilation. Respir Care 54: 198–208.
5. Zhu F, Liu ZL, Long X, Wu XD, Zhou J, et al. (2013) Effect of noninvasive positive pressure ventilation on weaning success in patients receiving invasive mechanical ventilation: a meta-analysis. Chin Med J (Engl) 126: 1337–1343.
6. Nozawa E, Azeka E, Ignêz ZM, Feltrim Z, Auler Júnior JO (2005) Factors associated with failure of weaning from long-term mechanical ventilation after cardiac surgery. Int Heart J 46: 819–831.
7. Glossop AJ, Shephard N, Bryden DC, Mills GH (2012) Non-invasive ventilation for weaning, avoiding reintubation after extubation and in the postoperative period: a meta-analysis. Br J Anaesth 109: 305–314.
8. Boles JM, Bion J, Connors A, Herridge M, Marsh B, et al. (2007) Weaning from mechanical ventilation. Eur Respir J 29: 1033–1056.
9. Teboul JL, Monnet X, Richard C (2010) Weaning failure of cardiac origin: recent advances. Crit Care 14: 211.
10. Ali ZA, Callaghan CJ, Ali AA, Sheikh AY, Akhtar A, et al. (2008) Perioperative myocardial injury after elective open abdominal aortic aneurysm repair predicts outcome. Eur J Vasc Endovasc Surg 35: 413–419.
11. Botto F, Alonso-Coello P, Chan MT, Villar JC, Xavier D, et al. (2014) Myocardial injury after noncardiac surgery: A large, international, prospective cohort study establishing diagnostic criteria, characteristics, predictors, and 30-day outcomes. Anesthesiology 120: 564–578.
12. Kidney Disease: Improving Global Outcomes (2012) KDIGO Clinical Practice Guideline for Acute Kidney Injury. Kidney International Supplements 2: 1–138.
13. Pinsky MR (2000) Breathing as exercise: the cardiovascular response to weaning from mechanical ventilation. Intensive Care Med 26: 1164–1166.
14. Monnet X, Teboul JL, Richard C (2007) Cardiopulmonary interactions in patients with heart failure. Curr Opin Crit Care 13: 6–11.
15. Naughton C, Feneck RO (2007) The impact of age on 6-month survival in patients with cardiovascular risk factors undergoing elective non-cardiac surgery. Int J Clin Pract 61: 768–776.

16. Mehta RH, Grab JD, O'Brien SM, Glower DD, Haan CK, et al. (2008) Clinical characteristics and in-hospital outcomes of patients with cardiogenic shock undergoing coronary artery bypass surgery: Insights from the Society of Thoracic Surgeons National Cardiac Database. Circulation 117: 876–885.
17. Carroll K, Majeed A, Firth C, Gray J (2003) Prevalence and management of coronary heart disease in primary care: population-based cross-sectional study using a disease register. J Public Health Med 25: 29–35.
18. Gupta B, Kant S, Mishra R, Verma S (2010) Nutritional status of chronic obstructive pulmonary disease patients admitted in hospital with acute exacerbation. J Clin Med Res 2: 68–74.
19. Porhomayon J, Papadakos P, Nader ND (2012) Failed weaning from mechanical ventilation and cardiac dysfunction. Crit Care Res Pract 2012: 173527.
20. Torres A, Gatell JM, Aznar E, el-Ebiary M, Puig de la Bellacasa J, et al. (1995) Re-intubation increases the risk of nosocomial pneumonia in patients needing mechanical ventilation. Am J Respir Crit Care Med 152: 137–141.
21. Hadda V, Khilnani GC, Dubey G, Nallan R, Kumar G, et al. (2014) Impact of ventilator associated pneumonia on outcome in patients with chronic obstructive pulmonary disease exacerbation. Lung India 31: 4–8.
22. Shi Z, Xie H, Wang P, Zhang Q, Wu Y, et al. (2013) Oral hygiene care for critically ill patients to prevent ventilator-associated pneumonia. Cochrane Database Syst Rev 8: CD008367.

4

Emergent Endovascular vs. Open Surgery Repair for Ruptured Abdominal Aortic Aneurysms

Chuan Qin, Lin Chen, Ying-bin Xiao*

The Department of Cardiovascular Surgery, Xinqiao Hospital, the Third Military Medical University, Chongqing, PR China

Abstract

Objectives: To systematically review studies comparing peri-operative mortality and length of hospital stay in patients with ruptured abdominal aortic aneurysms (rAAAs) who underwent endovascular aneurysm repair (EVAR) to patients who underwent open surgical repair (OSR).

Methods: The Medline, Cochrane, EMBASE, and Google Scholar databases were searched until Apr 30, 2013 using keywords such as abdominal aortic aneurysm, emergent, emergency, rupture, leaking, acute, endovascular, stent, graft, and endoscopic. The primary outcome was peri-operative mortality and the secondary outcome was length of hospital stay.

Results: A total of 18 studies (2 randomized controlled trials, 5 prospective studies, and 11 retrospective studies) with a total of 135,734 rAAA patients were included. rAAA patients who underwent EVAR had significantly lower peri-operative mortality compared to those who underwent OSR (overall OR = 0.62, 95% CI = 0.58 to 0.67, $P < 0.001$). rAAA patients with EVAR also had a significantly shorter mean length of hospital stay compared to those with OSR (difference in mean length of stay ranged from −2.00 to −19.10 days, with the overall estimate being −5.25 days (95% CI = −9.23 to −1.26, $P = 0.010$). There was no publication bias and sensitivity analysis showed good reliability.

Conclusions: EVAR confers significant benefits in terms of peri-operative mortality and length of hospital stay. There is a need for more randomized controlled trials to compare outcomes of EVAR and OSR for rAAA.

Editor: Vincenzo Lionetti, Scuola Superiore Sant'Anna, Italy

Funding: The authors have no support or funding to report.

Competing Interests: The authors have declared that no competing interests exist.

* E-mail: Xiaoyb@vip.sina.com

Introduction

An aortic aneurysm is defined as a permanent, localized focal dilation of the aorta with an aortic diameter of 30 mm or greater is defined as an aortic aneurysm [1,2]. Aortic aneurysms located under the diaphragm are classified as abdominal aortic aneurysms (AAA), occur more frequently than thoracic aortic aneurysms, and are responsible for approximately 15,000 deaths yearly [3,4]. AAAs are often asymptomatic, and the size of the aneurysm has been shown to correlate with the risk of rupture [5,6], which has a mortality rate of 85–95% [7]. Deaths from ruptured aneurysms are most effectively minimized by timely detection, followed by surveillance and open or endovascular repair of the aneurysm [8]. Although prophylactic, open surgical repair (OSR) of AAAs using a prosthetic graft was shown to reduce the mortality to 2–6% [6,7], data from meta-analyses studies showed that open repair for ruptured AAAs (rAAAs) had a mortality rate as high as 48.5% [9,10]. Efforts to reduce surgical insult, mortality and morbidity associated with open repair led to the development of minimally invasive endovascular aneurysm repair techniques (EVAR) [11–13]. A number of studies have reported that EVAR was associated with improved post-operative mortality rates compared to OSR [14–18]. Interestingly, although recent large randomized trials showed that EVAR was associated with a significantly lower operative mortality compared to OSR, it was also associated with higher rates of graft-related complications, and reintervention [5,15,16,19]. Retrospective data from the United States showed that the use of endovascular repair for rAAAs has significantly increased over the past 10 years and the use of OSR has decreased [20].

Although ethical considerations limit the randomization of patients for emergency procedures, there has been a recent focus on designing randomized trials to evaluate EVAR as an alternative to OSR in the treatment of rAAA patients. However, the benefits of using EVAR in these patients remain controversial. A meta-analysis of 23 studies which compared outcomes of OSR and EVAR for rAAAs concluded that EVAR was associated with a significant reduction in 30-day mortality and a reduction in the mean hospital stay [21]. However, the heterogeneity and associated bias in this study make these data difficult to interpret. EVAR was also shown to be feasible in patients with rAAAs who were unsuitable for OSR due to hemodynamic instability or morphologic criteria [22]. Other studies suggested that EVAR was not significantly superior to OSR for rAAAs [23–25]. Interestingly, clinical outcomes after EVAR were shown to be associated with gender, and women with rAAAs had a significantly lower survival after emergent EVAR compared to men [26]. Outcome was also associated with age except for patients who received elective EVAR [27].

Despite the volume of data comparing EVAR to open repair for elective as well as emergent procedures, there are wide variations in trial design between studies and the paucity of studies evaluating EVAR for emergent procedures could be due to practical and ethical considerations. In this meta-analysis, we reviewed studies comparing the clinical outcomes in patients who underwent emergent open surgical repair and those who underwent emergent endovascular repair for abdominal aortic aneurysms. We analyzed data from 18 studies which compared the peri-operative mortality and length of hospital stay between these two patient populations.

Methods

Study Selection and Search Strategy

In this meta-analysis, we performed a systematic analysis of randomized controlled trials, prospective studies (either single-center or multi-center) or retrospective multi-center studies (including analysis of a national registry or database, eg. Medicare), which compared outcomes between patients who received emergent EVAR with those who received emergent OSR. Inclusion criteria were 1) presence of ruptured or leaking AAA, 2) patients had interventions of OSR or EVAR, 3) The timing of intervention was at the time of the emergency, 4) Included studies had to compare outcomes between emergent open and endovascular approaches to ruptured AAA repair and 5) only English language publications were analyzed.

The exclusion criteria were 1) single-arm studies, 2) when the surgery was elective and not emergent, 3) publications which were Letters, Comments, Editorials or Case Reports, 4) retrospective, single-center studies, and 5) when the study did not provide numerical information for the targeted primary and secondary outcomes.

The Medline, Cochrane, EMBASE,and Google Scholar databases were searched (until Apr 30, 2013). Reference lists of relevant studies were manually searched with keywords including abdominal aortic aneurysm, emergent, emergency, rupture, ruptured, leaking, leak, acute, endovascular, stent, graft, and endoscopic. Studies were identified by two independent reviewers based on the above criteria. Where there was uncertainty regarding eligibility, a third reviewer was consulted.

Data Extraction

The following information/data were extracted from studies that met the inclusion criteria: the name of the first author, year of publication, study design, number of participants in each treatment group, participants' age and gender, mortality, and length of hospital stay.

After reviewing full text articles, we excluded 13 studies based on exclusion criteria listed in Figure 1.

Quality Assessment

The quality of primary studies was evaluated using the Newcastle-Ottawa Scale, which is a validated technique to assess the quality of nonrandomized studies [28]. The assessed outcomes for the 18 studies included in this meta-analysis are listed in Table 1.

Outcome Measures

The primary outcome in this study was peri-operative mortality, which included intra-operative mortality, in-hospital mortality, and 30-day mortality. The secondary outcome was length of hospital stay.

Statistical Analysis

The two outcomes used to compare the efficacy of the two surgical approaches in this meta-analysis were 1) peri-operative mortality and 2) length of hospital stay. Odds ratios (OR) with 95% confidence intervals (CI) were calculated for comparisons of peri-operative mortality rates between patients with rAAAs who underwent EVAR and those who underwent OSR; OR <1 indicates that the EVAR approach is favored. Difference in mean length of hospital stay with 95% CI was calculated for patients who underwent EVAR compared to those who underwent OSR. To analyze studies for which calculation of mean $\pm$ standard deviations (SD) was not possible, the mean and variance were estimated from the median, range, and sample size if these data were available [29]. Heterogeneity among the studies was assessed by calculating Cochran Q and the I^2 statistic. For the Q statistic, $P<0.10$ indicated statistically significant heterogeneity. The I^2 statistic indicates the percentage of the observed between-study variability caused by heterogeneity. Heterogeneity determined using the I^2 statistic was defined as follows: 0 to 24% = no heterogeneity; 25 to 49% = moderate heterogeneity; 50 to 74% = large heterogeneity; and 75 to 100% = extreme heterogeneity. If either the Q statistic ($P<0.1$) or I^2 statistic ($>50\%$) indicated that heterogeneity existed between studies, the random-effects model (DerSimonian-Laird method) was used. Otherwise, the fixed-effects model was used (Mantel-Haenszel method). Pooled OR or difference in means was calculated and a 2-sided P value <0.05 was considered statistically significant. Sensitivity analysis was performed for primary outcome based on the leave-one-out approach. Publication bias was assessed by constructing funnel plots for primary outcome and quantitatively detected by fail-safe N (NFS) and Egger's test. The absence of publication bias is indicated by the data points forming a symmetric funnel-shaped distribution, large NFS and $P>0.10$ in Egger's test. All statistical analyses were performed using the statistical software Comprehensive Meta-Analysis, version 2.0 (Biostat, Englewood, NJ, USA).

Results

Study Characteristics

The process used for selection of studies is depicted in Figure 1. This meta-analysis included a total of 18 studies and the basic characteristics of the studies are summarized in Table 1[18,20,22–24,26,27,30–40]. Of the 18 studies, there were 2 randomized controlled trials, 4 prospective studies, and 12 retrospective studies. A total of 140,707 patients with rAAA were enrolled, of which 13,231 patients underwent EVAR and 127,476 underwent OSR. The total number of patients in each of studies ranged from 32 to 48,865. In the group that underwent EVAR, peri-operative mortality ranged from 20.0% to 53.3% in the group that underwent EVAR and from 25.0% to 52.9% in the group that underwent OSR. In general, patients who underwent EVAR had a shorter mean or median length of hospital stay compared to those who underwent OSR.

Primary Outcome: Peri-operative Mortality

Since two of the selected studies did not have clear information regarding sample size [20] and peri-operative mortality [36], we only included a total of 16 studies in the meta-analysis. After pooling of data, we found significant heterogeneity among the studies ($Q=27.83$, $df=15$, $P=0.023$; $I^2=46.11\%$), making it necessary to use a random-effects model for the meta-analysis of peri-operative mortality. The combined OR showed significantly lower peri-operative mortality in patients with EVAR compared to those with OSR. Among the 16 studies, ORs ranged from 0.30 to

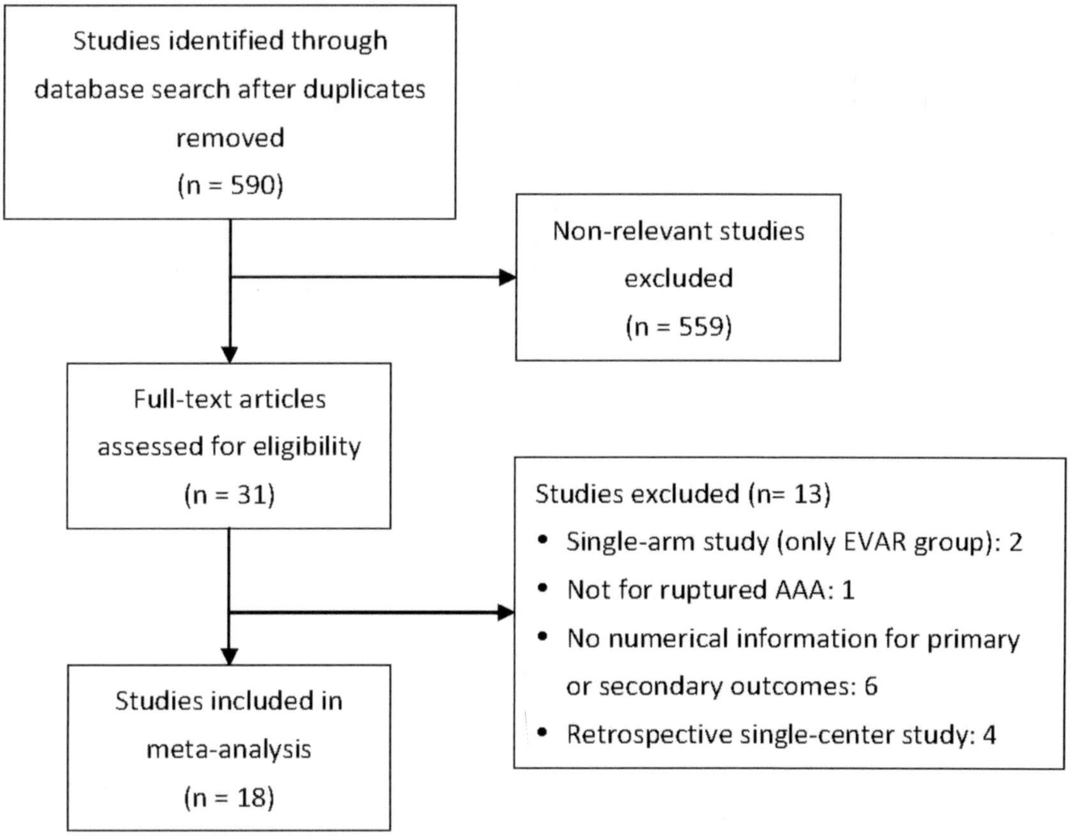

Figure 1. Flow chart for study selection. Abbreviation: EVAR, endovascular aneurysm repair; AAA, abdominal aortic aneurysm.

1.02, with the overall OR being 0.62 (95% CI = 0.57 to 0.67, $P < 0.001$, Figure 2).

Secondary Outcome: Length of Hospital Stay

Only 5 studies provided sufficient information to calculate the difference in mean length of hospital stay between the EVAR and OSR groups: two studies had mean ± SD for each group [[24,27]], while three studies estimated the mean and variance using the median, range, and sample size [[31,32,41]]. After pooling of data, we did not find a significant heterogeneity among the studies ($Q = 3.34$, $df = 4$, $P = 0.503$; $I^2 = 0.0\%$) and therefore used a fixed-effects model for the meta-analysis of the length of hospital stay. The combined difference in means showed a significantly shorter mean length of hospital stay in patients with EVAR compared to those with OSR. Among the 5 studies, the difference in mean length of stay ranged from −7.30 to 0.66 days, with the overall estimate being −1.96 days (95% CI = −3.06 to −0.86, $P < 0.001$, Figure 3).

Sensitivity Analysis

The results of sensitivity analysis, in which studies were omitted one at a time, are summarized in Figure 4. For peri-operative mortality, the direction and magnitude of the pooled estimate did not vary markedly with the removal of any study (Figure 4), indicating good reliability in this meta-analysis.

Publication Bias

The funnel plot for publication bias (standard error by log odds ratio of peri-operative mortality) demonstrated evidence of symmetry (Figure 5), indicating no evidence of publication bias. Additionally, the combined effect size for the 16 studies yielded a Z value of −17.23 and corresponding 2-tailed p-value of <0.0001. The NFS was 1221, indicating that we would need to locate and include 1221 'null' studies in order for the combined 2-tailed p-value to exceed 0.050. We also used the Egger's test to show that there was no publication bias for peri-operative mortality (Figure 5, $t = 0.345$, $P = 0.368$).

Discussion

In this meta-analysis of 18 studies, we compared peri-operative mortality and length of hospital stay in patients with rAAAs who underwent emergent EVAR to those who underwent emergent OSR. Our analysis showed that patients who underwent emergent EVAR had significantly lower peri-operative mortality rates and a significantly shorter hospital stay compared to those who underwent emergent OSR.

The use of EVAR for rAAAs has increased in the United States, especially in urban areas, likely because EVAR is associated with reduced mortality and a reduced complication rate compared to OSR [38,42]. However, there are conflicting data on the efficacy and outcomes of EVAR in patients with rAAAs due to wide variations in trial design. Data from some of the retrospective studies included in our analysis showed that 1) mortality rates have decreased in patients receiving emergent EVAR for rAAAs, while the rates have remained stable in patients who received emergent OSR, 2) high-volume institutions have lower mortality rates compared to low-volume institutions [31,35,37] and 3) in-hospital mortality for emergent AAA repairs is lower in hospitals with a

Table 1. Characteristics of studies included in the meta-analysis.

Author (Year)	Study type	Institute or database	Number of cases	Age (year), mean	Gender, male (%)	Hospital stay (days), mean	Peri-operative mortality (%)	Conversion to open surgery (%)	Study quality (maximum 9)‡
Alsac JM (2005) [22]	prospective	Henri-Mondor University Hospital, Créteil (France)	17 vs. 20	72.9 vs. 72.8	94 vs. 100	Median: 11.5 vs. 20	23.5 vs. 50.0	17.6	8
Davenport DL (2010) [30]	retrospective	American College of Surgeons National Surgical Quality Improvement Program database (USA)	99 vs. 328	72.1 vs. 73.6	80 vs. 77	NA	22.2 vs. 37.2	NA	8
Egorova NN (2011) [26]	retrospective	Medicare Inpatient Standard Analytical and Denominator files (USA)	2007 vs. 46858	Male: 77.5 vs. 75.9 Female: 78.8 vs.:78.2	75 vs. 77	NA	41.1 vs. 52.7	7	7
Giles KA (2009) [31]	retrospective	Healthcare Cost and Utilization Project Nationwide Inpatient Sample database (USA)	2323 vs. 26106	Median: 75 vs. 73	NA	Median: 7 vs. 9	32.6 vs. 41.5	NA	8
Giles KA (2009) [32]	retrospective	American College of Surgeons National Surgical Quality Improvement Program database (USA)	121 vs. 446	72.6 vs. 73.7	80 vs. 76	Median: 7 vs. 10	24.0 vs. 36.0	4.1	8
Greco G (2006) [20]	retrospective	The hospital discharge databases for the four states of California, Florida, New Jersey and New York (USA)	NA	NA	NA	13.4 vs. 19	39.3 vs. 47.7	N = 20	8
Hinchliffe RJ (2006) [23]	Prospective, randomized controlled	University Hospital, Nottingham (UK)	15 vs. 17	Median: 74 vs. 80	73 vs. 76	Median: 10 vs. 12	53.3 vs. 52.9†	13.3	N/A
Holt PJ (2010) [33]	retrospective	National Health Service Hospital Episode Statistics (UK)	335 vs. 4079	NA	NA	NA	32.2 vs. 47.4	NA	7
Vogel TR (2009) [34]	retrospective	Healthcare Cost and Utilization Project New Jersey State Inpatient Database (USA)	82 vs. 618	NA	NA	14.08 vs. 13.42	45.1 vs. 52.4	NA	8
Leon LR Jr (2005) [27]	retrospective	Illinois Hospital Association COMPdata database (USA)	55 vs. 2063	NA	75 vs. 77	11.7 vs. 13.1	36.4 vs. 42.4	NA	8
Lesperance K (2008) [35]	retrospective	Healthcare Cost and Utilization Project Nationwide Inpatient Sample database (USA)	949 vs. 8982	73.9 vs. 73.1	78 vs. 76	Median: 6 vs. 9	31.0 vs. 42.0	NA	8
Mandawat A (2012) [36]	retrospective	Healthcare Cost and Utilization Project Nationwide Inpatient Sample database (USA)	64 vs. 207	70.5 vs. 72	73 vs. 76	NA	<18.0 vs. 35.7	NA	8
McPhee J (2009) [37]	retrospective	Healthcare Cost and Utilization Project Nationwide Inpatient Sample database (USA)	3179 vs. 24571	74.3 vs. 73	77 vs. 77	NA	31.7 vs. 40.7	NA	7

Table 1. Cont.

Author (Year)	Study type	Institute or database	Number of cases	Age (year), mean	Gender, male (%)	Hospital stay (days), mean	Peri-operative mortality (%)	Conversion to open surgery (%)	Study quality (maximum 9)‡
Park BD (2013) [38]	retrospective	Healthcare Cost and Utilization Project Nationwide Inpatient *Sample database (USA)	3796 vs. 12761	NA	75 vs. 75	9.91 vs. 13	27.4 vs. 41.0	0.64	8
Peppelenbosch N (2006) [24]	prospective	The New ERA trial; ten hospitals in Europe and Canada	49 vs. 51	75.1 vs. 73.8	86 vs. 80	14.9 vs. 22.2	35.0 vs. 39.0	6.1	8
Reimerink JJ (2013) [39]	Prospective, randomized controlled	Academic Medical Center, Amsterdam (The Netherlands)	57 vs. 59	74.9 vs. 74.5	86 vs. 85	Median: 9 vs. 13	21.0 vs. 25.0†	8.8	N/A
		VU University Medical Center, Amsterdam(The Netherlands)							
		OnzeLieveVrouweGastnhuis, Amsterdam (The Netherlands)							
Ten Bosch JA (2012) [18]	prospective	Catharina Hospital, Eindhoven (The Netherlands)	25 vs. 104	72.2 vs. 73.7	88 vs. 89	Median: 9.5 vs. 16	20.0 vs. 45.2	NA	7
Visser JJ (2009) [45]	prospective	Atrium Medical Center, Heerlen (The Netherlands)	58 vs. 143	73.2 vs. 73.5	93 vs. 83	NA	26.0 vs. 40.0	15.5	8
		Catharina Hospital, Eindhoven (The Netherlands)							
		Erasmus Medical Center, Rotterdam (The Netherlands)							
		Medical Spectrum Twente, Enschede (The Netherlands)							
		Medical Center Rotterdam Zuid, Rotterdam (The Netherlands)							
		University Medical Center, Groningen (The Netherlands)							
		University Medical Center, Nijmegen (The Netherlands)							

†The peri-operative mortality for these studies was calculated on an intention to treat basis.
‡Stucy quality assessment performed using the Newcastle-Ottawa Scale.
Abbreviation: EVAR, endovascular repair; OSR, open surgical repair; AAA, abdominal aortic aneurysm.

Study name	Comparison	Odds ratio	Lower limit	Upper limit	Z-Value	P-Value	Relative Weight
Alsac JM (2005)	EVAR vs. OSR	0.31	0.07	1.27	-1.63	0.104	0.27
Davenport DL (2010)	EVAR vs. OSR	0.48	0.29	0.81	-2.73	0.006	1.83
Egorova NN (2011)	EVAR vs. OSR	0.62	0.57	0.68	-10.15	0.000	16.77
Giles KA (2009)a	EVAR vs. OSR	0.68	0.62	0.75	-8.32	0.000	16.83
Giles KA (2009)b	EVAR vs. OSR	0.56	0.35	0.89	-2.46	0.014	2.33
Hinchliffe RJ (2006)	EVAR vs. OSR	1.02	0.25	4.08	0.02	0.982	0.28
Holt PJ (2010)	EVAR vs. OSR	0.53	0.42	0.67	-5.29	0.000	6.79
Vogel TR (2009)	EVAR vs. OSR	0.75	0.47	1.19	-1.24	0.215	2.30
Leon LR Jr (2005)	EVAR vs. OSR	0.78	0.45	1.36	-0.89	0.375	1.64
Lesperance K (2008)	EVAR vs. OSR	0.62	0.54	0.72	-6.51	0.000	12.15
McPhee J (2009)	EVAR vs. OSR	0.68	0.62	0.73	-9.72	0.000	17.87
Park BD (2013)	EVAR vs. OSR	0.54	0.50	0.59	-15.02	0.000	17.81
Peppelenbosch N (2006)	EVAR vs. OSR	0.84	0.37	1.90	-0.41	0.679	0.80
Reimerink JJ (2013)	EVAR vs. OSR	0.80	0.33	1.90	-0.51	0.609	0.71
Ten Bosch JA (2012)	EVAR vs. OSR	0.30	0.11	0.87	-2.22	0.026	0.48
Visser JJ (2009)	EVAR vs. OSR	0.53	0.27	1.04	-1.86	0.063	1.14
combined		0.62	0.57	0.67	-12.70	0.000	

Heterogeneity test: Q = 27.83, df = 15, P = 0.023, I-square = 46.11%

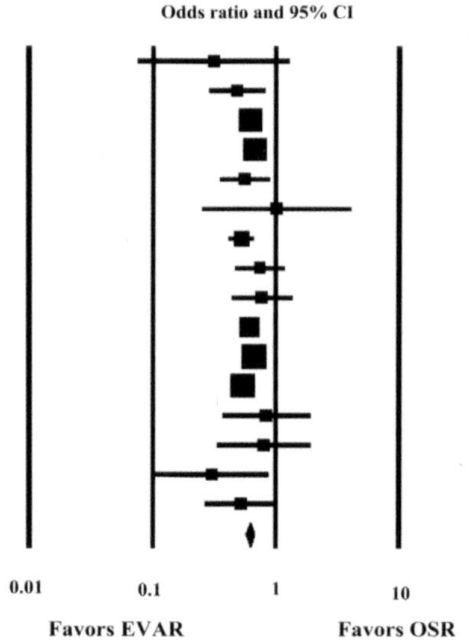

Figure 2. Forest plot showing results for the meta-analysis of peri-operative mortality: rAAA patients with EVAR vs. rAAA patients with OSR. Abbreviation: EVAR, endovascular aneurysm repair; OSR, open surgical repair; CI, confidence interval.

greater number of elective AAA repairs, possibly due to the higher numbers of specialist surgeons and vascular critical care facilities [33].

The ACS National Surgical Quality Improvement Program (ACS NSQIP) is the first nationally validated, risk-adjusted, outcomes-based program to measure and improve the quality of surgical care (http://www.facs.org/cqi/outcomes.html). Some retrospective studies analyzing the NSQIP database showed a significantly lower composite 30-day morbidity risk and a lower intraoperative transfusion requirement in patients with rAAAs after EVAR compared to open repair [30,32]. Data from two retrospective studies included in our analysis showed that 1) rAAA patients who received EVAR had a significant survival benefit compared to patients who received OSR [33] and 2) EVAR resulted in superior short-term outcomes compared to open repair in rAAA patients who are transferred to institutions with EVAR facilities [36]. Peppelenbosch et al. showed lower first-month mortality and lower blood loss in a prospectively enrolled group of patients with rAAAs when compared to a retrospective control group [41]. These studies were consistent with results from a recent meta-analysis of randomized and risk-adjusted observational studies comparing EVAR vs. open repair for rAAA, which showed that EVAR was associated with a significantly lower mortality rate compared to open repair [43]. Another recent meta-analysis of 41 studies showed that emergent EVAR was associated with a significantly lower risk of in-hospital mortality and respiratory, renal and cardiac complications compared to OSR [44].

However, these data contrast with studies showing that although patients who received emergent EVAR had better 30-day mortality rates compared to patients who received OSR, this was not statistically significant [39,40]. Data from a randomized controlled trial included in our analysis also did not show a significant benefit conferred by EVAR, which could be due to the small sample size of this study [23]. Additionally, a retrospective cohort study included in our analysis showed no survival benefit in patients who received emergent EVAR compared to those who received OSR. This was suggested to be due to a number of factors including the lack of well-established EVAR facilities and patient insurance constraints [34]. Our meta-analysis included data from a randomized trial in Amsterdam which showed no

Study name	Comparison	Difference in means	Lower limit	Upper limit	Z-Value	P-Value	Relative Weight
Giles KA (2009)a	EVAR vs. OSR	-2.00	-3.31	-0.69	-2.99	0.003	70.53
Giles KA (2009)b	EVAR vs. OSR	-3.00	-6.17	0.17	-1.86	0.063	12.10
Vogel TR (2009)	EVAR vs. OSR	0.66	-3.52	4.84	0.31	0.757	6.94
Leon LR Jr (2005)	EVAR vs. OSR	-1.40	-5.08	2.28	-0.75	0.456	8.96
Peppelenbosch N (2006)	EVAR vs. OSR	-7.30	-16.39	1.79	-1.57	0.115	1.47
Combined		-1.96	-3.06	-0.86	-3.49	0.000	

Heterogeneity test: Q = 3.34, df = 4, P = 0.503, I-square = 0.0%

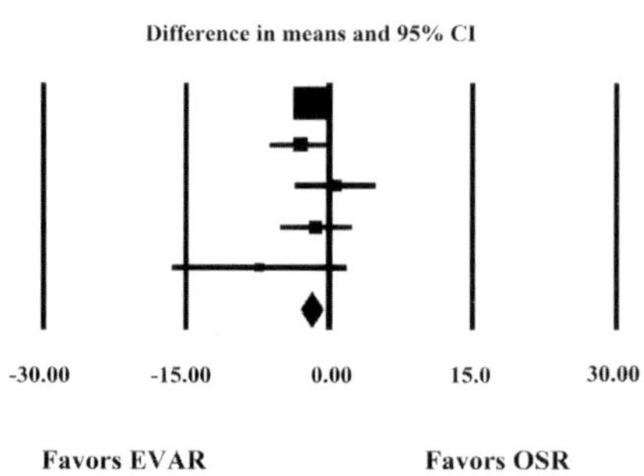

Figure 3. Forest plot showing results for the meta-analysis of length of hospital stay in rAAA patients with EVAR vs. rAAA patients with OSR. Abbreviation: EVAR, endovascular aneurysm repair; OSR, open surgical repair; CI, confidence interval.

Study name	Comparison	Statistics with study removed: Odds ratio	Lower limit	Upper limit	Z-Value	P-Value
Alsac JM (2005)	EVAR vs. OSR	0.62	0.58	0.67	-12.62	0.000
Davenport DL (2010)	EVAR vs. OSR	0.62	0.58	0.67	-12.41	0.000
Egorova NN (2011)	EVAR vs. OSR	0.62	0.56	0.67	-10.51	0.000
Giles KA (2009)a	EVAR vs. OSR	0.61	0.56	0.66	-12.35	0.000
Giles KA (2009)b	EVAR vs. OSR	0.62	0.57	0.67	-12.22	0.000
Hinchliffe RJ (2006)	EVAR vs. OSR	0.62	0.57	0.67	-12.56	0.000
Holt PJ (2010)	EVAR vs. OSR	0.63	0.58	0.68	-12.11	0.000
Vogel TR (2009)	EVAR vs. OSR	0.62	0.57	0.66	-12.51	0.000
Leon LR Jr (2005)	EVAR vs. OSR	0.62	0.57	0.66	-12.56	0.000
Lesperance K (2008)	EVAR vs. OSR	0.62	0.57	0.67	-11.24	0.000
McPhee J (2009)	EVAR vs. OSR	0.61	0.56	0.66	-12.34	0.000
Park BD (2013)	EVAR vs. OSR	0.65	0.62	0.68	-18.74	0.000
Peppelenbosch N (2006)	EVAR vs. OSR	0.62	0.57	0.67	-12.57	0.000
Reimerink JJ (2013)	EVAR vs. OSR	0.62	0.57	0.67	-12.49	0.000
Ten Bosch JA (2012)	EVAR vs. OSR	0.62	0.58	0.67	-12.83	0.000
Visser JJ (2009)	EVAR vs. OSR	0.62	0.57	0.67	-12.34	0.000

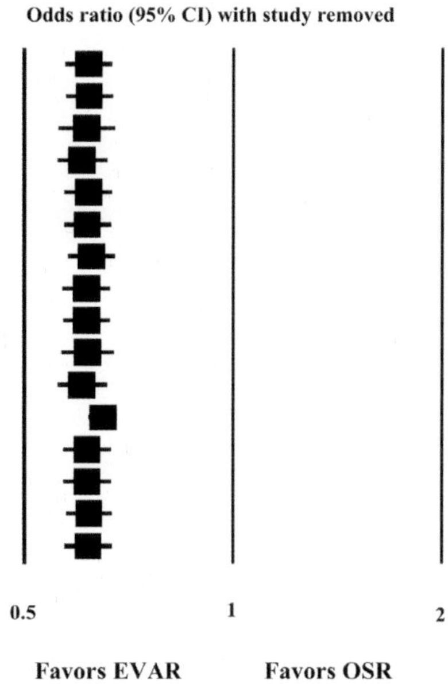

Figure 4. Results of sensitivity analysis to examine the influence of individual studies on pooled estimates of peri-operative mortality as determined by the "leave-one-out" approach. Abbreviation: EVAR, endovascular aneurysm repair; OSR, open surgical repair; CI, confidence interval.

significant difference in combined death or severe complications between patients who received emergent EVAR and those who received OSR. This was attributed to optimization of logistics and protocols, resulting in comparable outcomes with both procedures [39]. Although our data showed an overall benefit in terms of peri-operative mortality and length of hospital stay in rAAA patients compared to OSR, there is an urgent need to resolve such discrepancies with prospective randomized controlled trials performed on larger sample sizes.

It is important to note that in our present meta-analysis of 18 studies, only 7 were prospective studies and only 2 were randomized, controlled studies. Although we included multi-center, retrospective studies, we excluded single-center, retrospective studies in order to prevent selection bias. We are also aware that inclusion of two large population-based studies in this meta-analysis [26,37] is a limitation of this study, since they may incorporate duplications. The small number of qualified studies could reflect the practical and ethical considerations which limit

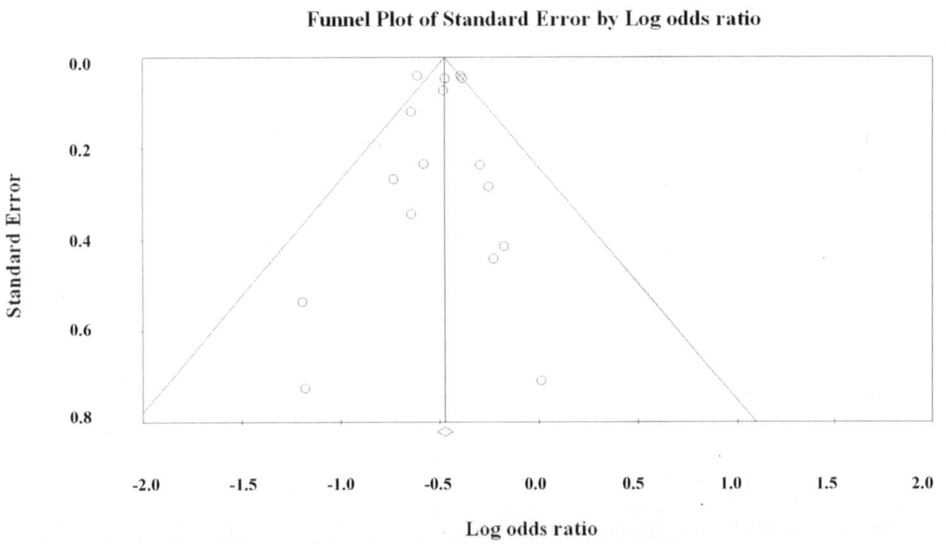

Figure 5. Funnel plot for evaluating publication bias while reporting peri-operative mortality. White circles represent published article and white rhombuses represent the actual combined effect sizes, respectively.

the design of randomized, controlled trials to compare EVAR and OSR for ruptured AAAs. These considerations include the endovascular expertise of the surgeons, the time required for a CT scan prior to EVAR and the time required for randomization [23,39]. However, since it was shown that CT scanning did not delay treatment, it is possible to recruit patients with ruptured AAAs to randomized trials to compare outcomes of EVAR and OSR [23]. After pooling data from 16 studies, we showed significantly lower peri-operative mortality rates in rAAA patients who received emergent EVAR compared to those who received OSR. We also used a random-effects model to analyze data from 5 studies and showed that rAAA patients who received EVAR had significantly shorter hospital stays compared to those who received OSR. It is possible that our data could be a reflection of the fact that emergent EVAR attenuates the inflammatory response, which could be advantageous in rAAA patients [21].

Dropping one study at a time from the meta-analysis did not significantly change the direction or magnitude of the pooled data, indicating the reliability of this analysis. We also used a funnel plot and the Egger's test to show that there was no publication bias in our meta-analysis.

In summary, we showed that EVAR conferred significant benefits in terms of peri-operative mortality and length of hospital stay in rAAA patients compared to OSR. A number of factors such as logistics and preoperative CT scanning could explain the dearth of prospective randomized controlled trials to compare EVAR and OSR in rAAA patients.

Author Contributions

Conceived and designed the experiments: YbX CQ. Performed the experiments: CQ LC. Analyzed the data: CQ LC. Contributed reagents/materials/analysis tools: YbX LC. Wrote the paper: CQ.

References

1. Ren S, Fan X, Ye Z, Liu P (2012) Long-term outcomes of endovascular repair versus open repair of abdominal aortic aneurysm. Ann Thorac Cardiovasc Surg 18: 222–227.
2. Takayama T, Yamanouchi D (2013) Aneurysmal disease: the abdominal aorta. Surg Clin North Am 93: 877–891, viii.
3. Cury M, Zeidan F, Lobato AC (2013) Aortic disease in the young: genetic aneurysm syndromes, connective tissue disorders, and familial aortic aneurysms and dissections. Int J Vasc Med 2013: 267215.
4. Upchurch GR Jr, Schaub TA (2006) Abdominal aortic aneurysm. Am Fam Physician 73: 1198–1204.
5. United Kingdom ETI, Greenhalgh RM, Brown LC, Powell JT, Thompson SG, et al. (2010) Endovascular versus open repair of abdominal aortic aneurysm. N Engl J Med 362: 1863–1871.
6. Dubost C, Allary M, Oeconomos N (1951) [Treatment of aortic aneurysms; removal of the aneurysm; re-establishment of continuity by grafts of preserved human aorta]. Mem Acad Chir (Paris) 77: 381–383.
7. Akkersdijk GJ, Puylaert JB, de Vries AC (1991) Abdominal aortic aneurysm as an incidental finding in abdominal ultrasonography. Br J Surg 78: 1261–1263.
8. Von Allmen RS, Powell JT (2012) The management of ruptured abdominal aortic aneurysms: screening for abdominal aortic aneurysm and incidence of rupture. J Cardiovasc Surg (Torino) 53: 69–76.
9. Hoornweg LL, Storm-Versloot MN, Ubbink DT, Koelemay MJ, Legemate DA, et al. (2008) Meta analysis on mortality of ruptured abdominal aortic aneurysms. Eur J Vasc Endovasc Surg 35: 558–570.
10. Bown MJ, Sutton AJ, Bell PR, Sayers RD (2002) A meta-analysis of 50 years of ruptured abdominal aortic aneurysm repair. Br J Surg 89: 714–730.
11. Yusuf SW, Whitaker SC, Chuter TA, Wenham PW, Hopkinson BR (1994) Emergency endovascular repair of leaking aortic aneurysm. Lancet 344: 1645.
12. Volodos NL, Shekhanin VE, Karpovich IP, Troian VI, Gur'ev Iu A (1986) [A self-fixing synthetic blood vessel endoprosthesis]. Vestn Khir Im I I Grek 137: 123–125.
13. Parodi JC, Palmaz JC, Barone HD (1991) Transfemoral intraluminal graft implantation for abdominal aortic aneurysms. Ann Vasc Surg 5: 491–499.
14. Greenhalgh RM, Brown LC, Kwong GP, Powell JT, Thompson SG, et al. (2004) Comparison of endovascular aneurysm repair with open repair in patients with abdominal aortic aneurysm (EVAR trial 1), 30-day operative mortality results: randomised controlled trial. Lancet 364: 843–848.
15. De Bruin JL, Baas AF, Buth J, Prinssen M, Verhoeven EL, et al. (2010) Long-term outcome of open or endovascular repair of abdominal aortic aneurysm. N Engl J Med 362: 1881–1889.
16. Lederle FA, Freischlag JA, Kyriakides TC, Padberg FT Jr, Matsumura JS, et al. (2009) Outcomes following endovascular vs open repair of abdominal aortic aneurysm: a randomized trial. JAMA 302: 1535–1542.
17. Schermerhorn ML, O'Malley AJ, Jhaveri A, Cotterill P, Pomposelli F, et al. (2008) Endovascular vs. open repair of abdominal aortic aneurysms in the Medicare population. N Engl J Med 358: 464–474.
18. Ten Bosch JA, Willigendael EM, Kruidenier LM, de Loos ER, Prins MH, et al. (2012) Early and mid-term results of a prospective observational study comparing emergency endovascular aneurysm repair with open surgery in both ruptured and unruptured acute abdominal aortic aneurysms. Vascular 20: 72–80.
19. Propper BW, Abularrage CJ (2013) Long-term safety and efficacy of endovascular abdominal aortic aneurysm repair. Vasc Health Risk Manag 9: 135–141.
20. Greco G, Egorova N, Anderson PL, Gelijns A, Moskowitz A, et al. (2006) Outcomes of endovascular treatment of ruptured abdominal aortic aneurysms. J Vasc Surg 43: 453–459.
21. Sadat U, Boyle JR, Walsh SR, Tang T, Varty K, et al. (2008) Endovascular vs open repair of acute abdominal aortic aneurysms–a systematic review and meta-analysis. J Vasc Surg 48: 227–236.
22. Alsac JM, Desgranges P, Kobeiter H, Becquemin JP (2005) Emergency endovascular repair for ruptured abdominal aortic aneurysms: feasibility and comparison of early results with conventional open repair. Eur J Vasc Endovasc Surg 30: 632–639.
23. Hinchliffe RJ, Bruijstens L, MacSweeney ST, Braithwaite BD (2006) A randomised trial of endovascular and open surgery for ruptured abdominal aortic aneurysm - results of a pilot study and lessons learned for future studies. Eur J Vasc Endovasc Surg 32: 506–513; discussion 514–505.
24. Peppelenbosch N, Geelkerken RH, Soong C, Cao P, Steinmetz OK, et al. (2006) Endograft treatment of ruptured abdominal aortic aneurysms using the Talent aortouniiliac system: an international multicenter study. J Vasc Surg 43: 1111–1123; discussion 1123.
25. Trial I, Powell JT, Thompson SG, Thompson MM, Grieve R, et al. (2009) The Immediate Management of the Patient with Rupture: Open Versus Endovascular repair (IMPROVE) aneurysm trial–ISRCTN 48334791 IMPROVE trialists. Acta Chir Belg 109: 678–680.
26. Egorova NN, Vouyouka AG, McKinsey JF, Faries PL, Kent KC, et al. (2011) Effect of gender on long-term survival after abdominal aortic aneurysm repair based on results from the Medicare national database. J Vasc Surg 54: 1–12 e16; discussion 11–12.
27. Leon LR Jr, Labropoulos N, Laredo J, Rodriguez HE, Kalman PG (2005) To what extent has endovascular aneurysm repair influenced abdominal aortic aneurysm management in the state of Illinois? J Vasc Surg 41: 568–574.
28. Wells GA, Shea B, O'Connell D, Peterson J, Welch,V, etal. (2000) The Newcastle-Ottawa Scale (NOS) for assessing the quality of nonrandomized studies in meta-analyses. The 3rd Symposium on Systematic Reviews: Beyond the Basics. Oxford, England.
29. Hozo SP, Djulbegovic B, Hozo I (2005) Estimating the mean and variance from the median, range, and the size of a sample. BMC Med Res Methodol 5: 13.
30. Davenport DL, O'Keeffe SD, Minion DJ, Sorial EE, Endean ED, et al. (2010) Thirty-day NSQIP database outcomes of open versus endoluminal repair of ruptured abdominal aortic aneurysms. J Vasc Surg 51: 305–309 e301.
31. Giles KA, Hamdan AD, Pomposelli FB, Wyers MC, Dahlberg SE, et al. (2009) Population-based outcomes following endovascular and open repair of ruptured abdominal aortic aneurysms. J Endovasc Ther 16: 554–564.
32. Giles KA, Pomposelli FB, Hamdan AD, Wyers MC, Schermerhorn ML (2009) Comparison of open and endovascular repair of ruptured abdominal aortic aneurysms from the ACS-NSQIP 2005–07. J Endovasc Ther 16: 365–372.
33. Holt PJ, Karthikesalingam A, Poloniecki JD, Hinchliffe RJ, Loftus IM, et al. (2010) Propensity scored analysis of outcomes after ruptured abdominal aortic aneurysm. Br J Surg 97: 496–503.
34. Vogel TR, Dombrovskiy VY, Haser PB, Graham AM (2009) Has the implementation of EVAR for ruptured AAA improved outcomes? Vasc Endovascular Surg 43: 252–257.
35. Lesperance K, Andersen C, Singh N, Starnes B, Martin MJ (2008) Expanding use of emergency endovascular repair for ruptured abdominal aortic aneurysms: disparities in outcomes from a nationwide perspective. J Vasc Surg 47: 1165–1170; discussion 1170–1161.

36. Mandawat A, Mandawat A, Sosa JA, Muhs BE, Indes JE (2012) Endovascular repair is associated with superior clinical outcomes in patients transferred for treatment of ruptured abdominal aortic aneurysms. J Endovasc Ther 19: 88–95.
37. McPhee J, Eslami MH, Arous EJ, Messina LM, Schanzer A (2009) Endovascular treatment of ruptured abdominal aortic aneurysms in the United States (2001–2006): a significant survival benefit over open repair is independently associated with increased institutional volume. J Vasc Surg 49: 817–826.
38. Park BD, Azefor N, Huang CC, Ricotta JJ (2013) Trends in treatment of ruptured abdominal aortic aneurysm: impact of endovascular repair and implications for future care. J Am Coll Surg 216: 745–754; discussion 754–745.
39. Reimerink JJ, Hoornweg LL, Vahl AC, Wisselink W, van den Broek TA, et al. (2013) Endovascular repair versus open repair of ruptured abdominal aortic aneurysms: a multicenter randomized controlled trial. Ann Surg 258: 248–256.
40. Visser JJ, van Sambeek MR, Hamza TH, Hunink MG, Bosch JL (2007) Ruptured abdominal aortic aneurysms: endovascular repair versus open surgery–systematic review. Radiology 245: 122–129.
41. Peppelenbosch N, Yilmaz N, van Marrewijk C, Buth J, Cuypers P, et al. (2003) Emergency treatment of acute symptomatic or ruptured abdominal aortic aneurysm. Outcome of a prospective intent-to-treat by EVAR protocol. Eur J Vasc Endovasc Surg 26: 303–310.
42. Piffaretti G, Caronno R, Tozzi M, Lomazzi C, Rivolta N, et al. (2006) Endovascular versus open repair of ruptured abdominal aortic aneurysms. Expert Rev Cardiovasc Ther 4: 839–852.
43. Takagi H, Umemoto T (2011) A meta-analysis of randomized and risk-adjusted observational studies of endovascular versus open repair for ruptured abdominal aortic aneurysm. Vasc Endovascular Surg 45: 717–719.
44. Antoniou GA, Georgiadis GS, Antoniou SA, Pavlidis P, Maras D, et al. (2013) Endovascular repair for ruptured abdominal aortic aneurysm confers an early survival benefit over open repair. J Vasc Surg 58: 1091–1105.
45. Visser JJ, Williams M, Kievit J, Bosch JL, Group AS (2009) Prediction of 30-day mortality after endovascular repair or open surgery in patients with ruptured abdominal aortic aneurysms. J Vasc Surg 49: 1093–1099.

5

The Application of Transcutaneous CO_2 Pressure Monitoring in the Anesthesia of Obese Patients Undergoing Laparoscopic Bariatric Surgery

Shijiang Liu[1], Jie Sun[2], Xing Chen[3], Yingying Yu[4], Xuan Liu[5], Cunming Liu[6]*

1 Department of Anesthesiology, The First Affiliated Hospital of Nanjing Medical University, Nanjing, China, **2** Department of Anesthesiology, The First Affiliated Hospital of Nanjing Medical University, Nanjing, China, **3** Department of Project Management, Jiangsu New Energy Development Company, Jiangsu Guoxin Investment Group, Nanjing, China, **4** Department of Anesthesiology, The First Affiliated Hospital of Nanjing Medical University, Nanjing, China, **5** Department of Anesthesiology, General Hospital of TISCO, TaiYuan, China, **6** Department of Anesthesiology, The First Affiliated Hospital of Nanjing Medical University, Nanjing, China

Abstract

To investigate the correlation and accuracy of transcutaneous carbon dioxide partial pressure ($P_{TC}CO_2$) with regard to arterial carbon dioxide partial pressure (P_aCO_2) in severe obese patients undergoing laparoscopic bariatric surgery. Twenty-one patients with BMI>35 kg/m^2 were enrolled in our study. Their P_aCO_2, end-tidal carbon dioxide partial pressure ($P_{et}CO_2$), as well as $P_{TC}CO_2$ values were measured at before pneumoperitoneum and 30 min, 60 min, 120 min after pneumoperitoneum respectively. Then the differences between each pair of values ($P_{et}CO_2$–P_aCO_2) and ($P_{TC}CO_2$–P_aCO_2) were calculated. Bland–Altman method, correlation and regression analysis, as well as exact probability method and two way contingency table were employed for the data analysis. 21 adults (aged 19–54 yr, mean 29, SD 9 yr; weight 86–160 kg, mean119.3, SD 22.1 kg; BMI 35.3–51.1 kg/m^2, mean 42.1,SD 5.4 kg/m^2) were finally included in this study. One patient was eliminated due to the use of vaso-excitor material phenylephrine during anesthesia induction. Eighty-four sample sets were obtained. The average P_aCO_2–$P_{TC}CO_2$ difference was 0.9±1.3 mmHg (mean±SD). And the average P_aCO_2–$P_{et}CO_2$ difference was 10.3±2.3 mmHg (mean±SD). The linear regression equation of P_aCO_2–$P_{et}CO_2$ is $P_{et}CO_2 = 11.58+0.57\times P_aCO_2$ ($r^2 = 0.64$, $P<0.01$), whereas the one of P_aCO_2–$P_{TC}CO_2$ is $P_{TC}CO_2 = 0.60+0.97\times P_aCO_2$ ($r^2 = 0.89$). The LOA (limits of agreement) of 95% average P_aCO_2–$P_{et}CO_2$ difference is 10.3±4.6 mmHg (mean±1.96 SD), while the LOA of 95% average P_aCO_2–P_{TC}CO2 difference is 0.9±2.6 mmHg (mean±1.96 SD). In conclusion, transcutaneous carbon dioxide monitoring provides a better estimate of $PaCO_2$ than $P_{et}CO_2$ in severe obese patients undergoing laparoscopic bariatric surgery.

Editor: Zhongcong Xie, Massachusetts General Hospital, United States of America

Funding: This study was supported by a project funded by the Priority Academic Program Development of Jiangsu Higher Education Institutions (PAPD). The funders had no role in study design, data collection and analysis, decision to publish, or preparation of the manuscript.

Competing Interests: Xing Chen is employed by Jiangsu New Energy Development Company, Jiangsu Guoxin Investment Group. There are no patents, products in development or marketed products to declare.

* E-mail: mingliu870@sohu.com

Introduction

Currently the "gold standard" technique for the measurement of arterial carbon dioxide partial pressure (P_aCO_2) is performed by direct analysis of arterial blood gases (ABG), but this method is invasive, intermittent and may cause iatrogenic anemia in infants. The end-tidal carbon dioxide partial pressure ($P_{et}CO_2$) measurement has been widely used for the continuous noninvasive monitoring of carbon dioxide in patients with tracheal intubation during general anesthesia, However, many factors may possibly affect the accuracy of $P_{et}CO_2$ monitoring, such as mismatch of ventilation to blood flow (V/Q ratio), chronic obstructive pulmonary disease, obstructive sleep apnea syndrome, surgery postures, smoking, ect. Recently, noninvasive transcutaneous carbon dioxide partial pressure ($P_{TC}CO_2$) monitoring has been used in infants and in adult patients with good accuracy [1–3].

Laparoscopic bariatric surgery is a quite common operation for the treatment of severe obese patients. Griffin J et al [4] reported that the $P_{TC}CO_2$ monitoring had a better accuracy than that of $P_{et}CO_2$ in estimate of P_aCO_2 for sever obesity undergoing open bariatric surgery, but the accuracy and correlation between P_aCO_2 measurements and $P_{TC}CO_2$ monitoring for patients with laparoscopic bariatric surgery is still unknown. We therefore designed the present study to evaluate the accuracy and correlation of estimating P_aCO_2 using a $P_{TC}CO_2$ monitor in severe obese patients undergoing laparoscopic bariatric surgery.

Materials and Methods

Ethics Statement

This study was approved by the ethic committee of Jiangsu Province Hospital. Before the study, oral informed consent was obtained from each participant. The Ethics Committee of Jiangsu Province Hospital approved oral informed consent because the study was to be of minimal risk.

We consulted with the Ethics Committee of Jiangsu Province Hospital before the experiment and were confirmed that the $P_{TC}CO_2$ monitor was capable of monitoring the CO_2 level noninvasively. Meanwhile, it was almost impossible to cause thermal injuries on the skin or skin allergy, which in turn made it a non-invasive medical instrument. So the monitor could be applied to the selected patients as long as their oral consents were obtained in the first place. We recorded the conversation of inquiries of those consents by note and were fully supported by the Ethics Committee.

Data

22 patients were collected from our hospital, who were ASA I–II and scheduled for laparoscopic bariatric surgery. Patients with history of severe trauma, operations, smoking, and severe cardiovascular or respiratory diseases, such as coronary heart disease, congestive heart failure, or chronic obstructive pulmonary disease were excluded from this study.

Anesthesia was induced with propofol (1–2 mg.kg^{-1}), fentanyl (2–4 μg.kg^{-1}), and rocuronium (0.6 mg.kg^{-1}) by the same anesthetist. After tracheal intubation, patients were ventilated with 100% oxygen (2 L/min) under the mode of intermittent positive pressure ventilation (IPPV), with a tidal volume of 6–10 ml/kg and an I:E ratio of 1:2. The ventilatory frequency and tidal volume were adjusted to maintain normocarbia ($P_{et}CO_2$, 35–45 mmHg). The $P_{et}CO_2$ was monitored by side stream spirpometry (Datex-Ohmeda, Finland, air pumping speed 150 ml.min^{-1}). $P_{TC}CO_2$ was monitored with a TCM-4 device (Radiometer, Copenhagen, Denmark). One of the authors calibrated, placed, and maintained the monitor. Before placement, the electrode was cleaned, a new membrane applied, and calibration done according to the manufacturer's recommendations. The working temperature of the electrode was set at 44°C and the electrode was placed on the chest. The area where the electrode was placed was swabbed with alcohol in order to to facilitate adhesion of the disk to the skin. Re-calibration was required once the position of the electrode was changed. The electrode was removed, adjusted, and replaced in a different location on the chest every 2 h to avoid thermal injury.

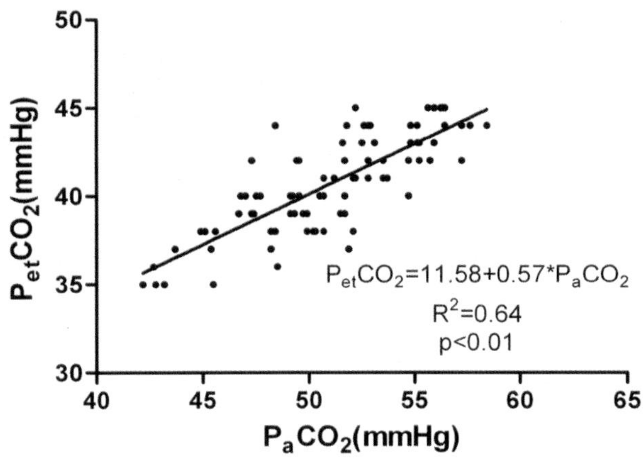

Figure 2. Linear regression analysis between $P_{et}CO_2$ and P_aCO_2. Linear regression analysis between the end tidal carbon dioxide partial pressure ($P_{et}CO_2$) and the arterial carbon dioxide partial pressure (P_aCO_2) in 21 severe obese patients during laparoscopic bariatric surgery. The linear regression equation: $P_{et}CO_2 = 11.58 + 0.57 \times P_aCO_2$, $r^2 = 0.64$, $P < 0.01$.

An AS/5 monitor (Datex-Ohmeda, Finland) was employed to monitor the patients' electrocardiography, pulse oxymetry, and noninvasive blood pressure. Before anesthesia, patients' heart rate (HR) and arterial blood pressure were both recorded as baseline. A 20-G or 22-G arterial catheter was inserted into the left radial artery under local anesthesia for ABG sampling. P_aCO_2 from the ABG was determined with an i-STAT Analyzer System with Disposable EG4-cartridges. Before ABG sampling was performed, the patients' blood pressure, HR, tidal volume, and respiratory rate were constant for at least 5 minutes to obtain the stable $P_{TC}CO_2$. $P_{TC}CO_2$ and $P_{et}CO_2$ were recorded simultaneously. Anesthesia was maintained with propofol (5–8 mg.kg^{-1}.h^{-1}), remifentanil (0.1–0.2 μg kg^{-1}.min^{-1}), and atracurium (0.6 mg.

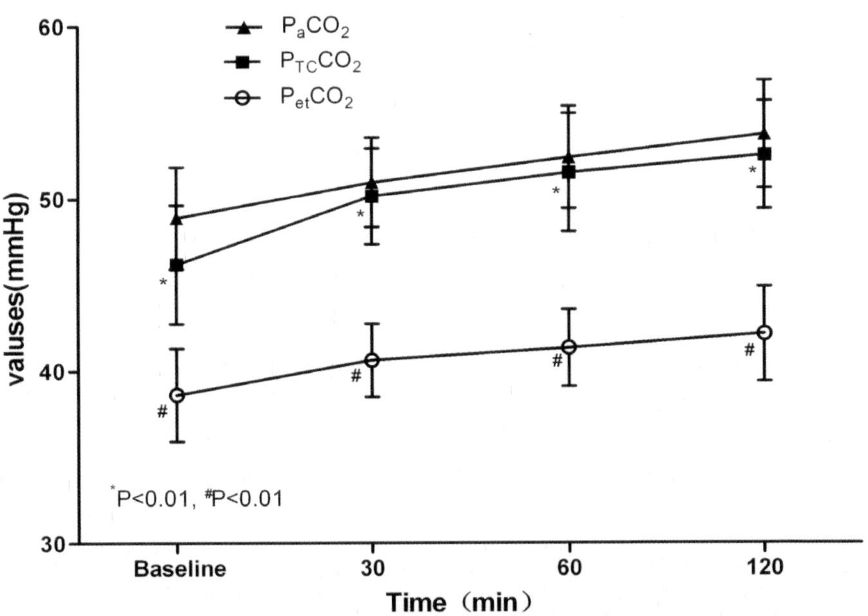

Figure 1. $P_{et}CO_2$, $P_{TC}CO_2$ and P_aCO_2 at different time points after CO_2 pneumoperitoneum. End tidal carbon dioxide partial pressure ($P_{et}CO_2$), transcutaneous carbon dioxide partial pressure ($P_{TC}CO_2$), and arterial carbon dioxide partial pressure (P_aCO_2) at baseline, 30 minutes after, 60 minutes after, and 120 minutes after CO_2 pneumoperitoneum. *$P < 0.01$, compared with P_aCO_2. #$P < 0.01$, compared with P_aCO_2.

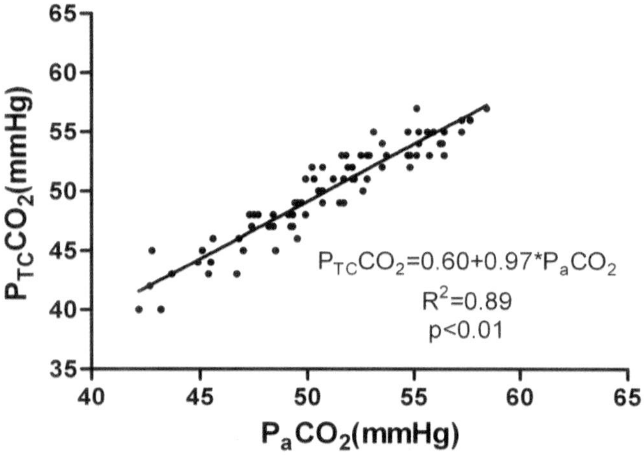

Figure 3. Linear regression analysis between $P_{TC}CO_2$ and P_aCO_2. Linear regression analysis between the transcutaneous carbon dioxide partial pressure ($P_{TC}CO_2$) and the arterial carbon dioxide partial pressure (P_aCO_2) in 21 severe obese patients during laparoscopic bariatric surgery. The linear regression equation: $P_{TC}CO_2 = 0.60 + 0.97 \times P_aCO_2$, $r^2 = 0.89$, P<0.01.

$kg^{-1}.h^{-1}$) to keep the variation of blood pressure and HR within 20% of baseline values. Those patients whose blood pressure drop was more than 20% baseline value or who needed a vasoconstrictor to maintain hemodynamics stable were excluded from the study. yet the data from them before hypotension occurred could still be used for the analysis. The patient's body temperature was continuously monitored nasopharyngeally and maintained at 36°C to 37°C. The room temperature was maintained at 23°C to 25°C. Pneumoperitoneum was established and intraperitoneal CO_2 infusion pressure was maintained at 12–14 mmHg during the surgery.

Statistic

Data were presented as mean±SD. Statistical analysis was performed by SPSS version 17.0(SPSS Inc, USA).We assessed the agreement between P_aCO_2 and $P_{TC}CO_2$ or P_aCO_2 and $P_{et}CO_2$ using Bland–Altman method. Pearson correlation coefficient and linear regression analysis were used to establish the relationship. The exact probability method and two way contingency table were employed to compare the difference of 5 mmHg or less and 3 mmHg or less between P_aCO_2 and the other two noninvasive variables. A P value of 0.05 or less was considered statistically significant.

Results

21 patients (8 men and 13 women; age from 19–55 yr, 29(9)yr; weight from 86 to 160 kg, 119.3(22.1)kg; BMI from 35.3 to 51.1 kg/m^2, 42.1(5.4) kg/m^2) were recruited into this study. All patients underwent laparoscopic bariatric surgery. The P_aCO_2, $P_{et}CO_2$, and $P_{TC}CO_2$ values were recorded at 4 time points. Eight-four samples were finally obtained. The mean values of these variables at different time points are presented in Table 1 and Figure 1. In these samples, $P_{TC}CO_2$ was correlated with P_aCO_2 at each time point (r = 0.90, 0.89, 0.93 and 0.90, respectively, P<0.01). $P_{et}CO_2$ was correlated with P_aCO_2 at each time point (r = 0.66, 0.71, 0.69 and 0.86, respectively, P<0.01). The P_aCO_2 values were ranging from 42.2 to 58.4 mmHg. The average P_aCO_2–$P_{et}CO_2$ difference was 10.3±2.3 mmHg and the

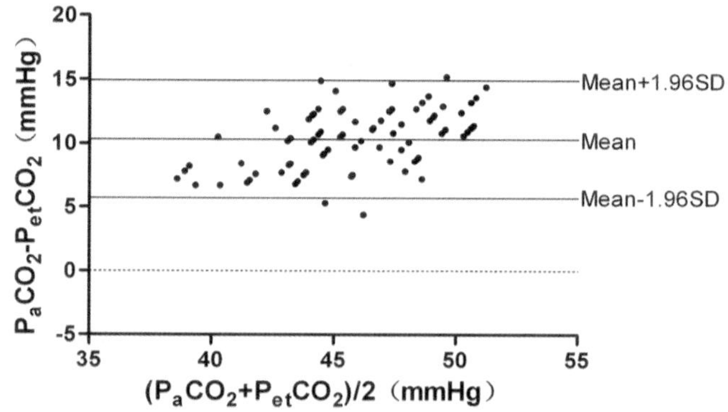

Figure 4. Agreement between $P_{et}CO_2$ and P_aCO_2. Agreement between $P_{et}CO_2$ and P_aCO_2 by the Bland-Altman method. Plot of the arterial carbon dioxide minus the end tidal carbon dioxide (y-axis) against the mean of the end tidal carbon dioxide and the arterial carbon dioxide (x-axis).The bias and precision are labeled. According to the Bland-Altman analysis, the 95% limits of agreement (LOA) of the average P_aCO_2–$P_{et}CO_2$ difference was 10.3±4.6 mmHg (mean±1.96 SD).

average P_aCO_2–$P_{TC}CO_2$ difference was 0.9±1.3 mmHg. In those samples, both $P_{et}CO_2$ and $P_{TC}CO_2$ were closely correlated with P_aCO_2. The linear regression equation between $P_{et}CO_2$ and P_aCO_2 was $P_{et}CO_2 = 11.58 + 0.57 \times P_aCO_2$, $r^2 = 0.64$, P<0.01(Figure 2); and $P_{TC}CO_2$ and P_aCO_2 was $P_{TC}CO_2 = 0.60 + 0.97 \times P_aCO_2$, $r^2 = 0.89$, P<0.01(Figure 3). In all samples, there wasn't a difference of 3 mmHg or less between P_aCO_2 and $P_{et}CO_2$, yet there was a difference of 3 mmHg or less between P_aCO_2 and $P_{TC}CO_2$ in 79 of the 84 samples (P<0.01). Only one $P_{et}CO_2$–P_aCO_2 difference (absolute value) was 5 mmHg or less while all values of $P_{TC}CO_2$–P_aCO_2 difference (absolute value) were 5 mmHg or less (P<0.01). According to Bland-Altman analysis, the 95% limits of agreement (LOA) of the average P_aCO_2–$P_{et}CO_2$ difference was 10.3±4.6 mmHg (mean±1.96 SD, Figure 4), while the 95% limits of agreement (LOA) of the average P_aCO_2–$P_{TC}CO_2$ difference was 0.9±2.6 mmHg (mean±1.96 SD, Figure 5).

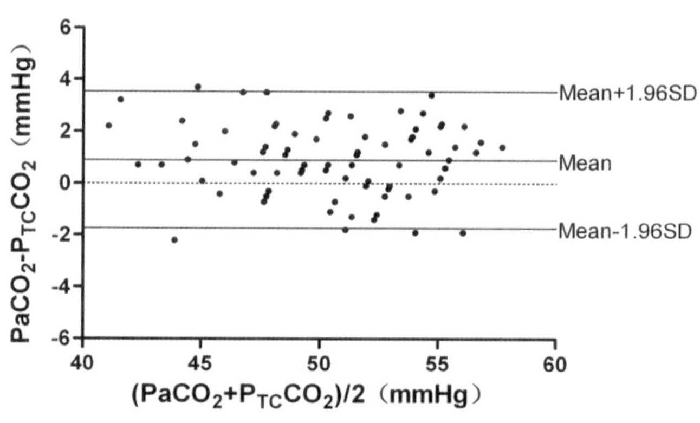

Figure 5. Agreement between $P_{TC}CO_2$ and P_aCO_2. Agreement between $P_{TC}CO_2$ and P_aCO_2 by the Bland-Altman method. Plot of the arterial carbon dioxide minus the transcutaneous carbon dioxide (y-axis) against the mean of the transcutaneous carbon dioxide and the arterial carbon dioxide (x-axis).The bias and precision are labeled. The 95% limits of agreement (LOA) of the average P_aCO_2–$P_{TC}CO_2$ difference was 0.9±2.6 mmHg (mean±1.96 SD).

Table 1. CO_2 Partial Pressure at Different Time Points (Mean±SD, n = 21).

	Before pneumoperitoneum		After pneumoperitoneum					
	Baseline (mmHg)	r	30 min (mmHg)	r	60 min (mmHg)	r	120 min (mmHg)	r
$PaCO_2$	46.89±2.97		50.95±2.59		52.40±2.97		53.73±3.12	
$PetCO_2$	38.62±2.69	0.66	40.62±2.13	0.71	41.33±2.24	0.69	42.14±2.76	0.86
$P_{TC}CO_2$	46.19±3.43	0.90	50.14±2.78	0.89	51.52±3.44	0.93	52.52±3.14	0.90

Correlation between end-tidal carbon dioxide partial pressure ($P_{et}CO_2$) and arterial carbon dioxide partial pressure (P_aCO_2) and transcutaneous carbon dioxide partial pressure ($P_{TC}CO_2$) and P_aCO_2 at 4 time points. P<0.01.

Discussion

The end-tidal carbon dioxide ($P_{et}CO_2$) measurement has been widely used in the anesthetic management. However, quite a number of factors may possibly affect the accuracy of $P_{et}CO_2$ measurement, including alveolar ventilation volume, V/Q ratio, chronic obstructive pulmonary disease, etc. Due to the effects of weight loss, remission of diabetes mellitus and improvement of health-related quality, bariatric surgery gets rapid development in clinical practice [5]. For those patients with severe obesity, the functional residual capacity (FRC) is reduced with increase of intrapulmonary shunt (10–25%), especially for those with abdominal obesity. And the CO_2 pneumoperitoneum results in the further decrease of FRC and greater degree of intrapulmonary shunt, which diminishes the accuracy of $P_{et}CO_2$. Nevertheless, $P_{TC}CO_2$ monitoring uses heated electrodes to improve local perfusion (capillary arterialisation), which facilitates the absorption of carbon dioxide into the heated electrodes via skin diffusion. The carbon dioxide inside the electrodes changes the internal pH value, which results in $P_{TC}CO_2$ signals. Reid CW et al [6] reported that the P_aCO_2–$P_{et}CO_2$ difference increased along with P_aCO_2 levels. In the patients undergoing bariatric surgery the $P_{et}CO_2$ is usually greater than 40 mmHg, and P_aCO_2 may be underestimated, while the $P_{TC}CO_2$ is still accurately reflect the P_aCO_2 levels. Especially after the extubation, $P_{et}CO_2$ monitor becomes unavailable. And it is highly likely that hypoxia and hypercapnia happens. $P_{TC}CO_2$ monitoring is particularly valuable. In our study, the average P_aCO_2–$P_{et}CO_2$ difference was 10.3±2.3 mmHg whereas the average P_aCO_2–$P_{TC}CO_2$ difference was 0.9±1.3 mmHg. Those findings are unanimous with the past study.

Previous studies reported that the CO_2 partial pressure was at its highest 30 minutes after pneumoperitoneum and was stable 60 minutes after pneumoperitoneum [7–9]. But Cuevlier et al [10] suggested that O_2 partial pressure was stable 5 minutes and CO_2 partial pressure got stable 20 minutes after pneumoperitoneum, resulting from accumulation of more CO_2 in vivo. Therefore, determination of $P_{TC}CO_2$ 30 minutes after pneumoperitoneum in our study was feasible for most patients. Xue Q et al [11] suggested that in prolonged laparoscopic surgery $P_{TC}CO_2$ monitor was more accurate than $P_{et}CO_2$, and the linear regression equations were $P_{TC}CO_2 = 0.74 \times P_aCO_2 + 11.07$, $r^2 = 0.71$, $P<0.0001$; $P_{et}CO_2 = 1.04 \times P_aCO_2 + 6.45$, $r^2 = 0.55$, $P<0.01$. However, the correlation of the $P_{TC}CO_2$ and P_aCO_2 is unknown more than 60 minutes after pneumoperitoneum. In this study, the laparoscopy was applied during the whole surgery process, and we found $P_{TC}CO_2$ and P_aCO_2 still demonstrated excellent correlation 120 minutes after pneumoperitoneum (r = 0.93).

Griffin J et al [4] found that carbon dioxide monitoring by using $P_{TC}CO_2$ was more accurate in patients with a BMI greater than 40 kg/m^2 undergoing transabdominal bariatric surgery. Maniscalco M et al [12] suggested that in patients (BMI, 43.7 kg/m^2) with chronic obstructive pulmonary disease (COPD), obstructive sleep apnea syndrome (OSAS), hypopnea syndrome (OHS) and respiratory failure (RF), $P_{TC}CO_2$ still accurately reflected the P_aCO_2,compared with the blood gas analysis. Our findings indicated that $P_{TC}CO_2$ was more accurate in reflecting the real levels of P_aCO_2 than $P_{et}CO_2$ in patients with BMI>35 kg/m^2 undergoing laparoscopic bariatric surgery. And only one $P_{et}CO_2$ readings was 5 mmHg or less from P_aCO_2 while all values of $P_{TC}CO_2$ were 5 mmHg or less.

The successful $P_{TC}CO_2$ monitoring depends on monitor and a series of patient factors. Although TC-CO_2 monitoring more accurately reflected P_aCO_2 in most of the patients in the previous studies, several technical factors may affect the accuracy of monitor, including trapped air bubbles, improper placement, damaged membranes, and inappropriate calibration techniques. Patient-related factors may also affect the accuracy, such as variations in skin thickness, the presence of edema, tissue hypoperfusion, or the use of vasoconstricting drugs and oxygen deficiency acidosis. Nishiyama T et al [13] found $P_{TC}CO_2$ and $P_{TC}O_2$ more precisely predict the P_aCO_2 and P_aO_2 when the electrodes were put on the chest, compared to the placement at the upper arm and forearm. Nishiyama T etc [14] found chest electrode was better than the ear electrode. We put the electrode on the left side chest (between nipple and clavicle), which was easy to be observe by the anesthesiologists and reduced the influence of electrode caused by the body movement during abdominal operation.

Electrode heating temperature can significantly affect the accuracy of the measurement results. Nishiyama T et al [15] suggested that the electrode should be heated to at least 43°C in adults patients, when $P_{TC}CO_2$ and $P_{TC}O_2$ could accurately estimate P_aCO_2 and P_aO_2 respectively. Sorensen LC et al [16] found that lower electrode temperature increased systematic error of measurements in premature and newborns. The higher the electrode temperature was, the greater the risk of burn injury was.Accordingly, in our study we set the electrode temperature at 44°C as manufactures recommedation, and no patient suffered from postoperative skin burn, while skin erythema occurred in 15 patients, and disappeared in 24 hours.

Skin tissue perfusion also affected the accuracy of the $P_{TC}CO_2$ monitoring. Lower environmental temperature resulted in skin vascular contraction, reduced blood flow, In this study temperature in the operating room always maintained above 23°C. Meanwhile, patients' exposure was reduced to the lowest possible level. Currently there are still disputes about the accuracy of $P_{TC}CO_2$ monitoring with the use of vasopressors, and past studies suggested vasopressors affected accuracy of $P_{TC}CO_2$ monitoring [16,17], whereas Berkenbosch JW [2] and Rodriguez P [18] found that vasopressors didn't affect the accuracy of the $P_{TC}CO_2$ monitoring. Most of general anesthetics have the effect of vasodilation. Propofol administration produced venodilation and peripheral vasodilation in humans [19]. Opioids (like fentanyl and remifentanil) produced concentration-dependent and endothelium-independent relaxations in human being radial artery rings [20]. In our study only one patient received vasoconstrictor during anesthesia induction and the other 21 patients not.

We all know that during jet ventilation (JV), $P_{et}CO_2$ may underestimate P_aCO_2 because of inadequate washout of the anatomical dead space by a small tidal volume and the relatively slow response time of infrared CO_2 analyzers. Especially during use of high frequency jet ventilation (HFJV) [21]. But the transcutaneous devices provide an effective method for non-invasive monitoring of P_aCO_2 in situations where continuous and precise control of CO_2 levels in perioperative with HFJV [22]. $P_{TC}CO_2$ monitoring especially useful during use of HFJV in obese patients which can avoid them in high risks of hypercapnia.

However, $P_{TC}CO_2$ can not substitute the $P_{et}CO_2$ monitoring completely as $P_{et}CO_2$ monitoring has many unique advantages, including the judgment of successful intubation, the warning of breathing circuit disconnected and indicator of pulmonary embolism, etc. In addition, the $P_{et}CO_2$ wave pattern had more clinical significance. The $P_{TC}CO_2$ monitoring was limited by many factors, including longer priming time, adjuscting before use, periodically electrode replacement, no CO_2 waveform and the risk of skin burn injury [23].

Conclusion

In conclusion, our study demonstrated that $P_{TC}CO_2$ can estimate the P_aCO_2 more accurately than $P_{et}CO_2$ in obese patients under laparoscopic bariatric surgery. Moreover, the application of $P_{TC}CO_2$ monitoring might improve the quality of the anesthesia management.

Acknowledgments

We sincerely thank Hui Liang in the Department of General Surgey at our hospital for his relentless support during this study, and we are indebted to Xiaoguang Guo in the Department of Anesthesiology at The First Affiliated Hospital of Zhengzhou University for his assistance in manuscript preparation.

Author Contributions

Conceived and designed the experiments: CML. Performed the experiments: SJL YYY XL. Analyzed the data: SJL JS. Contributed reagents/materials/analysis tools: SJL CML JS. Wrote the paper: SJL XC.

References

1. Rohling R, Biro P (1999) Clinical investigation of a new combined pulse oximetry and carbon dioxide tension sensor in adult anaesthesia. J Clin Monit Comput 15: 23–27.
2. Berkenbosch JW, Lam J, Burd RS, Tobias J (2001) Noninvasive monitoring of carbon dioxide during mechanical ventilation in older children: end-tidal versus transcutaneous techniques. Anesth Analg 92: 1427–1431.
3. Casati A, Squicciarini G, Malagutti G, Baciarello M, Putzu M, et al. (2006) Transcutaneous monitoring of partial pressure of carbondioxide in the elderly patient: a prospective, clinical comparison with end-tidal monitoring. J Clin Anesth 18: 436–440.
4. Griffin J, Terry BE, Burton RK, Ray TL, Keller BP, et al. (2003) Comparison of end-tidal and transcutaneous measures of carbon dioxide during general anaesthesia in severely obese adults. Br J Anaesth 91: 498–501.
5. Schroeder R, Garrison JM JR, Johnson MS (2011) Treatment of Adult Obesity with Bariatric Surgery. Am Fam Physician 84: 805–814.
6. Reid CW, Martineau RJ, Miller DR, Hull KA, Baines J, et al. (1992) A comparison of transcutaneous, end-tidal and arterial measurements of carbon dioxide during general anaesthesia. Can J Anaesth 39: 31–36.
7. Bozkurt P, Kaya G, Yeker Y, Tunali Y, Altintas F (1999) The caradiorespiratory effects of laparoscopic procedures in infants. Anesthesia 54: 831–834.
8. Gandara V, de Vega DS, Escriu N, Zorrilla G (1997) Acid-base balance alteration in laparoscopic cholecystectomy. Surg Endosc 11: 707–710.
9. Girardis M, Broi UD, Antonutto G, Pasetto A (1996) The effect of laparoscopic cholecystectomy on cardiovascular function and pulmonary gas exchange. Anesth Analg 83: 134–140.
10. Cuvelier A, Grigoriu B, Molano LC, Muir JF (2005) Limitations of transctaneous carbon dioxide measurements for assessing long-term mechanical ventilation. Chest 127: 1744–1748.
11. Xue QS, Wu XW, Jin J, Yu BW, Zheng MH (2010) Transcutaneous Carbon Dioxide Monitoring Accurately Predicts Arterial Carbon Dioxide Partial Pressure in Patients Undergoing Prolonged Laparoscopic Surgery. Anesth Analg 111: 417–420.
12. Maniscalco M, Zedda A, Faraone S, Carratu P, Sofia M (2008) Evaluation of a transcutaneous carbon dioxide monitor in severe obesity. Intensive Care Med 34: 1340–1344.
13. Nishiyama T, Nakamura S, Yamashita K (2006) Comparison of the transcutaneous oxygen and carbon dioxide tension in different electrode locations during general anaesthesia. Eur J Anaesthesiolgy 23: 1049–1054.
14. Nishiyama T, Kohno Y, Koishi K (2011) Comparison of ear and chest probes in transcutaneous carbon dioxide pressure measurements during general anesthesia in adults. J Clin Monit Comput 25: 323–328.
15. Nishiyama T, Nakamura S, Yamashita K (2006) Effects of the electrode temperature of a new monitor, TCM4, on the measurement of transcutaneous oxygen and carbon dioxide tension. J Anesth 20: 331–334.

16. Sorensen LC, Brage-Andersen L, Greisen G (2011) Effects of the transcutaneous electrode temperature on the accuracy of transcutaneous carbon dioxide tension. Scand J Clin Lab Invest 71: 548–552.
17. Rithalia SV, Ng YY, Tinker J (1982) Measurement of transcutaneous PCO2 in critically ill patients. Resuscitation 10: 13–18.
18. Rodriguez P, Lellouche F, Aboab J, Buisson CB, Brochard L (2006) Transcutaneous arterial carbon dioxide pressure monitoring in critically ill adult patients. Intensive Care Med 32: 309–312.
19. Muzi M, Berens RA, Kampine JP, Ebert TJ (1992) Venodilation Contributes to Propofol-Mediated Hypotension in Humans. Anesth Analg 74: 877–883.
20. Gursoy S, Baqcivan I, Yildirim MK, Berkan O, Kaya T (2006) Vasorelaxant effect of opioid analgesics on the isolated human radial artery. Eur J Anaesthesiol 23: 496–500.
21. Capan LM, Ramanathan S, Sinha K, Turndorf H (1985) Arterial to end-tidal CO_2 gradients during spontaneous intermittent positive-pressure ventilation and jet ventilation. Crit Care Med 13: 810–813.
22. Mizushima A, Nakamura A, Kawauchi Y, Miura K, Fujino S. et al. (2002) Transcutaneous carbon dioxide and oxygen measurement in patients undergoing microlaryngosurgery with high frequency jet ventilation. Masui 51: 1331–1335.
23. Tobias JD, Meyer DJ (1997) Noninvasive monitoring of carbon dioxided during respiratory, failure in toddlers and infants: end-tidal versus transcutaneous carbon dioxide. Anesth Analg 85: 55–58.

Risk for Hospital Readmission following Bariatric Surgery

Robert B. Dorman[1], Christopher J. Miller[2], Daniel B. Leslie[1], Federico J. Serrot[1], Bridget Slusarek[1], Henry Buchwald[1], John E. Connett[2], Sayeed Ikramuddin[1]*

1 Department of Surgery, University of Minnesota, Minneapolis, Minnesota, United States of America, **2** Division of Biostatistics, University of Minnesota, Minneapolis, Minnesota, United States of America

Abstract

Background and Objectives: Complications resulting in hospital readmission are important concerns for those considering bariatric surgery, yet present understanding of the risk for these events is limited to a small number of patient factors. We sought to identify demographic characteristics, concomitant morbidities, and perioperative factors associated with hospital readmission following bariatric surgery.

Methods: We report on a prospective observational study of 24,662 patients undergoing primary RYGB and 26,002 patients undergoing primary AGB at 249 and 317 Bariatric Surgery Centers of Excellence (BSCOE), respectively, in the United States from January 2007 to August 2009. Data were collected using standardized assessments of demographic factors and comorbidities, as well as longitudinal records of hospital readmissions, complications, and mortality.

Results: The readmission rate was 5.8% for RYGB and 1.2% for AGB patients 30 days after discharge. The greatest predictors for readmission following RYGB were prolonged length of stay (adjusted odds ratio [OR], 2.3; 95% confidence interval [CI], 2.0–2.7), open surgery (OR, 1.8; CI, 1.4–2.2), and pseudotumor cerebri (OR, 1.6; CI, 1.1–2.4). Prolonged length of stay (OR, 2.3; CI, 1.6–3.3), history of deep venous thrombosis or pulmonary embolism (OR, 2.1; CI, 1.3–3.3), asthma (OR, 1.5; CI, 1.1–2.1), and obstructive sleep apnea (OR, 1.5; CI, 1.1–1.9) were associated with the greatest increases in readmission risk for AGB. The 30-day mortality rate was 0.14% for RYGB and 0.02% for AGB.

Conclusion: Readmission rates are low and mortality is very rare following bariatric surgery, but risk for both is significantly higher after RYGB. Predictors of readmission were disparate for the two procedures. Results do not support excluding patients with certain comorbidities since any reductions in overall readmission rates would be very small on the absolute risk scale. Future research should evaluate the efficacy of post-surgical managed care plans for patients at higher risk for readmission and adverse events.

Editor: Mercedes Susan Mandell, University of Colorado, United States of America

Funding: The authors have no funding or support to report.

Competing Interests: The authors have declared that no competing interests exist.

* E-mail: ikram001@umn.edu

Introduction

The astonishing rise in obesity prevalence and the marked decline in perioperative mortality over the previous two decades have both contributed to the growing popularity of bariatric surgery. In the period from 1998 to 2003, the number of bariatric procedures performed increased 10-fold [1], and in 2009 alone, 220,000 bariatric surgeries were performed in the United States and Canada [2]. Despite the clinical benefits, the potential for serious and costly major adverse events deters many patients and payers from utilizing its advantages.

Bariatric surgery is safe with a 0.15% to 0.5% 30-day mortality rate [3–6], however an appreciable proportion of patients suffer at least one major adverse event within the first 30 days following either Roux-en-Y gastric bypass (RYGB) or adjustable gastric banding (AGB) that results in hospital readmission. A hospital readmission increases the average 180-day cost of a bariatric operation from approximately $27,000 to $65,000 [7]. In response to the high costs of hospital readmission, in 2008 the National Quality Forum indicated that hospital readmission rates would be a central factor in evaluating hospital performance with penalties being levied against hospitals with high readmission rates.

Identifying patient and surgical factors that increase perioperative risk of readmission would improve both the tenability of bariatric surgery for patients and the cost-effectiveness for payers. Comprehensive assessment of patient risks a priori would provide physicians with a framework for either tailoring the selection of intervention or identifying patients most in need of enhanced education or monitoring post-operatively, which could, in turn, reduce the frequency of readmission following bariatric surgery. We have utilized the Bariatric Outcomes Longitudinal Database (BOLD), the largest prospective database of bariatric patient outcomes worldwide, to identify predictors of serious postoperative complications requiring hospital readmission within 30 days of discharge.

Methods

Design Overview

We obtained patient data from BOLD collected between January 1, 2007 and August 31, 2009 at 450 Bariatric Surgery

Centers of Excellence (BSCOE). Data collection for BOLD was overseen by the Surgical Review Corporation (SRC). Written informed consent was obtained from all patients, and the protocols of this study were approved by the University of Minnesota institutional review board.

The American Society for Metabolic and Bariatric Surgery (ASMBS) founded SRC in 2003 as an independent, nonprofit research organization to oversee compliance and collect data on patient outcomes for accredited BSCOE hospitals. The criteria set forth by the ASMBS for BSCOE certification include: performing at least 125 bariatric surgeries per year in hospitals or 100 bariatric surgeries per year in surgery centers; surgeons must have completed 125 bariatric surgeries during their career and must continue to perform at least 50 bariatric surgeries per year; a multidisciplinary staff including a team of nurses, surgeons, dieticians and other consultants; onsite inspections of BSCOE must be performed every three years; and, hospitals must report their outcomes to the BOLD database.

BOLD, an internet-based database implemented in 2007, represents the largest repository of clinical bariatric patient surgery information in the world with 521 contributing BSCOE. BOLD collects standardized assessments of patient demographics, preoperative morbidities, medication use, surgical procedures, and post-surgical follow-up visits. Additional details regarding the operational procedures of BOLD have been reported previously [8]. Standard protocol for BSCOE requests that patients return to their operating physician for periodic follow-up visits including at least one visit one month post-operatively. At each follow-up visit, visit-specific information is recorded into BOLD on weight, complications, and readmissions since the previous follow-up visit regardless of whether the readmitting hospital was BSCOE-certified.

Setting and Participants

Enrollment and data entry for BOLD is ongoing, though we excluded surgeries which took place after August 31, 2009 to ensure that all patients had adequate opportunity to follow-up with their surgical center and BSCOE had sufficient time to submit patient data as of the most recent database closing on March 1, 2010. For each patient in the study, we extracted complete data on demographic information, comorbidities, inpatient data, and post-surgical follow-up, including data on readmissions, complications, and mortality. Self-reported data on demographics and comorbid conditions were complete for nearly all patients and suspect data entry errors were rare. Suspect BMI values were replaced with data from an alternate visit. Patients were eligible for inclusion if they underwent a non-revision RYGB or AGB and had complete follow-up through at least 30 days following discharge.

The 30-day follow-up rate among BOLD participants was 91.6% during the study period, however follow-up rates were variable across BSCOE. Analysis of the within-BSCOE relationship between the follow-up rate and readmission rate indicated that centers with lower follow-up rates tended to report lower readmission rates, suggesting that centers with lower follow-up rates underreported their true readmission rates. To ensure high accuracy of outcomes reporting, we excluded BSCOE reporting complete 30-day outcome data for fewer than 90% of their surgical patients. Statistically significant differences between patients from included and excluded BSCOE were observed for several baseline characteristics due to the large sample sizes and correspondingly small standard errors, but these differences were small in magnitude and not clinically relevant. Sensitivity analyses on the effect of restricting participants to highly compliant BSCOE were performed on the readmission and mortality rates under a wide variety of assumptions, but had little effect on the rates due to the relative rarity of the outcome.

Outcomes and Follow-up

Predictors of interest were demographic, health, and surgical variables. Clinical definitions of comorbid conditions are presented in Table 1. Prolonged length of stay was defined as a hospital stay ≥4 days for laparoscopic RYGB, ≥6 days for open RYGB and ≥2 days for AGB. Our outcome was all-cause hospital readmission within 30 days of discharge requiring hospitalization for >23 hours. We considered patients to be at risk for readmission on the day of discharge. No serious intraoperative complications requiring additional hospitalization were classified as readmissions. Patients were considered at risk for mortality on the day of surgery. Patients who were readmitted and died in the hospital within 30 days of surgery were classified as both readmissions and mortalities; patients who died outside a hospital were classified as mortalities but not readmissions.

Statistical Analysis

The demographic characteristics and medical histories of patients undergoing the two surgeries were compared with *t*-tests for continuous variables and chi-square tests for categorical variables, and Fisher's exact tests for rare counts. Risk factors for readmission were evaluated using a series of generalized linear mixed-effects models. Demographic, health, and surgical covariates were estimated as fixed effects and a random effect was estimated for BSCOE to account for variation between and correlation within BSCOE in their readmission rates. Those covariates significantly associated with readmission in univariate analysis at a significance level of 0.10 or greater were entered into a multivariate model with an iterative backward selection procedure that continued until all variables were significant at the 0.10 level.

We used expanded mixed-effects logistic models with interactions to examine mediation of risk factors by surgical approach. Readmission risk was higher among open surgeries, however the risk factors for open and laparoscopic RYGB approaches were not significantly different in the expanded models, so we controlled for the higher rate of readmission among open procedures with an additional fixed effect and did not stratify models by surgical approach. All P values are two-sided and are unadjusted for multiple comparisons. Statistical analyses were conducted in SAS version 9.2 (SAS Institute Inc., Cary, North Carolina) and graphs were generated in R version 2.14.0 (R Development Core Team, 2011).

Results

Patients

Figure 1 details the patient selection process. Among BSCOE eligible for analysis, 24,662 RYGB patients from 249 BSCOE and 26,002 AGB patients from 317 BSCOE were followed-up at 30 days. Bariatric surgery patients had a mean age of 45.9±11.9 years and were predominantly female (78.9%) and Caucasian (80.1%). Patients undergoing RYGB had higher BMI and higher prevalence of comorbidities than patients who underwent AGB (Table 2). The laparoscopic approach was employed for 90.7% of RYGB and 99.7% of AGB operations. Prior to discharge, 1,728 (7.7%) laparoscopic RYGB patients, 159 (7.0%) open RYGB patients, and 1,183 AGB patients (4.6%) had a prolonged length of stay.

Table 1. Clinical definitions of pre-existing conditions.

Condition	Clinical Definition
Abdominal hernia	Any history of symptomatic or asymptomatic abdominal hernia
Abdominal/skin pannus	Any current symptoms, including intertriginous irritation, interfering with ambulation, recurrent cellulitis, or ulceration
Alcohol use	Any current alcohol use
Angina	Any chest pain symptoms or angina regardless of exertion
Asthma	Any symptoms of asthma regardless of medication usage
Back pain	Has degenerative changes or positive objective findings, symptoms require narcotic treatment
Bipolar disorder	Confirmed diagnosis of bipolar disorder
Cholelithiasis	Has had gallstones with severe symptoms or has had a cholecystectomy
Congestive heart failure	Any history or symptoms of congestive heart failure (Class I, II, III, and IV)
Depression	At least moderate depression with significant impairment, undergoing medical or therapeutic treatment
DVT/PE	Any history of resolved or recurrent deep venous thrombosis or pulmonary embolism
Fibromyalgia	Any degree of fibromyalgia
Gastroesophageal reflux disease	Symptoms require the use of medical treatment (at least H2 blockers or low-dose proton pump inhibitor)
Gout/hyperuricemia	Has at least symptomatic or asymptomatic hyperuricemia
Hypertension	Requires medical treatment with multiple medications
Ischemic heart disease	Has at least abnormal electrocardiogram, regardless of active ischemia; may include history of myocardial infarction
Lipids	Heightened cholesterol requiring at least single medication
Liver disease	Any history of liver disease, including hepatomegaly or non-normal liver function test
Lower extremity edema	Has symptoms requiring treatment, diuretics, elevation, or hose
Musculoskeletal disease	Has pain with household ambulation, requires surgical intervention, or past joint replacement
Obesity hypoventilation syndrome	Any symptoms including hypoxemia or hypercarbia on room air
Obstructive sleep apnea	Sleep apnea requiring oral appliance, significant hypoxia, or oxygen-dependent
Panic disorder	Confirmed diagnosis of panic disorder
Peripheral vascular disease	Any symptoms of peripheral vascular disease
Personality disorder	Confirmed diagnosis of personality disorder
Psychosocial impairment	Any indicated psychosocial impairment, regardless of ability to perform primary tasks
Pseudotumor cerebri	Any symptoms of pseudotumor cerebri (at least headaches with dizziness, nausea, or pain behind the eyes) with or without visual symptoms
Psychosis	Confirmed diagnosis of psychosis
Pulmonary hypertension	Any symptoms associated with pulmonary hypertension (shortness of breath, dizziness, fainting)
Substance abuse	Any recent substance abuse
Stress urinary incontinence	Frequent stress urinary incontinence, regardless of severity
Tobacco use	Any recent tobacco use
Type-2 diabetes	Diabetes requiring insulin

Abbreviations: DVT, deep venous thrombosis; PE, pulmonary embolism.

Readmission and mortality

In the first 30 days after discharge, 1437 (5.8%) RYGB patients and 322 (1.2%) AGB patients were readmitted (Figure 2; $P<0.001$ for difference). Patients undergoing RYGB procedures with the laparoscopic approach had fewer readmissions than patients who underwent RYGB with an open approach (5.6% v. 7.9%, $P<0.001$). The most commonly reported complications at readmission were nausea/vomiting and dehydration for both procedures, though more than one reason could be recorded for a readmission (Table 3). For RYGB, other common complications at readmission were gastrointestinal bleeding, stricture, and obstruction; pneumonia, device-related infection, and obstruction were common complications reported at AGB readmissions.

Within the 30 days of the primary operation, 35 (0.14%) RYGB patients and 6 (0.02%) AGB patients died ($P<0.001$ for difference). For RYGB patients, causes of mortality were sepsis (n = 11), cardiac failure (n = 6), myocardial infarction (n = 4) respiratory failure (n = 4), stroke (n = 2), pulmonary embolus (n = 1), or could not be determined (n = 6). For AGB patients, causes of death were myocardial infarction (n = 3) or indeterminate (n = 3).

Predictors of readmission

Table 4 presents univariate and multivariate risk factor analyses for readmission. After adjusting for other significant covariates, prolonged length of stay more than doubled the odds of readmission for a RYGB patient and the open surgical approach nearly doubled odds of readmission. Patients with current symptoms of clinical depression or psychosocial impairment, peripheral vascular disease, pseudotumor cerebri, or those with a previous history of gallstones or cholecystecomy were more likely to be readmitted than those without those symptoms. The number of medications used preoperatively was also associated with higher

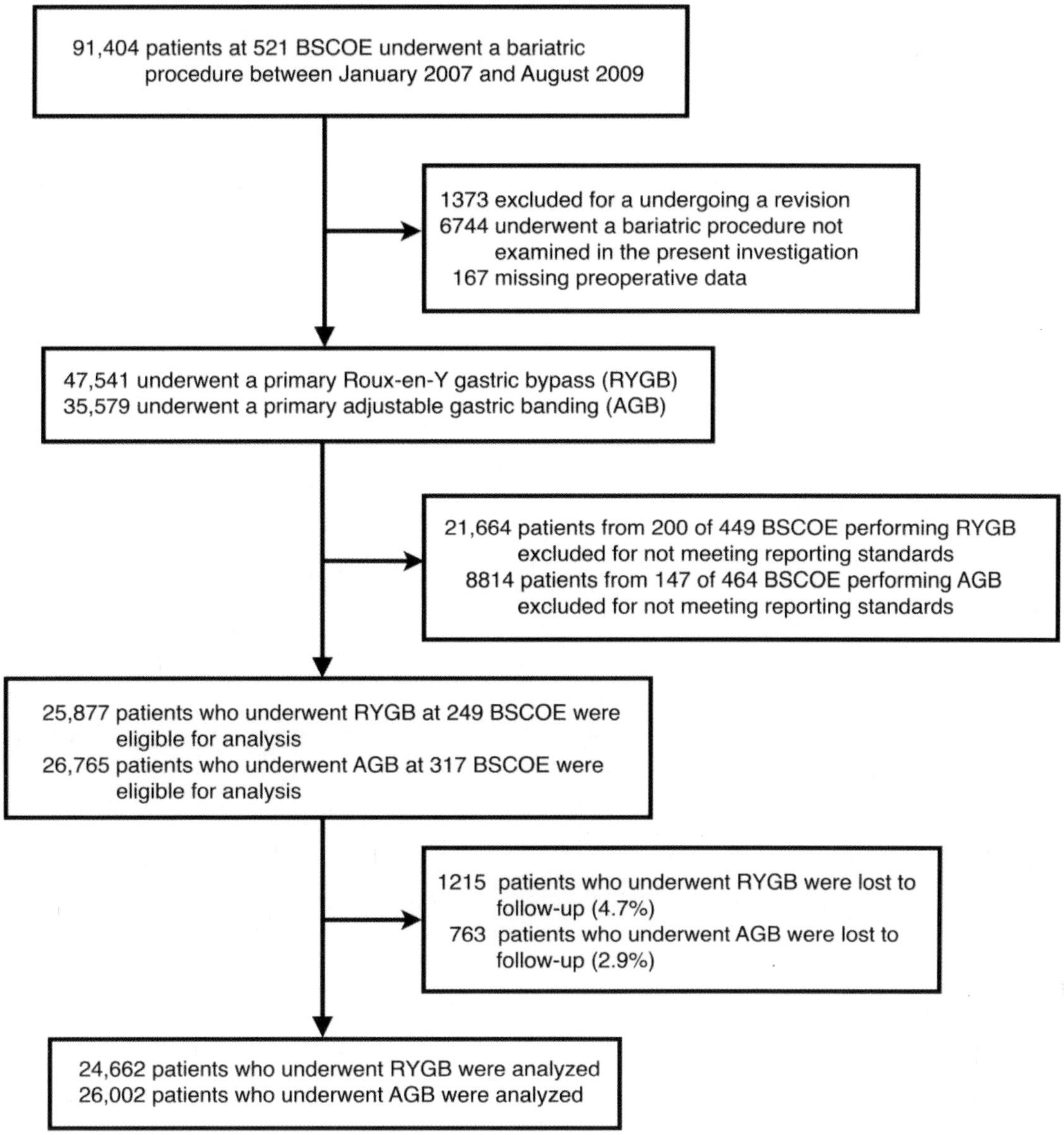

Figure 1. Flow diagram of patient selection.

readmission rates, and an African-American patient had 34% higher odds of readmission compared to a Caucasian individual holding other factors constant.

For AGB, prolonged length of stay also doubled a patient's odds of readmission. Male patients had nearly 50% greater odds of readmission than female patients, and disabled and retired employment statuses were more likely to have been readmitted than employed individuals after controlling for other significant demographic and health factors. Patients undergoing AGB with symptomatic asthma, gastroesophageal reflux disease (GERD), obstructive sleep apnea (OSA), or a history of deep venous thrombosis or pulmonary embolism (DVT/PE) had significantly higher odds of being readmitted within 30 days compared to patients without those medical complications.

Discussion

The overall reduction in mortality and the resolution of chronic diseases such as type 2 diabetes are substantial following bariatric surgery [9–15]. However, the potential for serious complications is a barrier for patients and payers to utilizing the long-term advantages offered by bariatric surgery. The penalizing of hospitals for early readmissions is already underway, and several states are imposing mandates that call for further reductions in readmissions. Primary care providers and surgeons alike will see substantial decreases in reimbursements for readmitted patients, and it is therefore imperative that systems be in place to prevent the occurrence of readmissions. In this study, we have identified factors predictive of severe events requiring hospital readmission within 30 days of RYGB or AGB in the largest prospective bariatric cohort to date and have established that short-term risk for readmission is low for both procedures and risk profiles are largely unique to each procedure.

We observed a RYGB readmission rate nearly five times higher than AGB. Previously reported hospital readmission rates for bariatric surgery vary widely in the literature [6,7,16–20]. Possible explanations for these disparities may be due to differences in the patient populations, the definition of a hospital readmission, the

Table 2. Characteristics of Study Participants by Surgery.

	Roux-en-Y Gastric Bypass	Adjustable Gastric Banding	
	(n = 24,662)	(n = 26,002)	
Variable	**Mean (SD)/No. (%)**	**Mean (SD)/No. (%)**	***P* value**[a]
Demographics			
Age	45.7 (11.6)	46.1 (12.1)	<0.001
Female sex	19,259 (78.1)	20,736 (79.8)	<0.001
Black race	2265 (9.2)	2890 (11.1)	<0.001
Caucasian race	19,973 (81.0)	20,590 (79.2)	<0.001
Disabled	2140 (8.7)	1192 (4.6)	<0.001
Private insurance	20,878 (84.7)	21,478 (82.6)	<0.001
Medicare/Medicaid	2919 (11.8)	2148 (8.6)	<0.001
Medical history			
BMI[b]	47.2 (8.3)	44.2 (6.7)	<0.001
Number of medications	3.8 (4.0)	2.8 (3.5)	<0.001
Comorbidities			
Abdominal hernia	1379 (5.6)	1032 (4.0)	<0.001
Abdominal/skin pannus	2097 (8.5)	1081 (4.2)	<0.001
Alcohol use	7469 (30.3)	7194 (27.7)	<0.001
Angina	914 (3.7)	576 (2.2)	<0.001
Asthma	3312 (13.4)	2707 (10.4)	<0.001
Back pain	2629 (10.7)	1926 (7.4)	<0.001
Bipolar disorder	490 (2.0)	350 (1.4)	<0.001
Cholelithiasis	4614 (18.7)	3843 (14.8)	<0.001
Congestive heart failure	703 (2.9)	435 (1.7)	<0.001
Depression	3589 (14.6)	3065 (11.8)	<0.001
DVT/PE	937 (3.8)	850 (3.3)	0.001
Fibromyalgia	908 (3.7)	694 (2.7)	<0.001
GERD	6473 (26.3)	5629 (21.7)	<0.001
Gout/hyperuricemia	1006 (4.1)	644 (2.5)	<0.001
Hypertension	5850 (23.7)	5051 (19.4)	<0.001
Ischemic heart disease	1299 (5.3)	1152 (4.4)	<0.001
Lipids	6750 (27.4)	6015 (23.1)	<0.001
Liver disease	2160 (8.8)	1102 (4.2)	<0.001
Lower extremity edema	3138 (12.7)	2342 (9.0)	<0.001
Musculoskeletal disease	2637 (10.7)	2137 (8.2)	<0.001
Obesity hypoventilation syndrome	578 (2.3)	506 (2.0)	0.002
Obstructive sleep apnea	7424 (30.1)	5811 (22.4)	<0.001
Panic disorder	2073 (8.4)	1520 (5.9)	<0.001
Peripheral vascular disease	327 (1.3)	227 (0.9)	<0.001
Personality disorder	189 (0.8)	59 (0.2)	<0.001
Psychosocial impairment	4321 (17.5)	3040 (11.7)	<0.001
Pseudotumor cerebri	446 (1.8)	278 (1.1)	<0.001
Psychosis	23 (0.1)	15 (0.1)	0.15
Pulmonary hypertension	1430 (5.8)	1051 (4.0)	<0.001
Substance abuse	105 (0.4)	71 (0.3)	0.004
Stress urinary incontinence	2859 (11.6)	2692 (10.4)	<0.001
Tobacco use	1805 (7.3)	1748 (6.7)	0.009
Type-2 diabetes requiring insulin	3029 (12.3)	2030 (7.8)	<0.001

Abbreviations: BSCOE, bariatric surgery center of excellence; DVT, deep venous thrombosis; GERD, gastroesophageal reflux disease; PE, pulmonary embolism.
[a] *P* values calculated using *t*-tests for continuous variables and Pearson's chi-squared tests or Fisher's exact tests for categorical variables.
[b] Body mass index (BMI) was calculated as weight in kilograms divided by height in meters squared.

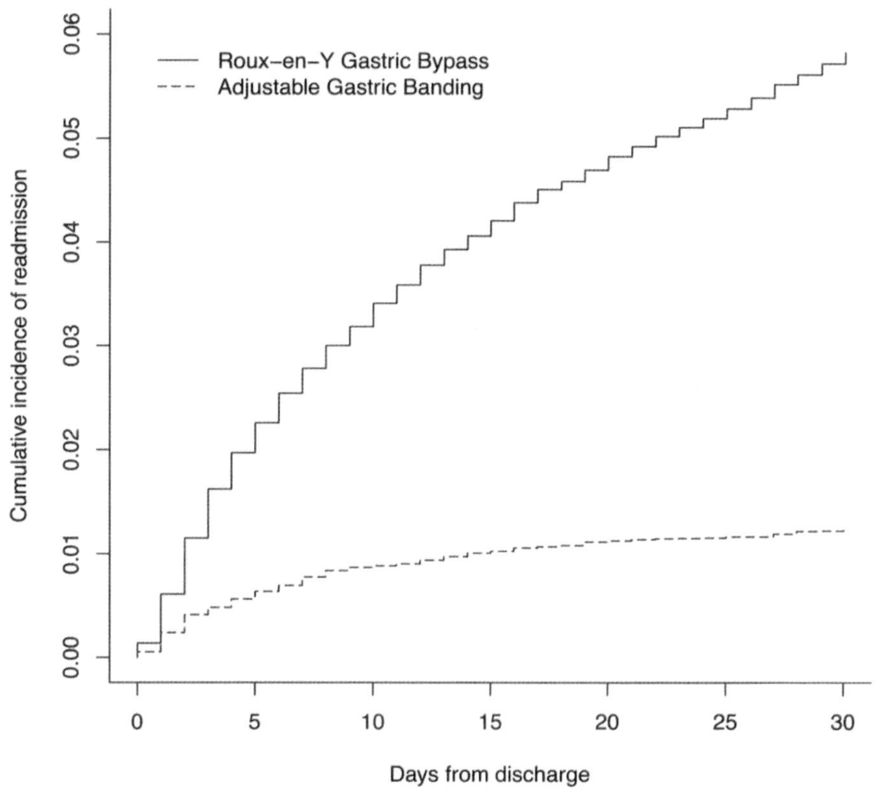

Figure 2. Cumulative incidence of 30-day readmission by surgery.

proportion of patients within a sample undergoing open versus laparoscopic procedures, or surgeon experience.

The higher readmission and mortality rates for RYGB relative to AGB might suggest that AGB is preferable, however such risks must be weighed with the treatment outcomes. RYGB has been shown to result in greater weight loss and superior improvement in comorbid illness [11,21–23]. Our group recently reported on greater one-year improvements among patients with type 2 diabetes with respect to weight loss, hemoglobin A_1C, medication scores, and rates of diabetes resolution for RYGB patients compared to matched AGB controls [11]. Short-term complications must be weighed against the long-term benefits and complications of each procedure.

The clearest predictors of readmission following RYGB were the use of the open surgical approach and prolonged length of stay. While open procedures are justified for certain complex cases

Table 3. Common Complications at Readmission by Surgery.

	Roux-en-Y Gastric Bypass		Adjustable Gastric Banding	
Most common complications reported at readmission	**Complication**	**No. (%)**	**Complication**	**No. (%)**
	Nausea/vomiting	346 (24.1)	Nausea/vomiting	57 (17.7)
	Dehydration	170 (11.8)	Dehydration	37 (11.5)
	Gastrointestinal bleeding	82 (5.7)	Device-related infection	27 (8.4)
	Stricture	79 (5.5)	Device-related obstruction	18 (5.6)
	(Internal) obstruction	76 (5.3)	Pneumonia	13 (4.0)
	Anastomotic leakage	58 (4.0)	Wound complication	13 (4.0)
	Wound complications	52 (3.6)	Device-related intolerance	12 (3.7)
	Intra-abdominal abscess	52 (3.6)	Deep venous thrombosis	11 (3.4)
30-day readmission rate		1437 (5.8)		322 (1.2)
30-day mortality rate		35 (0.14)		6 (0.02)

BSCOE could report more than one complication at readmission, so the reported percentages reflect the proportion of all readmissions involving those complications. This table lists the eight most-reported complications per surgery and does not add to 100%. A device-related obstruction was a complication of the device causing intestinal obstruction, whereas device-related intolerance is an unspecified complication due the device, implant, and graft.

Table 4. Univariate and Multivariate Models of Risk Factors for 30-Day All-Cause Hospital Readmission by Surgery.

	Roux-en-Y Gastric Bypass		Adjustable Gastric Banding	
	Univariate models	Multivariate model	Univariate models	Multivariate model
Variable	OR (95% CI)	OR (95% CI)	OR (95% CI)	OR (95% CI)
Age (5 years)	1.00 (0.98–1.03)	-	1.11 (1.06–1.17)	-
Male gender	0.94 (0.83–1.08)	-	1.68 (1.32–2.14)	1.45 (1.12–1.87)
Race (ref. Caucasian)				
Black/African American	1.32 (1.10–1.58)	1.34 (1.11–1.62)	0.63 (0.41–0.97)	-
Hispanic/Latino	1.01 (0.77–1.31)	1.05 (0.81–1.38)	0.97 (0.55–1.70)	-
Other	1.06 (0.74–1.51)	1.07 (0.74–1.53)	0.83 (0.44–1.55)	-
ASA classification[a] (ref. "1")				
2/3 – mild systemic disease	1.45 (0.81–2.61)	-	1.64 (0.77–3.47)	1.41 (0.66–2.99)
4/5 – severe disease	2.23 (1.20–4.16)	-	4.49 (1.88–10.7)	2.44 (1.01–5.89)
BMI[b] (ref. 45–49.9)				
30–34.9	1.07 (0.71–1.61)	-	0.81 (0.42–1.57)	-
35–39.9	1.02 (0.86–1.22)	-	1.25 (0.88–1.78)	-
40–44.9	0.98 (0.84–1.15)	-	1.19 (0.84–1.67)	-
50–54.9	1.12 (0.94–1.35)	-	1.48 (0.96–2.29)	-
55–59.9	1.15 (0.91–1.46)	-	1.93 (1.11–3.33)	-
60+	1.35 (1.10–1.66)	-	2.52 (1.47–4.33)	-
Employment status (ref. Employed)				
Disabled	1.55 (1.30–1.85)	-	2.82 (1.95–4.09)	1.79 (1.21–2.65)
Retired	1.18 (0.96–1.45)	-	1.98 (1.43–2.73)	1.43 (1.02–2.01)
Unemployed	1.26 (1.03–1.53)	-	1.15 (0.68–1.93)	1.02 (0.60–1.72)
Payment method (ref. private insurance)				
Self-payer	0.67 (0.46–0.97)	0.69 (0.48–1.01)	1.10 (0.72–1.69)	-
Medicare/Medicaid	1.46 (1.24–1.70)	1.12 (0.95–1.32)	2.22 (1.63–3.03)	-
Number of medications (5 med interval)	1.25 (1.17–1.34)	1.10 (1.02–1.19)	1.50 (1.30–1.72)	-
Open surgical method	1.93 (1.56–2.39)	1.78 (1.44–2.20)	2.48 (0.59–10.37)	-
Prolonged length of stay	2.47 (2.11–2.89)	2.28 (1.95–2.68)	3.08 (2.19–4.33)	2.32 (1.63–3.30)
Comorbidities				
Alcohol use	0.76 (0.66–0.87)	0.82 (0.71–0.94)	0.83 (0.63–1.08)	-
Angina	1.41 (1.09–1.83)	-	2.35 (1.43–3.85)	1.58 (0.95–2.63)
Asthma	1.26 (1.09–1.46)	-	1.77 (1.32–2.37)	1.52 (1.12–2.05)
Cholelithiasis	1.29 (1.13–1.48)	1.18 (1.03–1.36)	1.25 (0.93–1.68)	-
Depression	1.34 (1.15–1.56)	1.18 (1.01–1.39)	1.18 (0.85–1.65)	-
DVT/PE	1.49 (1.17–1.91)	1.24 (0.96–1.60)	2.79 (1.78–4.37)	2.09 (1.32–3.29)
GERD	1.22 (1.08–1.38)	-	1.54 (1.20–1.97)	1.30 (1.01–1.68)
Ischemic heart disease	1.49 (1.21–1.83)	1.21 (0.97–1.51)	1.86 (1.24–2.79)	-
Lower extremity edema	1.24 (1.06–1.45)	-	1.98 (1.45–1.90)	1.36 (0.99–1.89)
Obstructive sleep apnea	1.10 (0.98–1.24)	-	1.97 (1.56–2.49)	1.45 (1.13–1.87)
Psychosocial impairment	1.36 (1.17–1.57)	1.19 (1.02–1.39)	0.97 (0.69–1.38)	-
Pseudotumor cerebri	1.75 (1.20–2.55)	1.63 (1.11–2.39)	1.82 (0.79–4.22)	-
Peripheral vascular disease	1.78 (1.23–2.57)	1.44 (0.99–2.11)	1.28 (0.47–3.50)	-

Abbreviations: ASA, American Society of Anesthesiologists; CI, confidence interval; DVT, deep venous thrombosis; GERD, gastroesophageal reflux disease; OR, odds ratio; PE, pulmonary embolism. Ref denotes the reference group of a categorical variable. The variables for participation of surgical resident, COE volume, abdominal hernia, abdominal pannus, back pain, bipolar disorder, congestive heart failure, fibromyalgia, gout/hyperuricemia, hypertension, lipids, liver disease, musculoskeletal disease, obesity hypoventilation syndrome, panic disorder, personality disorder, psychosis, pulmonary hypertension, substance abuse, stress urinary incontinence, and type-2 diabetes were not significant at $P \leq .10$ in univariate analysis and/or not significant in either multivariate model for either surgery and are not shown. Dashes indicate that the variable was not included in the multivariate model because it was removed either for not meeting the significance threshold in the univariate model or for being removed in the backwards selection procedure.

Table 5. Comparison of RYGB Patients from Included and Excluded BSCOE.

	Included BSCOE	Excluded BSCOE	
	n = 25,877	**n = 21,664**	
Variable	**Mean (SD) or No. (%)**	**Mean (SD) or No. (%)**	***P* value**[a]
BSCOE	249 (55.5)	200 (44.5)	-
Age	45.6 (11.6)	45.1 (11.5)	<0.001
Female sex	20,162 (77.9)	17,051 (78.7)	0.04
Race			<0.001
Black	2406 (9.3)	2373 (11.0)	
Caucasian	20,909 (80.8)	15,808 (73.0)	
Hispanic/Latino	1789 (6.9)	1799 (8.3)	
Other	773 (3.0)	1684 (7.8)	
ASA Classification			<0.001
1 – normal, healthy	338 (1.3)	1337 (6.2)	
2/3 – mild systemic disease	24,072 (93.0)	19,276 (89.0)	
4/5 – severe/very severe disease	1467 (5.7)	1051 (4.9)	
BMI[b]	47.2 (8.3)	47.3 (8.3)	0.37
Employment status			<0.001
Employed	19,879 (76.8)	16,885 (77.9)	
Disabled	2273 (8.8)	1680 (7.8)	
Retired	1819 (7.0)	1425 (6.6)	
Unemployed	1906 (7.4)	1674 (7.7)	
Payment Information			0.10
Private insurance	21,876 (84.5)	18,467 (85.2)	
Self-payer	903 (3.5)	731 (3.4)	
Medicare/Medicaid	3098 (12.0)	2466 (11.4)	
Number of medications	3.8 (4.0)	3.2 (3.8)	<0.001
Comorbidities			
Abdominal hernia	1456 (5.6)	939 (4.3)	<0.001
Abdominal/skin pannus	2180 (8.4)	1111 (5.1)	<0.001
Alcohol use	7798 (30.1)	6167 (28.5)	<0.001
Angina	976 (3.8)	488 (2.3)	<0.001
Asthma	3477 (13.4)	2903 (13.4)	0.91
Back pain	2754 (10.6)	1982 (9.2)	<0.001
Bipolar disorder	521 (2.0)	446 (2.1)	0.74
Cholelithiasis	4836 (18.7)	3470 (16.0)	<0.001
Congestive heart failure	751 (2.9)	437 (2.0)	<0.001
Depression	3782 (14.6)	2890 (13.3)	<0.001
DVT/PE	971 (3.8)	612 (2.8)	<0.001
Fibromyalgia	949 (3.7)	670 (3.1)	<0.001
GERD	6781 (26.2)	5073 (23.4)	<0.001
Gout/hyperuricemia	1036 (4.0)	655 (3.0)	<0.001
Hypertension	6115 (23.6)	4587 (21.2)	<0.001
Ischemic heart disease	1374 (5.3)	917 (4.2)	<0.001
Lipids	7014 (27.1)	5562 (25.7)	<0.001
Liver disease	2264 (8.8)	1091 (5.0)	<0.001
Lower extremity edema	3287 (12.7)	2370 (10.9)	<0.001
Musculoskeletal disease	2766 (10.7)	2319 (10.7)	0.96
Obesity hypoventilation syndrome	608 (2.4)	525 (2.4)	0.60
Obstructive sleep apnea	7779 (30.1)	6474 (29.9)	0.67
Panic disorder	2175 (8.4)	1483 (6.9)	<0.001
Peripheral vascular disease	247 (1.3)	241 (1.1)	0.02

Table 5. Cont.

	Included BSCOE	Excluded BSCOE	
	n = 25,877	n = 21,664	
Variable	Mean (SD) or No. (%)	Mean (SD) or No. (%)	*P* value[a]
Personality disorder	196 (0.8)	52 (0.2)	<0.001
Psychosocial impairment	4544 (11.6)	3138 (14.5)	<0.001
Pseudotumor cerebri	467 (1.8)	635 (2.9)	<0.001
Psychosis	23 (0.1)	24 (0.1)	0.47
Pulmonary hypertension	1502 (5.8)	727 (3.4)	<0.001
Substance abuse	111 (0.4)	96 (0.4)	0.83
Stress urinary incontinence	2968 (11.5)	2683 (12.4)	0.002
Tobacco use	1910 (7.4)	1447 (6.7)	0.003
Type-2 diabetes	3172 (12.3)	2493 (11.5)	0.01

Abbreviations: BSCOE, bariatric surgery center of excellence; DVT, deep venous thrombosis; GERD, gastroesophageal reflux disease; PE, pulmonary embolism.
[a]*P* values calculated using a *t*-test for continuous variables and Pearson's chi-squared test or Fisher's exact test for categorical variables.
[b]Body mass index (BMI) was calculated as weight in kilograms divided by height in meters squared.

[24], our results, when considered with previous research [25], suggest that laparoscopic techniques should be preferred to open surgery in the absence of contraindications for laparoscopy. Patients with previous histories of bariatric surgery or other anatomical abnormalities may be best suited for open surgeries and would understandably be at higher risk for readmission. However, 7.6% of hospitals (19 of 249 BSCOE) conducted >80% of their RYGB procedures using the open approach and accounted for 46.6% of all open procedures in the database, suggesting that the open approach may be often dictated by surgeon preference in these hospitals rather than case difficulty.

The influence of serious comorbid disease on readmission risk for RYGB patients is expected, though the causal pathway of elevated risk for African-Americans is less clear. We suspect that the association with race may have been confounded by unmeasured variables such as surgical preparation, social support, economic status, or dietary intake. For AGB, readmission risk factors were quite different from those identified with RYGB with the exception of prolonged length of stay and severe ASA score: disability status, asthma, male gender, history of DVT/PE, and the presence of OSA or GERD.

Surprisingly, the profiles of risk factors for readmission were almost entirely distinct for the AGB and RYGB procedures. Prolonged length of stay following surgery was one of the only factors that significantly predicted readmissions in both surgical populations in multivariate analysis. That procedure-specific risk factors contrast so greatly between the two procedures is an important finding potentially overlooked by prior investigations. Previous studies have chosen to pool patients across procedures for analysis assuming that the underlying risk factors were the same [5,26]. While several of our results are complementary, the choice to aggregate surgical patients may account for some important differences in results. Some previous studies examining readmission rates have identified high BMI as a risk factor for readmission [5,17], while our own did not. Risk analyses that pooled patients from multiple procedures may have observed an artificial inflation of risk for high-BMI patients who tend to undergo RYGB, which has a significantly higher readmission rate than AGB. The relationship between BMI and readmission risk may also have been confounded by a less complete comorbidity profile in risk models, since many conditions are more prevalent among individuals of greater weight. The ability to examine the role of a very extensive list of comorbidities is a major strength of this analysis.

Many of the identified risk factors, while complex, multifactorial, and often not necessarily modifiable, provide an impetus to follow patients at higher risk for readmission more aggressively following discharge. Prolonged length of stay, for example, was identified as an important risk factor yet the reasons for the longer stay varied widely in BOLD; both preoperative and perioperative factors can interact to influence the duration of a patient's stay. Despite this heterogeneity, prolonged length of stay could be utilized as a prompt for enhanced post-discharge monitoring in patients at higher risk for readmission. Intervention studies are needed to determine if and how enhanced monitoring, adjunctive treatments, or additional education might reduce readmission rates for high-risk patients. Certainly, enhanced monitoring is unlikely to prevent more serious readmissions such as those in patients who develop gastrointestinal leaks or obstructions. Further, it is unknown at this time how much effort would need to be applied to significantly lower the current readmission rates that are already acceptably low. However, it may be possible to impact the most prevalent reasons for readmission, nausea and vomiting, by establishing infusion centers for patients suffering from a slow return of bowel function and dehydration.

It is important to recognize the magnitude of relative risk differences associated with the predictors of readmission in this analysis; primarily, comorbid conditions must be weighed with the absolute risk for each procedure. For example, a relative risk of 1.5 for a high-risk patient group compared to a group of typical patients would equate to an increase of the readmission rate from 5.8% to 8.7% for RYGB and from 1.2% to 1.8% for AGB, or absolute risk differences of 2.9% and 0.6%, respectively. Patients, payers, and practitioners alike may find these higher risks acceptable if outweighed by the benefits of surgery, which are often greatest among patients with more severe comorbidity profiles. For these reasons, we deem that the current results do not support patient selection, but rather highlight patient groups that could benefit from appropriate preventative or educational efforts, and possibly, closer post-discharge follow-up.

This study has several limitations. The exclusion of centers with low follow-up rates is the most important limitation, since it is

Table 6. Comparison of AGB Patients from Included and Excluded BSCOE.

	Included BSCOE	Excluded BSCOE	
	n = 26,765	n = 8814	
Variable	Mean (SD) or No. (%)	Mean (SD) or No. (%)	*P* value[a]
BSCOE	317 (68.3)	147 (31.7)	-
Age	46.1 (12.1)	46.5 (12.3)	0.01
Female sex	21,319 (79.7)	6919 (78.5)	0.02
Race			<0.001
Black/African American	2979 (11.1)	942 (10.7)	
Caucasian	21,171 (79.1)	6183 (70.2)	
Hispanic/Latino	1089 (4.1)	674 (7.7)	
Other	1526 (5.7)	1015 (11.5)	
ASA Classification			0.004
1 – normal, healthy	1388 (5.2)	381 (4.3)	
2/3 – mild systemic disease	24,635 (92.0)	8200 (93.0)	
4/5 – severe/very severe disease	742 (2.8)	233 (2.6)	
BMI[b]	44.2 (6.7)	44.2 (7.2)	0.62
Employment Status			<0.001
Employed	21,937 (82.0)	7132 (80.9)	
Disabled	1240 (4.6)	527 (6.0)	
Retired	2313 (8.6)	783 (8.9)	
Unemployed	1275 (4.8)	372 (4.2)	
Payment Information			<0.001
Private Insurance	22,085 (82.5)	7169 (81.3)	
Self-Payer	2447 (9.1)	652 (7.4)	
Medicare/Medicaid	2233 (8.3)	993 (11.3)	
Number of medications	2.8 (3.5)	3.1 (3.5)	<0.001
Comorbidities			
Abdominal hernia	1054 (3.9)	486 (5.5)	<0.001
Abdominal/Skin pannus	1107 (4.1)	381 (4.3)	0.44
Alcohol use	7407 (27.7)	2750 (31.2)	<0.001
Angina	596 (2.2)	158 (1.8)	0.01
Asthma	2788 (10.4)	893 (10.1)	0.45
Back pain	1999 (7.5)	626 (7.1)	0.25
Bipolar disorder	364 (1.4)	140 (1.6)	0.12
Cholelithiasis	3938 (14.7)	1146 (13.0)	<0.001
Congestive heart failure	445 (1.7)	140 (1.6)	0.66
Depression	3144 (11.8)	767 (8.7)	<0.001
DVT/PE	878 (3.3)	218 (2.5)	<0.001
Fibromyalgia	708 (2.7)	240 (2.7)	0.70
GERD	5783 (21.6)	1563 (17.7)	<0.001
Gout/hyperuricemia	661 (2.5)	414 (4.7)	<0.001
Hypertension	5197 (19.4)	1693 (19.2)	0.67
Ischemic heart disease	1197 (4.5)	359 (4.1)	0.12
Lipids	6192 (23.1)	2278 (25.9)	<0.001
Liver disease	1151 (4.3)	438 (5.0)	0.008
Lower extremity edema	2413 (9.0)	671 (7.6)	<0.001
Musculoskeletal disease	2219 (8.3)	814 (9.1)	0.02
Obesity hypoventilation syndrome	517 (1.9)	150 (1.7)	0.17
Obstructive sleep apnea	5993 (22.4)	1931 (21.9)	0.34
Panic disorder	1567 (5.9)	541 (6.1)	0.33
Peripheral vascular disease	234 (0.9)	89 (1.0)	0.24

Table 6. Cont.

	Included BSCOE	Excluded BSCOE	
	n = 26,765	n = 8814	
Variable	Mean (SD) or No. (%)	Mean (SD) or No. (%)	*P* value[a]
Personality disorder	62 (0.2)	10 (0.1)	0.04
Psychosocial impairment	3145 (11.8)	1034 (11.7)	0.96
Pseudotumor cerebri	290 (1.1)	88 (1.0)	0.55
Psychosis	15 (0.1)	6 (0.1)	0.62
Pulmonary hypertension	1084 (4.1)	167 (1.9)	<0.001
Substance abuse	73 (0.3)	35 (0.4)	0.07
Stress urinary incontinence	2748 (10.3)	833 (9.5)	0.03
Tobacco use	1813 (6.8)	568 (6.4)	0.28
Type-2 diabetes	2093 (7.8)	670 (7.6)	0.51

Abbreviations: BSCOE, bariatric surgery center of excellence; DVT, deep venous thrombosis; GERD, gastroesophageal reflux disease; PE, pulmonary embolism.
[a]*P* values calculated using a *t*-test for continuous variables and Pearson's chi-squared test or Fisher's exact test for categorical variables.
[b]Body mass index (BMI) was calculated as weight in kilograms divided by height in meters squared.

possible that BSCOE excluded for low follow-up rates may have been the hospitals with the highest readmission rates, as well. Our sensitivity analyses comparing included and excluded centers did not indicate that there were substantive clinical differences between the patient populations (Tables 5 and 6), and if such a bias were present, it is highly unlikely that an underestimation of readmission rates would have a considerable impact on the strength or direction of the risk factors themselves. Long-term follow-up in BOLD was limited and precluded the examination of readmissions occurring beyond 30 days. RYGB patients continue to require readmission up to and beyond one year, and the need for band revisions generally do not occur within the first 30 days of

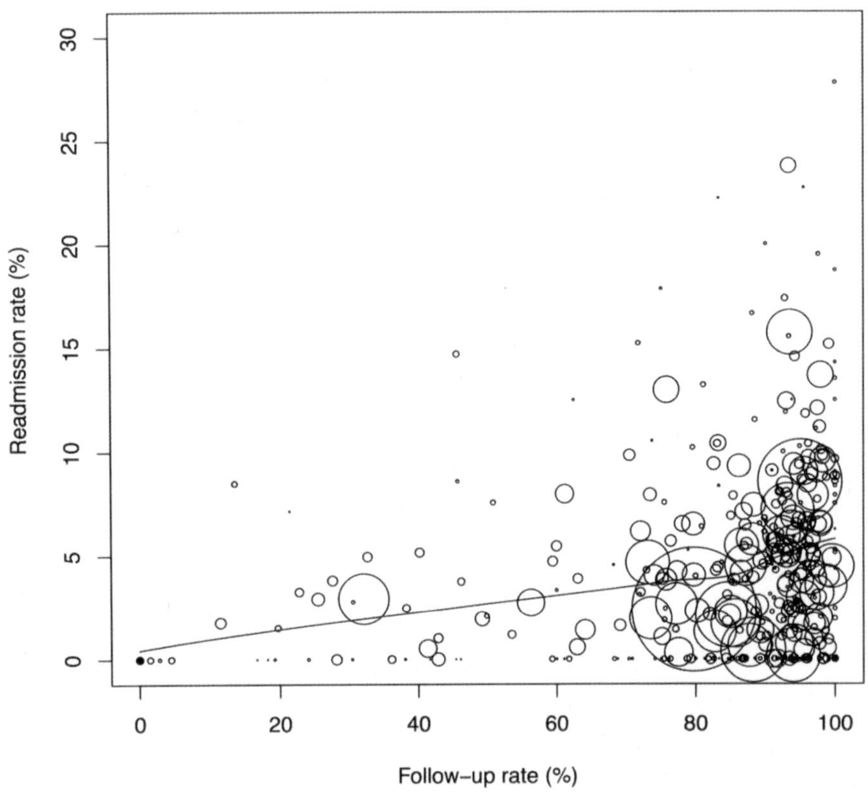

Figure 3. Loess plot of RYGB readmission rates on follow-up rates. Circles represent BSCOE hospitals with the size weighted by the number of patients who underwent the procedure in the hospital during the study period.

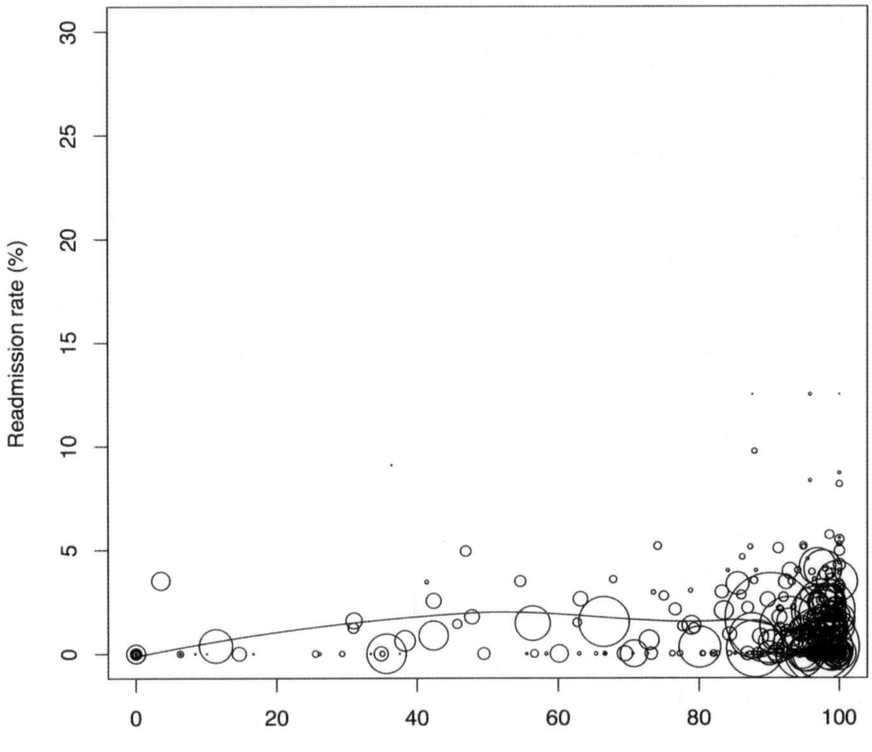

Figure 4. Loess plot of AGB readmission rates on follow-up rates. Circles represent BSCOE hospitals with the size weighted by the number of patients who underwent the procedure in the hospital during the study period.

surgery; however, the greatest proportion of readmissions occur within 30 days [17,18], so the current study likely captures the most important risk factors for readmission.

The present analysis was also unable to control for surgeon volume, an important factor in readmission [16,19,20]. however surgeons reporting to BOLD must log over 50 cases annually in order to maintain BSCOE certification. Also, the distribution of readmission rates was not consistent with a uniform rate across centers (Figures 3 and 4). An appreciable number of BSCOE, for AGB in particular, reported readmission rates considerably lower than would be expected under a constant rate across centers of varying surgical volume. We suspect that unusually low BSCOE readmission rates reflect unmeasured variables such as surgical experience, and those with high rates of readmission could be indicative of either surgeon inexperience, case difficulty, or surgeon preference for open procedures. Data entered into BOLD is self-reported by BSCOE, so post-discharge events are potentially underreported in the database, though our selection of centers with high follow-up rates was undertaken to offset potential underreporting in the larger database.

Finally, the observational nature of the study precludes causal inference about risk factors. Given that examination of factors influencing relatively rare events like readmissions requires thousands of patients to be adequately powered to assess differences in risk, it is unlikely that randomized studies of these factors will ever be performed. Therefore, decisions on patient selection and risk calculations will inevitably be based on large prospective observational databases like BOLD. Nested case-control studies, in which more extensive collection of possible explanatory variables is performed, may shed light on the problem of unmeasured confounders in the BOLD dataset.

In conclusion, we have characterized patterns of risk for readmission associated with patient and intraoperative factors for the two most common bariatric procedures in the largest prospective cohort of bariatric surgery patients to date. While the overall readmission rates for both procedures are low, the present results may prove to be an important clinical tool in the development of patient education programs, algorithms for procedure selection, and follow-up plans. In an effort to maximize patient benefit and cost-effectiveness of bariatric surgery and to reduce penalties from payers, primary care providers and surgeons should understand patient-specific risks to optimize clinical care for patients when both selecting for and immediately following their bariatric operation.

Acknowledgments

We would like to acknowledge Deborah Winegar and Bintu Sharif of the Surgical Review Corporation for their assistance in the review of the manuscript. We would also like to thank Barbara Sampson of the University of Minnesota Department of Surgery for her administrative and technical assistance and Avis Thomas of the University of Minnesota Division of Biostatistics for her intellectual contribution to the study design.

Author Contributions

Conceived and designed the experiments: RBD CJM DBL FJS BS HB JEC SI. Analyzed the data: RBD CJM JEC SI. Contributed reagents/materials/analysis tools: BS. Wrote the paper: RBD CJM JEC SI. Conducted statistical analyses: CJM JEC. Contributed to manuscript revisions: DBL FJS BS HB.

References

1. Santry HP, Gillen DL, Lauderdale DS (2005) Trends in bariatric surgical procedures. JAMA 294: 1909–1917.
2. American Society for Metabolic and Bariatric Surgery, Metabolic & Bariatric Surgery Fact Sheet (2011) Final report May 2011. Gainesville, FL: Media Press Kit, Available: http://s3.amazonaws.com/publicASMBS/MediaPressKit/MetabolicBariatricSurgeryOverviewJuly2011.pdf. Accessed 2011 August 25.
3. Buchwald H, Avidor Y, Braunwald E, Jensen MD, Pories W, et al. (2004) Bariatric surgery: a systematic review and meta-analysis. JAMA 292: 1724–1737.
4. Dorman RB, Abraham AA, Al-Refaie WB, Parsons HM, Ikramuddin S, et al. (2011) Bariatric Surgery Outcomes in the Elderly Population: An ACS NISQIP Study. J Gastrointest Surg 16: 35–44.
5. Flum DR, Belle SH, King WC, Wahed AS, Berk P, et al. (2009) Perioperative safety in the longitudinal assessment of bariatric surgery. NEJM 361: 445–454.
6. Zingmond DS, McGory ML, Ko CY (2005) Hospitalization before and after gastric bypass surgery. JAMA 294: 1918–1924.
7. Encinosa WE, Bernard DM, Chen CC, Steiner CA (2006) Healthcare utilization and outcomes after bariatric surgery. Med Care 44: 706–712.
8. DeMaria EJ, Pate V, Warthen M, Winegar DA (2010) Baseline data from American Society for Metabolic and Bariatric Surgery-designated Bariatric Surgery Centers of Excellence using the Bariatric Outcomes Longitudinal Database. Surg Obes Relat Dis 6: 347–355.
9. Adams TD, Gress RE, Smith SC, Halverson RC, Simper SC, et al. (2007) Long-term mortality after gastric bypass surgery. NEJM 357: 753–761.
10. Buchwald H, Estok R, Fahrbach K, Banel D, Jensen MD, et al. (2009) Weight and type 2 diabetes after bariatric surgery: systematic review and meta-analysis. Am J Med 122: 248–256.
11. Dorman RB, Serrot FJ, Miller CJ, Slusarek B, Sampson B, et al. (2012) Case-matched outcomes in bariatric surgery for the treatment of type 2 diabetes in the morbidly obese patient. Ann Surg 255: 287–293.
12. Pories WJ, MacDonald KG, Morgan EJ, Sinha MK, Dohm GL, et al. (1992) Surgical treatment of obesity and its effect on diabetes: 10-y follow-up. Am J Clin Nutr 55: 582S–585S.
13. Sjostrom L, Lindroos AK, Peltonen M, Torgerson J, Bouchard C, et al. (2004) Lifestyle, diabetes, and cardiovascular risk factors 10 years after bariatric surgery. NEJM 351: 2683–2693.
14. Sjostrom L, Narbro K, Sjostrom CD, Karason K, Larsson B, et al. (2007) Effects of bariatric surgery on mortality in Swedish obese subjects. NEJM 357: 741–752.
15. Vetter ML, Cardillo S, Rickels MR, Iqbal N (2009) Narrative review: effect of bariatric surgery on type 2 diabetes mellitus. Ann Intern Med 150: 94–103.
16. Birkmeyer NJ, Dimick JB, Share D, Hawasli A, English WJ, et al. (2010) Hospital complication rates with bariatric surgery in Michigan. JAMA 304: 435–442.
17. Kellogg TA, Swan T, Leslie DA, Buchwald H, Ikramuddin S (2009) Patterns of readmission and reoperation within 90 days after Roux-en-Y gastric bypass. Surg Obes Relat Dis 5: 416–423.
18. Saunders J, Ballantyne GH, Belsley S, Stephens DJ, Trivedi A, et al. (2008) One-year readmission rates at a high volume bariatric surgery center: laparoscopic adjustable gastric banding, laparoscopic gastric bypass, and vertical banded gastroplasty-Roux-en-Y gastric bypass. Obes Surg 18: 1233–1240.
19. Weller WE, Hannan EL (2006) Relationship between provider volume and postoperative complications for bariatric procedures in New York State. J Am Coll Surg 202: 753–761.
20. Weller WE, Rosati C, Hannan EL (2007) Relationship between surgeon and hospital volume and readmission after bariatric operation. J Am Coll Surg 204: 383–391.
21. Nguyen NT, Slone JA, Nguyen XM, Hartman JS, Hoyt DB (2009) A prospective randomized trial of laparoscopic gastric bypass versus laparoscopic adjustable gastric banding for the treatment of morbid obesity: outcomes, quality of life, and costs. Ann Surg 250: 631–641.
22. Weber M, Muller MK, Bucher T, Wildi S, Dindo D, et al. (2004) Laparoscopic gastric bypass is superior to laparoscopic gastric banding for treatment of morbid obesity. Ann Surg 240: 975–982. discussion 982-973.
23. Maggard MA, Shugarman LR, Suttorp M, Maglione M, Sugerman HJ, et al. (2005) Meta-analysis: surgical treatment of obesity. Ann Intern Med 142: 547–559.
24. Puzziferri N, Austrheim-Smith IT, Wolfe BM, Wilson SE, Nguyen NT (2006) Three-year follow-up of a prospective randomized trial comparing laparoscopic versus open gastric bypass. Ann Surg 243: 181–188.
25. Hutter MM, Randall S, Khuri SF, Henderson WG, Abbott WM, et al. (2006) Laparoscopic versus open gastric bypass for morbid obesity: a multicenter, prospective, risk-adjusted analysis from the National Surgical Quality Improvement Program. Ann Surg 243: 657–662.
26. Gupta PK, Franck C, Miller WJ, Gupta H, Forse RA (2011) Development and validation of a bariatric surgery morbidity risk calculator using the prospective, multicenter NSQIP dataset. J Am Coll Surg 212: 301–309.

7

CDK4 Amplification Predicts Recurrence of Well-Differentiated Liposarcoma of the Abdomen

Sanghoon Lee[1,9,¶], Hyojun Park[1,9,¶], Sang Yun Ha[2], Kwang Yeol Paik[3], Seung Eun Lee[2], Jong Man Kim[1], Jae Berm Park[1], Choon Hyuck David Kwon[1], Jae-Won Joh[1], Yoon-La Choi[2,4*†], Sung Joo Kim[1,4*†]

1 Department of Surgery, Samsung Medical Center, Sungkyunkwan University School of Medicine, Seoul, Korea, **2** Department of Pathology, Samsung Medical Center, Sungkyunkwan University School of Medicine, Seoul, Korea, **3** Department of Surgery, The Catholic University of Korea, Yeouido St. Mary's Hospital, Seoul, Korea, **4** SHIST, Samsung Medical Center, Sungkyunkwan University School of Medicine, Seoul, Korea

Abstract

Background: The absence of *CDK4* amplification in liposarcomas is associated with favorable prognosis. We aimed to identify the factors associated with tumor recurrence in patients with well-differentiated (WD) and dedifferentiated (DD) liposarcomas.

Methods: From 2000 to 2010, surgical resections for 101 WD and DD liposarcomas were performed. Cases in which complete surgical resections with curative intent were carried out were selected. *MDM2* and *CDK4* gene amplification were analyzed by quantitative real-time polymerase chain reaction (Q-PCR).

Results: There were 31 WD and 17 DD liposarcomas. Locoregional recurrence was observed in 11 WD and 3 DD liposarcomas. WD liposarcomas showed better patient survival compared to DD liposarcomas ($P<0.05$). Q-PCR analysis of the liposarcomas revealed the presence of *CDK4* amplification in 44 cases (91.7%) and *MDM2* amplification in 46 cases (95.8%). WD liposarcomas with recurrence after surgical resection had significantly higher levels of *CDK4* amplification compared to those without recurrence ($P=0.041$). High level of *CDK4* amplification (cases with *CDK4* amplification higher than the median 7.54) was associated with poor recurrence-free survival compared to low *CDK4* amplification in both univariate ($P=0.012$) and multivariate analyses ($P=0.020$).

Conclusions: Level of *CDK4* amplification determined by Q-PCR was associated with the recurrence of WD liposarcomas after surgical resection.

Editor: Anthony W. I. Lo, The Chinese University of Hong Kong, Hong Kong

Funding: The authors have no support or funding to report.

Competing Interests: The authors have declared that no competing interests exist.

* Email: kmhyj.kim@samsung.com (SJK); yla.choi@samsung.com (YLC)

9 These authors contributed equally to this work.

¶ These authors are co-first authors on this work.

† These authors also contributed equally to this work.

Introduction

Liposarcomas are the most common type of soft tissue sarcoma accounting for approximately 20% of all soft tissue sarcomas [1,2]. Well-differentiated (WD) liposarcomas are characterized by atypical but relatively mature adipocyte proliferation, while dedifferentiated (DD) liposarcomas consist of non-lipogenic spindle or pleomorphic cells with elevated mitotic activity [3,4]. These two histologic subtypes share a common genetic feature characterized by a supernumerary circular and/or giant rod chromosome containing a highly amplified sequence of genes from the 12q13-q21 region [5]. This region contains the *MDM2* and *CDK4*, which are known to play crucial roles in the control of the cell cycle progression [6]. *CDK4* amplification has been observed in several malignancies including glioma, breast cancer, lymphoma, melanoma, and sarcoma [7]. It has been suggested that an absence of *CDK4* amplification in WD and DD liposarcomas is associated with lower rate of recurrence and favorable prognosis [6].

In this study, we sought to identify factors associated with tumor recurrence and patient survival including the levels of *MDM2* and *CDK4* amplification in a homogeneous population of patients with WD and DD liposarcomas of the abdomen undergoing complete surgical resection.

Methods

Patient Selection

From December 2000 to December 2010, 139 patients underwent surgical resection for liposarcoma at Samsung Medical Center, Seoul, Korea. Among these patients, 101 cases were diagnosed as WD or DD liposarcomas. Retrospective review was performed for consideration of inclusion in the study. Cases referred to our institute from other centers for management of

Table 1. Primer sequence.

MDM2 (product size = 98 bp)
Forward primer 5′-CCG GAT GAT CGC AGG TG-3′
Reverse primer 5′-AAA AGC TGA GTC AAC CTG CCC-3′
CDK4 (product size = 103 bp)
Forward primer 5′-TTG CAT CGT TCA CCG AGA TC-3′
Reverse primer 5′-CTG GTA GCT GTA GAT TCT GGC CA-3′
Albumin (PCR product size = 81 bp)
Forward primer 5′-TGA AAC ATA CGT TCC CAA AGA GTT T-3′
Reverse primer 5′-CTC TCC TTC TCA GAA AGT GTG CAT AT-3′

bp, base pairs; PCR, polymerase chain reaction.

recurrent tumors were excluded from the analysis. Cases were selected for this analysis when complete surgical resections with curative intent were carried out for WD or DD liposarcomas of the retroperitoneum and peritoneal cavity. Complete surgical resection of the tumor was achieved when all of the following three criteria were met: no gross residual tumor in the surgical field as observed by the surgeon (pathologic R0 or R1 status), histologic confirmation of negative surgical margins and no radiologic signs of residual tumor in the first postoperative follow-up abdomen computed tomography (CT) scan, typically done between postoperative 1 to 4 weeks.

Common practice for surgical resection of abdominal liposarcomas was wide excision of the mass with combined resection of adjacent viscera when the organ is suspected to have direct tumor invasion by preoperative radiologic evaluation and inspection in the surgical field. A tissue expander was left in the space previously occupied by the tumor when adjuvant radiotherapy was planned.

Patients were followed at our outpatient clinic with abdominal CT scans and chest plain x-rays every 3 to 6 months. When local recurrence was suspected, abdominal CT scans were repeated after 1 month or positron emission tomography-CT (PET-CT) was done to confirm the presence of locoregional recurrence or distant metastases. When possible, surgical resection of the recurred tumor mass was attempted. Unresectable tumors or distant metastases to multiple sites were managed with systemic chemotherapy.

This research has been approved by the institutional review board at Samsung Medical Center (Seoul, Korea). All data collection and analysis were done anonymously, and written or verbal consent were not provided by the participants of this work. The lack of consent for this study was also approved.

MDM2 and CDK4 Quantitative Real-Time PCR

MDM2 and *CDK4* amplification was analyzed by quantitative real-time polymerase chain reaction (Q-PCR) performed on a PRISM 7500HT Fast Realtime PCR system (Applied Biosystems, Foster City, CA) by using a HotStart-IT SYBR Green qPCR Master mix (USB, Cleveland, OH). Ten nanograms of target DNA was dispensed into each sample with a final reaction volume of 10 μl. Each sample was amplified in triplicate. The PCR was carried out as follows: preheating at 50°C for 2 min and then at 95°C for 10 min, followed by 40 cycles at 95°C for 15 s and 60°C for 1 min. (Primer sequences for each gene are shown in Table 1.) *MDM2* and *CDK4* copy numbers were calculated by comparison to the reference gene (*ALB*) located at 4q11-q13, and were normalized to normal tissue genomic DNA as a calibrator. The level of amplification for *MDM2* or *CDK4* was calculated as follows: copy number of the target gene (*MDM2*, *CDK4*)/copy number of the reference gene (*ALB*). Each gene was considered to have positive amplification when the copy number was greater than 2 times that of the reference gene.

CDK4 Immunohistochemical Staining

Immunohistochemical (IHC) staining for CDK4 was performed on representative paraffin-embedded tumor material from the biopsy cut into 4 μm-thick sections and placed onto glass slides. For IHC staining, the slides were deparaffinized in xylene. Staining for CDK4 was performed automatically using the Leica Bond Max immunostainer with Bond Polymer Refine Detection Kits and heat-induced epitope retrieval pH 6.0 (Bond max ER1 (EDTA) solution, Australia) for 15 min. The CDK4 expression was analyzed using mouse monoclonal antibody specific for CDK4 protein (Clone DSC-31, dilution 1:50, Invitrogen, Carlsbad, CA, USA) [8]. Antibodies against CDK4 react inside the nucleus, so any specific nuclear weak to strong immunostaining was evaluated by microscopy. The cases were stratified into four categories by intensity of the nuclear staining and scores between 0 and 3 were given for each of the categories: negative (0), weak positivity (1), moderate positivity (2), and strong positivity (3). The percentage of tumor cell reactivity was determined, approximately, by visually inspecting the slides and counting 100 tumor cells, at medium/high power, in at least five different fields. The percentage of tumors stained was categorized and scored as follows: 1~25% (1), 26~50% (2), 51~75% (3) and 76~100% (4). The 2 scores for intensity and percentage given for each case were multiplied to yield the final score of the tumor. A cut-off point for positivity was set at the mean score (6) of the 48 cases analyzed, and a score higher than 6 was considered be indicative of positive expression of CDK4 [9,10]. Stains were evaluated by two individuals (SYH and YLC) and discordant cases were revised together.

Statistical Analysis

Chi-square tests (or Fisher's exact test, when necessary) were used to compare categorical variables. Pearson's correlation was used to measure the correlation between variables. The Cox proportional hazard model was used for survival and risk factor analysis. All analyses were done using IBM SPSS Statistics version 19 program. Results were considered to be significant when *P*-values were less than 0.05.

Results

Patient and Tumor Characteristics

One hundred thirty-nine patients were surgically treated for liposarcoma at our center during the study period. Pathologic examination of the resected tumors of 101 patients showed either WD or DD histologic subtype. Ninety-two tumors were found in the retroperitoneum or peritoneal cavity. Fifty-four patients had their first surgical treatment at our center and 48 had complete surgical resection of the tumor. The patient selection process for inclusion in this study is outlined in Figure 1.

The 48 patients who had complete tumor resection (29 male and 19 female) were included in this analysis. The median age of patients was 57 years (range 37~78 years). There were 31 WD and 17 DD liposarcomas. Tumors were located in the retroperitoneum in 43 cases, the mesentery in 4 cases and the pelvis in 1 case. Tumor size ranged from 6.8 cm to 60 cm (median 21 cm). The characteristics of the 48 patients and clinicopathological

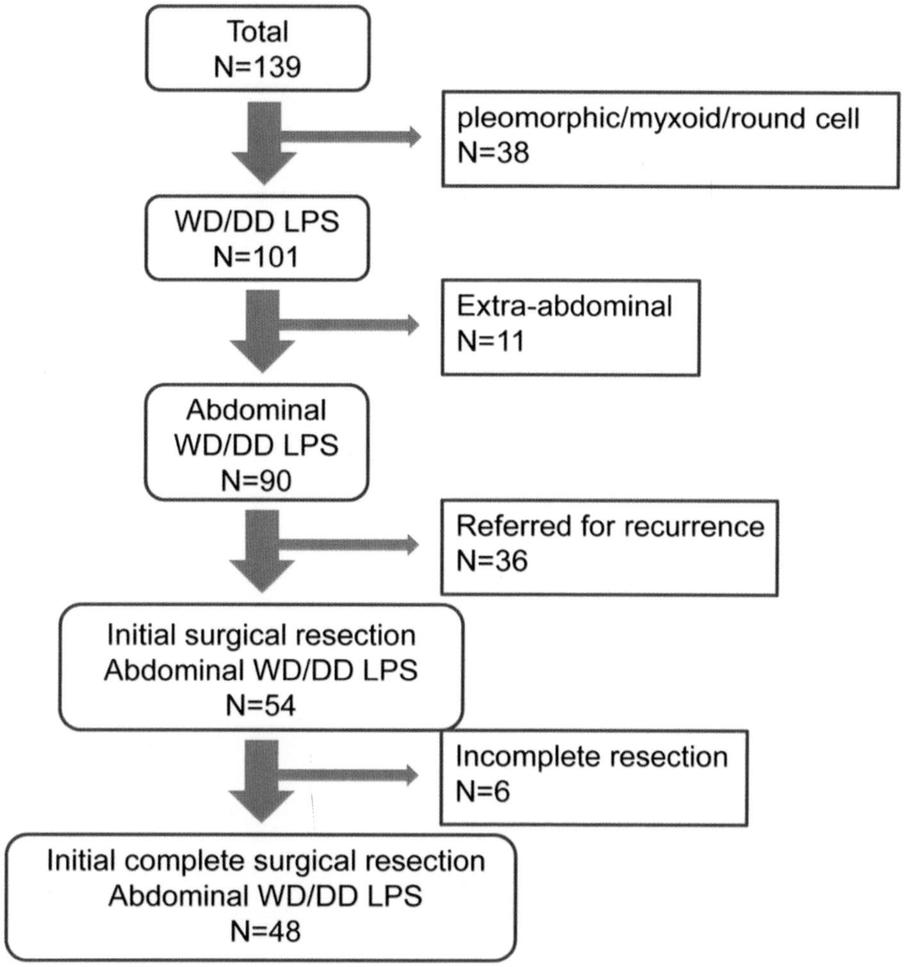

Figure 1. Synopsis of the patient inclusion and exclusion process. (WD, well-differentiated; DD, dedifferentiated; LPS, liposarcoma).

features of the liposarcomas according to histologic type are outlined in Table 2.

Surgical Treatment and Outcome of WD and DD Liposarcoma. Table 3 shows the surgical and pathological features of the 48 cases according to histologic type of the primary tumor. Combined resection of adjacent viscera was done in 21 of 31 WD and in 15 of 17 DD liposarcomas. An average 1.86 organs were surgically removed during surgery, and the kidney was the

Table 2. Clinicopathologic characteristics of well-differentiated and dedifferentiated liposarcomas.

	N = 48
Age, median (range)	57 (37~78)
Sex	
Male	29
Female	19
Histologic type	
Well-differentiated	31
Dedifferentiated	17
Tumor location	
Retroperitoneum	43
Pelvis	1
Mesentery	4
Tumor size, median (range), cm	21.0 (6.8~60.0)

Table 3. Clinicopathologic characteristics of well-differentiated and dedifferentiated liposarcomas.

	Primary tumor histology	
	Well-differentiated (N = 31)	**Dedifferentiated (N = 17)**
Extent of surgery		
Mass excision only	10 (32.3)	2 (11.8)
Combined organ resection	21 (67.7)	15 (88.2)
Tumor invasion of resected organ		
Yes*	7 (33.3)	10 (66.7)
No*	14 (66.7)	5 (33.3)
Microscopic resection margin		
Positive	13 (41.9)	11 (64.7)
Negative	11 (35.5)	3 (17.6)
Unknown	7 (22.6)	3 (17.6)
Adjuvant Radiotherapy		
Yes	6 (19.4)	4 (23.5)
No	25 (80.6)	13 (76.5)
Follow-up, median (months)	35.0	18.7
Recurrence		
Yes	11 (35.5)	9 (52.9)
No	20 (64.5)	8 (47.1)
Recurrence pattern		
Locoregional recurrence only**	11 (100)	3 (33.3)
Distant metastasis**	0	6 (66.7)

*p<0.05,
**p<0.01.

organ most often resected with the tumor. Invasion of the resected organ by the tumor was observed upon pathologic evaluation in 7 of 21 WD and 10 of 15 DD liposarcomas (33.3% vs. 66.7%, $p = 0.021$). Microscopic examination of the surgical margin was negative in 11 (35.5%) WD and 3 (17.6%) DD liposarcomas. Tumor recurrence after surgical resection with curative intent was observed in 20 patients (20/48, 41.7%); 11 were WD and 9 were DD liposarcomas (35.5% vs. 52.9%, $p = 0.144$). Recurrence was locoregionally limited in all 11 WD cases while 6 of the 9 DD liposarcomas recurred as distant metastases. A significant difference in recurrence pattern was observed between the 2 histologic subtypes ($p = 0.001$).

Figure 2a shows the disease-specific patient survival of the 48 patients after surgery. Patient survival was approximately 72% at postoperative 10 years. Patient survival according to histologic type is shown in Figure 2b. Kaplan-Meier survival curves showed better patient survival with WD liposarcoma compared to DD liposarcoma ($p<0.05$).

Lococregional Recurrence and Distant Metastasis of WD and DD Liposarcoma. Locoregional recurrence was observed in 11 WD and 3 DD liposarcoma cases. The median time interval

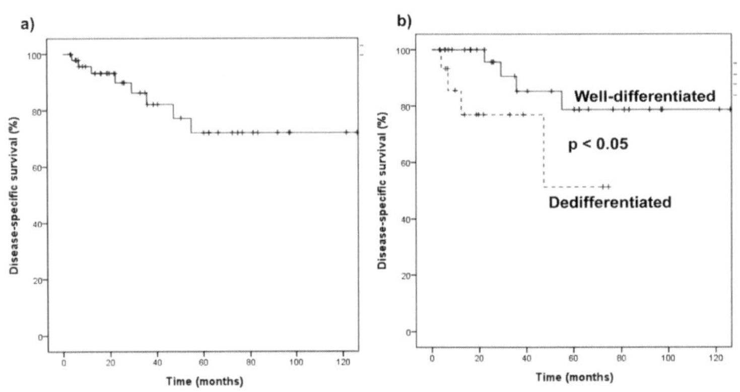

Figure 2. Overall patient survival, a), after surgical resection for well-differentiated and dedifferentiated liposarcoma of the abdomen, and b) Patient survival stratified by histologic subtype of liposarcoma. Well-differentiated liposarcoma group show better survival compared to dedifferentiated liposarcoma group (p<0.05).

Table 4. Locoregional recurrence of abdominal well-differentiated and dedifferentiated liposarcomas.

	Primary tumor histology	
	Well-differentiated (N = 11)	**Dedifferentiated (N = 3)**
Histologic type of recurred tumor		
Well-differentiated	6	0
Dedifferentiated	2	2
Pleomorphic	2	0
No pathologic evaluation	1	1
Time interval to 1st recurrence, median (range), months	13.5 (4~120)	11.8 (7~50)
Treatment of recurrence		
Surgery	4	2
Surgery + radiotherapy	5	0
No Treatment	1	1
Follow-up after recurrence, median (range), months	20.0 (10~68)	9.6 (4~22)
Outcome of recurrence		
Dead of disease	5	2
Alive with disease	4	1
No evidence of disease	2	0

between surgical resection and the occurrence of the first recurrence was 13.5 months and 11.8 months for WD and DD liposarcomas, respectively. Primary WD liposarcomas expressed variable histologic types in their recurrence lesions; pathologic analyses of the recurrent tumor specimen were WD in 6 cases, DD in 2 cases and pleomorphic in 1 case. All recurrences of primary DD liposarcomas were of the DD histologic subtype. Surgical resection of locoregional recurrence was done in 9 WD and 2 DD cases. Patients underwent an average of 2.0 surgical resections for recurrences (Table 4).

Six cases had distant metastases during their follow-up period (Table 5). Of these, the primary tumors were of the DD histologic

Table 5. Distant metastasis of abdominal dedifferentiated liposarcomas.

	N = 6
Site of metastasis	
Intraperitoneal metastasis	4
Liver	1
Lung	1
Thigh	1
Time interval to metastasis, median (months)	13.7
Metastatic tumor histology	
Dedifferentiated	2
No pathologic evaluation	4
Number of recurrences prior to metastasis	
0	4
1	2
Treatment of metastasis	
Surgery	2
Chemotherapy	1
No treatment	3
Median follow-up after metastasis, months (range)	22 (1~37)
Outcome of metastasis	
Dead of disease	4
Alive with disease	2

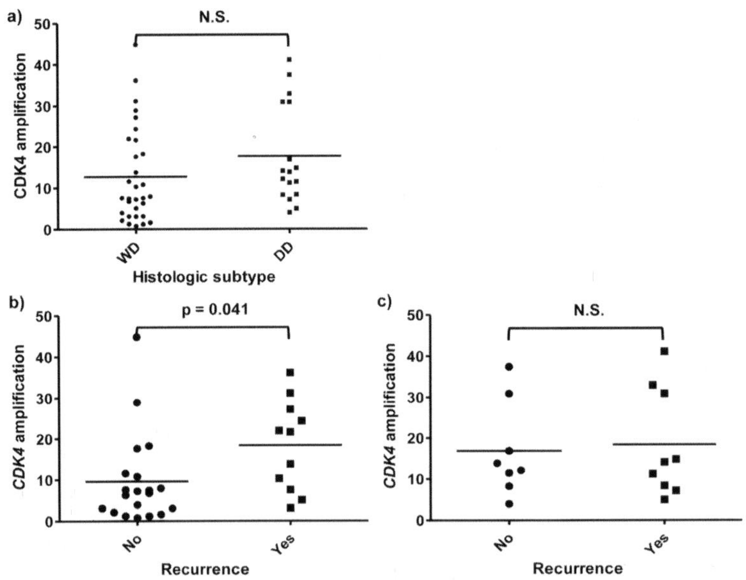

Figure 3. Quantitative real-time PCR results of *CDK4* amplification by a) well-differentiated (WD) and dedifferentiated (DD) liposarcomas: amplification levels were not different between the two histologic subtypes. Quantitative real-time PCR results of *CDK4* amplification in **b)** WD and **c)** DD liposarcomas according to tumor recurrence: amplification was higher in WD liposarcomas with recurrence after surgical resection, but not different in DD liposarcomas regardless of tumor recurrence.

type in all cases. The median time interval from surgical resection to detection of metastasis was 13.7 months. Metastatic spread was the first evidence of recurrence detected in 4 cases, while in 2 cases, locoregional recurrences were followed by distant metastases. The most common pattern of metastasis was as metastatic nodules in the peritoneal cavity in remote regions away from the primary site (intraperitoneal metastasis) were. One case of liver metastasis and 1 lung metastasis were observed. Metastasic tumor in the deep soft tissue of the thigh was observed in 1 case. Pathologic evaluation of the metastatic lesion was possible in 2 cases and all were DD liposarcomas.

Surgical resection of the metastatic tumor was carried out in 2 cases and systemic chemotherapy was done in 1 case. Metastatic liposarcoma was the cause of death in 4 patients. Patient survival after metastasis was 22.2% at 24 months.

CDK4 and MDM2 Gene Amplification and Immunohistochemistry Results

PCR analysis of the liposarcomas revealed the presence of *CDK4* amplification in 44 cases (91.7%) and *MDM2* amplification in 46 cases (95.8%). The levels of *CDK4* amplification were not different between the two histologic subtypes (Figure 3a). However, among WD liposarcomas, *CDK4* amplification was higher in the subgroup of cases which recurred after surgical resection compared to those without recurrence ($P = 0.041$, independent sample *t*-test, Figure 3b). The levels of *CDK4* amplification were not different in DD liposarcomas, regardless of tumor recurrence status (Figure 3c). *MDM2* amplification levels were not different regardless of histologic subtype or tumor recurrence (Figure 4).

CDK4 immunohistochemistry results were interpretable in all cases. Positive immunoreactivity for CDK4 was observed in 32 out of 48 cases (66.7%, Figure 5). However, positive CDK4 IHC immunoreactivity was not different according to tumor recurrence in all cases ($p = 0.363$), and in each histological subtypes ($p = 0.128$ in WD, $p = 0.576$ in DD; Table 6). The level of *CDK4* amplification by Q-PCR and CDK4 IHC immunoreactivity scores did not show a positive correlation in all cases ($r = 0.279$, $P = 0.07$), and also in each histological subtypes ($p = 0.581$ in WD, $p = 0.112$ in DD).

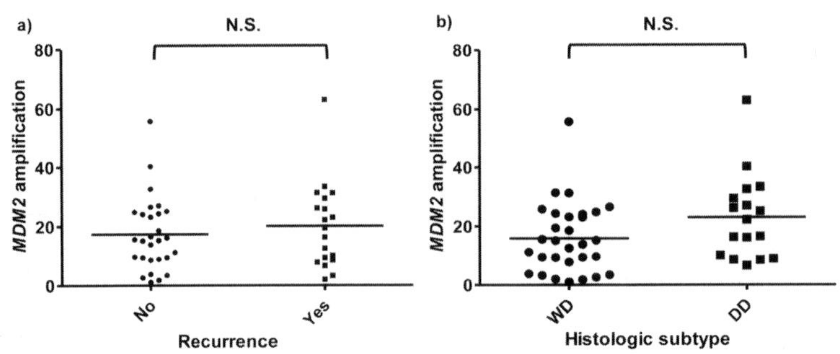

Figure 4. Quantitative real-time PCR results of *MDM2* amplification according to a) tumor recurrence, and b) histologic subtype: *MDM2* amplification levels were not different according to tumor recurrence or histologic subtype.

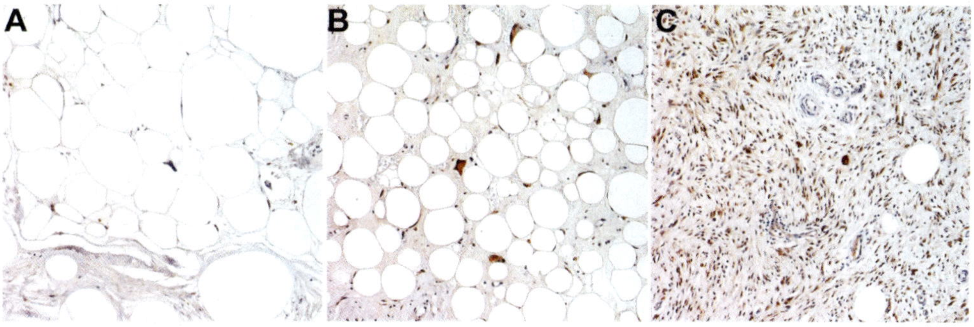

Figure 5. CDK4 immunohistochemistry staining. A. CDK4(−) well-differentiated liposarcoma, **B.** CDK4(+) well-differentiated liposarcoma, **C.** CDK4(+) dedifferentiated liposarcoma.

Predictors of Recurrence-Free Survival of Liposarcoma

Predictors of recurrence-free survival of WD liposarcoma are shown in Table 7. High level of *CDK4* amplification (cases with *CDK4* amplification higher than the median 7.54) was associated with poor recurrence-free survival compared to low *CDK4* amplification in both univariate ($P = 0.012$) and multivariate analyses ($P = 0.020$). Disease-specific survival and recurrence-free survival curves of WD liposarcoma patients are shown in Figure 6. Cases with *CDK4* amplification levels greater than 7.54 (*CDK4* high) had significantly inferior recurrence-free survival compared to cases with *CDK4* amplification less than 7.54 (*CDK4* low). None of the analyzed variables were found to significantly affect survival of DD liposarcoma patients.

Discussion

Amplification of chromosome 12q13-15 is a typical feature of WD and DD liposarcomas [11,12]. The two main genes in the amplified segment of chromosome 12, *MDM2* and *CDK4*, belong to distinct amplicons and no consistency exists in the amplified sequences between MDM2 and CDK4. It has been well documented that these two genes are involved in the oncogenesis and progression of WD and DD liposarcomas [13,14]. While *MDM2* amplification and overexpression is present in most WD and DD liposarcomas, *CDK4* amplification is absent in a small proportion of cases [6,15,16]. WD and DD liposarcomas with no *CDK4* amplification represent a distinct clinical subgroup with a lower recurrence rate and are more likely to be peripherally located [6]. A limitation of the previously cited study by Italiano *et al.* was the fact that the better prognosis observed in liposarcomas without *CDK4* amplification may have been confounded by these tumors more often being located in the extremities. Liposarcomas of the extremities are more likely to be resected with sufficient free surgical margin compared to those in the retroperitoneum. The liposarcomas included in the current study were limited to tumors arising in the retroperitoneum and peritoneal cavity. Q-PCR of the tumor specimens revealed varying levels of *MDM2* and *CDK4* amplification, with 44 cases (91.7%) and 46 cases (95.8%) showing positive amplification of *CDK4* and *MDM2* genes, respectively. Moreover, WD liposarcomas with recurrence after surgical resection had significantly higher levels of *CDK4* amplification compared to those without recurrence and the degree of *CDK4* amplification was an independent risk factor for recurrence of WD liposarcoma after complete excision. To the best of our knowledge, this study is the first to describe the correlation between *CDK4* amplification and WD liposarcoma recurrence in a quantitative manner. In accordance with the study by Italiano *et al.*, four cases in our series that were negative for CDK4 amplification are free of disease recurrence at median 25 months (range 16~39 months) after surgical resection.

In vitro data on the contribution of *CDK4* to DD liposarcoma progression was presented in a study by Barretina *et al.*, in which shRNA was used to knockdown *CDK4* in two DD liposarcoma cell lines. Sustained knockdown of *CDK4* led to inhibition of proliferation of the cell lines. In addition, pharmacological inhibition of *CDK4* with a selective *CDK4* inhibitor (PD0332991) induced G1 arrest in the same two cell lines [13]. The results of a phase II trial of this drug recently presented show promising prospects for CDK4 inhibition in patients with progressed WD and DD liposarcoma [17]. The results of the current study showed a higher rate of recurrence with increasing levels of amplification of the *CDK4* gene. Our study adds further

Table 6. CDK4 Immunohistochemistry Results According to Tumor Recurrence.

	Overall		WD liposarcoma		DD liposarcoma	
	N = 48	p-value	N = 31	p-value	N = 17	p-value
CDK4 IHC immunopositivity, n (%)						
Recurred	15 (75.0)	0.363	9 (81.8)	0.128	6 (66.7)	0.576
Non-recurred	17 (60.7)		10 (50.0)		7 (87.5)	
CDK4 IHC score, mean ± SD						
Recurred	1.88±2.49	0.745	1.18±2.13	0.758	3.38±2.67	0.251
Non-recurred	1.67±1.41		1.40±1.00		2.00±1.85	

WD, well-differentiated; DD, dedifferentiated; IHC immunohistochemistry.

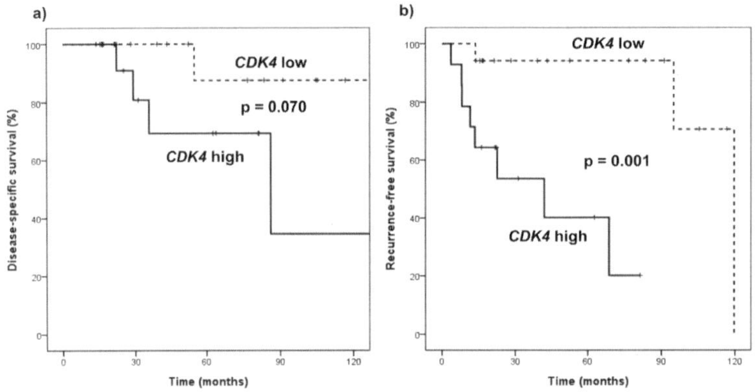

Figure 6. Disease-specific survival, a), and recurrence-free survival of patients, b), with well-differentiated liposarcoma stratified by level of *CDK4* amplification. Low *CDK4* amplification group (*CDK4*≤7.54) showed significantly better recurrence-free survival compared to high *CDK4* amplification group (*CDK4*>7.54).

rationale to the current body of evidence that the use of *CDK4* inhibitors in DD liposarcoma may prove to be beneficial.

Immunohistochemical analysis of CDK4 has been shown to be helpful in the differential diagnosis of liposarcomas and benign lipomatous tumors [9,18]. In this study, tumors showed positive CDK4 IHC staining in 66.7% of cases. Previous studies have reported positive immunoreactivity for CDK4 on IHC in approximately 68~70% of liposarcomas [9,10]. However, IHC results were not associated with histologic subtype of liposarcomas and no significant correlation was seen between CDK4 IHC findings and *CDK4* amplification by Q-PCR. These results suggest that translational or post-translational events function in fine tuning the final outcome of amplication and protein expression can be induced by other mechanism rather than amplication. Discrepancies between CDK4 IHC and Q-PCR findings were also observed in a study by Sirvent *et al.*, in which negative staining by IHC for CDK4 was observed despite the presence of amplification by Q-PCR in approximately 40% of cases of WD and DD liposarcomas [10]. MDM2 IHC analyses were not carried out because we have seen from past reports that *MDM2* was almost ubiquitously overexpressed in WD and DD liposarcomas and therefore did not affect tumor biology [13,18]. Our *MDM2* Q-PCR analysis results also showed *MDM2* amplification in 46 out of 48 cases in our liposarcoma specimens.

Our group previously analyzed 94 cases of liposarcomas in both the trunk and the extremities and concluded that high grade histologic subtype and positive margin status (microscopic and macroscopic) were independent risk factors for poor survival [19]. In the present study, we have seen consistent results with DD liposarcoma patients showing significantly worse survival compared to WD liposarcoma patients. However, we failed to observe a significant association between surgical margin status and patient outcome. The reason for this may be related to the fact that we have restricted the study population to patients who had achieved complete surgical resection without macroscopically residual tumor, and also the resultant small number of patients analyzed. Previous studies focusing on liposarcomas of the abdomen, particularly the retroperitoneum, emphasized the importance of complete tumor removal during the initial operation [20,21]. Grossly positive surgical margin was associated with poor disease-specific survival compared to negative surgical margin, while microscopically positive surgical margins did not negatively affect disease-specific survival [21].

In conclusion, the level of *CDK4* amplification determined by Q-PCR was associated with the recurrence of WD liposarcomas of the retroperitoneum and peritoneal cavity. Well-differentiated liposarcomas with higher level of amplification of *CDK4* (≥7.54) were more likely to recur after surgical resection. Utilization of Q-PCR for analysis of *CDK4* amplification may aid clinicians in the

Table 7. Predictors of Recurrence-free Survival for Well-differentiated Liposarcoma in Univariate and Multivariate Analyses.

	Univariate analysis		Multivariate analysis		
	HR	**p-value**	**HR**	**95% CI**	**p-value**
Older age	1.044	0.122	-	-	-
Tumor size	1.000	0.996	-	-	-
Combined organ resection	1.112	0.872	-	-	-
Adjacent organ involvement	2.912	0.076	-	-	-
Positive resection margin	0.363	0.182	1.491	0.178 ~ 12.515	0.713
Adjuvant radiotherapy	2.356	0.417	1.681	0.346 ~ 8.168	0.520
High *MDM2* amplification	22.397	0.638	-	-	-
High *CDK4* amplification	14.608	0.012	12.076	1.476 ~ 98.833	0.020

HR, hazard ratio; CI, confidence interval.

postoperative surveillance and management of patients with abdominal WD and DD liposarcomas.

Author Contributions

Conceived and designed the experiments: SL YLC SJK. Performed the experiments: SEL SYH. Analyzed the data: HP KYP JMK. Contributed reagents/materials/analysis tools: JBP CHDK JWJ. Wrote the paper: SL.

References

1. Dei Tos AP (2000) Liposarcoma: new entities and evolving concepts. Ann Diagn Pathol 4: 252–266.
2. Lewis JJ, Leung D, Woodruff JM, Brennan MF (1998) Retroperitoneal soft-tissue sarcoma: analysis of 500 patients treated and followed at a single institution. Ann Surg 228: 355–365.
3. Evans HL, Soule EH, Winkelmann RK (1979) Atypical lipoma, atypical intramuscular lipoma, and well differentiated retroperitoneal liposarcoma: a reappraisal of 30 cases formerly classified as well differentiated liposarcoma. Cancer 43: 574–584.
4. Hoffman A, Lazar AJ, Pollock RE, Lev D (2011) New frontiers in the treatment of liposarcoma, a therapeutically resistant malignant cohort. Drug Resist Updat 14: 52–66.
5. Pedeutour F, Suijkerbuijk RF, Forus A, Van Gaal J, Van de Klundert W, et al. (1994) Complex composition and co-amplification of SAS and MDM2 in ring and giant rod marker chromosomes in well-differentiated liposarcoma. Genes Chromosomes Cancer 10: 85–94.
6. Italiano A, Bianchini L, Gjernes E, Keslair F, Ranchere-Vince D, et al. (2009) Clinical and biological significance of CDK4 amplification in well-differentiated and dedifferentiated liposarcomas. Clin Cancer Res 15: 5696–5703.
7. Malumbres M, Barbacid M (2009) Cell cycle, CDKs and cancer: a changing paradigm. Nat Rev Cancer 9: 153–166.
8. Binh MB, Garau XS, Guillou L, Aurias A, Coindre JM (2006) Reproducibility of MDM2 and CDK4 staining in soft tissue tumors. Am J Clin Pathol 125: 693–697.
9. Aleixo PB, Hartmann AA, Menezes IC, Meurer RT, Oliveira AM (2009) Can MDM2 and CDK4 make the diagnosis of well differentiated/dedifferentiated liposarcoma? An immunohistochemical study on 129 soft tissue tumours. J Clin Pathol 62: 1127–1135.
10. Sirvent N, Coindre JM, Maire G, Hostein I, Keslair F, et al. (2007) Detection of MDM2-CDK4 amplification by fluorescence in situ hybridization in 200 paraffin-embedded tumor samples: utility in diagnosing adipocytic lesions and comparison with immunohistochemistry and real-time PCR. Am J Surg Pathol 31: 1476–1489.
11. Fletcher CD, Akerman M, Dal Cin P, de Wever I, Mandahl N, et al. (1996) Correlation between clinicopathological features and karyotype in lipomatous tumors. A report of 178 cases from the Chromosomes and Morphology (CHAMP) Collaborative Study Group. Am J Pathol 148: 623–630.
12. Meis-Kindblom JM, Sjogren H, Kindblom LG, Peydro-Mellquist A, Roijer E, et al. (2001) Cytogenetic and molecular genetic analyses of liposarcoma and its soft tissue simulators: recognition of new variants and differential diagnosis. Virchows Arch 439: 141–151.
13. Barretina J, Taylor BS, Banerji S, Ramos AH, Lagos-Quintana M, et al. (2010) Subtype-specific genomic alterations define new targets for soft-tissue sarcoma therapy. Nat Genet 42: 715–721.
14. Oliner JD, Kinzler KW, Meltzer PS, George DL, Vogelstein B (1992) Amplification of a gene encoding a p53-associated protein in human sarcomas. Nature 358: 80–83.
15. Italiano A, Bianchini L, Keslair F, Bonnafous S, Cardot-Leccia N, et al. (2008) HMGA2 is the partner of MDM2 in well-differentiated and dedifferentiated liposarcomas whereas CDK4 belongs to a distinct inconsistent amplicon. Int J Cancer 122: 2233–2241.
16. Louis-Brennetot C, Coindre JM, Ferreira C, Perot G, Terrier P, et al. (2011) The CDKN2A/CDKN2B/CDK4/CCND1 pathway is pivotal in well-differentiated and dedifferentiated liposarcoma oncogenesis: an analysis of 104 tumors. Genes Chromosomes Cancer 50: 896–907.
17. Dickson MA, Keohan ML, Tap WD, Antonescu C, Landa J, et al. (2012) Phase II trial of the CDK4 inhibitor PD0332991 in CDK4-amplified liposarcoma. J Clin Oncol 30 (Suppl): abstr 10002.
18. Pilotti S, Della Torre G, Mezzelani A, Tamborini E, Azzarelli A, et al. (2000) The expression of MDM2/CDK4 gene product in the differential diagnosis of well differentiated liposarcoma and large deep-seated lipoma. Br J Cancer 82: 1271–1275.
19. Kim HS, Lee J, Yi SY, Jun HJ, Choi YL, et al. (2009) Liposarcoma: exploration of clinical prognostic factors for risk based stratification of therapy. BMC Cancer 9: 205.
20. Neuhaus SJ, Barry P, Clark MA, Hayes AJ, Fisher C, et al. (2005) Surgical management of primary and recurrent retroperitoneal liposarcoma. Br J Surg 92: 246–252.
21. Singer S, Antonescu CR, Riedel E, Brennan MF (2003) Histologic subtype and margin of resection predict pattern of recurrence and survival for retroperitoneal liposarcoma. Ann Surg 238: 358–370; discussion 370–351.

8

Lymphangiogenesis and Angiogenesis in Abdominal Aortic Aneurysm

Masaki Sano[1,7], Takeshi Sasaki[2], Satoshi Hirakawa[3], Junichi Sakabe[3], Mikako Ogawa[4], Satoshi Baba[5], Nobuhiro Zaima[6,8], Hiroki Tanaka[1,7], Kazunori Inuzuka[1,7], Naoto Yamamoto[1,7], Mitsutoshi Setou[6], Kohji Sato[2], Hiroyuki Konno[7], Naoki Unno[1,7]*

1 Division of Vascular Surgery, Applied Medical Photonics Laboratory, Medical Photonics Research Center, Hamamatsu City, Shizuoka, Japan, **2** Department of Anatomy and Neuroscience, Applied Medical Photonics Laboratory, Medical Photonics Research Center, Hamamatsu City, Shizuoka, Japan, **3** Department of Dermatology, Applied Medical Photonics Laboratory, Medical Photonics Research Center, Hamamatsu City, Shizuoka, Japan, **4** Department of Molecular Imaging, Applied Medical Photonics Laboratory, Medical Photonics Research Center, Hamamatsu City, Shizuoka, Japan, **5** Department of Diagnostic Pathology, Hamamatsu University School of Medicine, Hamamatsu, Shizuoka, Japan, **6** Department of Cell Biology and Anatomy, Hamamatsu University School of Medicine, Hamamatsu, Shizuoka, Japan, **7** Second Department of Surgery, Hamamatsu University School of Medicine, Hamamatsu, Shizuoka, Japan, **8** Department of Applied Biological Chemistry, Kinki University, Osaka, Japan

Abstract

The pathogenesis of abdominal aortic aneurysm (AAA) is characterized to be inflammation-associated degeneration of vascular wall. Neovascularization is regularly found in human AAA and considered to play critical roles in the development and rupture of AAA. However, little is known about lymphangiogenesis in AAA. The purpose of this study was to demonstrate both angiogenesis and lymphangiogenesis in AAA. Abdominal aortic tissue was harvested either from autopsy (control group) and during open-repair surgery for AAA (AAA group). Adventitial lymphatic vasa vasorum was observed in both groups, but seemed to be no significant morphological changes in AAA. Immunohistochemical studies identified infiltration of lymphatic vessel endothelial hyaluronan receptor (LYVE) −1, vascular endothelial growth factor (VEGF)-C, and matrix metalloproteinase (MMP)-9-positive macrophages and podoplanin and Prox-1-positive microvessels in the intima/media in AAA wall, where hypoxia-inducible factors (HIF)-1α was expressed. VEGF-C and MMP-9 were not expressed in macrophages infiltrating in the adventitia. Intraoperative indocyanine green fluorescence lymphography revealed lymph stasis in intima/medial in AAA. Fluorescence microscopy of the collected samples also confirmed the accumulation of lymph in the intima/media but not in adventitia. These results demonstrate that infiltration of macrophages in intima/media is associated with lymphangiogenesis and angiogenesis in AAA. Lymph-drainage appeared to be insufficient in the AAA wall.

Editor: Utpal Sen, University of Louisville, United States of America

Funding: This work was supported partly by a Grant-in-Aid for Scientific Research (C) (22591400) (to N.U.) from Japan Society for the Promotion of Science (JSPS) for purchasing reagents or analysis tools. No additional external funding was received for this study. The funder had no role in study design, data collection and analysis, decision to publish, or preparation of the manuscript.

Competing Interests: The authors have declared that no competing interests exist.

* E-mail: unno@hama-med.ac.jp

Introduction

Abdominal aortic aneurysm (AAA) is a common disease among elderly people. AAA affects 5–10% of men over 65 years and is the tenth leading cause of death in men over the age of 55 years in the United States [1]. When surgical treatment is inapplicable, AAA progress to rupture with a high mortality (30–50%). An effective nonsurgical therapy is currently not available, because the precise mechanisms of AAA pathogenesis is yet to be identified. The degeneration of vascular wall has been considered as one of the main causes of AAA onset and rupture. Previous studies have demonstrated infiltration of inflammatory cells, such as macrophages, T cells, neutrophils and dendric cells, into the aortic wall [2,3]. These inflammatory cells are considered to contribute to the pathogenesis of AAA through the secretion of inflammatory mediators, including cytokines, chemokines, and MMPs [4]. In AAA, an intraluminal thrombus prevents luminal perfusion of oxygen, allowing only the adventitial vasa vasorum (VV) to deliver oxygen and nutroents to the aortic wall. We have recently demonstrated the arteriosclerotic degeneration of VV and tissue ischemia in AAA wall [5]. These inflammatory and hypoxic environment are potential stimuli for angiogenesis as previously reported [6]. Angiogenesis is thought to contribute to destructive processes within the AAA wall and plays a key role in aortic aneurysm development and rupture [7]. In various chronic inflammatory situations such as asthma, atopic dermatitis, rheumatoid arthritis, and inflammatory bowel diseases, both angiogenesis and lymphangiogenesis occur simultaneously to glow neovessels to remodel vascular structure [8–10]. However, little is known about lymphangiogenesis in AAA. Here, we investigated the presence of lymphanagiogenesis and major drivers of angiogenesis and lymphangiogenesis such as VEGF-A and VEGF-C in AAA wall using AAA samples which were obtained during open repair of AAA surgery.

Materials and Methods

Sample collection

All procedures used in this study and the use of samples obtained at autopsy were approved by the Ethics Committee of Clinical Research of the Hamamatsu University School of Medicine. We enrolled 20 consecutive patients who underwent elective open surgery to repair infrarenal AAAs at the Division of Vascular Surgery, Hamamatsu University School of Medicine, between May 2010 and August 2013 and obtained written informed consent for use of the sample from each patient. The aortic tissue was dissected during surgery. Longitudinal tissue strips were resected from the infrarenal aortic neck to the bifurcation.

Twenty aorta obtained at autopsy were used as controls. Written informed consent was also obtained from the donor-family for use of the sample with approval of the Ethics Committee of Clinical Research of the Hamamatsu University School of Medicine. The mid-portion of the abdominal aorta between the renal artery and the bifurcation was resected and collected from routine autopsies between October 2011 and February 2013 in the Department of Pathology, Hamamatsu University Hospital. Autopsy specimens from patients with collagen disease, aortic aneurysm/dissection, or under the age of 18 years were excluded.

Atherosclerotic risk factors (hypertension, hypercholesterolemia, hypertriglyceridemia, diabetes, and smoking) were investigated in AAA patients and autopsy cases. The definition of each item was as follows: hypertension (medication for hypertension or a systolic blood pressure $\geq$140 mmHg and/or a diastolic blood pressure $\geq$90 mmHg), hypercholesterolemia (medication for hypercholesterolemia or total cholesterol concentration in the serum of $\geq$220 mg/dL), hypertriglyceridemia (medication for hypertriglyceridemia or total triglyceride in the serum of $\geq$150 mg/dL), diabetes (present or past medication for diabetes), smoking (present or past smoking history).

Resected aortic tissues were immersed in 10% neutral buffered formalin for at least 24 h for histological and immunohistochemical staining. These samples were embedded in paraffin; 4 μm sections were cut and mounted onto MAS-coated slides (Matsunami, Osaka, Japan). The aortic tissue was frozen in liquid nitrogen, and fresh frozen tissue was stored at −80°C for quantitative real-time polymerase chain reaction analysis and near-infrared fluorescence microscopy, and immunohistochemical staining.

Histological and immunohistochemical staining

Paraffin sections were deparaffinized in xylene, rehydrated in solutions of decreasing alcohol concentration, and stained routinely with elastica van Gieson (EVG) staining. Immunohistochemical staining for podoplanin, CD31, vascular endothelial growth factor (VEGF)-A, VEGF-C, vascular endothelial growth factor receptor (VEGFR)-1, VEGFR-2, VEGFR-3, Ki-67, human hypoxia-inducible factor 1 alpha (HIF-1α), macrophages, CD3, CD19, and myeloperoxidase (MPO) were performed. The following primary antibodies were used: mouse monoclonal antibody clone D2-40 (1:200, DakoCytomation, Glostrup, Denmark) to identify podoplanin in lymphatic endothelial cells, rabbit polyclonal antibody against a synthetic peptide corresponding to the C-terminus of CD31 (1:100, AnaSpec, CA, USA) to identify vascular endothelial cells, mouse monoclonal antibody against human VEGF-A (1:50, Abcam, Tokyo, Japan), rabbit polyclonal antibody against human VEGF-C (1:50, Abcam, Tokyo, Japan), rabbit monoclonal antibody against human VEGFR-1 (1:100, Epitomics, CA, USA), rabbit polyclonal antibody against human VEGFR-2 (1:200, Abcam, Tokyo, Japan), rabbit polyclonal antibody against human VEGFR-3 (1:400, Santa Cruz Biotechnology, CA, USA), rabbit polyclonal antibody against Ki-67 (1:500, Novus Biologicals, CO, USA), mouse monoclonal antibody against human HIF-1α (1:100, Novus Biologicals, CO, USA), mouse monoclonal antibody against human macrophages (1:100, AbD Serotec, Oxford, UK), mouse monoclonal antibody against human CD3 (1:100, LifeSpan Biosciences, Seatle, WA), mouse monoclonal against human CD19 (1:50, Santa Cruz Biotechnology, CA, USA), and mouse monoclonal antibody against human myeloperoxidase (MPO) (1:50, Santa Cruz Biotechnology, CA, USA). The sections were deparaffinized, dehydrated, and boiled in a pressure cooker in 0.01 M citric acid buffer (pH 6.0) for 20 min. The sections were washed with phosphate-buffered saline and incubated with 3% H_2O_2 in absolute methanol for 5 min to inhibit any endogenous peroxidase activity. Sections were preincubated with 3% normal goat serum for 20 min to minimize nonspecific binding to the primary antibody, and incubated with the primary antibodies at 4°C overnight in a moist chamber. The sections were washed with phosphate-buffered saline and then incubated with the appropriate secondary antibody for 30 min at room temperature. Staining was visualized with Vector DAB (3,3′-diaminobenzidine, Vector Laboratories, CA, USA), and sections were then counterstained with hematoxylin.

Immunohistochemical staining was also performed on frozen sections. Aortic tissues were embedded in Tissue-Tek OCT compound (Miles Inc., Elkhart, IN, USA), frozen in liquid nitrogen, and stored at −80°C. Frozen sections of 5-μm thickness were prepared using a cryostat (Microm HM560 cryostat, Thermo Scientific, Bremen, Germany), and mounted onto MAS-coated slides (Matsunami, Osaka, Japan). The sections were fixed for 10 min with 4% paraformaldehyde phosphate buffer solution (Wako, Osaka, Japan) and washed with phosphate-buffered saline. The sections were incubated with 3% H_2O_2 in absolute methanol for 5 min to inhibit any endogenous peroxidase activity, preincubated with 3% normal goat serum for 20 min to minimize nonspecific binding to the primary antibody, and incubated with the primary antibodies at 4°C overnight in a moist chamber. The sections were washed with phosphate-buffered saline and then incubated with the appropriate secondary antibody for 30 min at room temperature. Staining was visualized with Vector DAB (3,3′-diaminobenzidine, Vector Laboratories, CA, USA), and sections were then counterstained with hematoxylin.

Double immunofluorescence staining

Colocalization studies were performed with double immunofluorescence staining methods. The following primary antibodies were used: mouse monoclonal antibody against podoplanin (1:200, DakoCytomation, Glostrup, Denmark), rabbit polyclonal antibody against Prox-1 (1:2000, Millipore, MA, USA), rabbit polyclonal antibody against the N-terminus of human alpha smooth muscle isoform of actin (1:25, Thermo Scientific Japan, Tokyo, Japan), mouse monoclonal antibody against human HIF-1α (1:100, Novus Biologicals, CO, USA), rabbit monoclonal antibody against human CD11b (1:250, Millipore, MA, USA), mouse monoclonal antibody against human macrophages (1:100, AbD Serotec, Oxford, UK), rabbit polyclonal antibody against human LYVE-1 (1:100, Relia Tech, Braunschweig, Germany), rabbit polyclonal antibody against human VEGF-C (1:50, Abcam, Tokyo, Japan), rabbit polyclonal antibody against human matrix metalloproteinase (MMP)-9 (1:100, Abnova, Taipei, Taiwan), mouse monoclonal antibody against human CD3 (1:100, LifeSpan Biosciences, Seattle, WA), mouse monoclonal antibody against human CD19 (1:50, Santa Cruz Biotechnology, CA, USA), mouse monoclonal antibody against human myeloperoxidase (MPO) (1:50, Santa

Cruz Biotechnology, CA, USA), rabbit polyclonal antibody against transforming growth factor beta-1 (TGF-β1) (1:50, Abbiotec, CA, USA), rabbit polyclonal antibody against human interleukin-4 (IL-4) (1:50, Biozol, Munich, Germany), rabbit polyclonal antibody against human interleukin-8 (IL-8) (1:50, Abnova, Taipei, Taiwan), rabbit polyclonal antibody against human macrophage inflammatory protein-1α (MIP-1α) (1:50, Spring bioscience, CA, USA), rabbit polyclonal antibody against human interferon-γ (IFN-γ) (1:50, Santa Cruz Biotechnology, CA, USA), and rabbit polyclonal antibody against human monocyte chemotactic protein-1 (MCP-1) (1:50, Abnova, Taipei, Taiwan). The sections were deparaffinized, dehydrated, and boiled in a pressure cooker in 0.01 M citric acid buffer (pH 6.0) for 20 min. The sections were washed with phosphate-buffered saline and incubated with 3% H_2O_2 in absolute methanol for 5 min to inhibit any endogenous peroxidase activity, preincubated with 3% normal chicken serum for 20 min to minimize nonspecific binding to the primary antibody, and incubated with the primary antibodies at 4°C overnight in a moist chamber. Immunoreactivity was visualized using Alexa Fluor 488-conjugated anti-mouse IgG, Alexa Fluor 594-conjugated anti-mouse IgG, Alexa Fluor 488-conjugated anti-rabbit IgG, and Alexa Fluor 594-conjugated anti-rabbit IgG (Life Technologies, CA, USA). All Alexa Fluor-conjugated secondary antibodies were diluted 200-fold for use. The slides were mounted in glycerol-based Vectashield medium containing the nucleus stain DAPI (Vector Laboratories, CA, USA).

Morphometric analysis

Immunohistochemical staining for podoplanin was performed to detect lymphatic vessels. Podoplanin was expressed in aortic intima and some podoplanin-positive cells formed microvessels. Lymphatic microvessel (LMV) density and lymphatic microvessel area in the intima were counted per microscopic field [11,12]. The 10 areas with the highest podoplanin-positive areas within the intima ('hot spots') were selected at low magnification (×40) [13]. Lymphatic microvessel density was then determined by counting all immunostained microvessels per ×200 microscopic field using a computerized image analysis system (Lumina Vision version 3.0, Mitani Corp. Tokyo, Japan). The percentage of lymphatic microvessel area, consisting of the podoplanin-positive cells plus the vessel lumen, per ×200 microscopic field (corresponding to an examination area of 0.136 mm^2) was also measured using the computerized image analysis system [11,12,14,15].

Near-infrared fluorescence lymphography and microscopy of aneurysmal walls

In AAA patients, near-infrared fluorescence lymphography of the AAA wall was performed intraoperatively. The method was performed as previously described [16].Before open surgical aneurysm repair, 0.3 mL of indocyanine green (ICG; Daiichi Pharmaceutical, Tokyo, Japan; 5 mg/mL saline solution) was subcutaneously injected into the dorsum of each foot. Laparotomy was performed, and the AAA wall was observed with Photodynamic Eye near-infrared camera system (PDE-neo, Hamamatsu Photonics, Hamamatsu, Japan) 2 h after ICG injection. Portions of AAA walls were resected and frozen in liquid nitrogen, and 10 μm frozen sections were cut. The following near-infrared fluorescence microscopy procedure was performed with the use of an upright epifluorescence microscope (Eclipse 80i, Nikon Instruments Inc., NY, USA) with a microscopic near-infrared camera system (Photometrics Evolve 512, Nippon Roper, Tokyo, Japan) to evaluate lymphatic fluid in AAA walls. Fluorescence images were obtained with the ICG fluorescence filter (ICG-B-000, excitation wavelength 769±20.5 nm, emission wavelength 832±18.5 nm, Opto-Line, Tokyo, Japan), antifade reagent (ProLong Gold antifade reagent with DAPI, Life Technologies Japan, Tokyo, Japan), and exposure time 200 μseconds. Pseudo-color images were generated using a computerized image analysis system (Lumina Vision version 3.0, Mitani Corp. Tokyo, Japan). Serial frozen sections of 5 μm thickness were prepared using a cryostat. EVG staining and immunohistochemical staining for podoplanin and macrophages were also performed.

Quantitative real-time polymerase chain reaction analysis for VEGF and VEGFR gene products

Aortic walls were frozen in liquid nitrogen and stored at −80°C. Fresh frozen aortic tissues were placed into TRIzol reagent (Life Technologies, CA, USA), and homogenized with a mechanical rotor for 1 min. Total mRNA was isolated and purified using the PureLink RNA Mini Kit (Life technologies, CA, USA) according to the protocol for using TRIzol with the PureLink RNA Mini Kit as recommended by the manufacturer. The total RNA concentration of individual sample was determined by spectrophotometer analysis (Nano-drop Technologies, DE, USA) at 260 nm. Reverse transcription was performed using TaqMan Reverse Transcription Reagents (Life Technologies Japan, Tokyo, Japan), and cDNA was prepared from 1000 μg total RNA. Real-time quantitative polymerase chain reaction (PCR) of each sample was carried out with TaqMan Gene Expression Assays and an ABI Prism 7700 Sequence Detection System (Applied Biosystems, CA, USA), based on methods described previously [17]. The Taqman assays used were VEGF-A (Hs00900055_m1), VEGF-C (Hs00153458_m1), c-fos induced growth factor (VEGF-D, Hs01128657_m1), fms-related tyrosine kinase 1 (VEGFR-1, Hs01052961_m1), kinase insert domain receptor (a type III receptor tyrosine kinase, VEGFR-2, Hs00911700_m1), and fms-related tyrosine kinase 4 (VEGF-3, Hs01047677_m1) from Applied Biosystems. Data were analyzed by comparative Ct method [18]. For each sample, the Ct value was divided by that of the housekeeping gene, actin beta (Hs01060665_g1), to generate the standardized Ct value.

Statistical analysis

Lymphatic microvessel density and the percentage of lymphatic microvessel area in the intima are expressed as means ± SE. Differences between normal aorta and AAA were analyzed by Student's t-test.

Categorical variables were reported as frequencies with percentages, and compared between control and AAA groups using Fisher's exact test to obtain P-values. All continuous data were expressed as mean value ± SE, and compared between control and AAA groups using Student's t-test. Statistical significance of differences was defined as a P-value of <0.05. All statistical analyses were performed using SPSS 17.0 for Windows (SPSS Inc., IL, USA).

Results

Patient characteristics

Twenty AAA cases (16 male, 4 female; age 68.7±1.5 y) and 20 autopsy specimens (11 male, 9 female; age 66.5±3.0 y) were included in this study (Table 1). Male sex was more common among AAA patients compared with controls, but this difference was not statistically significant. Neither age nor BMI significantly differed between the AAA and control groups. The diameter of the abdominal aorta was larger in the AAA group than in the control group. The prevalence of hypertension, hypercholesterolemia, and

Table 1. Baseline characteristics of the AAA group and control group.

Category	Aneurysm (n = 20)	Control (n = 20)	*P* value
Sex (M/F)	16/4	11/9	0.176
Age	68.7±1.5	66.5±3.0	0.528
BMI	21.8±0.7	21.2±0.7	0.619
Diameter of abdominal aorta	49.8±2.7	18.0±0.7	<0.001
Hypertension (+/−)	15 (75%)/5 (25%)	11 (55%)/9 (45%)	0.320
Hypercholesterolemia (+/−)	9 (45%)/11 (55%)	5 (25%)/15 (75%)	0.320
Hypertriglyceridemia (+/−)	7 (35%)/13 (65%)	8 (40%)/12 (60%)	1.000
Diabetes (+/−)	3 (15%)/17 (85%)	4 (20%)/16 (80%)	1.000
Smoking (+/−)	15 (75%)/5 (25%)	11 (55%)/9 (45%)	0.320

The definition of each item: hypertension (medication for hypertension or a systolic blood pressure ≥140 mmHg and/or a diastolic blood pressure ≥90 mmHg), hypercholesterolemia (medication for hypercholesterolemia or total cholesterol concentration in the serum of ≥220 mg/dL), hypertriglyceridemia (medication for hypertriglyceridemia or total triglyceride in the serum of ≥150 mg/dL), diabetes (present or past medication for diabetes), smoking (present or past smoking history).

cigarette smoking were more common in AAA group compared with the control group, but these differences were not statistically significant. The prevalence of hypertriglyceridemia, and diabetes mellitus were not statistically different between the AAA and control groups.

Lymphatic microvessels in the intima of abdominal aortic aneurysm

Elastica van Gieson (EVG) staining of AAA walls revealed intimal thickening and degradation of the wavy structure of elastin fibers in media compared with normal aorta (Fig. 1A, B). Immunohistochemical staining indicated that podoplanin was rarely expressed in the intima of normal aorta and frequently expressed in that of AAA (Fig. 1C, D). Additionally, some podoplanin-positive cells in the intima of AAA formed vessels (Fig. 1E).

Double immunofluorescence staining revealed that the nuclei of vessel-forming, podoplanin-positive cells in the intima of AAA expressed Prox-1 (Fig. 1F–I). Colocalization of podoplanin and the alpha smooth muscle isoform of actin was not detected in the intima of AAA (Fig. 1J–M).

Immunohistochemical staining indicated that podoplanin was expressed in the adventitia of normal aorta and AAA. Immunohistochemical staining of adventitial lymphatic vessels seemed indicate no morphological changes between the walls of normal aorta and AAA (Fig. 1N, O).

Lymphatic microvessel density in the intima was 243.0±59.3 (vessels/10 fields) in the control group and 938.4±85.7 (vessels/10 fields) in AAA group ($P<0.001$; Fig. 1P). The percentage of lymphatic microvessel area was 1.3±0.4% in the control group and 4.5±0.4% in the AAA group ($P<0.001$; Fig. 1Q).

Lymphangiogenesis and angiogenesis in AAA

EVG staining of AAA walls showed degradation of the wavy structure of elastin fibers in the media, where numerous microvessels were distributed from intima to media (Fig. 2A, B). Podoplanin-positive microvessels and CD31-positive microvessels were present (Fig. 2C, D). Furthermore, expressions of vascular endothelial growth factor receptor (VEGFR)-1, VEGFR-2, and VEGFR-3 increased in the microvessels (Fig. 2E–G). VEGF-A or VEGF-C- positive cells were also seen within and around the microvessels (Fig. 2H, I). The nuclei of microvessel cells demonstrated strong expression of Ki-67 (Fig. 2J). These microvessels were not seen in adventitia of AAA. Real-time quantitative PCR analysis indicated that mRNA expression of VEGF-A, VEGF-C, and VEGFR-1, VEGFR-2, and VEGFR-3 was upregulated in AAA tissue, while that of VEGF-D was not significantly different, in comparison with expression levels in normal aortic tissues (Fig. 2K).

Infiltration of inflammatory cells into AAA walls

Comparison between normal aorta and AAA walls revealed marked degradation of elastin fibers in the media (Fig. 3A, C). Immunohistochemical staining showed both nuclear and cytoplasmic expression of hypoxia-inducible factor (HIF)-1α in the intima/media of AAA walls (Fig. 3D), while HIF-1α expression was not detected in that of normal aorta (Fig. 3B). Double immunofluorescence staining demonstrated infiltration of CD11b-positive macrophages with strong nuclear/cytoplasmic expression of HIF-1α into the intima/media of AAA(Fig. 3E). Those macrophages with strong nuclear/cytoplasmic expression of HIF-1α also expressed VEGF-C and MMP-9 (Fig. 3F,G)

Using EVG and immunohistochemical staining of AAA walls, lymphatic microvessels were observed in the intima/media with degradation of elastin fibers (Fig. 4A,B). Inflammatory cells, such as macrophages, CD3-positive T lymphocytes, CD19-positive B lymphocytes, and neutrophils infiltrated in the surrounding intima/media andadventitia (Fig. 4C–F). Infiltration of these inflammatory cells was more prominent in the surrounding intima/media microvessels. Large macrophages were observed in the surrounding intima/media microvessels, while small macrophages were observed in the adventitia of AAA (Fig. 4G–M). Double immunofluorescence staining indicated that both types of macrophages (large macrophages in intima/media and small macrophages in adventitia) were positive for CD11b (Fig. 4G). However, only the large macrophages observed in the intima/media were positive for LYVE-1 (Fig. 4H). Similarly, large macrophages in the intima/media but not small macrophages in adventitia expressed VEGF-C, MMP-9, TGF-β1, IL-4, IL-8, MIP-1α, and MCP-1 (Fig. 4I, J, K, L, M, N, P). IFN-γ was not expressed either large macrophages in the intima/media or small macrophages in adventitia (Fig. 4P). CD3-positive T lymphocytes in the intima/media did not express either VEGF-C, MMP-9, IL-8, or MIP-1α, but expressed TGF-β1, IL-4, IFN-γ(Fig. 4Q).CD19-positive B lymphocytes and MPO-positive neutrophils in the intima/media did not express either VEGF-C, MMP-9, TGF-β1, IL-4, IL-8, MIP-1α, IFN-γ, and MCP-1(Fig. 4R,S).

Lymph stasis in AAA walls

During open surgical repair of infra-renal AAA, ICG fluorescence lymphography was observed intraoperatively with a near-infrared camera after exposure of the retroperitoneal space to investigate lymph stasis, and strong ICG fluorescence signals were observed in the aneurysmal wall (Fig. 5 A–C). The pattern of the fluorescence-signal distribution was heterogeneous. ICG fluorescence lymphography was performed in all 17 patients with AAA. ICG fluorescence signals were identified in the AAA wall of all patients. Fluorescence lymphography of cross-sections of the aneurysmal wall in resected samples macroscopically localized the fluorescence signals to the intima/media area of the AAA wall (Fig. 5D–F). Near-infrared fluorescence microscopy also localized ICG fluorescence in the intima/media but not in adventitia,

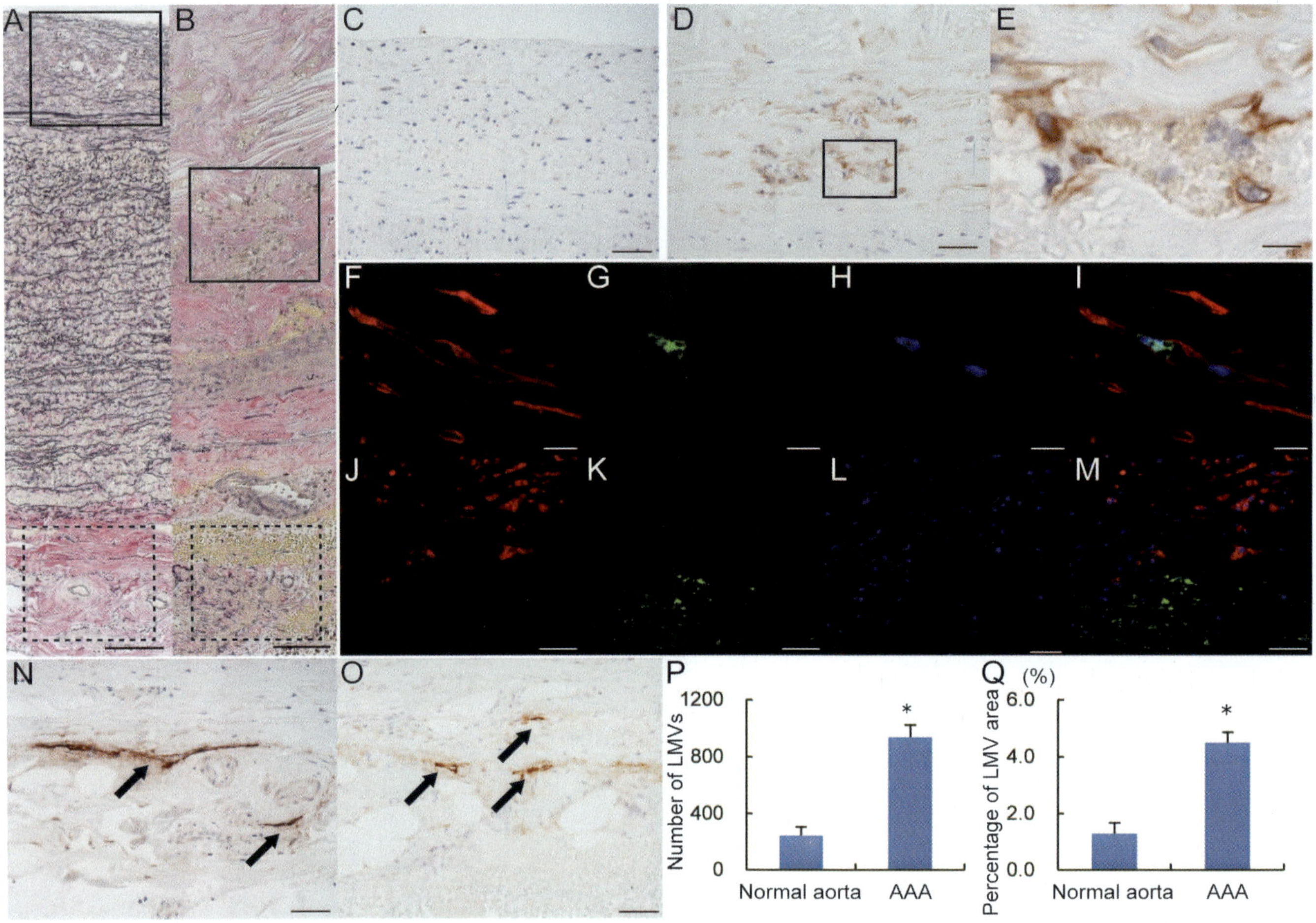

Figure 1. Lymphatic microvessels in intima of abdominal aortic aneurysm. EVG staining of normal aorta (**A**) and abdominal aortic aneurysm (AAA) wall (**B**). Immunohistochemistry for podoplanin corresponding to the areas outlined with a solid line in **A** and **B** (**C**, normal aorta; **D**, AAA). Podoplanin-positive microvessels were markedly increased in the intima in AAA wall. **E**, Higher magnification of the outlined area in **D**. Double immunofluorescence staining of lymphatic vessels in intima of AAA (**F–I**). **F**, Podoplanin (red); **G**, Prox-1 (green); **H**, DAPI (blue); **I**, merge of podoplanin, Prox-1, and DAPI. Double immunofluorescence staining of smooth muscle cells in intima of AAA (**J–M**). **J**, podoplanin (red); **K**, alpha smooth muscle isoform of actin (green), **L**, DAPI (blue); **M**, merge of podoplanin, alpha smooth muscle isoform of actin, and DAPI. Immunohistochemistry for podoplanin corresponding to the areas outlined with a dotted line in **A** and **B** (**N**; normal aorta, **O**; AAA). Lymphatic vasa vasorum was observed in adventitia in both normal aorta (**N**) and AAA (**O**) (black arrow: LVV). Scale bars indicate 100 μm (**A, B**), 50 μm (**C, D, J–M, N, O**), and 10 μm (**E–I**). Lymphatic microvessel density; the mean number of lymphatic microvessel (LMVs) in 10 microscopic fields at high magnification (×200) (**P**). Percentage of lymphatic microvessel area in 10 microscopic fields at high magnification (×200) (**Q**). Lymphatic microvessel density and percentage of lymphatic microvessel area were compared between normal aorta and AAA. (*$P<0.001$).

suggesting that lymph stasis occurred in the intima/media (Fig. 5G, H). Immunohistochemical staining revealed both extensive infiltration of macrophages and the presence of lymphatic microvessels in the intima/media of the AAA wall with lymph stasis (Fig. 5I–L).

Discussion

Lymph transportation network in aortic wall tissue is largely unknown. Recently, Drozdz et al. first reported the presence of adventitial LVV in human aorta with an immunohistological technique [19]. In the present study, we also demonstrated the presence of adventitial LVV in both autopsied normal aorta and AAA. There seemed to be no morphological differences in adventitial LVV in AAA. The LVV is an innate vascular structure for lymph transportation, although the detailed role of LVV in aortic tissue is yet to be identified. Immunohistological examination also revealed intimal/medial lymphangiogenesis in the AAA wall, particularly in the area where medial elastin was marketly degraded. While lymphatic vessels are usually absent from normal aortic intima and media, podoplanin-positive microvessels significantly increased in AAA intima/media. Podoplanin is specifically expressed by lymphatic endothelial cells but not blood vascular endothelial cells [20]. Podoplanin has also been reported in normal cells other than lymphatic endothelial cells, such as peritoneal mesothelial cells, osteocytes, glandular myoepithelial cells, ependymal cells, stromal reticular cells and follicular dendritic cells [21], and was observed in intimal smooth muscle cells in atherosclerotic aorta [22]. In the present study, podoplanin expression was seen in the intima/media of AAA, but not co-localized with smooth muscle cells. The nuclei of podoplanin-positive cells that formed vessels expressed Prox-1. Therefore, we speculated that the podoplanin-positive microvessels were lymphatic microvessels arising from lymphangiogenesis.

Lymphangiogenic factors such as VEGF-C and VEGFR-3 were also present in the areas in which podoplanin-positive microvessels were observed. CD11b-positive macrophages were observed

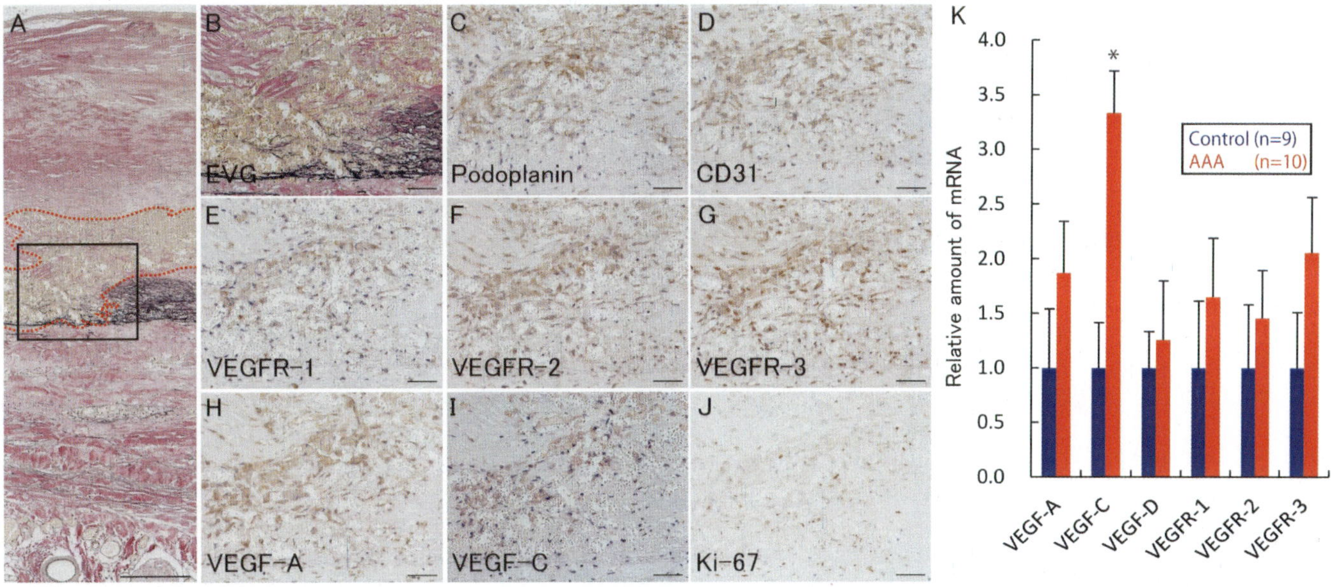

Figure 2. Lymphangiogenesis and angiogenesis in abdominal aortic aneurysm walls. A, Elastica van Gieson staining of the abdominal aortic aneurysm (AAA) wall. Microvessels in the intima/media are encircled by a red dotted-line. **B**, Higher magnification of the area outlined with a solid line in **A**. Immunohistochemistry for podoplanin (**C**), CD31 (**D**), VEGFR-1 (**E**), VEGFR-2 (**F**), VEGFR-3 (**G**), VEGF-A (**H**), VEGF-C (**I**), and Ki-67 (**J**) in the area outlined with a solid line in **A**. The microvessels encircled by the red dotted-line consisted of podoplanin-positive cells (**C**) and CD31-positive cells (**D**). These microvessels were positive for VEGFR-1, VEGFR-2, and VEGFR-3 (**E–G**). Expression of VEGF-A and C was increased within and around these microvessels (**H, I**). The nuclei of these microvessels were positive for Ki-67 (**H**). **K**, Comparison of mRNA expression of VEGF-A, VEGF-C, VEGF-D, VEGFR-1, VEGFR-2, and VEGFR-3 between normal aorta and AAA. Data were obtained from 10 AAA patients and 9 autopsied cases (controls). Data were analyzed by comparative Ct method. All of the mRNAs except VEGF-D were upregulated in AAA tissues. Standard deviation is indicated by bar errors. * indicates $p<0.05$ vs control. Scale bars indicated 200 μm (**A**), 50 μm (**B–J**).

within and around lymphatic microvessels in both intima and adventitia of AAA walls. However, LYVE-1-positive macrophages were only observed in intima, not in adventitia. Previous studies have reported that macrophages are related to lymphangiogenesis in pathological processes such as malignant tumors [23], inflammation [24–26], and transplantation [27]. Macrophages are thought to support lymphangiogenesis in two ways: by transdifferentiation into lymphatic endothelial cells [23,25–27], and by stimulating preexisting local lymphatic endothelial cells via release of lymphangiogenic factors [24,25].Although LYVE-1 is regarded to be specifically expressed by lymphatic endothelial cells [20], LYVE-1-positive macrophages have also been reported in

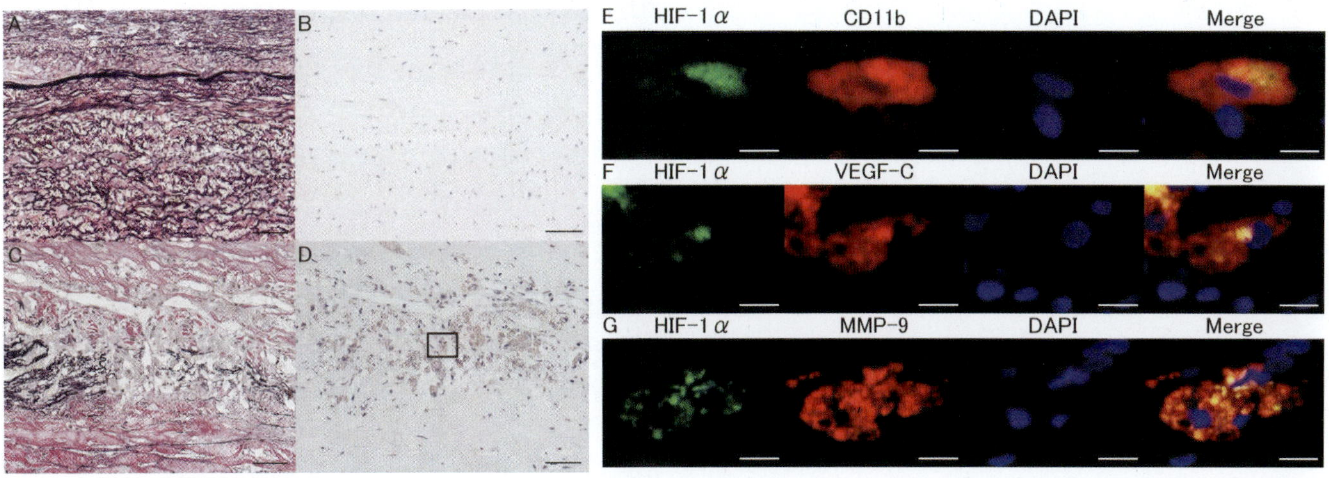

Figure 3. HIF-1 expression in normal aorta and AAA. Elastica van Gieson staining of the intima/media in normal aorta (**A**) and abdominal aortic aneurysm (AAA) wall (**C**). Immunohistochemistry for HIF-1α in normal aorta (**B**) and AAA (**D**). Nuclear and cytoplasmic expression of HIF-1α was observed in intima/media in AAA (**D**). **E**, Double immunofluorescence staining for HIF-1α (green), CD11b (red), DAPI (blue), and the merged image of the outlined in **D**. **F**, Double immunofluorescence staining for HIF-1α (green), VEGF-C(red), DAPI(blue), and the merged image of the outlined in **D**. **G**, Double immunofluorescence staining for HIF-1α(green), MMP-9 (red), DAPI (blue), and the merged image of the outlined in **D**. Expression of HIF-1α was increased in CD11b positive macrophages. VEGF-C and MMP-9 were expressed in the HIF-1α–positive macrophages. Scale bars indicated 50 μm (**A–D**) and 10 μm (**E–G**).

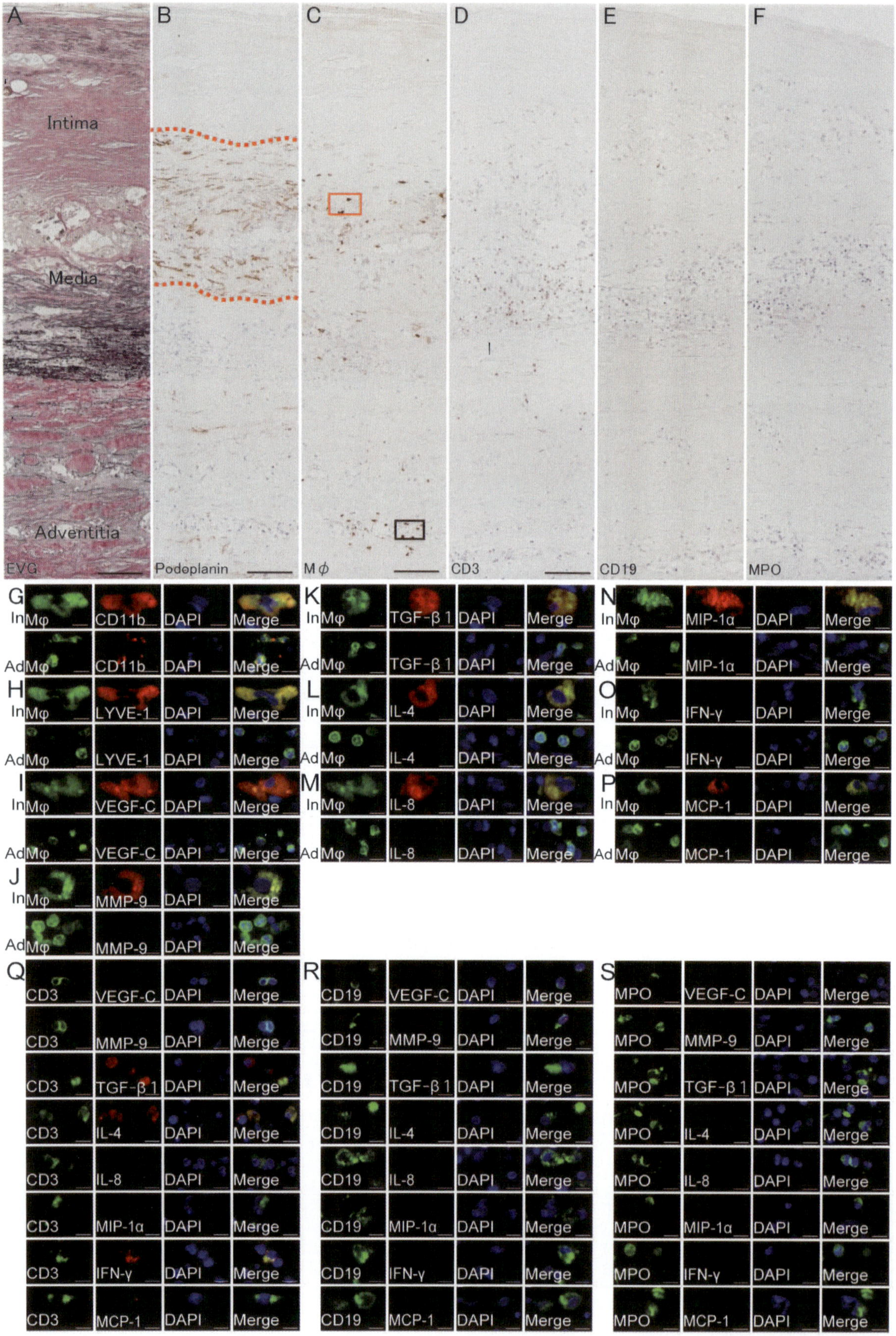
A
Intima
Media
Adventitia
EVG
B
Podoplanin
C
M φ
D
CD3
E
CD19
F
MPO
G
In Mφ CD11b DAPI Merge
Ad Mφ CD11b DAPI Merge
H
In Mφ LYVE-1 DAPI Merge
Ad Mφ LYVE-1 DAPI Merge
I
In Mφ VEGF-C DAPI Merge
Ad Mφ VEGF-C DAPI Merge
J
In Mφ MMP-9 DAPI Merge
Ad Mφ MMP-9 DAPI Merge
K
In Mφ TGF-β 1 DAPI Merge
Ad Mφ TGF-β 1 DAPI Merge
L
In Mφ IL-4 DAPI Merge
Ad Mφ IL-4 DAPI Merge
M
In Mφ IL-8 DAPI Merge
Ad Mφ IL-8 DAPI Merge
N
In Mφ MIP-1α DAPI Merge
Ad Mφ MIP-1α DAPI Merge
O
In Mφ IFN-γ DAPI Merge
Ad Mφ IFN-γ DAPI Merge
P
In Mφ MCP-1 DAPI Merge
Ad Mφ MCP-1 DAPI Merge
Q
CD3 VEGF-C DAPI Merge
CD3 MMP-9 DAPI Merge
CD3 TGF-β 1 DAPI Merge
CD3 IL-4 DAPI Merge
CD3 IL-8 DAPI Merge
CD3 MIP-1α DAPI Merge
CD3 IFN-γ DAPI Merge
CD3 MCP-1 DAPI Merge
R
CD19 VEGF-C DAPI Merge
CD19 MMP-9 DAPI Merge
CD19 TGF-β 1 DAPI Merge
CD19 IL-4 DAPI Merge
CD19 IL-8 DAPI Merge
CD19 MIP-1α DAPI Merge
CD19 IFN-γ DAPI Merge
CD19 MCP-1 DAPI Merge
S
MPO VEGF-C DAPI Merge
MPO MMP-9 DAPI Merge
MPO TGF-β 1 DAPI Merge
MPO IL-4 DAPI Merge
MPO IL-8 DAPI Merge
MPO MIP-1α DAPI Merge
MPO IFN-γ DAPI Merge
MPO MCP-1 DAPI Merge

Figure 4. Macrophage infiltration of AAA microvessels. A, Elastica van Gieson staining of abdominal aortic aneurysm (AAA). Immunohistochemistry for podoplanin (**B**) and macrophages (**C**), CD19 (**E**), and myeloperoxidase (MPO) of the AAA wall. **B**, Lymphatic microvessels in the intima/media of the AAA (red dotted line encircling lymphatic microvessels). **C**, Macrophages infiltration around/within lymphatic microvessels in the intima/media or in adventitia (red square: macrophages in intima/media, black square: macrophages in adventitia). **D**, CD3-positive T cells infiltration around/within lymphatic microvessels in the intima/media or in adventitia. **E**, CD19-positive B cells infiltration around/within lymphatic microvessels in the intima/media or in adventitia. **F**, MPO-positive neutrophils infiltration in the intima/media or in adventitia. **G–P**, Double immunofluorescence staining of macrophages infiltrating the intima/media (In) and adventitia (Ad). **G–P**, Macrophage: green, CD11b (**G**)/LYVE-1 (**H**)/ VEGF-C (**I**)/MMP-9 (**J**)/TGF-β1 (**K**)/IL-4 (**L**)/IL-8 (**M**)/MIP-1α (**N**)/IFN-γ (**O**)/MCP-1 (**P**): red, DAPI: blue. LYVE-1, VEGF-C, MMP-9, TGF-β1, IL-4, IL-8, MIP-1α, and MCP-1 were expressed in the CD11b-positive macrophages in the intima/media, but not by macrophages in adventitia. **Q**, Double immunofluorescence staining of T-cells in intima/media and inflammatory cytokines. CD3: green, VEGF-C/MMP-9/TGF-β1/IL-4/IL-8/MIP-1α/IFN-γ/MCP-1: red, DAPI: blue. TGF-β1, IL-4, and IFN-γ were expressed in CD3-positive T lymphocytes in the intima/media. **R**, Double immunofluorescence staining of B lymphocytes in the intima/media and inflammatory cytokines. CD19: green, VEGF-C/MMP-9/TGF-β1/IL-4/IL-8/MIP-1α/IFN-γ/MCP-1: red, DAPI: blue. These inflammatory cytokines were not expressed in CD19-positive B lymphocytes. **S**, Double immunofluorescence staining of neutrophils in intima/media and inflammatory cytokines. MPO: green, VEGF-C/MMP-9/TGF-β1/IL-4/IL-8/MIP-1α/IFN-γ/MCP-1: red, DAPI: blue. These inflammatory cytokines were not expressed in MPO-positive neutrophils. Scale bars indicated 100 μm (**A–F**) and 10 μm (**G–S**).

inflammatory tissue and malignant tumors [23,26,27]. Maruyama et al. recently reported that CD11b positive macrophages expressed LYVE-1 under inflammatory conditions in the cornea of mice. These macrophages aggregated and formed vessel-like structures, that expressed lymphatic endothelial cell markers, such as LYVE-1, Prox-1, and podoplanin [26]. CD11b and LYVE-1-positive macrophages may transdifferentiate into lymphatic endothelial cells. These macrophages could be derived from the circulation and transmigrate through the connective tissues, contributing to de novo lymphangiogenesis [25–27].

In the present study, overexpression of HIF-1α was observed in the intima/media of AAA, and large macrophages infiltrated hypoxic areas in the region. As we mentioned previously, the infrarenal aortic wall is susceptible to hypoxia. The presence of intraluminal thrombus (ILT) may prevent luminal perfusion of oxygen, allowing only the adventitial VV to deliver oxygen and nutrients to the aortic wall. Moreover, we recently reported that adventitial VV becomes stenotic due to the intimal hyperplasia, which causes malperfusion of the AAA wall and tissue hypoxia [5]. Notably, the tissue in the intima/media of AAA with thick ILT is farthest from both luminal perfusion and VV perfusion, so those layers are particularly prone to hypoxia. Vorp et al. also reported that thicker ILT was associated with localized tissue hypoxia, neovascularization, and inflammation in the AAA wall [28]. We therefore speculate that LYVE-1-positive macrophages may be induced by hypoxia in aortic intima/media and may transdifferentiate into lymphatic endothelial cells following lymphangiogenesis.

Macrophages can also promote lymphangiogenesis by producing lymphangiogenic factors, thereby stimulating the preexistent lymphatic endothelial cells in inflammatory tissue or in malignant tumors [23,24]. The development of lymphatic vessels is regulated either by lymphangiogenesis-specific or angiogenesis-nonspecific factors in malignant tumors [24,29]. Macrophage infiltration stimulates lymphatic endothelial cells by releasing VEGF-C. VEGF-C/VEGFR-3 signaling plays a critical role in the growth and survival of lymphatic endothelial cells in inflammation or in malignant tumors [25,29]. In the present study, lymphatic microvessels were observed in the intima/media of AAA walls, where mRNA expressions of both VEGF-C and VEGFR-3 were more prominent. Expression of VEGF-C was also increased in HIF-1α positive macrophages infiltrating the intima/media but not in adventitial macrophages. Furthermore, the expression of VEGFR-3 was increased in areas of neovascularization in the intima/media of AAA walls. Taken together, these results suggested that hypoxia-induced infiltration of macrophages in intima/media may release VEGF-C, stimulating the lymphatic endothelial cells and thus contributing to lymphangiogenesis.

In this study, VEGF-A positive cells were also observed within and around the microvessels in both intima and media of AAA walls. The mRNA expression of VEGF-A and VEGFR-1 was more prominent than that in normal aorta. Kaneko et al. also reported VEGF-A overexpression in the macrophages infiltrating AAA walls [30]. Because VEGF-A is not only a potent angiogenic factor but also promotes lymphangiogenesis [24,29], the VEGF-A/VEGFR-1 signaling pathway may also play an important role in both angiogenesis and lymphangiogenesis in the AAA wall.

Infiltration of inflammatory cells such as macrophages, T and B lymphocytes, and neutrophils, have been identified in AAA specimens [31]. In atherosclerotic lesions, monocyte-derived macrophages and T lymphocytes were observed most often [32,33]. During each phase of atherogenesis, the inflammatory response is mediated by monocyte-derived macrophages and specific subtypes of T lymphocytes [34]. With regard to macrophages, Stoger et al. reported that, atherosclerotic lesions contain foamy large macrophages expressing M1 markers in the intimal plaque, while adventitial small macrophages express M2 signature karkers [35]. Similarly, in AAA specimens, both macrophages and several subtypes of T lymphocytes also have been identified [31]. In this study, the infiltration of large macrophages and T lymphocytes was confirmed in the intima/media, while small macrophages and T lymphocytes were observed in the adventitia of AAA. Only large macrophages in the intima/media of AAA expressed VEGF-C and MMP-9. Large macrophages may be associated with hypoxia in the intima/media, contributing to lymphangiogenesis and the progression of AAA. On the other hand, T lymphocytes and adventitial small macrophages did not express either VEGF-C or MMP-9, suggesting that T lymphocytes might not play a major role in involved in lymphangiogenesis in AAA walls. Infiltration of T and B lymphocytes and neutrophils was markedly observed around lymphatic microvessels, suggesting that formation of lymphatic microvessels may introduce these inflammatory cells into the intima/media. Macrophages in the intima/media expressed not only VEGF-C and MMP-9 but also TGF-β1, IL-4, IL-8, and MIP-1α. These cytokines are known to cause further recruitment of macrophages and neutrophils, potentiating inflammation [31,36]. On the other hand, T lymphocytes expressed TGF-β1, IL-4, and IFN-γ but not VEGF-C and MMP-9, which suggested that T lymphocytes might accelerate macrophage recruitment in the region, but not directly contribute to the lymphangiogenesis [37,38]. Inflammatory cytokines such as TGF-β1, IL-4, IL-8, and IFN-γ were reported to promote lymphangiogenesis in various diseases [39] [40] [41] [42]. Therefore, cytokines such as TGF-β1, IL-4, IL-8, and IFN-γ may also contribute to lymphangiogenesis in AAA. With regard to B lymphocytes in the intima/media, neither VEGF-C, MMP-9, TGF-β1, IL-4, IL-8, MIP-1α, IFN-γ,

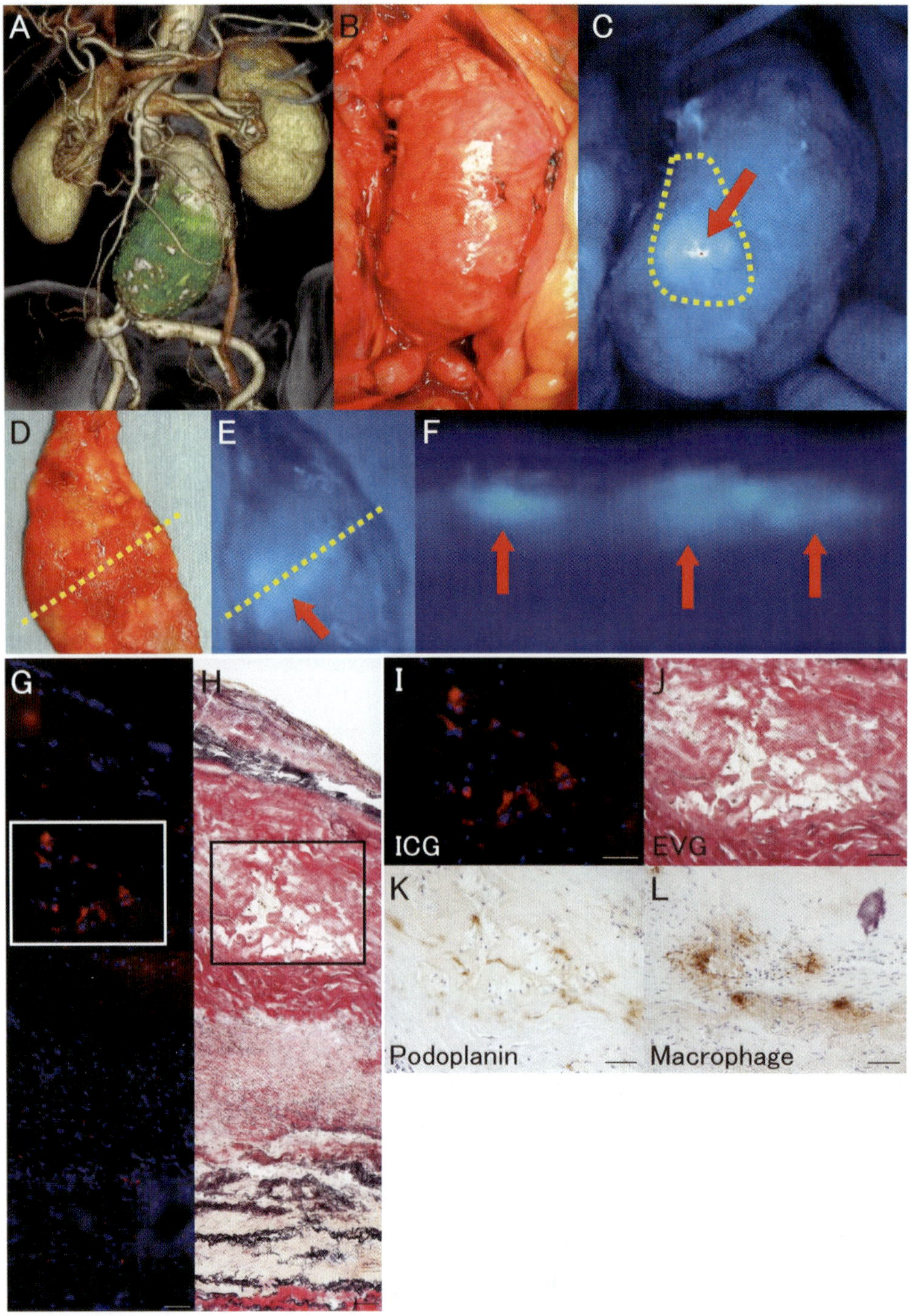

Figure 5. Fluorescence lymphography and microscopy of abdominal aortic aneurysm. A, Three dimensional CT image of an infrarenal abdominal aortic aneurysm (AAA). **B**, Intraoperative photography of an infrarenal AAA. **C**, Intraoperative near-infrared fluorescence lymphography of indocyanine green (ICG) (red arrow: ICG fluorescence, yellow dotted-line: sample resection line). **D**, Macroscopic findings of the resected sample observed from the luminal side (yellow dotted line: cross-section line of the harvested sample). **E**, Near-infrared fluorescence lymphography of ICG in the resected aneurysmal wall observed from the luminal side (red arrow: ICG fluorescence, yellow dotted line: cross-section line of the harvested sample). **F**, Near-infrared fluorescence lymphography of ICG in the cross-sectioned AAA wall (red arrow: ICG fluorescence, up: luminal side, bottom: adventitial side). **G**, Fluorescence microscopy of ICG in the AAA wall (ICG: red, DAPI: blue). **H**, Serial frozen section with Elastica van Gieson staining. **I**, Higher magnification of the outlined area in **G**. **J**, Higher magnification of the outlined area in **H**. **K**, Immunohistochemistry for podoplanin in the outlined area in **G** and **H**. **L**, Immunohistochemistry to label macrophages in the outlined area in **G** and **H**. Scale bars indicate 50 μm (**G–L**).

nor MCP-1 were expressed, which suggested that B cells may not play a major role in lymphangiogensis in AAA walls. Neutrophils did not express either VEGF-C and MMP-9, suggesting that neutrophils may contribute to macrophage recruitment rather than lymphangiogensis itself.

We investigated lymph stasis in AAA patients using ICG fluorescence lymphography. ICG fluorescence lymphography is an emerging technique to enable intraoperative observation of lymphatic flow [43,44]. In the present study, ICG fluorescence dye, which was subcutaneously injected bilaterally into the dorsum of the foot, stagnated in the AAA wall. Intraoperative ICG lymphography using a near-infrared camera visualized marked fluorescence signals in the AAA wall after exposure of the retroperitoneal space. Freshly harvested samples of the cross-sectioned AAA walls also demonstrated fluorescence signals in the intima/media, which was later confirmed using ICG fluorescence microscopy. These results suggest that lymph stasis occurred in the intima/media of AAA wall. This suggested that neovascularized lymph vessels were a less efficient lymph-transport pathway, causing lymph stasis in the intima/media of AAA wall. In the harvested samples, the lymphedematous regions in the AAA wall also demonstrated marked infiltration of macrophages. Previous studies have associated chronic lymph stasis with tissue inflammation [45]. Recently, Zampell et al. reported that lymph stasis causes infiltration of mononuclear cells and tissue fibrosis in a lymphatic fluid stasis model using rat tails [46,47]. Therefore, AAA wall lymphatic dysfunction causes lymph fluid stasis, which may contribute to the medial inflammation in the AAA wall [47]. Hypoxia-induced lymphangiogenesis could also be enhanced by lymph stasis [48]. However, the role of lymphangiogenesis in the AAA wall is unknown. Angiogenesis is thought to contribute to destructive processes within the AAA wall and plays a key role in aortic aneurysm development and rupture [7]. Therefore, various anti-angiogenic agents have been studied in animal models for potential treatment of AAA [30,49,50]. Maruyama et al. reported that down-regulation of VEGFR-3 and subsequent inhibition of lymphangiogenesis delayed diabetic wound healing in a mouse model [51]. Moreover, Zhou et al. reported that administration of VEGF-C and increased lymphangiogenesis improved lymph drainage and inhibited inflammation in a rat model of chronic arthritis [52]. Thus, inflammation has been widely accepted to stimulates lymphangiogenesis as a compensatory mechanism to enhance the clearance of inflammatory products. Therefore, lymphanagiogenesis in the AAA wall may be a rational response against loss of adventitial LVV and lymph stasis. However, as we demonstrated in the present study using ICG fluorescence lymphography, the newly formed lymphatic vessels may not fully function to drain lymph. Then, the insufficient lymph drainage may provoke further inflammation.

In conclusion, macrophage infiltration may be associated with lymphangiogenesis and angiogenesis in the intima/media. Lymph-drainage appeared to be insufficient in the AAA wall, which may become a new therapeutic target for non-surgical treatment of AAA by improving lymph flow.

Acknowledgments

We thank the staff of the Second Department of Surgery of the Hamamatsu University School of Medicine.

Author Contributions

Conceived and designed the experiments: NU M. Sano TS SH MO. Performed the experiments: M. Sano TS SH JS NZ HT. Analyzed the data: M. Setou KS HK NU. Contributed reagents/materials/analysis tools: SH JS SB KI NY. Wrote the paper: M. Sano NU. Patients recruit and registration: KI NY.

References

1. Baxter BT, Terrin MC, Dalman RL (2008) Medical management of small abdominal aortic aneurysms. Circulation 117: 1883–1889.
2. Kajimoto K, Miyauchi K, Kasai T, Shimada K, Kojima Y, et al. (2009) Short-term 20-mg atorvastatin therapy reduces key inflammatory factors including c-Jun N-terminal kinase and dendritic cells and matrix metalloproteinase expression in human abdominal aortic aneurysmal wall. Atherosclerosis 206: 505–511.
3. Lindeman JH, Abdul-Hussien H, van Bockel JH, Wolterbeek R, Kleemann R (2009) Clinical trial of doxycycline for matrix metalloproteinase-9 inhibition in patients with an abdominal aneurysm: doxycycline selectively depletes aortic wall neutrophils and cytotoxic T cells. Circulation 119: 2209–2216.
4. Bruemmer D, Collins AR, Noh G, Wang W, Territo M, et al. (2003) Angiotensin II-accelerated atherosclerosis and aneurysm formation is attenuated in osteopontin-deficient mice. J Clin Invest 112: 1318–1331.
5. Tanaka H, Zaima N, Sasaki T, Hayasaka T, Goto-Inoue N, et al. (2013) Adventitial vasa vasorum arteriosclerosis in abdominal aortic aneurysm. PLoS One 8: e57398.
6. Holmes DR, Liao S, Parks WC, Thompson RW (1995) Medial neovascularization in abdominal aortic aneurysms: a histopathologic marker of aneurysmal degeneration with pathophysiologic implications. J Vasc Surg 21: 761–771; discussion 771–762.
7. Swedenborg J, Mayranpaa MI, Kovanen PT (2011) Mast cells: important players in the orchestrated pathogenesis of abdominal aortic aneurysms. Arterioscler Thromb Vasc Biol 31: 734–740.
8. Baluk P, Tammela T, Ator E, Lyubynska N, Achen MG, et al. (2005) Pathogenesis of persistent lymphatic vessel hyperplasia in chronic airway inflammation. J Clin Invest 115: 247–257.
9. Danese S, Sans M, de la Motte C, Graziani C, West G, et al. (2006) Angiogenesis as a novel component of inflammatory bowel disease pathogenesis. Gastroenterology 130: 2060–2073.
10. Thairu N, Kiriakidis S, Dawson P, Paleolog E (2011) Angiogenesis as a therapeutic target in arthritis in 2011: learning the lessons of the colorectal cancer experience. Angiogenesis 14: 223–234.
11. Schoppmann SF, Birner P, Studer P, Breiteneder-Geleff S (2001) Lymphatic microvessel density and lymphovascular invasion assessed by anti-podoplanin immunostaining in human breast cancer. Anticancer Res 21: 2351–2355.
12. Nakayama Y, Matsumoto K, Nagato M, Inoue Y, Katsuki T, et al. (2007) Significance of lymphangiogenesis as assessed by immunohistochemistry for podoplanin in patients with esophageal carcinoma. Anticancer Res 27: 619–625.
13. Weidner N, Semple JP, Welch WR, Folkman J (1991) Tumor angiogenesis and metastasis–correlation in invasive breast carcinoma. N Engl J Med 324: 1–8.
14. Fox SB, Leek RD, Weekes MP, Whitehouse RM, Gatter KC, et al. (1995) Quantitation and prognostic value of breast cancer angiogenesis: comparison of microvessel density, Chalkley count, and computer image analysis. J Pathol 177: 275–283.
15. Vermeulen PB, Gasparini G, Fox SB, Toi M, Martin L, et al. (1996) Quantification of angiogenesis in solid human tumours: an international consensus on the methodology and criteria of evaluation. Eur J Cancer 32A: 2474–2484.
16. Unno N, Nishiyama M, Suzuki M, Yamamoto N, Inuzuka K, et al. (2008) Quantitative lymph imaging for assessment of lymph function using indocyanine green fluorescence lymphography. Eur J Vasc Endovasc Surg 36: 230–236.
17. Bustin SA (2000) Absolute quantification of mRNA using real-time reverse transcription polymerase chain reaction assays. J Mol Endocrinol 25: 169–193.
18. Schmittgen TD, Livak KJ (2008) Analyzing real-time PCR data by the comparative C(T) method. Nat Protoc 3: 1101–1108.
19. Drozdz K, Janczak D, Dziegiel P, Podhorska M, Piotrowska A, et al. (2012) Adventitial lymphatics and atherosclerosis. Lymphology 45: 26–33.
20. Ordonez NG (2012) Immunohistochemical endothelial markers: a review. Adv Anat Pathol 19: 281–295.
21. Schacht V, Dadras SS, Johnson LA, Jackson DG, Hong YK, et al. (2005) Up-regulation of the lymphatic marker podoplanin, a mucin-type transmembrane glycoprotein, in human squamous cell carcinomas and germ cell tumors. Am J Pathol 166: 913–921.
22. Hatakeyama K, Kaneko MK, Kato Y, Ishikawa T, Nishihira K, et al. (2012) Podoplanin expression in advanced atherosclerotic lesions of human aortas. Thromb Res.
23. Schledzewski K, Falkowski M, Moldenhauer G, Metharom P, Kzhyshkowska J, et al. (2006) Lymphatic endothelium-specific hyaluronan receptor LYVE-1 is expressed by stabilin-1+, F4/80+, CD11b+ macrophages in malignant tumours and wound healing tissue in vivo and in bone marrow cultures in vitro: implications for the assessment of lymphangiogenesis. J Pathol 209: 67–77.
24. Cursiefen C, Chen L, Borges LP, Jackson D, Cao J, et al. (2004) VEGF-A stimulates lymphangiogenesis and hemangiogenesis in inflammatory neovascularization via macrophage recruitment. J Clin Invest 113: 1040–1050.
25. Kerjaschki D (2005) The crucial role of macrophages in lymphangiogenesis. J Clin Invest 115: 2316–2319.

26. Maruyama K, Ii M, Cursiefen C, Jackson DG, Keino H, et al. (2005) Inflammation-induced lymphangiogenesis in the cornea arises from CD11b-positive macrophages. J Clin Invest 115: 2363–2372.
27. Kerjaschki D, Huttary N, Raab I, Regele H, Bojarski-Nagy K, et al. (2006) Lymphatic endothelial progenitor cells contribute to de novo lymphangiogenesis in human renal transplants. Nat Med 12: 230–234.
28. Vorp DA, Lee PC, Wang DH, Makaroun MS, Nemoto EM, et al. (2001) Association of intraluminal thrombus in abdominal aortic aneurysm with local hypoxia and wall weakening. J Vasc Surg 34: 291–299.
29. Tammela T, Enholm B, Alitalo K, Paavonen K (2005) The biology of vascular endothelial growth factors. Cardiovasc Res 65: 550–563.
30. Kaneko H, Anzai T, Takahashi T, Kohno T, Shimoda M, et al. (2011) Role of vascular endothelial growth factor-A in development of abdominal aortic aneurysm. Cardiovasc Res 91: 358–367.
31. Rizas KD, Ippagunta N, Tilson MD 3rd (2009) Immune cells and molecular mediators in the pathogenesis of the abdominal aortic aneurysm. Cardiol Rev 17: 201–210.
32. Ross R, Glomset JA (1976) The pathogenesis of atherosclerosis (first of two parts). N Engl J Med 295: 369–377.
33. Ross R, Glomset JA (1976) The pathogenesis of atherosclerosis (second of two parts). N Engl J Med 295: 420–425.
34. Fenyo IM, Gafencu AV (2013) The involvement of the monocytes/macrophages in chronic inflammation associated with atherosclerosis. Immunobiology 218: 1376–1384.
35. Stoger JL, Gijbels MJ, van der Velden S, Manca M, van der Loos CM, et al. (2012) Distribution of macrophage polarization markers in human atherosclerosis. Atherosclerosis 225: 461–468.
36. Wolpe SD, Davatelis G, Sherry B, Beutler B, Hesse DG, et al. (1988) Macrophages secrete a novel heparin-binding protein with inflammatory and neutrophil chemokinetic properties. J Exp Med 167: 570–581.
37. Schroder K, Hertzog PJ, Ravasi T, Hume DA (2004) Interferon-gamma: an overview of signals, mechanisms and functions. J Leukoc Biol 75: 163–189.
38. Deshmane SL, Kremlev S, Amini S, Sawaya BE (2009) Monocyte chemoattractant protein-1 (MCP-1): an overview. J Interferon Cytokine Res 29: 313–326.
39. Choi I, Lee YS, Chung HK, Choi D, Ecoiffier T, et al. (2013) Interleukin-8 reduces post-surgical lymphedema formation by promoting lymphatic vessel regeneration. Angiogenesis 16: 29–44.
40. Shi VY, Bao L, Chan LS (2012) Inflammation-driven dermal lymphangiogenesis in atopic dermatitis is associated with CD11b+ macrophage recruitment and VEGF-C up-regulation in the IL-4-transgenic mouse model. Microcirculation 19: 567–579.
41. Suzuki Y, Ito Y, Mizuno M, Kinashi H, Sawai A, et al. (2012) Transforming growth factor-beta induces vascular endothelial growth factor-C expression leading to lymphangiogenesis in rat unilateral ureteral obstruction. Kidney Int 81: 865–879.
42. James JM, Nalbandian A, Mukouyama YS (2013) TGFbeta signaling is required for sprouting lymphangiogenesis during lymphatic network development in the skin. Development 140: 3903–3914.
43. Sharma R, Wendt JA, Rasmussen JC, Adams KE, Marshall MV, et al. (2008) New horizons for imaging lymphatic function. Ann N Y Acad Sci 1131: 13–36.
44. Unno N, Yamamoto N, Suzuki M, Tanaka H, Mano Y, et al. (2013) Intraoperative lymph mapping with preoperative vein mapping to prevent postoperative lymphorrhea following paramalleolar bypass surgery in patients with critical limb ischemia. Surg Today.
45. Sugaya M, Kuwano Y, Suga H, Miyagaki T, Ohmatsu H, et al. (2012) Lymphatic dysfunction impairs antigen-specific immunization, but augments tissue swelling following contact with allergens. J Invest Dermatol 132: 667–676.
46. Zampell JC, Aschen S, Weitman ES, Yan A, Elhadad S, et al. (2012) Regulation of adipogenesis by lymphatic fluid stasis: part I. Adipogenesis, fibrosis, and inflammation. Plast Reconstr Surg 129: 825–834.
47. Xu X, Lu H, Lin H, Ni M, Sun H, et al. (2009) Lymphangiogenesis promotes inflammation and neointimal hyperplasia after adventitia removal in the rat carotid artery. Int J Cardiol 134: 426–427.
48. Zampell JC, Yan A, Elhadad S, Avraham T, Weitman E, et al. (2012) CD4(+) cells regulate fibrosis and lymphangiogenesis in response to lymphatic fluid stasis. PLoS One 7: e49940.
49. Miwa K, Nakashima H, Aoki M, Miyake T, Kawasaki T, et al. (2005) Inhibition of ets, an essential transcription factor for angiogenesis, to prevent the development of abdominal aortic aneurysm in a rat model. Gene Ther 12: 1109–1118.
50. Vijaynagar B, Bown MJ, Sayers RD, Choke E (2013) Potential role for anti-angiogenic therapy in abdominal aortic aneurysms. Eur J Clin Invest 43: 758–765.
51. Maruyama K, Asai J, Ii M, Thorne T, Losordo DW, et al. (2007) Decreased macrophage number and activation lead to reduced lymphatic vessel formation and contribute to impaired diabetic wound healing. Am J Pathol 170: 1178–1191.
52. Zhou Q, Guo R, Wood R, Boyce BF, Liang Q, et al. (2011) Vascular endothelial growth factor C attenuates joint damage in chronic inflammatory arthritis by accelerating local lymphatic drainage in mice. Arthritis Rheum 63: 2318–2328.

9

Adipose Stem Cells Promote Smooth Muscle Cells to Secrete Elastin in Rat Abdominal Aortic Aneurysm

Xiaohong Tian[1], Jun Fan[1], Miao Yu[1], Yu Zhao[2], Yan Fang[3], Shuling Bai[1]*, Weijian Hou[1], Hao Tong[1]

1 Department of Tissue Engineering, College of Basic Medical Sciences, China Medical University, Shenyang, Liaoning, P. R. China, **2** Department of Plastic Surgery, Shengjing Hospital of China Medical University, Shenyang, Liaoning, P. R. China, **3** Department of Anatomy, Liaoning Medical University, Jinzhou, Liaoning, P. R. China

Abstract

Background: Abdominal aortic aneurysm (AAA) is a life-threatening disease and its prevalence rate increases with social aging. The degradation of elastic is an important factor in the formation of AAA.

Methods: Adipose derived stem cells (ADSCs) and bone marrow mesenchymal stem cells (BMSCs) were isolated from rats, and identified by Oil red O and alizarin red staining after adipogenesis and osteogenesis induction. In addition, ADSCs were also identified by flow cytometry with CD markers. AAA model in rats was established, and smooth muscle cells (SMCs) were isolated from AAA aortic wall and identified by immunohistochemistry. ADSCs or BMSCs were co-cultured with AAA aortic wall for in vitro experiment, and ADSCs were injected into AAA model for in vivo test. Then orcein staining was used for observing the morphology of elastic fiber, Western blot and real-time PCR were used respectively to detect the protein and gene expression of elastin, gelatinases spectrum analysis was used to detect the activity of matrix metalloproteinase-2 (MMP-2) and MMP-9.

Results: Lots of red lipid droplets were visible by Oil red O staining after adipogenesis induction, and black calcium nodules appeared by alizarin red staining after osteogenesis induction. The results of flow cytometry showed that ADSCs expressed CD44 and CD105, but exhibited negligible expression of CD31 and CD45. SMCs exhibited spindle-like morphology and α-actin protein was positive in cytoplasm. After co-cultured with ADSCs or BMSCs, the elastic fiber recovered normal winding shape, both the gene and protein expression of elastin increased, and the activity of MMP-2 decreased. The in vivo result was similar to that of in vitro.

Conclusions: ADSCs promote the expression of elastin in SMCs and contribute to the reconstruction of elastic fiber, which may provide new ideas for treating AAA.

Editor: Hiromi Yanagisawa, UT-Southwestern Med Ctr, United States of America

Funding: The study was supported by National Natural Science Foundation of China (30772215) and Liaoning Education Department (serial number: 051525). The funders had no role in study design, data collection and analysis, decision to publish, or preparation of the manuscript.

Competing Interests: The authors have declared that no competing interests exist.

* Email: shuling_bai@126.com

These authors contributed equally to this work.

Introduction

Aortic aneurysm is a life-threatening disease and its prevalence rate increases with social aging [1]. The localized abdominal aorta expansion, which exceeds more than 50% of the normal vessel diameter, is called abdominal aortic aneurysm (AAA). The tunica media accounts for more than 90% of the abdominal aortic wall, and mainly composed of smooth muscle cells (SMCs) as well as the elastic fiber. Many factors are possibly involved in the formation of AAA, such as chronic inflammation, increase of proteolytic pathways, oxidative stress and the decrease of matrix in the aortic wall [2]. It has also been demonstrated that inflammation may play an important role in aneurysm progression, through the elastin breakdown and SMCs apoptosis mediated by inflammatory cells infiltration and activation of matrix metalloproteinases (MMPs) [3]. It has also been found that AAA could be eased by limiting proinflammatory signals in rats, and the expansion of AAA was positively correlated to inflammatory infiltration [4].

The traditional treatment methods for AAA are medical follow-up and surgical procedure. For large, high fracture risk of AAA, open surgery or endovascular repair is now widely accepted [5]. However, most of the AAA is small and does not reach the standard for operation. On the other hand, surgical mortality and high risk of complications for surgeons and patients are both serious challenge, so we must pay attention to the non-surgical treatment method [6]. It has been reported that some drug receptors could control the development of the AAA in experimental model, and part have been clinically tested. However, the results of clinical trials were not satisfying [7]. With the progress of stem cell research, using stem cells to treat AAA become an increasingly important idea. This kind of cell population is easily separated, and can differentiate into bone, cartilage, heart, etc. under certain conditions, like bone marrow mesenchymal stem cells (BMSCs). Furthermore, ADSCs has some advantages over BMSCs, such as widespread, easily accessible, small trauma, so it becomes a new hotspot of current research. In addition, ADSCs have the effect of the anti-infection and promoting wound healing [8–10]. It hasn't been reported so far that ADSCs were used for treating AAA.

In the present study, we have investigated the effect of rat ADSCs on elastin secretion of SMCs in AAA model in vitro or in vivo. Then the study provided a base for the therapy of AAA by ADSCs.

Materials and Methods

Ethics Statement

This study was carried out in strict accordance with the recommendations in the Guide for the Care and Use of Animal Research Committee of China Medical University. The protocol was approved by the Animal Research Committee of National Defense Medical Center (IACUC-11-051). All surgery was performed under sodium pentobarbital anesthesia, and all efforts were made to minimize suffering. Animals were housed individually, and were controlled daily by the research team and the animal house staff.

Isolation, culture and identification of ADSCs

Male SD rats weighing 120 g–150 g were selected and anesthetized by intraperitoneal injection of 3% sodium pentobarbital (30 mg/kg), then disinfected in 75% alcohol. The rat skin was cut along the belly line, muscle tissue was separated and groin subcutaneous fat was cut off. Sterile phosphate buffer solution (PBS) was used to remove blood cells, then adipose tissue was transferred into a small dish and cut into pieces with an eye scissors (volume of debris <1 mm^3). The debris was digested with 0.1% collagenase solution of type I (Gibco-BRL, Paisley, UK) for 40–50 min at 37°C, then digestion was terminated with DMEM/F12 (DMEM; Gibco-BRL) containing 10% fetal bovine serum (FBS, Gibco-BRL) and centrifuged at 4°C, 1500 rpm for 5 min. The supernatant was discarded, sediment was suspended with DMEM/F12 containing 10% FBS and filtrated with strainer of 200 mesh. Then the filter liquor was centrifuged at 4°C, 1500 rpm for 5 min, and the sediment was resuspended in DMEM-FBS, then transferred into dish and cultured at 37°C with 5% CO_2 and saturated humidity conditions.

After the third passage, the ADSCs were digested with 0.25% trypsin, and the cell concentration was adjusted to 0.5×10^5 cells/ml. The cells were then inoculated onto 6-well plates and replaced with inducing medium when cell fusion reached 90%. The adipogenesis inducing medium including 0.5 mM isobutyl-methylxanthine (IBMX), 1 μM dexamethasone, 10 μM insulin, 200 μM indomethacin, 1% antibiotic/antimycotic. The osteogenesis inducing medium including 0.01 μM 1,25-dihydroxyvitamin D3, 50 μM ascorbate-2-phosphate, 10 mM β-glycerophosphate, 1% antibiotic/antimycotic [11]. After 2 weeks of adipogenesis induction, oil red O staining was conducted; after 4 weeks of osteogenesis induction, alizarin red staining was conducted.

In addition, the ADSCs expanded to passage three were examined for surface marker expression using flow cytometry. Briefly, the cultured ADSCs were harvested and washed twice with cold PBS. After centrifugation and removal of the supernatants, the cells were resuspended and incubated with blocking buffer for 30 min at 4°C. Following washing with PBS, the cells were incubated for 30 min at 4°C in the dark with PE -conjugated monoclonal antibodies against CD31、CD44、CD45、CD105 (eBioscience). Flow cytometry analysis was performed with a FACSCalibur cytometer (BD Biosciences) and data were analyzed using CellQuest software.

Isolation, culture and identification of BMSCs

Male SD rats weighing 120 g–150 g were selected and anesthetized by intraperitoneal injection of 3% sodium pentobarbital (30 mg/kg), then disinfected in 75% alcohol. Then the femur was separated from muscle and fascia, and the two ends were cut off. All the contents of bone marrow were transferred to culture dish by injection syringe containing DMEM/F12 plus 10% FBS, then cultured at 37°C with 5% CO_2 and saturated humidity conditions. After 3–5 days, the BMSCs grew adherent to the wall while hematopoietic cell suspended in medium because of its characteristic, so changing the medium could remove these nonadherent cells and retain BMSCs. The medium was changed twice weekly and subculture was done when cells reached 80% confluence.

After the third passage, the BMSCs were digested with 0.25% trypsin, and the cell concentration was adjusted to 0.5×10^6 cells/ml. The cells were then inoculated onto 6-well plates and replaced with inducing medium when cell fusion reached 90%. The adipogenesis inducing medium including basic high-glucose DMEM supplemented with 1.0 μM dexamethasone, 0.5 mM IBMX, 10 μM insulin, 200 μM indomethacin, 10% FBS, 1% penicillin G-streptomycin, and 5.6 mg/L of amphotericin B. The osteogenesis inducing basic high-glucose DMEM supplemented with 100 nM dexamethasone, 10 mM β-glycerophosphate, 0.05 mM ascorbic acid-2-phosphate, 10% FBS, 1% penicillin G-streptomycin, and 5.6 mg/L of amphotericin B [11]. After 2 weeks of adipogenesis induction, oil red O staining was conducted; after 4 weeks of osteogenesis induction, alizarin red staining was conducted.

AAA model

The experimental AAA model was established by $CaCl_2$ infiltration, whereas saline was used in the control group [12]. Rats were first anesthetized by intraperitoneal injection of 3% sodium pentobarbital (30 mg/kg), then sheared and disinfected in the supine position. An incision was made on the abdominal median, and the abdominal cavity was exposed. Then the abdominal aortic below the renal artery and above the iliac artery was dissociated out, and covered by a polyethylene sponge containing 0.75 M $CaCl_2$ solution or saline. Meanwhile, the surrounding tissue was protected from the calcium salt infiltration by the sponge encapsulated with sterile rubber strips. After 30 minutes, the sponge and rubber strips were removed and the peritoneal cavity was washed with saline for three times. The incision was sutured layer by layer. Four weeks after the operation, animals were anesthetized and abdominal aorta was isolated for the following assays.

The co-culture of ADSCs or BMSCs and aortic wall of AAA model

The SD rats of AAA model were anesthetized and abdominal cavity was opened. Then cut off the aorta begin from beneath the diaphragm to the common iliac artery bifurcation, washed the blood with precooling PBS, and co-cultured with ADSCs or BMSCs for 7, 14 and 21 d. The AAA aortic wall cultured alone was used as the control group. Each group had 5 samples, and all experiments were repeated for three times. After that, the AAA aortic wall was fixed in 4% formaldehyde or preserved at −80°C for the follow-up test.

The primary culture and identification of vascular SMCs

The aorta of AAA model was cut off according to the previous method. Then cut into pieces and transferred them into culture dish. The tissue pieces distributed and adhered to the bottom of dish after culturing for 4 h. Then high glucose DMEM (H-DMEM) plus 20% FBS was added, and cultured at 37°C with 5% CO_2 and saturated humidity conditions. After 4 days, cells freed out around the tissue and subculture was done when cells reached 80% confluence. After the third passage, the SMCs were conducted with immunohistochemical staining for α-actin.

In vivo experiments

After the third passage, the ADSCs were adjusted to 4×10^6 cells/ml and implanted into the artery through the common carotid artery with a 1-ml syringe (0.5 ml per rat). The group that underwent implantation with the ADSCs, saline and PBS were defined respectively as the ADSCs group, sham-operated group and control group. Each group had six rats. After transplantation for 28 d, the abdominal aortic wall was taken out by surgery for gelatin enzyme spectrum analysis, orcein staining and Western blot detection.

Orcein staining

Orcein staining was used to observe the morphology of elastin. The AAA aortic wall was fixed in 4% formaldehyde for 24 h, dehydrated successively in 10%, 20%, 30% sucrose, then frozed rapidly in liquid nitrogen, embedded with embedding medium and prepared for slices of 8 μm. After placed at room temperature for 1 h, the slices were stained with orcein dye solution for 2 h, then immersed in 95% alcohol for 2 to 3 min and washed off excess dye solution. After dehydration, transparent and seal, the slices were observed with microscope.

Western blot

After co-cultured with ADSCs or BMSCs for 0, 7, 14 and 21 d in vitro, or injection of ADSCs into AAA model for 28 d, the AAA aortic wall was washed off with PBS, cut into pieces, lysed with RIPA buffer and determined protein concentration by the Bradford method. Equal amounts of protein (40 μg) were used for Western blot analysis with rabbit polyclonal antibodies to anti-elastin (abcam, ab23747, 1:1000 dilution). Specific antibody binding was detected by horseradish peroxidase-conjugated goat anti-rabbit antibodies and visualized with ECL reagent (Santa cruz) according to the manufacturer's protocol. Antibody to β-actin was used to evaluate protein loading in each lane.

Gelatin zymogram

Expression of MMP-2 and MMP-9 were assessed using a gelatin zymogram [13]. After co-cultured with ADSCs in vitro or injected with ADSCs in vivo, the AAA aortic wall was isolated and washed with PBS, then cut into pieces in the ice and homogenized (12000 g for 30 min) at 4°C. Protein concentration was determined using a BCA assay, and 50 μg of protein was loaded onto 7.5% Tris-glycine gels with 1 g/L gelatin. Following electrophoresis, gels were washed with distilled water and placed in 2.5% Triton X-100 for washing out SDS, and then incubated at 37°C with gelatinases buffer for 16 h. Gels were stained with 0.1% coomassie blue R-250 and then destained and qualified. A mixture of human MMP-2 and MMP-9 (Chemicon, Temecula, CA, USA) was utilized as standard control. The width and brightness of negative dyed stripe reflected the enzyme activity of gelatin.

Quantitative real-time polymerase chain reaction (qRT-PCR)

The gene expression of MMP-2, MMP-9 and elastin in SMCs were detected by qRT-PCR after co-culture with ADSCs. The co-culture of SMCs and ADSCs was performed in a transwell system. For that 6×10^4 ADSCs were seeded onto a polyester membrane transwell-clear insert (Corning, 0.4 μm) while SMCs were seeded onto the bottom of a six-well cell culture plate in the same cell density. After co-cultured for 24, 48 and 72 h respectively, total RNA was isolated from SMCs using the Trizol plus Kit (Life Technologies, Carlsbad, CA, USA) and quantitated using NanoDrop 1000 (NanoDrop, Wilmington, DE). Then the RNA was reverse transcribed into cDNA using PrimeScript RT reagent Kit With gDNA Eraser (TaKaRa). QRT-PCR was performed using SYBR Premix Ex TaqTM II (TaKaRa) on ABI 7500 Real-Time PCR System (Applied Biosystems). Sequences of the primers for MMP 2 were 5′- GATACAGGTGTGCCAAGGTG- 3′ (forward) and 5′- AAAGGGCAAACAAAGCAAAC -3′ (reverse), MMP 9 were 5′- CTGCAGTGCCCTTGAACTAA -3′ (forward) and 5′- TATCCGGCAAACTAGCTCCT-3′ (reverse), elastin were 5′- CATCGGTGGCTTAGGAGTCT-3′ (forward) and 5′- GAAGACCGACACCAGGAACT -3′ (reverse). Sequences of the primers for GAPDH were 5′- AGGCCGGTGCTGAGTATGTC -3′ (forward) and 5′- TGCCTGCTTCACCACCTTCT -3′ (reverse). The PCR amplification was done at: 95°C for 30 sec; 95°C for 5 sec, 60°C for 34 sec for 40 cycles. The relative changes in gene expression data were analyzed by the 2-ΔΔCT method. GAPDH was used as an internal control. Triplicates were run for each sample in three independent experiments.

Statistical analysis

The results were presented as Mean ± Standard deviation (S.D.) of triplicate determinations. The data were processed using the Statistical Package for the Social Sciences, version 16.0 (SPSS Inc., Chicago, IL, USA). One-way ANOVA was performed for comparison between different groups. Comparisons between groups were conducted using the Tukey Bonferroni test. P values of <0.05 were considered as statistically significant.

Results

The morphology of ADSCs in primary culture and differentiation

During the first day after plating, ADSCs adhered to the plastic surfaces of 6-well plates, as a small population of polygonal or spindle-shaped cells (Fig. 1a). Then ADSCs propagated rapidly in vitro, and showed a homogenous fibroblast-like morphology at 7 d. These cells need to be passaged two to three times in a week, after achieving a confluence of 80–90% (Fig. 1b). After adipogenesis induction, a lot of red lipid droplets were clearly visible by Oil red O staining (Fig. 1c). At 14 d of osteogenesis induction, cells begin to deformation, gathered together, and radiate out. At 28 d, nodular cells mass was visible, as well as red and black calcium, by alizarin red staining (Fig. 1d). Flow cytometry analyses demonstrated that ADSCs expressed CD44 and CD105, but exhibited negligible expression of CD31 and CD45 (Fig. 1e, f, g, h). After statistical analysis, the results were shown as Table 1.

The morphology of BMSCs in primary culture and differentiation

Primary cultured BMSCs grew slowly and showed pleomorphism shape (Fig. 2a). At day 10, cells exhibited a fibroblast shape with a unique vortex arrangement at 90% confluence (Fig. 2b).

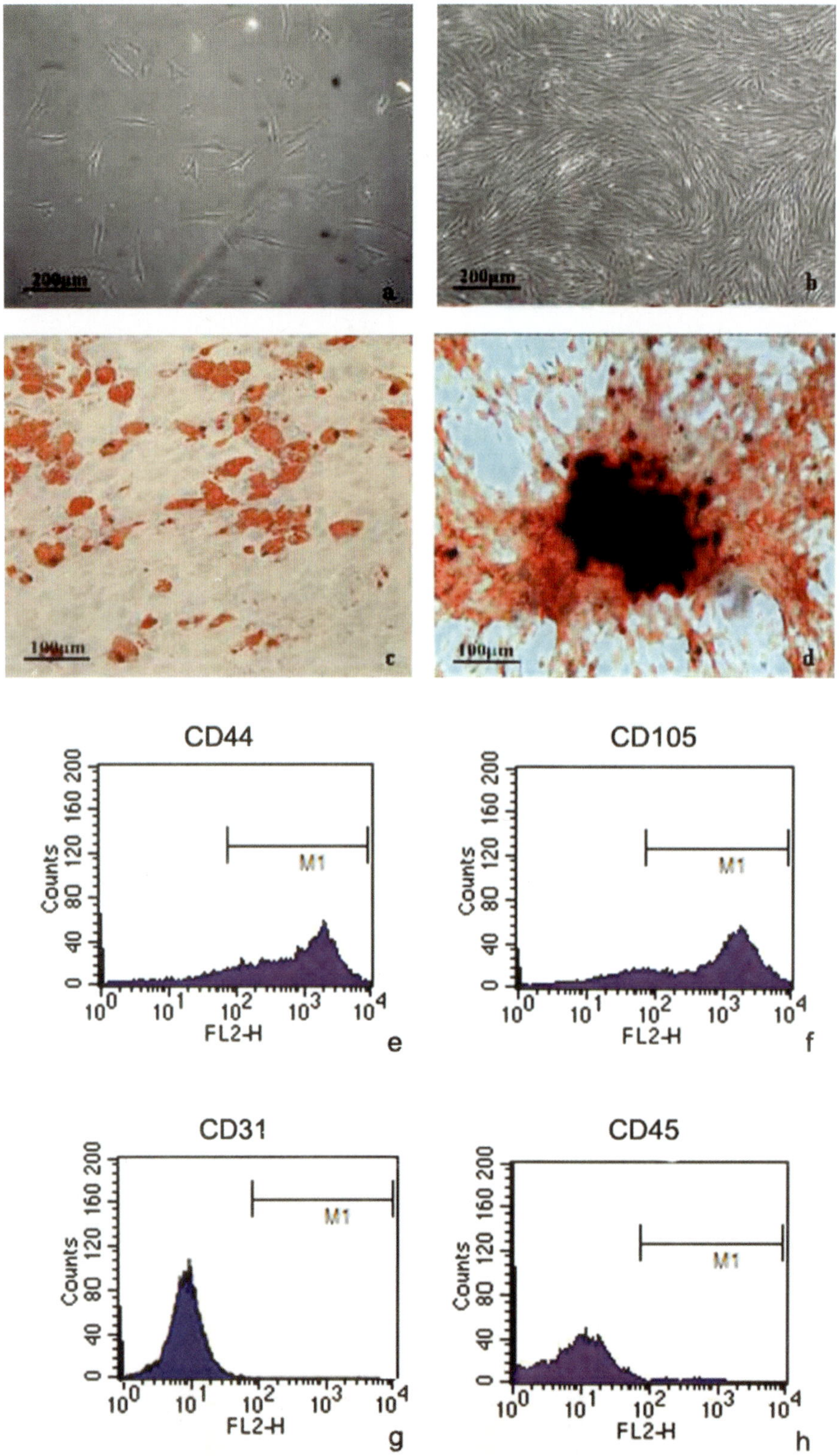

Figure 1. The primary culture and identification of ADSCs. (a) The morphology of ADSCs after plating for 24 h. Bar = 200 μm. (b) ADSCs achieved a confluence of 80–90% after plating for 7 d. Bar = 200 μm. (c) ADSCs were stained by Oil red O after adipogenesis induction. Bar = 100 μm. (d) ADSCs were stained by alizarin red at 14 d of osteogenesis induction. Bar = 100 μm. (e, f, g, h) Flow cytometry histograms of three passaged ADSCs for CD44, CD105, CD31 and CD45 markers.

Table 1. Cell surface phenotype of ADSCs.

Cell surface markers	Positive rate (%)
CD44	88.05±2.00
CD105	83.82±2.28
CD31	1.45±0.48
CD45	1.03±0.69

Values are the mean ± SD.

After subculture for three passages or more, BMSC cultures were homogenous populations. At 10 d after adipogenesis induction, cells had morphological changes, gradually in square shape, and red lipid droplets in the cell were visible by Oil red O staining (Fig. 2c). At about 28 d of osteogenesis induction, black calcium nodules appeared by alizarin red staining (Fig. 2d).

The morphology change of elastic fiber in aortic wall

After co-cultured with ADSCs or BMSCs for 0, 7, 14 and 21 d in vitro, AAA aortic wall was stained with orcein. The AAA aortic wall without co-culture was used as control group. In co-cultured group, the elastic fiber arranged closely and showed winding shape at 14 d and 21 d, which was similar to the structure of normal aortic wall (Fig. 3a1–a4, 3b1–b4). There was no significant difference between ADSCs and BMSCs group. The results of orcein staining showed that elastic fiber in control group became flat and straight (Fig. 3c1–c4). In vivo experiment, the elastic fiber also appeared wavy shape after injection of ADSCs, while that in control group or sham-operated group was straight and thinner (Fig. 3d, e, f).

ADSCs contribute to the protein expression of elastin in vitro or in vivo

The result of Western blot showed that the protein expression of elastin gradually increased with time after co-cultured with ADSCs or BMSCs compared with that of control group, and that in ADSCs co-culture group was significantly greater than that in BMSCs co-culture group at 21 d (Fig. 4a, c, P=0.001). The

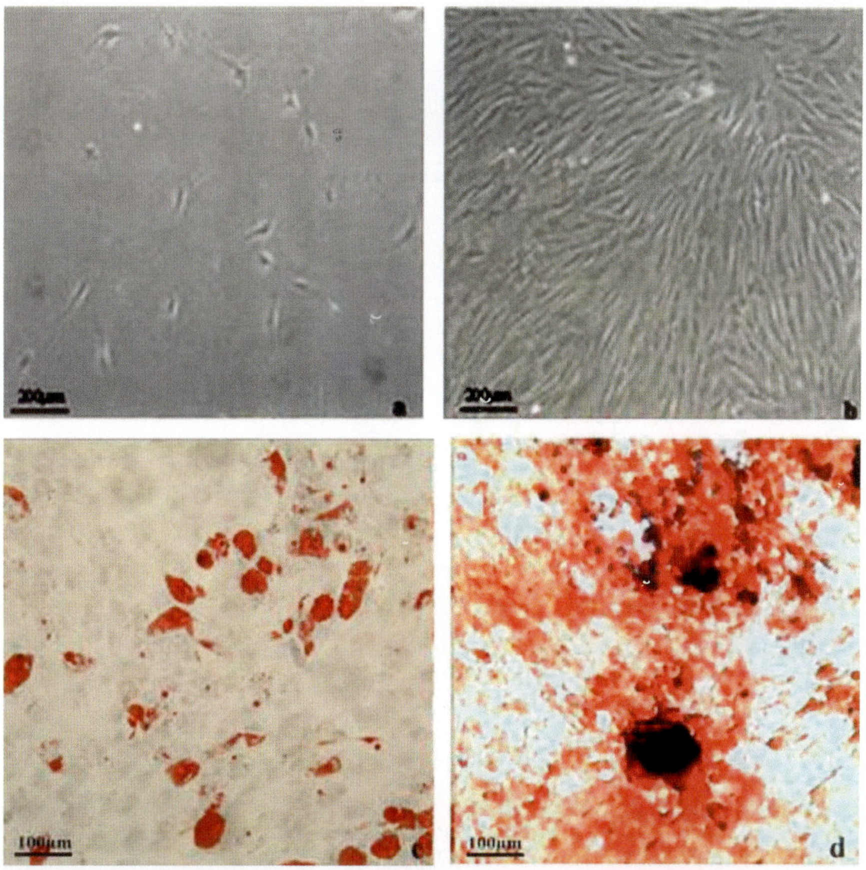

Figure 2. The primary culture and identification of BMSCs. (a) The morphology of BMSCs after plating for 48 h. Bar =200 µm. (b) BMSCs achieved a confluence of 80% after plating for 10 d. Bar =200 µm. (c) BMSCs were stained by Oil red O after adipogenesis induction. Bar =100 µm. (d) BMSCs were stained by alizarin red after osteogenesis induction. Bar =100 µm.

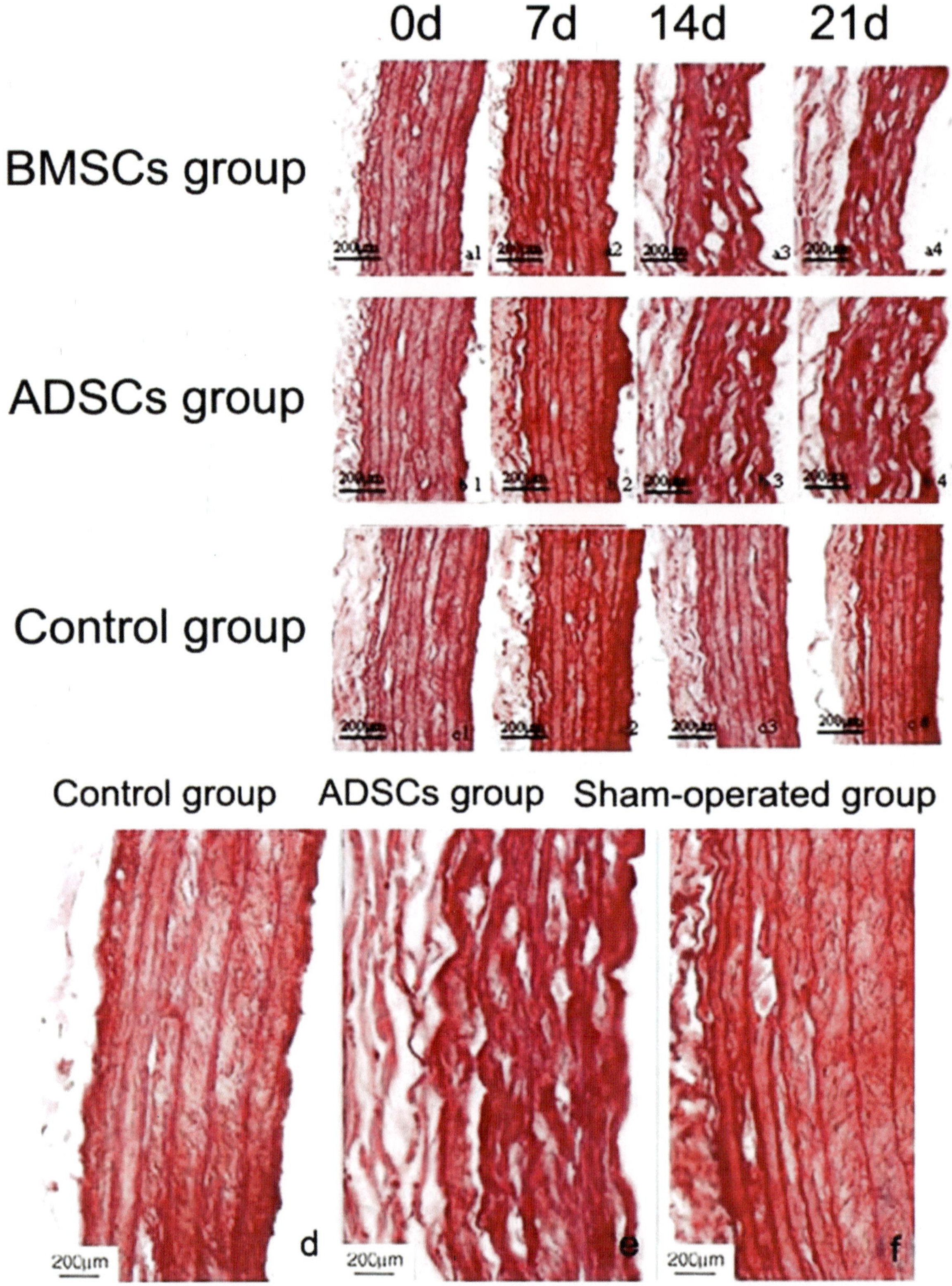

Figure 3. The morphology of elastic fiber after orcein staining. (a, b, c) were the in vitro result and (d, e, f) were the in vivo result. (a1–a4) The morphology of elastic fiber after co-cultured with BMSCs for 0, 7, 14 and 21 d. (b1–b4) The morphology of elastic fiber after co-cultured with ADSCs for 0, 7, 14 and 21 d. (c1–c4) The morphology of elastic fiber in control group. (d, e, f) The morphologies of elastic fiber in control group, ADSCs group and sham-operated group.

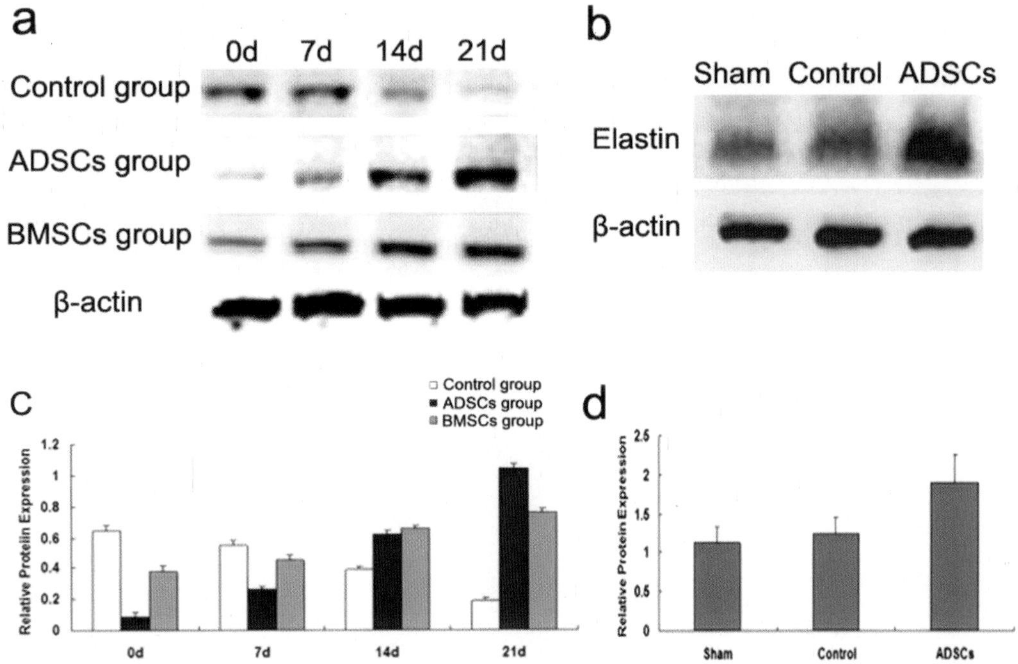

Figure 4. The results of Western blot. (a, c) were the in vitro result and (b, d) were the in vivo result. (a) The protein expression of elastin in control group, ADSCs and BMSCs co-cultured group at 0, 7, 14 and 21 d. β-actin was loading control. (b) The protein expression of elastin in sham-operated group, control group and ADSCs group at 28 d. (c, d) The bar graphs showed mean ± SD of the ratio elastin/β-actin band intensity. $P<0.05$.

relative protein expression of elastin in ADSCs group was 1.04±0.03 at 21 d, while that in BMSCs group was 0.76±0.02 (Fig. 4c). However, the protein expression of elastin gradually decreased with time in control group (Fig. 4a, c). In vivo experiment, the protein expression of elastin increased significantly in ADSCs group, compared with sham-operated group or control group (Fig. 4b, d, $P=0.011$, $P=0.013$).

ADSCs inhibited the expression of MMP-2 and MMP-9 in vitro or in vivo

The result of gelatinases spectrum analysis showed that the expression of pro-MMP-2 (72KD) and active MMP-2 (62KD) gradually decreased along with time in ADSCs co-culture group (Fig.5a). By contrast, the expression of MMP-2 gradually increased with time in control group, especially the active MMP-2 (Fig. 5b). In vivo experiment, the expression of pro-MMP-9 (92 kD), active MMP-9 (83KD), pro-MMP-2 and active MMP-2 in ADSCs group was less than that in sham-operated group or control group (Fig. 5c), especially MMP-2. Therefore we speculated that the increase of gelatinase activity in this experimental aneurysm was mainly MMP-2, rather than MMP-9, and MMP-2 might play a more important role than MMP-9 in aneurysm formation.

The morphology of SMCs in primary culture and identification

After 4 d of primary culture, cells were visible around tissue blocks (Fig. 6a). At day 7 of plating, SMCs exhibited the typical spindle-like morphology under optical microscope (Fig. 6b), which was similar to the morphology of SMCs in normal aortic wall (Fig. 6d). The result of immunohistochemistry for α-actin showed brown protein in cytoplasm (Fig. 6c).

The gene expression of elastin, MMP-2 and MMP-9 in SMCs

QRT-PCR was used to detect the gene expression of elastin, MMP-2 and MMP-9 in SMCs after co-cultured with ADSCs for 24, 48, 72 and 96 h. The result showed that the melting curves of GAPDH, elastin, MMP-2 and MMP-9 were standard single peak, indicating specific amplification products (Fig.7a). In co-culture with ADSCs group, the gene expression of MMP-2 and MMP-9 increased and reached a climax at 48 h, and decreased after that, especially at 96 h. The gene expression of MMP-2 and MMP-9

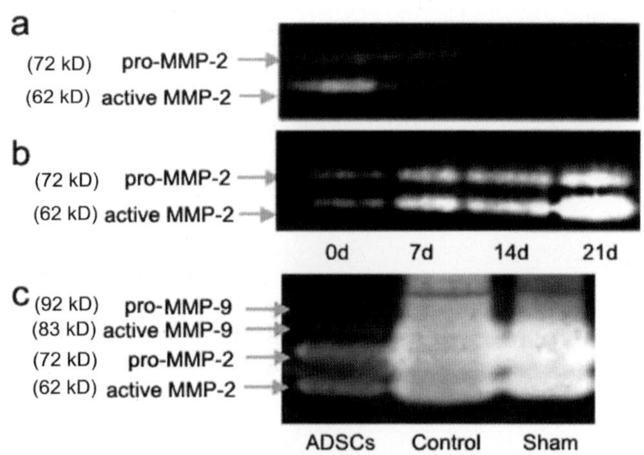

Figure 5. The results of gelatinases spectrum analysis. (a, b) were the in vitro result and (c) was the in vivo result. (a) The expression of pro-MMP-2 and active MMP-2 in ADSCs co-cultured group. (b) The expression of pro-MMP-2 and active MMP-2 in control group. (c) The expression of pro-MMP-9, active MMP-9, pro-MMP-2 and active MMP-2 in ADSCs group, control group and sham-operated group.

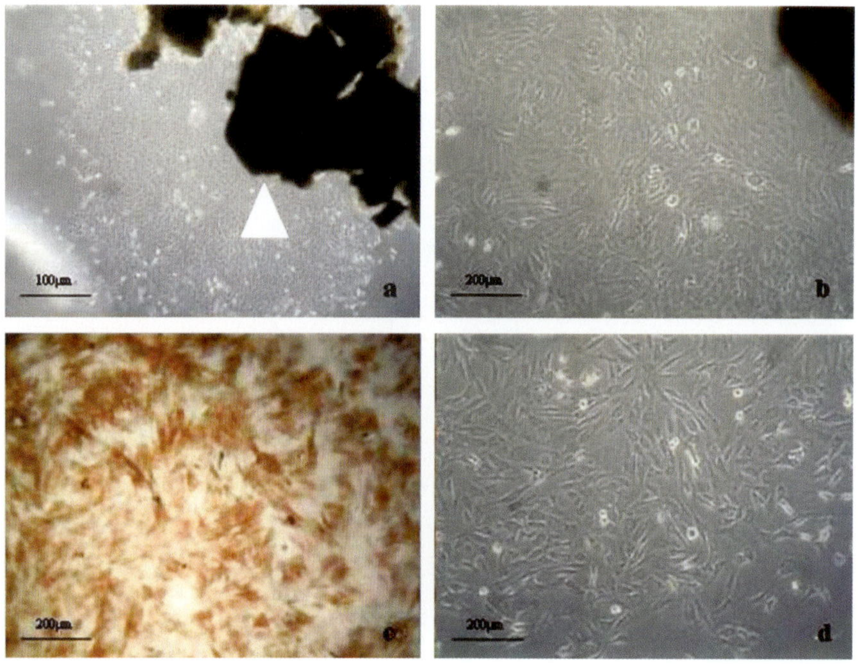

Figure 6. The primary culture and identification of SMCs. (a) At 4 d of primary culture. The arrow points at tissue blocks of AAA aortic wall. Bar = 100 μm. (b) The morphology of SMCs at 7 d of plating. Bar = 200 μm. (c) The result of immunohistochemistry for α-actin. Bar = 200 μm. (d) The morphology of SMCs in normal aortic wall. Bar = 200 μm.

had no significant difference in normal control group, while that increased with time in AAA control group (Fig.7b, $P = 0.009$, $P = 0.027$). However, the gene expression of elastin increased with time in ADSCs co-cultured group (Fig.7b, $P = 0.00$), while that in normal control group and AAA control group had no significant difference (Fig. 7b, $P = 0.052$, $P = 0.073$).

Discussion

AAA is usually a localized expansion associated with atherosclerosis, and its incidences increase with age [14]. Conventional treatment method is replacing diseased blood vessels with artificial blood vessels. But the accompanying risk factors such as leakage as well as re-intervention rate are higher than that in open surgery [15]. In AAA, the elastic plate of middle lamella of artery was damaged, the number of SMCs decreased, and the invasion of inflammatory cells led to the expansion of arterial wall. The foundation of extracellular matrix remodeling include the steady state of extracellular matrix synthesis in arterial wall of SMCs, the quantity and normal function of SMCs and the protease produced by inflammatory cells, which maintain normal morphology of arterial wall. The causes of aneurysms involved a variety of factors, but if the balance among them was broken, AAA occurred.

According to reports, the decrease of elastin in AAA was related to the excessive secretion of inflammatory cytokines and MMPs, both in the clinical field [16] or in animal models [17]. MMPs are large family, named dependent on zinc and other metal ions, and controlled by tissue inhibitors of metalloproteinase (TIMPs) [18]. The imbalance of excessive elastin degradation is the main cause of aneurysms. Therefore, inhibiting MMPs or increasing the secretion of TIMPs or a combination of both would be a way to limit the development of aneurysms. In fact, MMPs inhibitors applied in vivo have been reported [19]. In recent years, studies have shown that ADSCs could inhibit tumor necrosis factor-α (TNF-α) and promoted the secretion of anti-inflammatory cytokines-interleukin-10 [20]. Whether ADSCs can inhibit secretion of MMPs or not hasn't been reported. In this experiment, we co-cultured AAA aortic wall and ADSCs in vitro, injected ADSCs into rat model of AAA in vivo, then extracted protein from aortic wall and conducted gelatin zymography detection, and the results showed that the activity of MMP-2 and MMP-9 significantly reduced. In addition, SMCs were isolated from AAA aortic wall and co-cultured with ADSCs, the result showed that the gene expression of MMP-2 and MMP-9 also decreased significantly, which demonstrated that ADSCs inhibited the secretion of MMPs and might affect the development of AAA.

Elastin is a kind of extracellular matrix protein and plays an indispensable role in maintaining vascular elasticity. The content of elastin is the most abundant among all proteins in aorta wall [21], and gradually degenerated with age [22]. In animal models, the degradation of elastic plate led to expansion, sclerosis and dysfunction of arterial wall, and ultimately resulted in aneurysm formation or rupture of blood vessels [23]. Although pathological features of aortic aneurysms varied with different positions (ie, thoracic or abdominal aorta), the degradation of elastin was their common characteristics. In this background, it may be a strategy for treating AAA by promoting SMCs secreting elastin and inhibiting proteases meanwhile, including MMPs. In recent years, it has been reported that BMSCs could inhibit inflammatory cytokines and promote the survival of elastin in AAA, but so far there is no report about whether ADSCs can promote the synthesis and secretion of elastin in SMCs. In this experiment, we co-cultured the AAA aortic wall with ADSCs or BMSCs in vitro, then conducted frozen sections and stained with orcein, and found that elastic plate recovered to winding shape again, which was similar to that of normal arterial wall. This phenomenon demonstrated that ADSCs and BMSCs were able to promote the reconstruction of elastic plates. Then we detected the protein expression by Western blot, found that elastin content in ADSCs

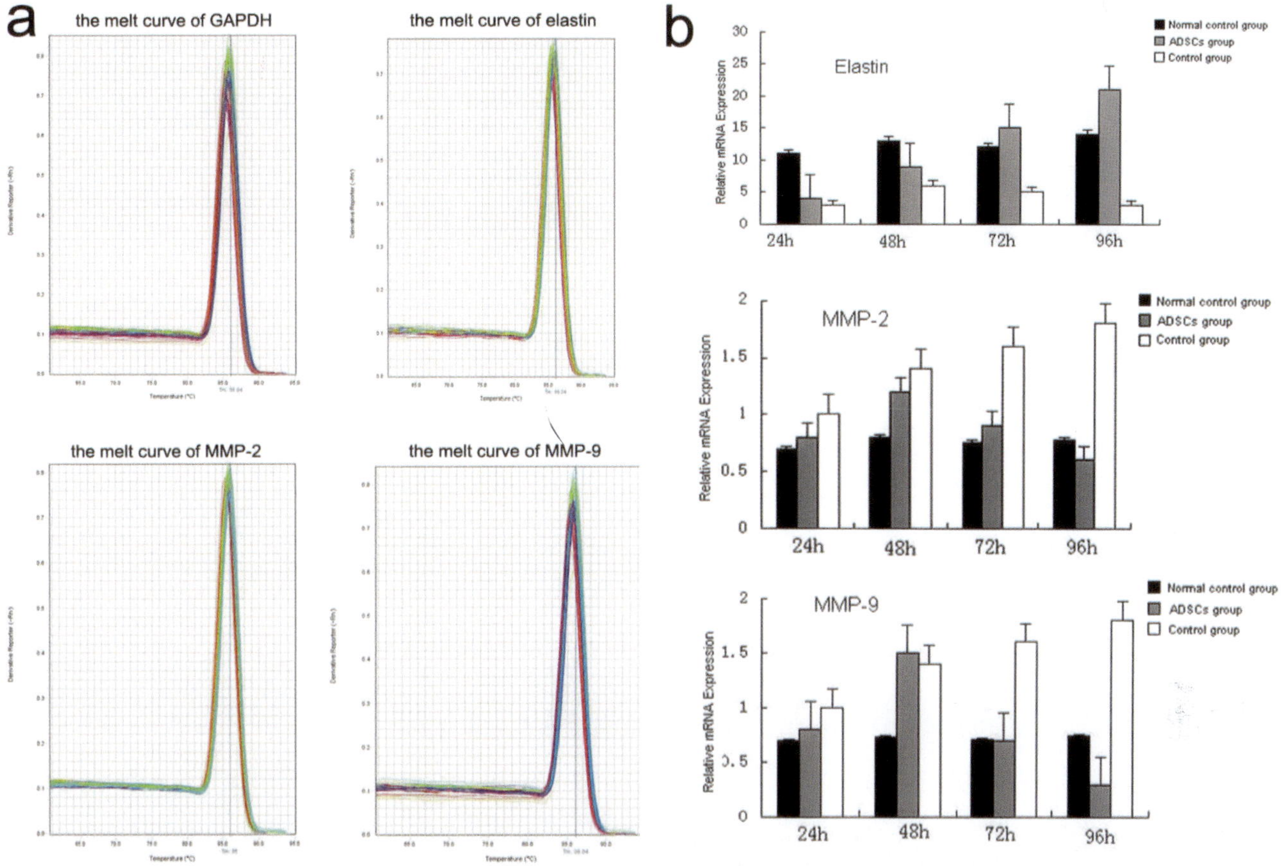

Figure 7. The results of Real-Time PCR. (a) The melting curves of GAPDH, elastin, MMP-2 and MMP-9. (b) The gene expression of elastin, MMP-2 and MMP-9 normal control group, ADSCs group and control group at 24, 48, 72 and 96 h.

or BMSCs co-culture group was significant higher than that in control group, and the former was higher that the latter. The findings suggested that both ADSCs and BMSCs could promote the reconstruction of the elastic plate. The in vivo result also verified this conclusion. Therefore it indicated that ADSCs might promote the secretion and synthesis elastin in SMCs, which was likely to provide new ideas for treating AAA. But the related mechanisms in this process are not very clear, which depends on subsequent trials.

Acknowledgments

The authors wish to thank Experimental Technology Center, Department of Developmental Biology, Department of Pharmacology, and Department of Pathophysiology in China Medical University. We also deeply thank all people who help us.

Author Contributions

Conceived and designed the experiments: XHT JF SLB. Performed the experiments: XHT JF MY YF. Analyzed the data: YZ. Contributed reagents/materials/analysis tools: WJH HT YF. Wrote the paper: XHT SLB.

References

1. Nordon IM, Hinchliffe RJ, Loftus IM, Thompson MM (2011) Pathophysiology and epidemiology of abdominal aortic aneurysms. Nat Rev Cardiol 8: 92–102.
2. Hashizume R1, Yamawaki-Ogata A, Ueda Y, Wagner WR, Narita Y, (2011) Mesenchymal stem cells attenuate angiotensin II-induced aortic aneurysm growth in apolipoprotein E-deficient mice. J Vasc Surg 54: 1743–52.
3. Lesauskait V, Epistolato MC, Castagnini M, Urbonavicius S, Tanganelli P (2006) Expression of matrix metalloproteinases, their tissue inhibitors and osteopontin in the wall of thoracic and abdominal aortas with dilatative pathology. Hum Pathol 27: 1076–1084.
4. Wang YI, Schulze J, Raymond N, Tomita T, Tam K, et al. (2011) Endothelial inglammation correlates with subjecr reifflycerides and waist size after a high-fat meal. Am J Physiol Heart Circ Physiol 300: 784–791.
5. Gu YQ, Guo LR, Qi LX, Yu HX, Li XF, et al (2013) Outcomè comparison of open versus endovascular techniques in the treatment of abdominal aortic aneurysms. Natl Med J China 93: 644–649.
6. Tan Z, Tan X, Peng MH, Li LQ, Yang DH (2006) Clinical analysis of abdominal aortic aneurysm surgery. JOURNAL OF GUANGXI MEDICAL UNIVERSITY 23: 786–788.
7. Fu XM, Yamawaki-Ogata A, Oshima H, Ueda Y, Usui A, et al. (2013) Intravenous administration of mesenchymal stem cells prevents angiotensin II-induced aortic aneurysm formation in apolipoprotein E-deficient mouse. J Transl Med 11: 175.
8. Wang JQ, Fan J, Gao JH, Zhang C, Bai SL (2013) Comparison of in vivo adipogenic capabilities of two different extracellular matrix microparticle scaffolds. Plast Reconstr Surg 131: 174e–187e.
9. Fang Y, Tian X, Bai S, Fan J, Hou W, et al. (2012) Autologous transplantation of adipose-derived mesenchymal stem cells ameliorates streptozotocin-induced diabetic nephropathy in rats by inhibiting oxidative stress, pro-inflammatory cytokines and the p38 MAPK signaling pathway. Int J Mol Med 30: 85–92.
10. Fang Y, Bai SL, Tian XH, Zeng RX, Shan W (2013) Inhibition of adipose derived stem cells on oxidative stress response of rats with diabetic nephropathy. Chinese Journal of Anatomy 36: 896–900.
11. Monaco E, Bionaz M, Sobreira de Lima A, Hurley WL, Loor JJ, et al. (2010) Selection and reliability of internal reference genes for quantitative PCR verification of transcriptomics during the differentiation process of porcine adult mesenchymal stem cells. Stem Cell Research & Therapy 1: 7.

12. Tanaka A, Hasegawa T, Chen Z, Okita Y, Okada K (2009) A novel rat model of abdominal aortic aneurysm using a combination of intraluminal elastase infusion and extraluminal calcium chloride exposure. J Vasc Surg 50: 1423e32.
13. Zuo W, Chen J, Zhang S, Tang J, Liu H, et al. (2014) IMM-H004 prevents toxicity induced by delayed treatment of tPA in a rat model of focal cerebral ischemia involving PKA-and PI3K-dependent Akt activation. Eur J Neurosci 39: 2107–18.
14. Hsieh HL, Yen MH, Jou MJ, Yang CM (2004) Intracellular signalings underlying bradykinin-induced matrix metalloproteinase-9 expression in rat brain astrocyte-1. Cell Signal 16: 1163–1176.
15. De Bruin JL, Baas AF, Buth J, Prinssen M, Verhoeven EL, et al. (2010) Long-term outcome of open or endovascular repair of abdominal aortic aneurysm. N Engl J Med 362: 1881–9.
16. Yamashita A, Noma T, Nakazawa A, Saito S, Fujioka K, et al. (2001) Enhanced expression of matrix metalloproteinase-9 in abdominal aortic aneurysms. World J Surg 25: 259–65.
17. Longo GM, Xiong W, Greiner TC, Zhao Y, Fiotti N, et al. (2002) Matrix metalloproteinases 2 and 9 work in concert to produce aortic aneurysms. J Clin Invest 110: 625–32.
18. Visse R, Nagase H (2003) Matrix metalloproteinases and tissue inhibitors of metalloproteinases: structure, function, and biochemistry. Circ Res 92: 827–39.
19. Yamawaki-Ogata A, Hashizume R, Satake M, Kaneko H, Mizutani S, et al. (2010) A doxycycline loaded, controlled-release, biodegradable fiber for the treatment of aortic aneurysms. Biomaterials 31: 9554–64.
20. Fan Y, Wang JJ, Wei F, Fan XH, Ma AQ (2014) Effect of adipose-derived mesenchymal stem cell transplantation on inflammatory response and ventricular remodeling after myocardial infarction. Journal of Clinical Rehabilitative Tissue Engineering Research 18: 900–905.
21. Thompson RW, Geraghty PJ, Lee JK (2002) Abdominal aortic aneurysms:basic mechanisms and clinical implications. Cur Probl Surg 39: 110–230.
22. Collins MJ, Dev V, Strauss BH, Fedak PW, Butany J (2008) Variation in the histopathological features of patients with ascending aortic aneurysms: a study of 111 surgically excised cases. J Clin Pathol 61: 519–23.
23. Pezet M1, Jacob MP, Escoubet B, Gheduzzi D, Tillet E, et al. (2008) Elastin haploinsufficiency induces alternative aging processes in the aorta. Rejuvenation Res 11: 97–112.

Long-Term Effect of Bariatric Surgery on Liver Enzymes in the Swedish Obese Subjects (SOS) Study

Maria Antonella Burza[1], Stefano Romeo[1,2], Anna Kotronen[3], Per-Arne Svensson[1], Kajsa Sjöholm[1], Jarl S. Torgerson[4], Anna-Karin Lindroos[5], Lars Sjöström[1], Lena M. S. Carlsson[1], Markku Peltonen[3]*

1 Department of Molecular and Clinical Medicine and Center for Cardiovascular and Metabolic Research, Sahlgrenska Academy, University of Gothenburg, Gothenburg, Sweden, **2** Clinical Nutrition Unit, Department of Medical and Surgical Sciences, University Magna Graecia, Catanzaro, Italy, **3** Department of Chronic Disease Prevention, National Institute for Health and Welfare, Helsinki, Finland, **4** Department of Health Care, Regional Secretariat, Västra Götaland Region, Gothenburg, Sweden, **5** Nutrition Department, National Food Administration, Uppsala, Sweden

Abstract

Background and Aim: Obesity is associated with elevated serum transaminase levels and non-alcoholic fatty liver disease and weight loss is a recommended therapeutic strategy. Bariatric surgery is effective in obtaining and maintaining weight loss. Aim of the present study was to examine the long-term effects of bariatric surgery on transaminase levels in obese individuals.

Methods: The Swedish Obese Subjects (SOS) study is a prospective controlled intervention study designed to compare the long-term effects of bariatric surgery and usual care in obese subjects. A total of 3,570 obese participants with no excess of alcohol consumption at baseline (1,795 and 1,775 in the control and surgery group, respectively) were included in the analyses. Changes in transaminase levels during follow-up were compared in the surgery and control groups.

Results: Compared to usual care, bariatric surgery was associated with lower serum ALT and AST levels at 2- and 10- year follow up. The reduction in ALT levels was proportional to the degree of weight loss. Both the incidence of and the remission from high transaminase levels were more favorable in the surgery group compared to the control group. Similarly, the prevalence of ALT/AST ratio <1 was lower in the surgery compared to the control group at both 2- and 10-year follow up.

Conclusions: Bariatric surgery results in a sustained reduction in transaminase levels and a long-term benefit in obese individuals.

Editor: Giovanni Targher, University of Verona, Ospedale Civile Maggiore, Italy

Funding: This study was supported by grants from the Swedish Research Council (K2012-55X-22082-01-3, K2010-55X-11285-13, K2008-65x-20753-01-4), the Swedish Foundation for Strategic Research to Sahlgrenska Centre for Cardiovascular and Metabolic Research, the Swedish federal government under the LUA/ALF agreement. The funders had no role in study design, data collection and analysis, decision to publish, or preparation of the manuscript.

Competing Interests: The authors have declared that no competing interests exist.

* E-mail: markku.peltonen@thl.fi

Introduction

Elevated serum transaminase levels are frequently associated with obesity [1–3] and with progression to chronic liver disease [4,5], including non-alcoholic liver disease (NAFLD). Bariatric surgery is the most effective strategy to obtain and maintain weight loss in obese individuals [6]. Results from uncontrolled studies [7–13] and two small controlled studies [14,15] indicate that weight loss obtained by bariatric surgery reduces transaminases and NAFLD. Previous studies have shown the favorable effect of weight loss obtained by bariatric surgery on transaminase levels, however, data from large controlled studies with long-term follow up, are not available [16]. The aim of the current report was to examine the long-term effects of bariatric surgery on serum transaminases in the prospective, controlled study, the Swedish obese subjects (SOS) study.

Materials and Methods

The Swedish Obese Subjects (SOS) Study

The SOS study is a non-randomized, matched, prospective, controlled, intervention trial that compares the long-term effects of bariatric surgery and usual care in obese subjects. The SOS study and its inclusion and exclusion criteria have been previously described [17] and they were identical for the two treatment groups. Briefly, from September 1st 1987 to January 31st 2001, a total of 4,047 obese individuals were recruited: 2,010 individuals who selected surgical treatment constituted the bariatric surgery group and a matched control group of 2,037 individuals was enrolled based on 18 matching variables.

Individuals in the surgery group underwent either nonadjustable or adjustable banding (n = 376), vertical banded gastroplasty (n = 1369) or gastric bypass (n = 265). Subjects in the control group received the conventional treatment for obesity at their center of registration (advanced lifestyle modification, other or no treatment). Inclusion criteria were age between 37 to 60 years and BMI of ≥34 kg/m^2 for men and ≥38 kg/m^2 for women. The exclusion criteria were: earlier bariatric surgery, earlier surgery for gastric or duodenal ulcer, gastric ulcer during the past six months, ongoing malignancy, active malignancy during the past five years, myocardial infarction during the past six months, bulimic eating pattern, psychiatric or cooperative problems contraindicating bariatric surgery, regular use of cortisone or non-steroidal anti-inflammatory treatment; excess of alcohol intake and alcohol or drug abuse, and other severe illnesses. The current and past health status was assessed by extensive questionnaires, completed by patients, and subsequently by health examination. The daily alcohol consumption was collected from the validated SOS dietary questionnaire [18].

The baseline examination took place approximately four weeks before the date of bariatric surgery for both the surgery patients and the matched control individuals. At baseline examination and after 2 and 10 years, anthropometric, clinical and biochemical parameters were measured. Blood samples were obtained in the morning after an overnight fast and analyzed at the Central Laboratory of Sahlgrenska University Hospital (accredited according to European Norm 45001).

In the current report, changes in serum transaminase levels and body weight were calculated as the difference between follow up (2 or 10 years) and baseline values. In addition, incidence of high transaminase during follow-up, as well as remission from high transaminase at baseline were analyzed. Specifically, the high transaminase group was defined by AST levels ≥33 U/L or 29 U/L and ALT levels ≥43 U/L or 30 U/L in men or women, respectively, as cut-offs. These transaminase cut-off levels have been shown to define NAFLD, indicated as liver fat content >5.6% by proton magnetic resonance spectroscopy in individuals with alcohol intake ≤20 (men) or ≤10 g/day (women) [19]. To be consistent with this previous report, SOS study participants with baseline self-reported alcohol consumptions of >20 g/day (men) or >10 g/day (women) were not included (n = 427) in the current analyses. Furthermore, individuals lacking data on baseline AST and ALT levels (n = 50) were also excluded from the analyses resulting in a total of 3,570 subjects examined in the current report. The ALT/AST ratio was calculated in the follow up as an index of severe liver damage [20]. Follow-up data were available for 3,102 (87%) persons after 2 years, and for 2,157 (60%) after 10 years. The cut-off date for our current analysis was March 20th, 2009.

Ethics Statement

SOS trial has been registered in the ClinicalTrials.gov registry (NCT01479452, http://clinicaltrials.gov/ct2/show/NCT01479452?term = NCT01479452&rank = 1). Written informed consent has been obtained by all the study participants. The study was approved by all the relevant ethics review boards in Sweden.

Statistical Analyses

Characteristics of the study population are showed as number and percentage for categorical variables or as means and standard deviations (SD) for continuous variables. Changes in anthropometric and laboratory variables between the treatment groups were compared with analysis of covariance (ANCOVA), adjusting for age, gender, baseline BMI and the baseline value of the respective variable. Results are presented as mean difference in changes between the surgery and control groups, together with corresponding 95% confidence intervals. Spearman rank correlation tests were performed to determine the relationship between transaminase and weight changes. For incidence and remission calculations, logistic regression models were used, adjusting for age, gender and baseline BMI. The prevalence of the ALT/AST ratio <1 in the control and in the surgery group was compared by Fisher's exact test. Analyses were performed with the statistics package Stata version 9.2 [21].

Results

Baseline Characteristics

A total of 3,570 individuals (control group, n = 1,795; surgery group, n = 1,775) from the overall SOS study population were included in the current analyses. Baseline characteristics of the surgery and control groups are described in Table 1. Individuals in the surgery group were younger than individuals in the control group. Furthermore, the surgery group had higher body weight, BMI, blood pressure, glucose and liver transaminase levels compared to the control group. No differences in other parameters including alcohol consumption and use of lipid- and blood glucose-lowering medications were observed in the two treatment groups. For incidence and remission calculations, the SOS individuals were stratified in groups with low (LT) and high serum transaminase (HT) levels. The baseline characteristics of these subgroups are shown in Table S1. At baseline, the prevalence of HT levels was 46% (n = 818) in the surgery group and 36% (n = 645) in the control group (P value<0.001). In both groups, individuals in the surgery group were younger and had higher body weight, BMI, blood pressure, glucose compared to the

Table 1. Baseline characteristics of the individuals from the SOS study included in this report.

	Control	Surgery	P value
N	1795	1775	
Gender F, %	72	73	0.82
Age, years	49±6	47±6	<0.001
Body weight, kg	115±16	121±17	<0.001
BMI, kg/m^2	40.2±4.7	42.4±4.5	<0.001
Systolic blood pressure, mmHg	138±18	145±19	<0.001
Diastolic blood pressure, mmHg	85±11	90±11	<0.001
Blood glucose, mmol/L	4.9±1.8	5.2±2.0	<0.001
Total cholesterol, mmol/L	5.6±1.1	5.9±1.1	<0.001
Triglycerides, mmol/L	1.99±1.34	2.24±1.58	<0.001
HDL cholesterol, mmol/L	1.34±0.33	1.34±0.32	0.92
ALT, U/L	33±26	37±23	<0.001
AST, U/l	23±12	25±14	<0.001
Alcohol consumption, g/day	3.2±4.3	3.3±4.2	0.38
Diabetes, %	13	18	<0.001
Glucose-lowering medication, %	7	8	0.06
Lipid-lowering medication, %	2	2	0.44

Data are shown as mean ± SD, or proportion.
Abbreviations: SOS, Swedish obese subjects; N, number; F, female; BMI, body mass index; HDL, high density lipoprotein; ALT, alanine transferase; AST, aspartate transferase.

control group, reflecting the overall population characteristics (Table 1).

Changes in Serum Transaminase Levels and Body Weight

Bariatric surgery was associated with a significant and sustained decrease in body weight compared to the control group [6].

After two years, both ALT and AST were reduced in the surgery group, while there was no change in the control group (Figure 1A). After ten years, this pattern remained for ALT, while there was an increase in AST, which was significantly smaller in the surgery group than in the control group (Figure 1B). Moreover, serum transaminase level changes were positively correlated to body weight changes at both 2- (ALT: $r = 0.500$, P value<0.001; AST: $r = 0.289$, P value<0.001) and 10- year (ALT: $r = 0.357$, P value<0.001; AST: $r = 0.160$, P value<0.001) follow up when the surgery and control groups were pooled (Figure 2A and B; Figure S1 and S2). There was a continuous reduction in ALT levels with increasing weight loss for both the 2- and 10-year follow-up. Similarly, serum AST level were related to weight loss, however, there was no further reduction in AST levels beyond weight loss of more than 10 kg at 2-year follow-up (Figure 2A). At 10-year follow up, the AST levels were associated with weight change, but compared to baseline there was no reduction in the AST levels irrespective of the weight change categories (Figure 2B). Weight gain was associated with increased serum transaminases at both 2- and 10-year follow-up (Figure 2A and B).

Incidence of and Remission from HT

The incidence of HT was lower in the surgery compared to the control group at both 2-year (6% and 21%, for surgery and control groups, respectively P value<0.001) and at 10-year (18% and 27%, $p<0.001$) follow up (Figure 3A). A reduced risk for HT onset was observed in the surgery group at 2 and 10 years (OR: 0.26 (95% confidence interval 0.18–0.36, P value<0.001) and 0.61 (95% confidence interval 0.46–0.81, P value<0.001, respectively). Moreover, remission from HT was more common in the surgery group compared to the control group (80% and 39%, for surgery and control groups, respectively after 2-years, P value<0.001, and 63% and 47%, respectively after 10-years, P value<0.001) (Figure 3B). An increased probability for HT remission was observed at 2- and 10- year follow up in the surgery group (OR: 6.55 (95% CI 5.0–8.5) and 1.80 (95% CI 1.35–2.40) at 2- and 10-year follow up, both P values<0.001).

Finally, the proportion of individuals with an ALT/AST ratio <1 was calculated in the control and in the surgery group in the follow-up (Figure 4). The prevalence of ALT/AST ratio <1 was lower in the surgery compared to the control group at both 2-year (14% vs. 25% respectively, P value <0.001) and 10-year follow up (31 vs. 38% respectively, P value = 0.001).

Discussion

Elevated serum transaminase levels are commonly associated with obesity [1–3] and with progression to chronic liver disease. Bariatric surgery is the most effective strategy to achieve and maintain weight loss [6]. In the present report, the long-term effect of bariatric surgery on serum transaminases has been examined.

A sustained reduction up to 10 years of both ALT and AST levels was observed in the surgery compared to the control group. Several studies investigating the effect of bariatric surgery on liver enzymes and NAFLD have shown an improvement of serum transaminases and hepatic histologic features after surgery [7–15]. The novelty of the current report is the observation of a beneficial effect of bariatric surgery on serum transaminases that is maintained up to 10 years after surgery. These data suggest that bariatric surgery has a long-term protective effect against chronic liver damage. The effects after 10 years were smaller than after 2 years and this is likely due to the weight regain observed 10 years after bariatric surgery [22]. Furthermore, analysis of the relation between changes in transaminase levels and changes in body weight showed that weight gain was associated with a significant increase of transaminase levels. ALT showed a continuous linear

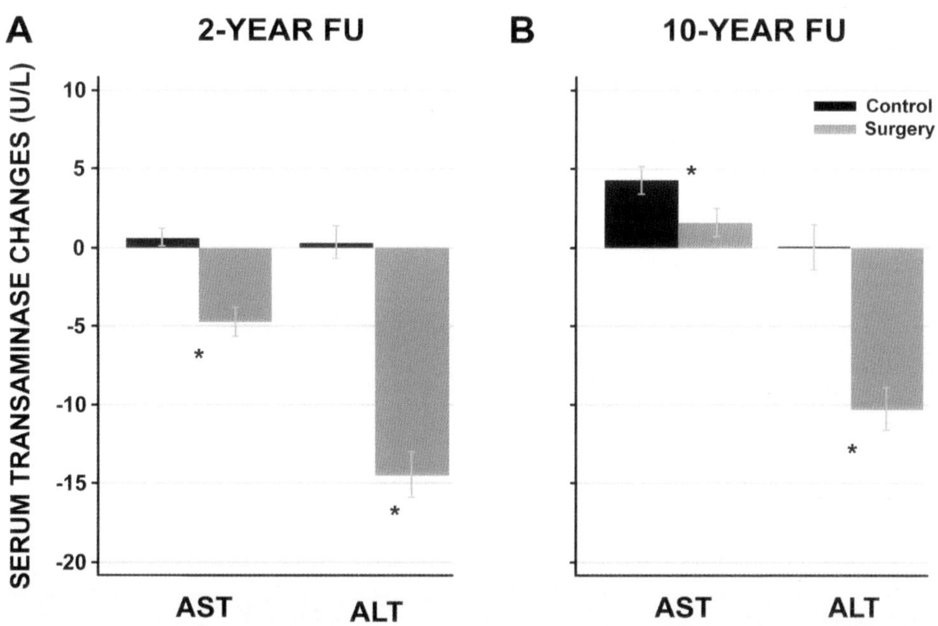

Figure 1. Serum transaminase changes in the surgery and control groups at 2- and 10-year follow up. The serum transaminase changes are expressed as mean and 95% confidence intervals. Changes are calculated as the difference between follow up (2 or 10 year) and baseline values. *P value <0.001, surgery vs. control group. *Abbreviations:* FU, follow up; AST, aspartate transferase; ALT, alanine transferase.

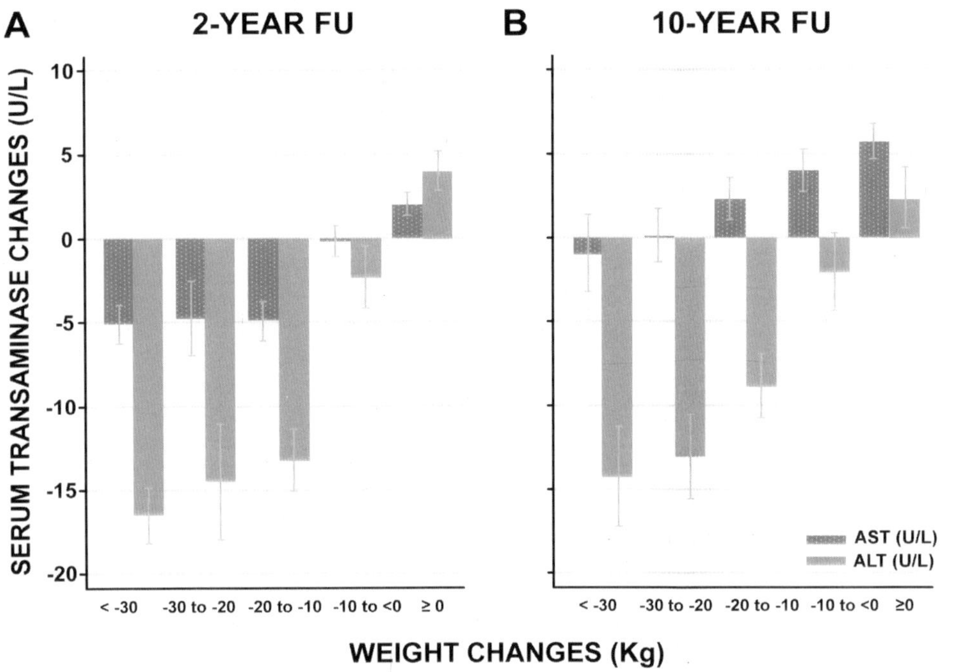

Figure 2. Serum transaminase changes and their relation to body weight changes at 2- and 10-year follow up. The serum transaminase changes are expressed as mean and 95% confidence intervals. The surgery and control groups are pooled. Changes are calculated as the difference between follow up (2 or 10 year) and baseline values. *Abbreviations:* FU, follow up; AST, aspartate transferase; ALT, alanine transferase.

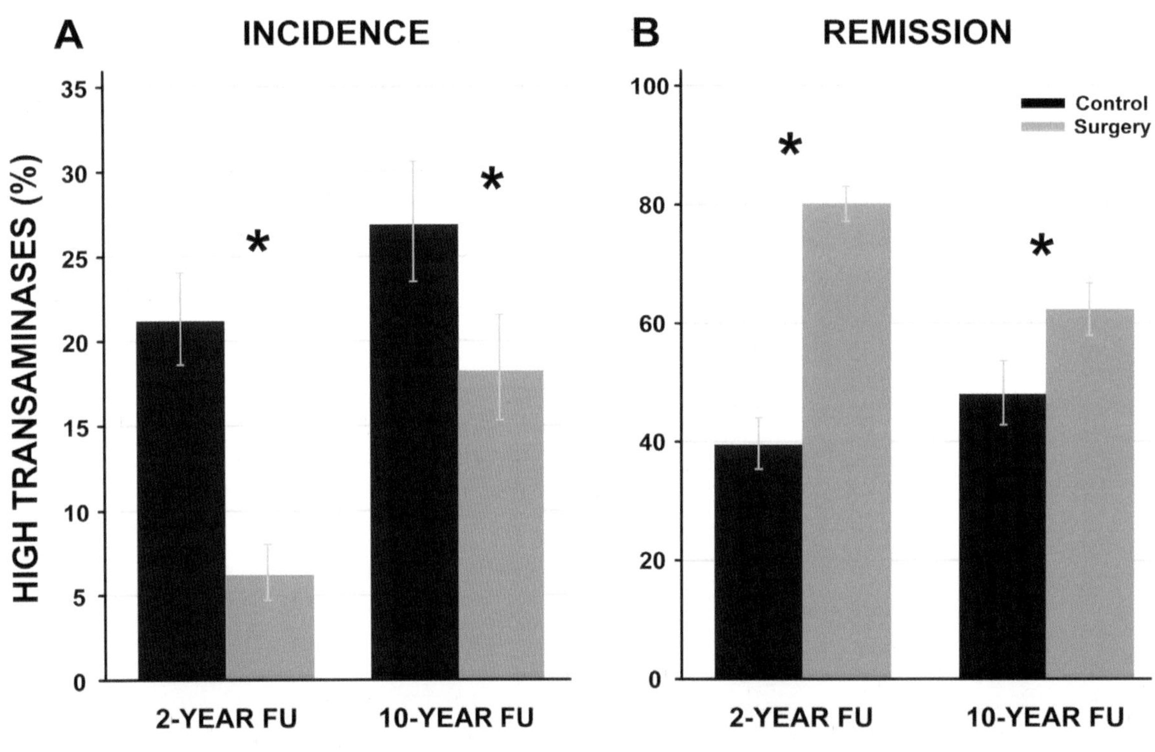

Figure 3. High transaminase (HT) incidence and remission in the surgery and the control groups at 2- and 10-year follow up. HT group was defined if one or both transaminase levels were above the following cut-offs: AST ≥33 U/L (men) and 29 U/L (women) ALT levels ≥43 U/L (men) and 30 U/L (women). Incidence and remission are expressed as proportion of individuals; the bars indicate the 95% confidence intervals. *P value <0.001, surgery vs. control group. A. Control n = 916 and 621 at 2- and 10-year FU; Surgery n = 857 and 618 at 2- and 10 -year FU. B. Control n = 519 and 332 at 2- and 10-year FU; Surgery n = 731 and 491 at 2- and 10-year FU. *Abbreviations:* FU, follow up; HT, high transaminase; AST, aspartate transferase; ALT, alanine transferase.

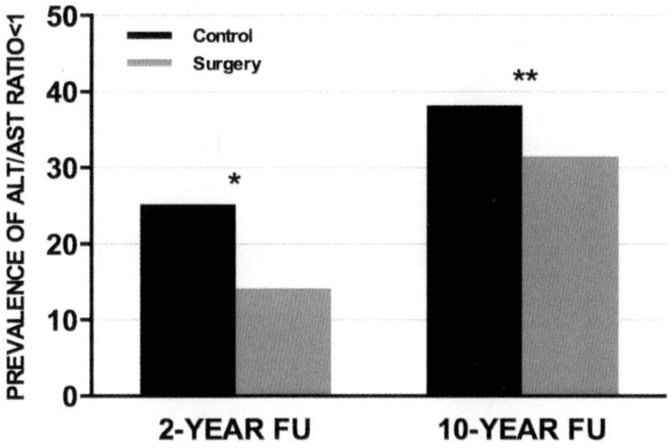

Figure 4. Prevalence of ALT/AST ratio <1 in the surgery and the control groups at 2- and 10-year follow up. The prevalence of ALT/AST ratio <1 is expressed as proportion of individuals. The differences in the prevalence of ALT/AST ratio<1 between the control and the surgery group has been analyzed by Fisher's exact test. Prevalence of ALT/AST ratio <1 was: 25% (n = 368, control group) and 14% (n = 231, surgery group) at 2-year follow-up; 38% (n = 381, control group) and 31% (n = 366, surgery group) at 10-year follow-up. *P value <0.001, surgery vs. control group. **P value = 0.001, surgery vs. control group. *Abbreviations*: ALT, alanine transferase; AST, aspartate transferase; FU, follow up.

reduction with increasing weight loss at the 2-year follow up which was maintained at the 10 year follow up. These data indicate that sustained weight loss has a beneficial long-term effect on chronic liver damage and that this effect is proportional to the weight loss reduction.

When changes in AST levels were examined, a reduction related to weight loss was observed at the 2-year but not at the 10-year follow up. The reason for this unexpected finding is unknown but it may be due to factors that have changed over time (e.g., age, environmental factors, lifestyle habits, medications) and influenced transaminase differently [23]. Nonetheless, it is worth noting that despite the absence of reduction at 10-year follow up, the AST levels remained lower in the surgery when compared to the control group.

Furthermore, the long-term effect of bariatric surgery on HT incidence and remission was examined. The incidence of and the remission from HT at both 2- and 10-year follow up were significantly more favorable in the surgery group compared to the control group. Similarly, the prevalence of an ALT/AST ratio <1, an index of severe liver disease [20], was lower in the surgery group compared to the control group at both 2- and 10-year follow up.

Taken as a whole, these data suggest that weight reduction has a positive effect on liver transaminases and chronic liver damage.

Strength of the present report is that we examined the effect of bariatric surgery on liver transaminase in a large obese cohort with a long-term follow up. Previous reports with different study design and shorter follow up have shown that both weight loss induced by lifestyle intervention and bariatric surgery reduce serum transaminase levels and NAFLD [7–15]. Our data confirm these short-term effects in a matched, controlled, prospective study including more than 3,000 obese individuals and also show that the effects are sustained during a 10-year follow up. A limitation of the present report is that the effect of bariatric surgery on transaminase levels was not a predefined endpoint of the SOS study, although the transaminase level measurements were performed prospectively. Thus, our analyses should be considered exploratory. Another limitation is that even though no clinical diagnosis of advanced chronic liver disease was present, we cannot exclude the presence of relevant liver injury at baseline.

Taken all this together it may be speculated that sustained weight loss obtained by bariatric surgery reduces liver damage and may possibly prevent hepatic long-term sequelae. Further longitudinal studies, using more sensitive techniques to assess chronic liver disease, are warranted to confirm these data. In conclusion, this report shows that bariatric surgery is associated with long-term reduction of serum transaminases in obese individuals.

Supporting Information

Figure S1 Association between weight and ALT level changes at 2- and 10-year follow up. Changes are calculated as the difference between follow up (2 or 10 years) and baseline values. The surgery and control groups are pooled. Spearman rank correlation tests were performed to determine the relationship between transaminase and weight changes. ALT level changes correlate to body weight changes at both 2- (ALT: r = 0.500, P value<0.001) and 10-year (ALT: r = 0.357, P value<0.001) follow up. *Abbreviations:* ALT, alanine transferase.

Figure S2 Association between weight and AST level changes at 2- and 10-year follow up. Changes are calculated as the difference between follow up (2 or 10 years) and baseline values. The surgery and control groups are pooled. Spearman rank correlation tests were performed to determine the relationship between transaminase and weight changes. AST level changes correlate to body weight changes at both 2- (AST: r = 0.289, P value<0.001) and 10-year (AST: r = 0.160, P value<0.001) follow up. *Abbreviations:* AST, aspartate transferase.

Table S1 Baseline characteristics of SOS individuals with LT and HT. Data are shown as mean ± SD, or proportions. *Abbreviations*: SOS, Swedish obese subjects; LT, low transaminase; HT, high transaminase; N, number; F, female; BMI, body mass index; HDL, high density lipoprotein; ALT, alanine transferase; AST, aspartate transferase.

Acknowledgments

We thank the staff members at 480 primary health-care centers and 25 surgical departments in Sweden that participated in the study. Moreover, Gerd Bergmark, Christina Torefalk and Lisbeth Eriksson are acknowledged for the precious administrative support.

Author Contributions

Conceived and designed the experiments: MP SR LMSC. Performed the experiments: MP MAB AK. Analyzed the data: MP MAB SR LMSC PAS KS. Contributed reagents/materials/analysis tools: MP LMSC LS SR. Wrote the paper: MAB SR AK PAS KS JST AKL LS LMSC MP.

References

1. Clark JM, Brancati FL, Diehl AM (2003) The prevalence and etiology of elevated aminotransferase levels in the United States. Am J Gastroenterol 98: 960–967.
2. Torgerson JS, Lindroos AK, Sjöström CD, Olsson R, Lissner L, et al. (1997) Are elevated aminotransferases and decreased bilirubin additional characteristics of the metabolic syndrome? Obes Res 5: 105–114.

3. Wanless IR, Lentz JS (1990) Fatty liver hepatitis (steatohepatitis) and obesity: an autopsy study with analysis of risk factors. Hepatology 12: 1106–1110.
4. Adams LA, Lymp JF, St Sauver J, Sanderson SO, Lindor KD, et al. (2005) The natural history of nonalcoholic fatty liver disease: a population-based cohort study. Gastroenterology 129: 113–121.
5. Ekstedt M, Franzén LE, Mathiesen UL, Thorelius L, Holmqvist M, et al. (2006) Long-term follow-up of patients with NAFLD and elevated liver enzymes. Hepatology 44: 865–873.
6. Sjöström L, Lindroos AK, Peltonen M, Torgerson J, Bouchard C, et al. (2004) Lifestyle, diabetes, and cardiovascular risk factors 10 years after bariatric surgery. N Engl J Med 351: 2683–2693.
7. Dixon JB, Bhathal PS, O'Brien PE (2006) Weight loss and non-alcoholic fatty liver disease: falls in gamma-glutamyl transferase concentrations are associated with histologic improvement. Obes Surg 16: 1278–1286.
8. Del Genio F, Del Genio G, De Sio I, Marra M, Alfonsi L, et al. (2009) Noninvasive evaluation of abdominal fat and liver changes following progressive weight loss in severely obese patients treated with laparoscopic gastric bypass. Obes Surg 19: 1664–1671.
9. Silvestre V, Ruano M, Domínguez Y, Castro R, García-Lescun MC, et al. (2004) Morbid obesity and gastric bypass surgery: biochemical profile. Obes Surg 14: 1227–1232.
10. Stratopoulos C, Papakonstantinou A, Terzis I, Spiliadi C, Dimitriades G, et al. (2005) Changes in liver histology accompanying massive weight loss after gastroplasty for morbid obesity. Obes Surg 15: 1154–1160.
11. Mathurin P, Hollebecque A, Arnalsteen L, Buob D, Leteurtre E, et al. (2009) Prospective study of the long-term effects of bariatric surgery on liver injury in patients without advanced disease. Gastroenterology 137: 532–540.
12. Wolf AM, Beisiegel U (2007) The effect of loss of excess weight on the metabolic risk factors after bariatric surgery in morbidly and super-obese patients. Obes Surg 17: 910–919.
13. Mathurin P, Gonzalez F, Kerdraon O, Leteurtre E, Arnalsteen L, et al. (2006) The evolution of severe steatosis after bariatric surgery is related to insulin resistance. Gastroenterology 130: 1617–1624.
14. Johansson HE, Haenni A, Ohrvall M, Sundbom M, Zethelius B (2009) Alterations in proinsulin and insulin dynamics, HDL Cholesterol and ALT after gastric bypass surgery. A 42-months follow-up study. Obes Surg 19: 601–607.
15. Pontiroli AE, Pizzocri P, Librenti MC, Vedani P, Marchi M, et al. (2002) Laparoscopic adjustable gastric banding for the treatment of morbid (grade 3) obesity and its metabolic complications: a three-year study. J Clin Endocrinol Metab 87: 3555–3561.
16. Chavez-Tapia NC, Tellez-Avila FI, Barrientos-Gutierrez T, Mendez-Sanchez N, Lizardi-Cervera J, et al. (2010) Bariatric surgery for non-alcoholic steatohepatitis in obese patients. Cochrane Database Syst Rev: CD007340.
17. Sjostrom L, Larsson B, Backman L, Bengtsson C, Bouchard C, et al. (1992) Swedish obese subjects (SOS). Recruitment for an intervention study and a selected description of the obese state. Int J Obes Relat Metab Disord 16: 465–479.
18. Lindroos AK, Lissner L, Sjöström L (1993) Validity and reproducibility of a self-administered dietary questionnaire in obese and non-obese subjects. Eur J Clin Nutr 47: 461–481.
19. Kotronen A, Yki-Järvinen H, Männistö S, Saarikoski L, Korpi-Hyövälti E, et al. (2010) Non-alcoholic and alcoholic fatty liver disease - two diseases of affluence associated with the metabolic syndrome and type 2 diabetes: the FIN-D2D survey. BMC Public Health 10: 237.
20. Angulo P, Keach JC, Batts KP, Lindor KD (1999) Independent predictors of liver fibrosis in patients with nonalcoholic steatohepatitis. Hepatology 30: 1356–1362.
21. StataCorp: Stata Statistical Software. Release 9.0. College Station, TX: StataCorp LP 2005.
22. Sjöström L, Narbro K, Sjöström CD, Karason K, Larsson B, et al. (2007) Effects of bariatric surgery on mortality in Swedish obese subjects. N Engl J Med 357: 741–752.
23. Siest G, Schiele F, Galteau MM, Panek E, Steinmetz J, et al. (1975) Aspartate aminotransferase and alanine aminotransferase activities in plasma: statistical distributions, individual variations, and reference values. Clin Chem 21: 1077–1087.

11

Enhanced Recovery after Elective Open Surgical Repair of Abdominal Aortic Aneurysm: A Complementary Overview through a Pooled Analysis of Proportions

Sanderland J. T. Gurgel[1]*, Regina El Dib[2], Paulo do Nascimento, Jr.[3]

1 Department of Anesthesiology, Faculdade de Medicina de Botucatu, UNESP, Univ Estadual Paulista, Brazil; and UNINGÁ University, Maringá, Paraná, Brazil, **2** Department of Anesthesiology, Faculdade de Medicina de Botucatu, UNESP, Univ Estadual Paulista, Brazil; and McMaster Institute of Urology, McMaster University, Canada, **3** Department of Anesthesiology, Faculdade de Medicina de Botucatu, UNESP, Univ Estadual Paulista, Brazil

Abstract

Objectives: To evaluate the efficacy and safety of enhanced recovery after surgery (ERAS) programs in elective open surgical repair (OSR) of abdominal aortic aneurysm (AAA).

Background: Open surgical repair of AAA is associated with high morbidity and mortality, prolonged hospital stay and high costs. ERAS programs contribute to the optimization of treatment by reducing hospital stay and improving clinical outcomes.

Methods: A review of PubMed, EMBASE and LILACS databases was conducted. As only one randomized controlled trial was found, a pooled analysis of proportions from case series was conducted, considering it a complementary overview of the topic. Inclusion criteria were case series with more than five cases reported, adult patients who underwent an elective OSR of AAA and use of an ERAS program. ERAS was compared to conventional perioperative care. The pooled proportion and the confidence interval (CI) are shown for each outcome. The overlap of the CI suggests similar effect of the interventions studied.

Results: Thirteen case series studies with ERAS involving 1,250 patients were compared to six case series with conventional care with a total of 1,429 patients. The pooled, respective proportions for ERAS and conventional care were: mortality, 1.51% [95% CI: 0.0091, 0.0226] and 3.0% [95% CI 0.0183, 0.0445]; and incidence of complications, 3.82% [95% CI 0.0259, 0.0528] and 4.0% [95% CI 0.03, 0.05].

Conclusion: This review shows that ERAS and conventional care therapies have similar mortality and complication rates in OSR of AAA.

Editor: Giovanni Landoni, San Raffaele Scientific Institute, Italy

Funding: The authors have no support or funding to report.

Competing Interests: The authors have declared that no competing interests exist.

* E-mail: drsanderland@hotmail.com

Introduction

Elective open surgical repair of the abdominal aortic aneurysm (AAA) has been the most effective treatment to prevent its rupture when considering anatomically more complex aneurysms with a diameter greater than 5.5 cm. On the other hand, currently, endovascular aortic aneurysm repair is progressively replacing open surgical repair for the treatment of infrarenal AAA and now accounts for more than half of all AAA repairs [1]. The open surgical repair is a major procedure with extended surgical incisions that involves opening the abdomen for several hours and aortic clamping for graft interposition, requiring prolonged anesthetic/surgery time and, sometimes, blood transfusions. As a result, there may be an increased incidence of cardiorespiratory complications and prolonged intensive care unit length of stay, and a long period before returning to routine activities [2].

Recently, a more systematic perioperative approach targeting the reduction of costs and the improvement of outcomes, consisting of multimodal strategies has replaced conventional perioperative care. These new strategies involve a combination of various different treatments, i.e., a reduced fasting time, less invasive surgical procedures, a better strategy for postoperative pain control, use of short-acting anesthetics, ileus control and the rational use of invasive monitoring and intensive care treatment [3]. These strategies have been adopted mainly for colorectal surgeries [4], but also for nephrectomy [5], thyroidectomy [6] and hip arthroplasty [7] and are called enhanced recovery after surgery (ERAS) programs.

Due to a lack of clinical trials on comparing the use of ERAS with the conventional perioperative care for elective open surgical repair of AAA, a pooled analysis of proportions from case series studies [8,9] was performed to enable comparison of the available scientific evidence. This study sought to improve current practice and outline new potential directions for future research and the development of randomized controlled trials [10–12].

The rationale for this study is that a perioperative strategy to reduce costs and to improve short-term outcomes seems to be a very sensible choice when an elective open surgical repair of an AAA is performed.

Methods

A review of clinical case series with pooled analysis of proportions of patients in elective open surgical repair of AAA with the use of an ERAS program was performed. The method used in this study to perform the pooled analysis of proportions from case series was previously described in detail by El Dib et al., 2013 [13]. A database search with no language restriction was made on the following sources (last update July 2013): Pubmed (1966–2013), EMBASE (1980–2013) and LILACS (1982–2013). The search aimed to identify all case series concerning the use of ERAS programs or perioperative conventional care. The following comprehensive search strategy was used: ((ERAS OR enhanced recovery after surgery OR fast track OR multimodal rehabilitation OR hospital length of stay) AND (abdominal aortic aneurysm OR aortic aneurysm OR aortic surgery OR aortic repair)). The search strategy was adapted for each database to achieve more sensitivity.

The reference lists of all relevant papers and published review articles were searched. The online trials registers www.clinicaltrials.gov and www.controlled-trials.com for published and unpublished studies were also searched. After removing duplicates, the articles were selected to evaluate the title and abstract. Two reviewers (SJTG and PNJ) independently evaluated the titles and abstracts, and in the case of disagreement, a third reviewer (RED) was consulted for resolution. In case of a non-English written manuscript, a language expert was consulted for translation.

The following inclusion criteria were used: (i) case series studies with more than five reported cases with at least a 30-day follow-up; (ii) patients older than 18 years who underwent an elective open surgical repair of AAA; (iii) use of an ERAS program, defined as the use of at least four out of a total of 15 previously established items aiming to reduce hospital length of stay and hospital costs, or perioperative conventional care [14]; and (iv) a reported 30-day mortality, as the primary outcome.

Secondary outcome was the rate of complications or morbidity, defined as the absolute number of patients with at least one postoperative complication (acute myocardial infarction, characterized by electrocardiographic elevation of the ST segment above 0.1 mV in 2 leads, or biochemical elevation of CK-MB mass or troponin enzymes; renal failure, characterized by the need for renal replacement therapy; and stroke, defined as the change in consciousness or motor level developed postoperatively or proof of injury by brain imaging.

Due to the difficulty in defining conventional perioperative care, and although the comparison between endovascular repair and elective open surgical repair was not the focus of this systematic review, it was decided to use results for patients undergoing open surgical repair of AAA in studies where there was randomization and comparison with endovascular repair. This approach verified that the perioperative care provided to patients who underwent open surgical repair had not employed an ERAS strategy, but rather represented conventional care based on the best-available medical practice. Six randomized controlled trials were published between 2004 and 2011 comparing endovascular repair with open surgical repair. These data were summarized in a recently published meta-analysis [15].

If there were more than one published study on the same group of patients, the articles were analyzed to verify whether they reported different outcomes or not. If they presented the same outcome data, the data were extracted from the most recent or most complete article. The mean age and follow-up calculated in this study were based on the mean age and follow-up of each case series included in this review.

Statistical analysis

The morbidity and mortality rates for the case series studies were treated as dichotomous variables with their respective confidence intervals (CI) of 95%. Because of clear differences between the included studies and several uncontrollable variables, a random-effects model was used to perform the pooled analysis of proportions [16]. The program used to perform the meta-analysis was the StatsDirect (StatsDirect Ltd, UK) [8].

Forest plot charts were presented to summarize the data. Each horizontal line on the graph represents a case series included in the meta-analysis. The estimated effect is marked with a solid black square, and the size of the square represents the weight of the corresponding study plotted in the meta-analysis. The combined total estimate is marked with an unfilled diamond at the bottom of the forest plot. Combined proportionality and the 95% CIs are presented. The presence of an overlap of the confidence intervals from the two interventions, ERAS and conventional perioperative care, suggests similar effect of the interventions on the outcome. On the other hand, non-overlapping CIs suggest different effects from the interventions studied.

Results

The search was conducted until July 2013 and identified 1,440 titles. After screening by title and then abstract, we obtained full paper copies of 49 studies on ERAS and conventional perioperative care that were potentially eligible for inclusion in the review. However, most of these studies were either retrospective, animal studies, reviews, or did not evaluate a relevant clinical outcome. A total of 13 case series studies with 1,250 patients met all inclusion criteria and were selected for the pooled analysis of proportions (Figure 1).

The demographic characteristics and perioperative data are presented in Tables 1 and 2, respectively, for patients in which ERAS was performed. Data from the control group involving 1,429 patients treated with conventional perioperative care are shown in Table 3. The year of publication of the ERAS case series ranged from 1999 to 2011. The studies were distributed across North America, Europe and Asia. The mean patient age was 70 years, 84% were male, 62% were smokers, 63% had hypertension, 42% had prior heart disease and 11% were diabetic. The domains associated with ERAS programs are described in Table 4.

The pooled proportion in ERAS group from 13 case series studies with a total of 1,250 patients and in conventional perioperative care from six studies with a total of 1,429 patients were, respectively, and for each outcome (Figure 2): mortality, 1.51% [95% CI 0.0091, 0.0226] and 3% [95% CI 0.0183, 0.0445]; and incidence of complications (morbidity), 3.82% [95% CI 0.0259, 0.0528] and 4% [95% CI 0.03, 0.05].

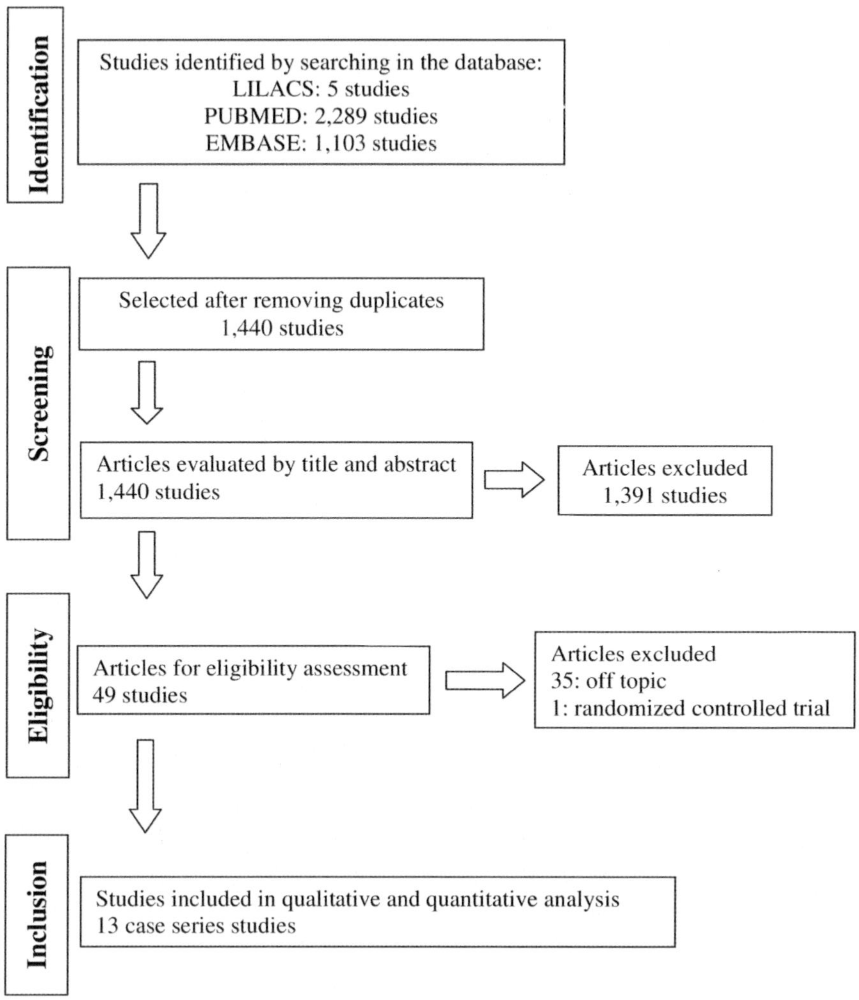

Figure 1. Flow chart showing the number of abstracts and articles identified and evaluated during the review process.

Subgroup analysis for incidence of complications is presented in Figure 3. The pooled proportion in ERAS group from 13 case series studies with a total of 1,250 patients and in conventional perioperative care from six studies with a total of 1,429 patients were, respectively: acute myocardial infarction, 1.77% [95% CI 0.0103, 0.0270] and 2.9% [95% CI 0.019, 0.042]; renal failure, requiring renal replacement therapy, 2.79% [95% CI 0.0159, 0.0432] and 0.69% [95% CI 0.0030, 0.0123]; stroke, 0.26% [95% CI 0.0005, 0.0063] and 1.8% [95% CI 0.0091, 0.0299].

Discussion

Systematic reviews of randomized controlled trials on therapeutic interventions are the best study design for decision-making in clinical practice. However, they often provide inconsistent evidence or uncertain conclusions, especially when there is a lack of randomized controlled trials [17,18]. For this reason, other strategies to deal with the absence of randomized controlled trials have become necessary.

In our search, just one randomized controlled trial comparing ERAS in elective open surgical repair of AAA to conventional perioperative care was identified [19]. Due to the lack of randomized controlled trials in this topic, we performed a pooled analysis of proportions from case series studies [8,9,13] as a complementary overview of this topic. The pooled analysis of proportions from case series provide support for clinical practice until high-quality primary studies are conducted, although clinical and methodological heterogeneity is observed due to the nature of case series studies [8,9,13].

This review identified 13 case series studies in which ERAS was used with the aim of accelerating postoperative recovery. A total of 1,250 individuals underwent ERAS programs, and their comorbidities correspond to those reported in the literature [20]. The difficulty in obtaining conventional perioperative care case series led our group decide to use the open surgical repair branch of studies randomized for comparison with endovascular aortic aneurysm repair. These data were summarized in a recently published meta-analysis [15], and their results with a 30-day follow-up were used in the present study. These patients' demographics were comparable to those of the ERAS case series (Tables 1 and 3).

The fact that the case series were reported in recent publications (1999 to 2011) along with their geographical distribution (five studies in North America, seven in Europe and one in Asia) demonstrates a global concern regarding the need to change the perioperative approach in AAA. Therefore, the study of case series due to the lack of randomized controlled trials in this field seems to

Table 1. Demographic data of case series studies of ERAS programs included in this review.

Study	Year	Country	n	Age, years mean (range)	Gender, male/female n/n	Smokers n (%)	Hypertension n (%)	Cardiac disease n (%)	Diabetes n (%)
Abularrage et al. [28]	2005	USA	30	68 (66–70)	25/5	23 (77%)	24 (80%)	14 (47%)	4 (13%)
Brustia et al. [29]	2007	Italy	323	70 (50–87)	294/29	–	–	–	–
Callaghan et al. [30]	2005	UK	178	72 (66–77)	156/22	57 (38%)	73 (48%)	45 (29%)	12 (8%)
Chang et al. [31]	2003	USA	240	69 (60–80)	171/69	208 (87%)	167 (70%)	113 (47%)	29 (12%)
Hafez et al. [32]	2011	UK	83	73 (61–87)	77/6	11 (13%)	48 (58%)	47 (57%)	13 (16%)
Ko et al. [33]	2004	China	10	73 (63–89)	7/3	–	8 (80%)	–	2 (20%)
Löhr et al. [34]	2008	Germany	35	71 (59–83)	31/4	–	–	–	–
Moniaci et al. [35]	2011	Italy	94	71 (63–79)	84/10	80 (85%)	84 (89%)	–	9 (10%)
Mukherjee et al [36]	2008	USA	30	67 (60–88)	25/5	–	–	–	–
Murphy et al. [37]	2007	UK	30	73 (50–89)	26/4	–	–	–	–
Podore et al. [38]	1999	USA	50	64 (40–88)	34/16	37 (74%)	26 (52%)	24 (48%)	3 (6%)
Renghi et al. [39]	2001	Italy	58	66 (55–75)	–	–	–	–	–
Rigberg et al. [40]	2004	USA	89	73	71/18	58 (65%)	58 (65%)	37 (42%)	13 (15%)
Total values, n (range or %)			1,250	70 (40–89)	1001 (84%)/191 (16%)	474 (62%)	488 (63%)	280 (42%)	85 (11%)

Table 2. Perioperative data from the case series studies included in review.

Study	Aortic diameter, cm (range)	Surgery length, min mean	Extubation site	ICU* length of stay, days mean	Morbidity rate† n (%)	Acute myocardial infarction n (%)	Renal failure n (%)	Stroke n (%)	Mortality rate n (%)	Hospital length of stay, days mean (range)
Abularrage et al. [28]	N/A‡	157	LMA§, OR‖	N/A	4 (13)	0	1 (3)	0	1 (3)	3 (1–7)
Brustia et al. [29]	N/A	175	OR	1	16 (5)	6 (2%)	10 (3)	0	8 (2%)	3 (1–21)
Callaghan et al. [30]	N/A	N/A	OR	1	85 (56)	N/A	10 (7)	0	2 (1)	12 (2–28)
Chang et al. [31]	5.9 (5.1–10)	150	OR	1	44 (18)	3 (1%)	2 (1%)	0	1 (0.5)	8 (4–28)
Hafez et al. [32]	6.8 (5.5–9)	N/A	ICU	1	18 (22%)	2 (2%)	2 (2%)	1 (1%)	2 (2%)	4 (2–88)
Ko et al. [33]	N/A	160	OR	N/A	0	0	0	0	0	5 (3–8)
Löhr et al. [34]	6.1 (5–8.5)	175	N/A	1	5 (15%)	1 (3%)	1 (3%)	0	0	N/A
Moniaci et al. [35]	N/A	N/A	OR	1	14 (15%)	1 (1%)	1 (1%)	0	2 (2%)	4 (2–17)
Mukherjee et al [36]	6.5 (5.5–8.4)	140	OR	1	2 (7%)	0	2 (7%)	0	1 (3%)	3 (3–7)
Murphy et al. [37]	N/A	N/A	PACU¶	N/A	18 (54%)	N/A	N/A	N/A	0	5 (2–12)
Podore et al [38]	6.1 (6.3–5.9)	216	OR	1	6 (12%)	1 (2%)	N/A	0	0	3 (2–8)
Renghi et al. [39]	5.5 (4.3–6.8)	151	LMA, OR	N/A	1 (2%)	0	0	0	0	7.6 (5–10)
Rigberg et al. [40]	N/A	N/A	N/A	N/A	7 (8%)	N/A	N/A	N/A	0	5 (2–11)
Total values n (range, mean or %)	6.15 (4.3–10)	165.5		1	220 (18%)	14 (1%)	29 (2%)	1 (0.1%)	17 (1%)	5.21 (1–88)

*ICU = intensive care unit;
†Morbidity rate = absolute number of patients with at least one complication described in the included article;
‡N/A = not applicable;
§LMA = laryngeal mask airway;
‖OR = operating room;
¶PACU = post anesthetic care unit.

Table 3. Perioperative data and demographics of patients submitted to elective open surgical repair of AAA from comparative studies with endovascular repair of AAA and submitted to conventional perioperative care.

Study	n	Age, years mean	Gender (male/female) n/n	Smokers n (%)	Hypertension n (%)	Cardiac disease n (%)	Diabetes n (%)	Aortic diameter, cm mean	Hospital length of stay, days mean	ICU[‖] length of stay, days mean	Mortality rate n
ACE[*] [41]	149	70	146/3	146 (98%)	95 (64%)	65 (44%)	29 (20%)	5.56	10.4	N/A[¶]	1
DREAM[†] [42–44]	178	70	161/17	161 (90%)	97 (55%)	83 (47%)	17 (10%)	6	10	1	8
EVAR-1[‡] [45–47]	626	74	570/56	580 (91%)	N/A	261 (42%)	68 (11%)	6.5	N/A	N/A	24
OVER[§] [48]	437	70	435/2	413 (94%)	330 (75%)	185 (42%)	100 (23%)	5.7	7	4	10
Soulez et al., 2005 [49]	20	71	20/0	16 (80%)	10 (50%)	14 (60%)	5 (25%)	5.1	11.5	1	0
Lottman et al., 2004 [50]	19	69	16/3	N/A	N/A	N/A	N/A	5.6	11	1	1
Total values n (range, mean or %)	1,429	70.6	1,348 (94%)/81 (6%)	1,316 (93%)	532 (68%)	608 (43%)	219 (15%)	5.7	10	1.7	44 (3%)

[*] ACE = Aneurysme de l'aorte abdominale; Chirurgie versus Endoprothese;
[†] DREAM = Dutch randomized Endovascular aneurysm management;
[‡] EVAR-1 = Endovascular aneurysm repair;
[§] OVER = Open versus endovascular repair;
[‖] ICU = intensive care unit;
[¶] N/A = not applicable.

Table 4. Description of the domains of the ERAS program for each included study.

Studies	1	2	3	4	5	6	7	8	9	10	11	12	13	14	15
Abularrage et al. [28]					X		X	X	X			X	X	X	X
Brustia et al. [29]	X			X		X	X	X	X	X		X	X	X	X
Callaghan et al. [30]	X						X			X		X			
Chang et al. [31]	X						X		X			X		X	X
Hafez et al. [32]	X						X		X			X	X	X	X
Ko et al. [33]							X	X				X	X	X	X
Löhr et al. [34]			X		X		X	X	X			X	X	X	X
Moniaci et al. [35]	X			X			X	X	X	X		X	X	X	X
Mukherjee et al. [36]	X				X		X	X	X			X	X	X	X
Murphy et al. [37]	X					X	X		X			X		X	X
Podore et al. [38]								X				X	X	X	X
Renghi et al. [39]	X			X		X	X	X		X		X		X	X
Riǵberg et al. [40]							X	X	X			X	X	X	X

1. Oral and written preadmission counseling and information.
2. Lack of routine preoperative bowel preparation.
3. Reduced fasting time plus carbohydrate loading.
4. Short-acting preanesthetic medication.
5. Prophylaxis against thromboembolism.
6. Antimicrobial prophylaxis.
7. Short-acting opioids/Epidural analgesia.
8. Prevention and treatment of postoperative nausea and vomiting.
9. Less invasive surgical incisions.
10. Prevention of intraoperative hypothermia.
11. Standardization of perioperative fluid management.
12. Judicious use of drains and catheters.
13. Prevention of postoperative ileus.
14. Postoperative nutritional care.
15. Early mobilization.

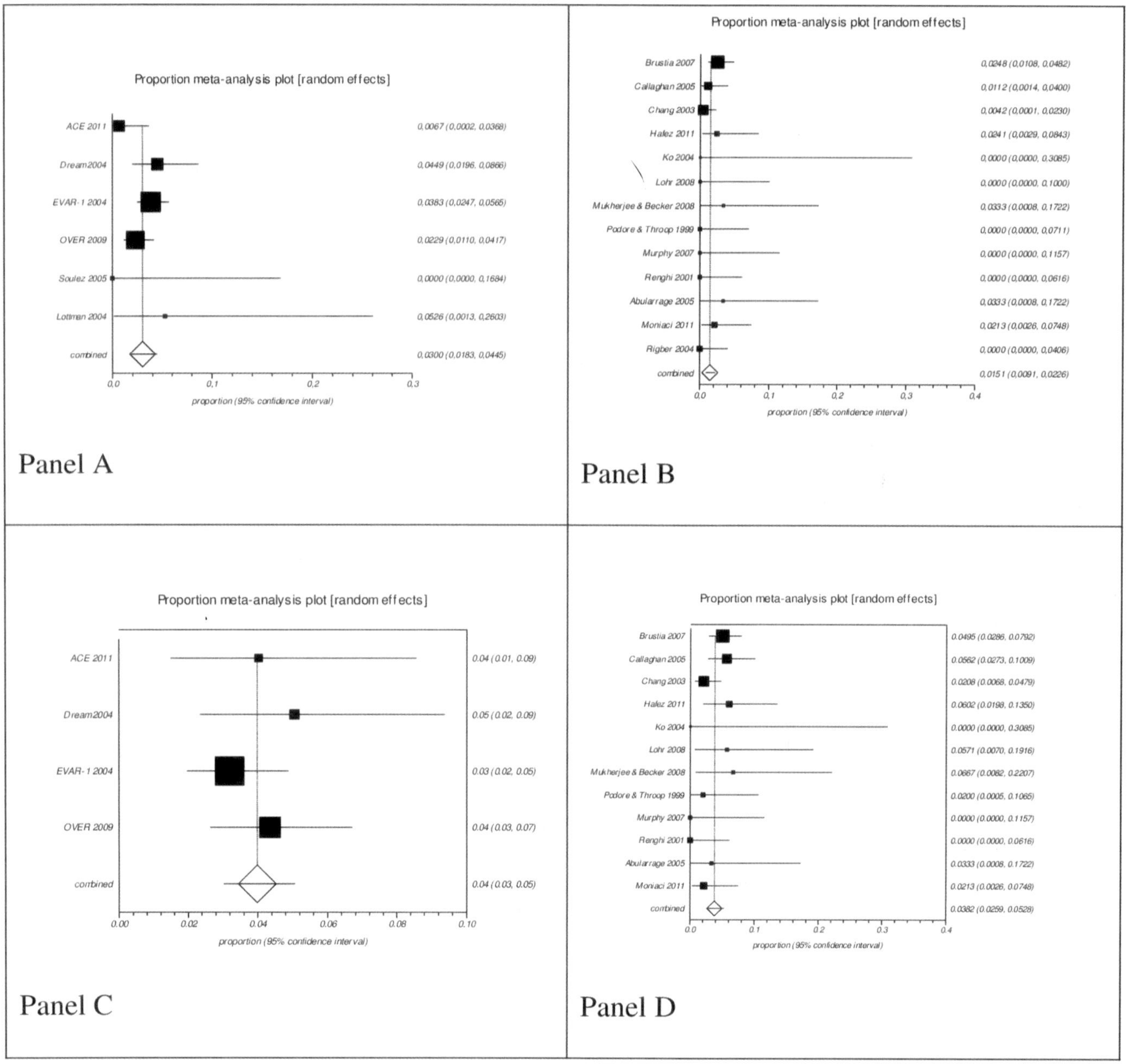

Figure 2. Pooled analysis of proportions from case series. Panel A: Conventional care series mortality; Panel B: ERAS series mortality; Panel C: Conventional care series morbidity; Panel D: ERAS series morbidity. Morbidity results are shown as the absolute number of patients with at least one complication, including acute myocardial infarction, renal failure and stroke. No effect differences were seen due to the overlap of the 95% confidence intervals.

be appropriate and allows a more comprehensive analysis of the collected available evidence.

The mean number of ERAS items for each of the 13 case series studies was eight, ranging from four to 13. Although the use of more items was suggested, only those formally described in the methodology of each study were used. The multimodal approach for enhanced recovery after surgery targets the reduction of overall stress, i.e., social, psychological and physical during the perioperative period, and reduces the time required for recovery [3,21,22].

AAA rupture is a catastrophic event with mortality rates reaching 80% [23]. The most commonly used predictor of rupture is the maximum diameter of the aneurysm (above 5.5 cm) [24]. Elective surgery together with a program to enhance recovery seems to be very rational as a better result at a lower cost would favor patients and health care system. The results of the pooled proportions showed a lower combined proportion in mortality rate in favor of ERAS (1.51%) compared to conventional perioperative care (3%). However, due to the overlap of their respective 95% confidence intervals, probably the effect of ERAS and conventional perioperative care on mortality rate is not different. The same observation is made for the overall incidence of complications. No effect difference was seen between ERAS (3.82%) and conventional perioperative care (4%). When analyzing the perioperative complications, it was verified that there was no

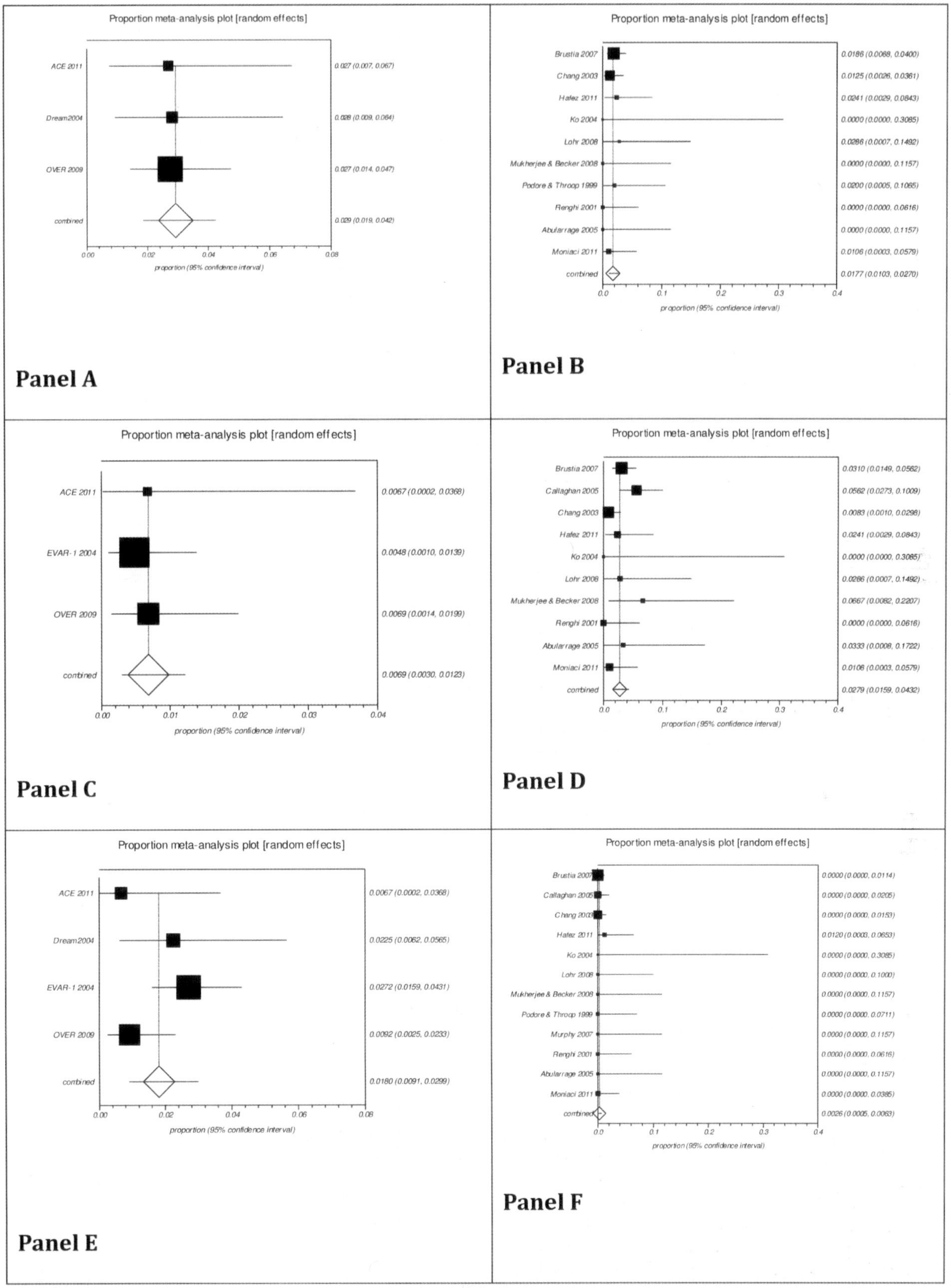

Figure 3. Pooled analysis of proportions from case series related to stratified morbidity. Panel A: Acute myocardial infarction, Conventional care series; Panel B: Acute myocardial infarction, ERAS case series; Panel C: Renal failure, Conventional care series; Panel D: Renal failure, ERAS case series; Panel E: Stroke, Conventional care series; Panel F: Stroke, ERAS case series. An effect difference was seen due to the non-overlap of the 95% confidence intervals in relation to renal failure (favoring conventional care) and stroke (favoring ERAS). No effect difference was seen due to the overlap of the 95% confidence interval considering incidence of acute myocardial infarction.

effect difference of the interventions on the incidence of acute myocardial infarction due to the overlap of the 95% confidence interval. On the other hand, an effect difference due to the non-overlap of the confidence intervals favored conventional perioperative care on renal failure incidence, but favored the ERAS group on stroke incidence.

The StatsDirect software used in the present study to perform the pooled analysis of proportions does not plot continuous variables and, for this reason, we were not able to analyze the effects of ERAS and conventional care on the hospital length of stay. An overview of this variable is shown on Tables 2 and 3.

Major surgeries such as elective open AAA repair are performed worldwide each year and account for a high utilization of financial resources, especially in developed countries [25]. The demand for the highest quality of health care, combined with the need for the rational use of both public and private resources, have become a challenge to the professionals to ensure quality and patient safety at the lowest cost [26]. As a result, ERAS programs tend to gradually replace the so-called conventional perioperative care, providing a more rational treatment.

Potential biases and high heterogeneity most likely occur in nonrandomized studies, and their results should be interpreted with caution. Particularly in our analysis, one potential source of bias is that ERAS series are reports of consecutive cases done by different groups of doctors, with a high chance of heterogeneity among individuals. On the other hand, the conventional perioperative care group (control group) was selected from randomized controlled trials and probably less heterogeneity in these subjects has occurred. When comparing very different and heterogeneous subjects, conclusions have to be made cautiously and the readers must be aware of this issue. Different subjects not randomly selected and not blinded to treatment may respond very differently to the same intervention, decreasing the external validity of the results. Then, the possibility of high heterogeneity in our study may have influenced the results. Due to the nature of the procedure, i.e., AAA repair, the patients tend to have the same clinical profile (age, gender, comorbidities) and probably similar diameter of the aorta, one of the criteria for surgical selection. We were careful when analyzing clinical characteristics of patients from both groups and verified that they had similar profile, tending to reduce the potential heterogeneity. We also considered the number of participants in both groups adequate for the comparison we proposed to do, understanding that the number of subject does not mean quality and homogeneity.

We are aware that this methodology, i.e., pooled analysis of proportions from case series and the estimate of the interventions results according to the overlap of the 95% confidence interval is not strong. Nonetheless, it is a strategy to analyze available data from case series. Some other reasons encourage performing a pooled analysis of proportions from case series studies [27]: support further randomized controlled trials evaluating the potential weaknesses of the topic under discussion, including the identification of relevant subgroups; provide evidence of either beneficial or harmful effects of an intervention that cannot be randomized; and provide evidence of either beneficial or harmful effects that cannot adequately be studied in randomized controlled trials, such as rare conditions or outcomes, and those requiring long follow-ups.

The pooled analysis of proportions from case series is an alternative approach for clinical research until well-conducted clinical trials are conducted. The health care professionals shoud weigh the benefits/risks profile of this approach and also take into consideration the patients' values and preferences.

Conclusions

The present pooled analysis of proportions from case series shows that ERAS programs and conventional perioperative care therapies are similar considering 30-day mortality and overall complication rates in elective open surgical repair of AAA. However, further and well-conducted randomized controlled trials are necessary to determine the real value of ERAS in elective open AAA surgery.

Author Contributions

Conceived and designed the experiments: STG RED PN. Performed the experiments: STG RED PN. Analyzed the data: STG RED PN. Contributed reagents/materials/analysis tools: STG RED PN. Wrote the paper: STG RED PN.

References

1. Chaikof EL, Brewster DC, Dalman RL, Makaroun MS, Illig KA, et al. (2009) SVS practice guidelines for the care of patients with an abdominal aortic aneurysm: executive summary. J Vasc Surg 50: 880–896.
2. Hirsch AT, Haskal ZJ, Hertzer NR, Bakal CW, Creager MA, et al. (2006) ACC/AHA 2005 Practice Guidelines for the management of patients with peripheral arterial disease (lower extremity, renal, mesenteric, and abdominal aortic): a collaborative report from the American Association for Vascular Surgery/Society for Vascular Surgery, Society for Cardiovascular Angiography and Interventions, Society for Vascular Medicine and Biology, Society of Interventional Radiology, and the ACC/AHA Task Force on Practice Guidelines (Writing Committee to Develop Guidelines for the Management of Patients With Peripheral Arterial Disease): endorsed by the American Association of Cardiovascular and Pulmonary Rehabilitation; National Heart, Lung, and Blood Institute; Society for Vascular Nursing; TransAtlantic Inter-Society Consensus; and Vascular Disease Foundation. Circulation 113: e463–654.
3. Kehlet H, Dahl JB (2003) Anaesthesia, surgery, and challenges in postoperative recovery. Lancet 362: 1921–1928.
4. Kehlet H (2008) Fast-track colorectal surgery. Lancet 371: 791–793.
5. Firoozfard B, Christensen T, Kristensen JK, Mogensen S, Kehlet H (2003) Fast-track open transperitoneal nephrectomy. Scand J Urol Nephrol 37: 305–308.
6. Sahai A, Symes A, Jeddy T (2005) Short-stay thyroid surgery. Br J Surg 92: 58–59.
7. Bertin KC (2005) Minimally invasive outpatient total hip arthroplasty: a financial analysis. Clin Orthop Relat Res: 154–163.
8. El Dib R, Touma NJ, Kapoor A (2012) Cryoablation vs radiofrequency ablation for the treatment of renal cell carcinoma: a meta-analysis of case series studies. BJU Int 110: 510–516.
9. El Dib RP, Touma N, Kapoor A (2012) A new approach to deal with the absence of clinical trials in systematic reviews: a meta-analysis of case series studies. 20th Cochrane Colloquium, New Zealand, Australia.
10. Albrecht J, Werth VP, Bigby M (2009) The role of case reports in evidence-based practice, with suggestions for improving their reporting. J Am Acad Dermatol 60: 412–418.
11. Albrecht J, Meves A, Bigby M (2005) Case reports and case series from Lancet had significant impact on medical literature. J Clin Epidemiol 58: 1227–1232.
12. Jenicek M (2008) Clinical case reports and case series research in evaluating surgery. Part II. The content and form: uses of single clinical case reports and case series research in surgical specialties. Med Sci Monit 14: RA149–162.
13. El Dib R, Nascimento Junior P, Kapoor A (2013) An alternative approach to deal with the absence of clinical trials: a proportional meta-analysis of case series studies. Acta Cir Bras 28: 870–876.
14. Lassen K, Soop M, Nygren J, Cox PB, Hendry PO, et al. (2009) Consensus review of optimal perioperative care in colorectal surgery: Enhanced Recovery After Surgery (ERAS) Group recommendations. Arch Surg 144: 961–969.
15. Dangas G, O'Connor D, Firwana B, Brar S, Ellozy S, et al. (2012) Open versus endovascular stent graft repair of abdominal aortic aneurysms: a meta-analysis of randomized trials. JACC Cardiovasc Interv 5: 1071–1080.
16. DerSimonian R, Laird N (1986) Meta-analysis in clinical trials. Control Clin Trials 7: 177–188.

17. Villas Boas PJ, Spagnuolo RS, Kamegasawa A, Braz LG, Polachini do Valle A, et al. (2013) Systematic reviews showed insufficient evidence for clinical practice in 2004: what about in 2011? The next appeal for the evidence-based medicine age. J Eval Clin Pract.
18. El Dib RP, Atallah AN, Andriolo RB (2007) Mapping the Cochrane evidence for decision making in health care. J Eval Clin Pract 13: 689–692.
19. Muehling B, Schelzig H, Steffen P, Meierhenrich R, Sunder-Plassmann L, et al. (2009) A prospective randomized trial comparing traditional and fast-track patient care in elective open infrarenal aneurysm repair. World J Surg 33: 577–585.
20. Lederle FA, Johnson GR, Wilson SE, Gordon IL, Chute EP, et al. (1997) Relationship of age, gender, race, and body size to infrarenal aortic diameter. The Aneurysm Detection and Management (ADAM) Veterans Affairs Cooperative Study Investigators. J Vasc Surg 26: 595–601.
21. Wilmore DW, Kehlet H (2001) Management of patients in fast track surgery. BMJ 322: 473–476.
22. Kehlet H, Wilmore DW (2002) Multimodal strategies to improve surgical outcome. Am J Surg 183: 630–641.
23. Nordon IM, Hinchliffe RJ, Loftus IM, Thompson MM (2011) Pathophysiology and epidemiology of abdominal aortic aneurysms. Nat Rev Cardiol 8: 92–102.
24. Norris EJ, Beattie C, Perler BA, Martinez EA, Meinert CL, et al. (2001) Double-masked randomized trial comparing alternate combinations of intraoperative anesthesia and postoperative analgesia in abdominal aortic surgery. Anesthesiology 95: 1054–1067.
25. Weiser TG, Regenbogen SE, Thompson KD, Haynes AB, Lipsitz SR, et al. (2008) An estimation of the global volume of surgery: a modelling strategy based on available data. Lancet 372: 139–144.
26. Haynes RB (1998) Using informatics principles and tools to harness research evidence for patient care: evidence-based informatics. Stud Health Technol Inform 52 Pt 1: suppl 33–36.
27. Deeks JJ, Dinnes J, D'Amico R, Sowden AJ, Sakarovitch C, et al. (2003) Evaluating non-randomised intervention studies. Health Technol Assess 7: iii–x, 1–173.
28. Abularrage CJ, Sheridan MJ, Mukherjee D (2005) Endovascular versus "fast-track" abdominal aortic aneurysm repair. Vasc Endovascular Surg 39: 229–236.
29. Brustia P, Renghi A, Fassiola A, Gramaglia L, Della Corte F, et al. (2007) Fast-track approach in abdominal aortic surgery: left subcostal incision with blended anesthesia. Interact Cardiovasc Thorac Surg 6: 60–64.
30. Callaghan CJ, Lynch AG, Amin I, Fazel M, Lindop MJ, et al. (2005) Overnight intensive recovery: elective open aortic surgery without a routine ICU bed. Eur J Vasc Endovasc Surg 30: 252–258.
31. Chang JK, Calligaro KD, Lombardi JP, Dougherty MJ (2003) Factors that predict prolonged length of stay after aortic surgery. J Vasc Surg 38: 335–339.
32. Hafez H, Makhosini M, Abbassi-Ghadi N, Hill R, Bentley M (2011) Transverse minilaparotomy for open abdominal aortic aneurysm repair. J Vasc Surg 53: 1514–1519.
33. Ko PJ, Hsieh HC, Liu YH, Liu HP (2004) Experience with early postoperative feeding after abdominal aortic surgery. Chang Gung Med J 27: 210–216.
34. Lohr G, Keller H, Kutscher J, Huber R (2008) [Fast-track rehabilitation after open aorto-iliac vascular procedures]. Zentralbl Chir 133: 344–348.
35. Moniaci D, Brustia P, Renghi A, Casella F, De Simeis L, et al. (2011) Abdominal aortic aneurysm treatment: minimally invasive fast-track surgery and endovascular technique. Vascular 19: 233–241.
36. Mukherjee D, Becker TE (2008) An update on the 'fast-track' abdominal aortic aneurysm repair. Int J Angiol 17: 93–97.
37. Murphy MA, Richards T, Atkinson C, Perkins J, Hands LJ (2007) Fast track open aortic surgery: reduced post operative stay with a goal directed pathway. Eur J Vasc Endovasc Surg 34: 274–278.
38. Podore PC, Throop EB (1999) Infrarenal aortic surgery with a 3-day hospital stay: A report on success with a clinical pathway. J Vasc Surg 29: 787–792.
39. Renghi A, Gramaglia L, Ciarlo M, Cerioli S, Albani A (2001) [Fast track in abdominal aortic surgery]. Minerva Anestesiol 67: 441–446.
40. Rigberg DA, Dorafshar A, Sridhar A, Quinones-Baldrich W, Moore WS (2004) Abdominal aortic aneursym: stent graft vs clinical pathway for direct retroperitoneal repair. Arch Surg 139: 941–944; discussion 945–946.
41. Becquemin JP, Pillet JC, Lescalie F, Sapoval M, Goueffic Y, et al. (2011) A randomized controlled trial of endovascular aneurysm repair versus open surgery for abdominal aortic aneurysms in low- to moderate-risk patients. J Vasc Surg 53: 1167–1173 e1161.
42. Blankensteijn JD, de Jong SE, Prinssen M, van der Ham AC, Buth J, et al. (2005) Two-year outcomes after conventional or endovascular repair of abdominal aortic aneurysms. N Engl J Med 352: 2398–2405.
43. De Bruin JL, Baas AF, Buth J, Prinssen M, Verhoeven EL, et al. (2010) Long-term outcome of open or endovascular repair of abdominal aortic aneurysm. N Engl J Med 362: 1881–1889.
44. Prinssen M, Verhoeven EL, Buth J, Cuypers PW, van Sambeek MR, et al. (2004) A randomized trial comparing conventional and endovascular repair of abdominal aortic aneurysms. N Engl J Med 351: 1607–1618.
45. EVAR trial participants (2005) Endovascular aneurysm repair versus open repair in patients with abdominal aortic aneurysm (EVAR trial 1): randomised controlled trial. Lancet 365: 2179–2186.
46. Greenhalgh RM, Brown LC, Kwong GP, Powell JT, Thompson SG, et al. (2004) Comparison of endovascular aneurysm repair with open repair in patients with abdominal aortic aneurysm (EVAR trial 1), 30-day operative mortality results: randomised controlled trial. Lancet 364: 843–848.
47. United Kingdom ETI, Greenhalgh RM, Brown LC, Powell JT, Thompson SG, et al. (2010) Endovascular versus open repair of abdominal aortic aneurysm. N Engl J Med 362: 1863–1871.
48. Lederle FA, Freischlag JA, Kyriakides TC, Padberg FT Jr, Matsumura JS, et al. (2009) Outcomes following endovascular vs open repair of abdominal aortic aneurysm: a randomized trial. JAMA 302: 1535–1542.
49. Soulez G, Therasse E, Monfared AA, Blair JF, Choiniere M, et al. (2005) Pain and quality of life assessment after endovascular versus open repair of abdominal aortic aneurysms in patients at low risk. J Vasc Interv Radiol 16: 1093–1100.
50. Lottman PE, Laheij RJ, Cuypers PW, Bender M, Buth J (2004) Health-related quality of life outcomes following elective open or endovascular AAA repair: a randomized controlled trial. J Endovasc Ther 11: 323–329.

12

Culture-Independent Evaluation of the Appendix and Rectum Microbiomes in Children with and without Appendicitis

Hope T. Jackson[1¶], Emmanuel F. Mongodin[2¶], Katherine P. Davenport[1¤a¤b], Claire M. Fraser[2], Anthony D. Sandler[3], Steven L. Zeichner[4,5*]

1 Sheikh Zayed Institute for Pediatric Surgical Innovation Children's National Medical Center, Washington DC, United States of America, **2** Institute for Genome Sciences, University of Maryland School of Medicine, Baltimore, Maryland, United States of America, **3** Department of Pediatric Surgery, and the Sheikh Zayed Institute for Pediatric Surgical Innovation Children's National Medical Center, Washington DC, United States of America, **4** Center for Cancer and Immunology Research, Children's Research Institute, Children's National Medical Center, Washington DC, United States of America, **5** Departments of Pediatrics and Microbiology, Immunology, and Tropical Medicine George Washington University, Washington DC, United States of America

Abstract

Purpose: The function of the appendix is largely unknown, but its microbiota likely contributes to function. Alterations in microbiota may contribute to appendicitis, but conventional culture studies have not yielded conclusive information. We conducted a pilot, culture-independent 16S rRNA-based microbiota study of paired appendix and rectal samples.

Methods: We collected appendix and rectal swabs from 21 children undergoing appendectomy, six with normal appendices and fifteen with appendicitis (nine perforated). After DNA extraction, we amplified and sequenced 16S rRNA genes and analyzed sequences using CLoVR. We identified organisms differing in relative abundance using ANOVA ($p<0.05$) by location (appendix vs. rectum), disease (appendicitis vs. normal), and disease severity (perforated vs. non-perforated).

Results: We identified 290 taxa in the study's samples. Three taxa were significantly increased in normal appendices vs. normal rectal samples: *Fusibacter* ($p=0.009$), *Selenomonas* ($p=0.026$), and *Peptostreptococcus* ($p=0.049$). Five taxa were increased in abundance in normal vs. diseased appendices: *Paenibacillaceae* ($p=0.005$), *Acidobacteriaceae GP4* ($p=0.019$), *Pseudonocardinae* ($p=0.019$), *Bergeyella* ($p=0.019$) and *Rhizobium* ($p=0.045$). Twelve taxa were increased in the appendices of appendicitis patients vs. normal appendix: *Peptostreptococcus* ($p=0.0003$), *Bilophila* ($p=0.0004$), *Bulleidia* ($p=0.012$), *Fusobacterium* ($p=0.018$), *Parvimonas* ($p=0.003$), *Mogibacterium* ($p=0.012$), *Aminobacterium* ($p=0.019$), *Proteus* ($p=0.028$), *Actinomycineae* ($p=0.028$), *Anaerovorax* ($p=0.041$), *Anaerofilum* ($p=0.045$), *Porphyromonas* ($p=0.010$). Five taxa were increased in appendices in patients with perforated vs. nonperforated appendicitis: *Bulleidia* ($p=0.004$), *Fusibacter* ($p=0.005$), *Prevotella* ($p=0.021$), *Porphyromonas* ($p=0.030$), *Dialister* ($p=0.035$). Three taxa were increased in rectum samples of patients with appendicitis compared to the normal patients: *Bulleidia* ($p=0.034$), *Dialister* ($p=0.003$), and *Porphyromonas* ($p=0.026$).

Conclusion: Specific taxa are more abundant in normal appendices compared to the rectum, suggesting that a distinctive appendix microbiota exists. Taxa with altered abundance in diseased and severely diseased (perforated) samples may contribute to appendicitis pathogenesis, and may provide microbial signatures in the rectum useful for guiding both treatment and diagnosis of appendicitis.

Editor: Daniel Paredes-Sabja, Universidad Andres Bello, Chile

Funding: This work was supported in part by grants DE021570 from NIDCR, NIH, AI090571 from NIAID, NIH,CA157417 from NCI, NIH, and the District of Columbia Developmental Center for AIDS Research P30AI087714, from NIAID, NIH. The funders had no role in study design, data collection and analysis, decision to publish, or preparation of the manuscript.

Competing Interests: The institutions employing the authors of the paper have filed a provisional patent application (Composition and Methods for Diagnosing Appendicitis; US Provisional Patent Application Serial No. 61/938,447) covering the discoveries reported in this manuscript. The institutions have not yet licensed the intellectual property and there are no products currently under development. The institutions employing the authors of the paper have intellectual property policies in place that say that inventors will be given a share of any income the institutions get from the inventions. There are no further patents, products in development or marketed products to declare.

* E-mail: zeichner@gwu.edu

¶ These authors contributed equally to this work.

¤a Current address: Department of Pediatric Surgery, Rady Children's Hospital San Diego, San Diego, California, United States of America
¤b Current address: Department of Surgery, University of California San Diego, San Diego, California, United States of America

Introduction

The physiologic function of the human appendix is largely unknown. Some hypotheses hold that the appendix plays a critical role in the education, development and maturation of the immune system [1,2]. Other studies suggest that the appendix may serve as a reservoir for beneficial components of the GI microbiome that can repopulate the GI tract following acute illness [3,4]. While these theories are intriguing, the detailed function of the appendix remains poorly understood, but likely involves interactions between the lymphoid tissue that exists in abundance in the appendix and the microbiota contained within the appendix. Shifts in the appendiceal microbiota are believed to play a key role in the pathophysiology of acute appendicitis, a common pediatric and adult disorder.

Acute appendicitis is a classic disease of the modern medical era. It is a paradigm for the application of increasingly sophisticated diagnostic, medical, and surgical technology. Appendicitis was one of the first acute non-traumatic disorders effectively cured by surgery [5]. Later, once it became available, antimicrobial therapy demonstrated great efficacy for the complications of perforated appendicitis [6]. Appendicitis affects ~77,000 patients/year in the US, with annual costs estimated at $680 million/year [7]. The lifetime risk of appendicitis has been estimated at 7% [8], with peak incidence occurring between 10 and 30 years of age, although as patients age, the characteristics of the disease may be clouded by other similarly presenting disorders. The incidence of appendicitis varies in different populations, in different regions, and over time [8,9,10]. The changing incidence has been attributed to a variety of environmental and behavioral factors that include general hygiene, parasitic infections, enteric infections resulting in GI lymphoid hyperplasia and variations in consumption of dietary fiber, but the definitive causes of appendicitis remain poorly understood.

The pathogenesis of appendicitis is classically thought to result, in part, from obstruction of the appendiceal lumen. Obstruction has been attributed to lymphoid hyperplasia, anatomic position, tumors and fecaliths, which are found in 11–52% of patients with acute appendicitis [11,12,13]. Obstruction is then thought to lead to an accumulation of undrained secretions, alteration and overgrowth of appendiceal microbes, compromised perfusion, and epithelial damage [9,14,15,16]. The precise sequence of events is not definitively established, but most authors count microbial overgrowth or distortion of the appendiceal microbial flora as key elements of the pathogenic cascade.

Several reports over many years have described the bacteriology of appendicitis [17,18,19,20,21,22,23]. These studies initially focused on using conventional culture techniques to study the bacteriology of the diseased appendix, the peritoneum and the surgical wound following appendiceal rupture. While some information has been published concerning the bacteriology of the diseased appendix, the bacteriology of the normal appendix is even less well understood, particularly at the complete microbiome level using culture-independent approaches. One study of quantitative bacterial colony counts using conventional techniques showed no differences between normal and inflamed appendices [20]. Another study identified *Bilophilia sp* as a new microbe from cultures of appendicitis samples, while another study identified *Fusobacterium sp* as the major microbe responsible for acute appendicitis using rRNA-based fluorescence in situ hybridization (FISH) [21,23]. A recent study [22] provided a culture-independent survey of the appendix using gene sequencing. This study examined seven patients presenting with signs and symptoms of appendicitis. The study found that the notable taxa in the appendix were *Firmicutes, Proteobacteria, Bacteroidetes, Actinobacteria, and Fusobacteria*, but only looked at those patients with suspected appendicitis. None of these studies have been extensively replicated.

While traditional, culture-based techniques have been used to characterize microbial populations [24,25], these conventional culture studies have not yielded conclusive information about the contribution of the appendix microbiota to health and disease. This is likely, at least in part, because standard culturing approaches do not furnish a complete picture of prokaryotic diversity, as more than 90–99% of the microbes are not culturable by standard techniques [26]. Based on the observation that 16S ribosomal RNA (rRNA) genes are highly conserved within species and among species of the same genus, knowledge of microbial diversity has expanded enormously as a result of applying recently developed 16S rRNA-gene sequencing-based culture-independent approaches [27,28,29].

We conducted a pilot study using a culture-independent 16S rRNA gene-based examination of the appendix microbiota in pediatric patients, with corresponding matched rectal samples from each patient. We studied both patients diagnosed as having appendicitis and patients undergoing appendectomy incidental to abdominal surgery for another indication. We catalogued and compared the relative abundance of bacterial genera in both healthy and diseased appendix samples, and in matched rectal samples. We found that the appendix microbiota significantly differs from the rectal microbiota, that the microbiota of the diseased appendix differs from the microbiota of the healthy appendix, and further that the microbiota of the appendix in appendicitis patients with a perforated appendix differs from the microbiota of the appendix in non-perforated appendicitis. Interestingly, we also found that the bacterial profile observed in the rectum differed between patients with normal appendices and appendicitis patients. Therefore, it may be possible that culture-independent microbial identification, particularly in rectal samples, could improve management of appendicitis, and suggest a new approach for possible appendicitis molecular diagnostics.

Materials and Methods

Study Participants

Following approval of the Children's National Medical Center IRB, we collected, with written consent from the parent or guardian, appendix and rectal swabs from 21 children undergoing appendectomy. The ages of participants ranged from 5 months to 18 years (8 males and 13 females) (Figure 1). Six patients had normal appendices and fifteen patients had appendicitis, nine of which were categorized as perforated based on pathology report. Seventeen patients underwent an appendectomy with an established or presumed diagnosis of acute appendicitis. The remaining four patients received an appendectomy incidental to another condition. Incidental appendectomies are common practice in the pediatric population, and in some situations considered a standard-of-care to help clarify a diagnosis or eliminate appendicitis from the differential diagnosis in a patient with a history of abdominal complaints or abnormal gastrointestinal anatomy. The most common presenting symptoms for the group of patients with appendicitis were nausea, vomiting, anorexia and abdominal pain. All participants, including patients who underwent incidental appendectomies, were given antibiotics within 24 hours of arrival at the hospital up until the time of surgery. See Figure 1 for a list of patient demographics and clinical data, including the antibiotics given to the patients.

Race	African-American: 3	Caucasian: 7	Hispanic: 6	Asian: 2	Other: 2	Not Documented: 11

	0-2	***3-5***	***6-10***	***11-15***	***16-18***
Age Range (years)	1	1	11	6	2

Gender	Male: 8	Female: 13
Most Common Presenting Symptoms	Abdominal pain, nausea, vomiting, anorexia	
Diagnostic Imaging Used	Computed Tomography: 9 Ultrasound: 9 None: 2 (incidental appendectomy) Upper GI: 1 (to diagnose malrotation, leading to incidental appendectomy)	
Average Length of Stay	2.8 days (range <24 hours to 6 days)	

Antibiotic Used	***Appendix Pathology***		
	Normal	Non-perforated	Perforated
Ertapenem (Invanz)	5	5	8
Ampicillin-Sulbactam (Unasyn)	–	1	1
Cefazolin (Ancef)	1	–	–

Figure 1. Participant demographics and clinical data. Of note, in those patients where an upper GI or no diagnostic imaging was performed, appendicitis was not the preoperative diagnosis and the appendectomy was incidental.

Sample Acquisition

Once each patient was taken to the operating room and placed under anesthesia, an internal swab of the patient's rectum was performed and stored using the Copan ESwab (Copan Diagnostics) collection and preservation system. After the appendix was resected, it was inspected and opened with Metzenbaum scissors. The full length of the opened appendix was swabbed with an ESwab and the swab was then placed in the transport container. The specimens were stored at −80 C until analysis.

Pathological Diagnosis

The diagnosis of appendicitis was established with pathological reports, which included both macro and microscopic examination of the appendix. Operative reports were reviewed for surgeon commentary on the macroscopic condition of the appendix (inflamed, injected, grossly perforated, normal). The clinical assessment of appendicitis of the surgeon and the pathologic diagnosis of appendicitis agreed in all cases.

DNA Extraction and 16S rRNA Gene Sequencing

Total genomic DNA was extracted using a protocol developed at the University of Maryland Institute for Genome Sciences and previously described [30]. Briefly, samples were thawed on ice, incubated in an enzymatic cocktail containing lysozyme, mutanolysin, proteinase K and lysostaphin, after which the microbial cells were lysed using bead beating with the FastPrep instrument (MBio, Santa Ana, CA). The DNA was then further extracted and purified using the Zymo Fecal DNA kit (Zymogen).

The variable regions V1–V3 of the 16S rRNA gene were PCR amplified using barcoded 27F and 338R 16S primers, as described previously [30]. Negative controls without a template were included for each barcoded primer pair. The presence of PCR amplicons was then confirmed by gel electrophoresis on a 2% agarose gel and staining with ethidium bromide. PCR products were quantified using the Quant-iT PicoGreen dsDNA assay, and equimolar amounts (100 ng) of PCR amplicons were pooled prior to pyrosequencing [30]. This 16S amplicon pool was sequenced by 454 FLX Titanium sequencing technology using 454 Life Sciences primer A by the Genomics Resource Center at the Institute for Genome Sciences, University of Maryland School of Medicine, using protocols recommended by the manufacturer as amended by the Center.

16S sequence analysis and Statistical Analyses

The pipeline CloVR-16S version 1.1 within the CLoVR system (www.CLoVR.org) [31] was used to bin the raw 16S reads using the sample-specific barcode sequences, then trim the barcode and primer sequences, and process the resulting sequences for phylogenetic analyses (for more information about the CLoVR-16S workflow, see http://clovr.org/methods/clovr-16s/). The average read length after barcode and primer trimming was 368 bp. Statistical analysis of differentially abundant bacterial taxa in the 16S rRNA sequence dataset was performed using the METASTATS tool within CLoVR (http://clovr.org/docs/metastats/). We identified organisms that differed significantly (ANOVA, $p<0.05$) in relative abundance by anatomic location (appendix vs. rectum), disease state (appendicitis vs. normal) and disease severity (perforated vs. non-perforated).

The 16S sequencing data for all the samples analyzed in this study was submitted to the Sequence Read Archive (SRA; http://www.ncbi.nlm.nih.gov/Traces/sra/), under accession SRP035179.

Results

In this pilot study aimed at characterizing the microbiota associated with the appendix, matched appendix and rectal swabs were collected from 21 children (age range: 5 months–18 years), six with normal appendices and 15 with appendicitis, out of which nine were perforated. A total of 42 samples were processed and DNA extracted. rRNA gene sequences were PCR amplified using the 27F and 338R bacterial primers, and the PCR amplicons were sequenced using 454 Titanium pyrosequencing. Out of these 42 samples, 5 samples did not yield enough PCR amplicons, and were subsequently removed from the analysis. From the remaining 37 samples that were successfully PCR-amplified and sequenced, we obtained a total of 325,342 non-chimeric sequences (8,793±3888 reads on average per sample) that were assigned to a total of 13,751 unique operational taxonomic units (OTUs) using a cutoff of 95% sequence identity. The CloVR-16S v. 1.1 (http://clovr.org/methods/clovr-16s/) automated analysis pipeline was used to process the raw 454 pyrosequencing reads, perform taxonomic assignments and calculate microbial diversity and richness indices.

Median values of bacterial community richness and diversity calculated for samples groups are displayed in Table 1 (for individual values by samples, see Figure S1 in File S1). The observed number of OTUs (sobs calculator in mothur) was the highest for the rectal samples, compared to appendix (median values: 446 *vs.* 237 OTUs). Among the rectal samples, the bacterial communities associated with perforated appendicitis were characterized by the highest number of observed OTUs (478 OTUs), compared to non-perforated appendicitis rectal samples (411 OTUs), and rectal samples from subjects with a normal appendix (220 OTUs). Among the appendix samples, the number of observed OTUs was the highest for the appendix samples from subjects with perforated appendicitis (344 OTUs), appendix samples from patients with non-perforated appendicitis had 228 OTUs. Appendix samples from patients with a normal appendix had 237 OTUs. According to these observations, severity in diagnosis of appendicitis seems to be characterized by a greater observed bacterial richness (sobs calculator), for both appendix and rectal bacterial communities.

In order to further characterize the bacterial biodiversity of the samples analyzed in this study, richness and diversity estimators were calculated. These ecological indices have classically been used to gain insight about bacterial community structures when using 16S rRNA gene datasets. Community richness, through the use of the Chao1 and ACE estimators, provides information about the estimated number of OTUs present in the samples. Measure of the community diversity, through the use of the Shannon and Simpson indices, provide information about the composition of a given bacterial community, e.g. not only a measure of richness but also take into account the relative abundance of OTUs (or evenness). The Chao1 and ACE richness estimators confirmed the observations previously made using the sobs calculator: sample richness was higher for rectal samples compared to appendix, and for perforated appendicitis rectal and appendix samples compared to normal rectal and appendix samples (Table 1). The Shannon diversity index displayed a similar trend with rectal samples displaying a higher diversity compared to appendix samples, and with diversity being the highest for increasing severity of appendicitis diagnosis, for both rectal and appendix samples (Table 1). The Simpson index showed an opposite trend, as expected.

The similarity in microbial composition among the samples analyzed in the present study was further compared using the Bray-Curtis algorithm [32,33], an abundance-weighted measure of how similar two communities are in terms of their taxonomic composition. Communities were clustered using an average-linkage algorithm, and the results are presented in the cluster dendogram in Figure 2. Out of the 37 samples analyzed (16 rectal samples and 20 appendix samples), 13 appendix samples clustered together (green box in Figure 2). The appendix cluster was composed almost entirely (12 samples out of 13 samples belonging to that cluster) of samples from patients with appendicitis, both non-perforated and perforated appendicitis, suggesting that the appendix microbiota associated with appendicitis differs from the normal appendix. A second group of 10 samples, composed entirely of rectal samples (blue oval in Figure 2), clustered separately. For the rectal sample cluster, 8 samples out of 10 samples belonging to that cluster were from appendicitis samples, from patients with both non-perforated and perforated appendicitis, suggesting that an alteration in the appendix microbiota of patients with appendicitis is reflected in an corresponding

Table 1. Diversity and Richness Estimators (median values).

	N	Observed Number of OTUs (sobs calculator)	Chao1 (Richness)	ACE (Richness)	Shannon (Diversity)	Simpson
Appendix	20	237	507.621	911.130	2.742	0.150
Rectal	17	446	957.621	1371.363	3.534	0.083
Appendix: Normal	5	237	463.622	804.885	2.742	0.150
Appendix: Non Perforated Appendicitis	6	228	542.096	921.922	2.557	0.178
Appendix: Perforated Appendicitis	9	344	750.978	1241.873	3.041	0.100
Rectal: Normal Appendix	5	220	373.867	604.679	2.312	0.206
Rectal: Non Perforated Appendicitis	6	411	884.560	1363.194	3.779	0.056
Rectal: Perforated Appendicitis	6	478	1101.720	1680.009	3.756	0.078

Microbial diversity and richness indices. Median values of bacterial community richness and diversity calculated for samples groups are displayed. The observed number of OTUs was highest for the rectal samples, compared to appendix. Among the rectal samples, samples from subjects with perforated appendicitis had the highest number of observed OTUs (478 OTUs), compared to non-perforated appendicitis (411 OTUs) and subjects with normal appendix (220 OTUs). Similarly, with respect to the appendix samples, samples from subjects with perforated appendicitis had the highest number of observed OTUS (344 OTUs), compared to non-perforated appendicitis and normal appendix (228 and 237 OTUs, respectively). This suggests that severity in diagnosis of appendicitis seems to be characterized by a higher number of observed OTUs, compared to normal appendices. The rectal samples from patients with appendicitis also had a larger number of OTUs than samples from patients with normal appendices. Rectal samples from patients with perforated appendicitis had a larger number of OTUs than samples from patients with non-perforating appendicitis. The Chao1 and ACE richness estimators also showed that sample richness was higher for rectal samples compared to appendix samples. Chao1 and ACE richness estimators also showed greater richness for rectal samples from patients with appendicitis than samples from patients with normal appendices. The richness estimators for the rectal samples were higher for patients with perforating appendicitis than for patients with non-perforating appendicitis. The Shannon diversity index displayed a similar trend with rectal samples displaying a higher diversity compared to appendix samples, and with diversity was highest for samples from patients with the most severe form of appendicitis, for both rectal and appendix samples.

alteration in the microbiota of the rectum. There was only one pair of rectal-appendix samples from the same subject, who did not have appendicitis (subject 10; red arrows in Figure 2) that clustered together. None of the other paired appendix and rectal samples from other patients clustered together, reinforcing the observation that the appendix and rectal microbiota have significant differences.

Taxonomic assignments of the 16S sequences revealed 290 different bacterial taxa across all the samples (Tables 1–5). The relative Phyla and Genus abundance in each sample are shown in Figures S2 and S3 in File S1. The Metastats program was used for detection of differentially abundant taxa between the appendix and rectal sites, between the appendix of patients with and without appendicitis, and between the rectum of patients with and without appendicitis (Table 2). In patients without appendicitis we observed three taxa with a statistically significant increased presence in the normal appendix compared to corresponding rectal samples: *Fusibacter* ($p = 0.009$), *Selenomonas* ($p = 0.026$), and *Peptostreptococcus* (0.049). In patients without appendicitis we also observed a statistically significant increase in abundance in seven taxa in the rectum compared to the appendix: *Frankineae* ($p = 0.019$), *Dyadobacter* ($p = 0.019$), *Actinomycineae* ($p = 0.033$), *Curvibacter* ($p = 0.042$), *Melissococcus* ($p = 0.042$), *Variovorax* ($p = 0.042$) and *Larkinella* ($p = 0.042$).

In comparing patients with and without appendicitis, we found that five taxa showed a statistically significant increase in the normal appendix when compared to diseased appendices: *Paenibacillaceae* ($p = 0.005$), *Acidobacteriaceae* GP4 ($p = 0.019$), *Pseudonocardinae* ($p = 0.019$), *Bergeyella* ($p = 0.019$) and *Rhizobium* ($p = 0.045$) (Table 3). When comparing normal appendices to diseased samples, we found twelve taxa with increased abundance in appendicitis: *Peptostreptococcus* ($p = 0.0003$), *Bilophila* ($p = 0.0004$), *Bulleidia* ($p = 0.012$), *Fusobacterium* ($p = 0.018$), *Parvimonas* ($p = 0.003$), *Mogibacterium* ($p = 0.012$), *Aminobacterium* ($p = 0.019$), *Proteus* ($p = 0.028$), *Actinomycineae* ($p = 0.028$), *Anaerovorax* ($p = 0.041$), *Anaerofilum* ($p = 0.045$), *Porphyromonas* ($p = 0.010$) (Table 3).

Comparing the taxa found in the rectal samples between the patients with and without appendicitis, we found three taxa with increased abundance in the rectal samples of those with appendicitis: *Bulleidia* ($p = 0.034$), *Dialister* ($p = 0.003$) and *Porphyromonas* ($p = 0.026$) (Table 4). These taxa overlap with those taxa identified in the appendix, and the finding suggests that there may be a microbial signal evident in rectal samples indicative of appendicitis.

Looking more closely at the appendicitis cases, we compared non-perforated and perforated samples to determine whether any flora were over or under-represented in the most severe form of appendicitis, perforated appendicitis. We found that five genera showed a significant increase in the perforated group: *Bulleidia* ($p = 0.004$), *Fusibacter* ($p = 0.005$), *Prevotella* ($p = 0.021$), *Porphyromonas* ($p = 0.030$), *Dialister* ($p = 0.035$) (Table 5). The observation that taxa found to have increased abundance in the most severe form of appendicitis includes taxa that were also found to be increased in abundance in the rectums of appendicitis patients compared to the rectums of patients without appendicitis further strengthens the model that microbial analysis of rectal samples can provide helpful diagnostic insights into disease in the appendix.

Figure 3 shows a schematic of the genera showing significant differences comparing the appendix and rectal sites and comparing patients with and without appendicitis. We found no significant differences in relative abundance across gender, race or age.

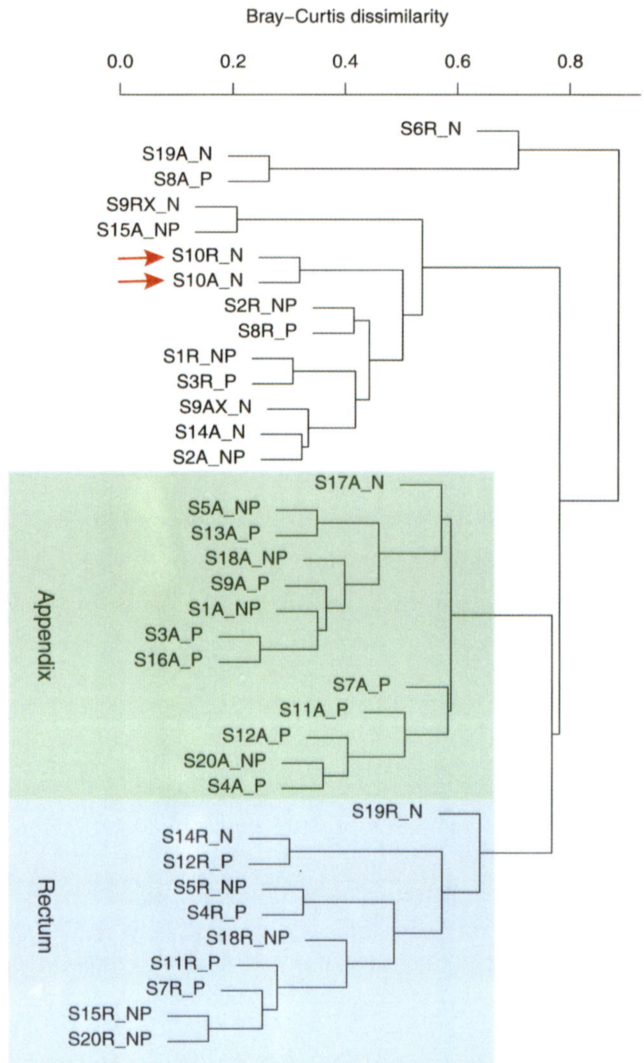

Figure 2. Bray-Curtis Cluster Dendogram. This abundance-weighted measures how similar two communities are in terms of their genus composition using the Bray-Curtis metric [32,33]. 37 samples were analyzed (16 rectal samples and 20 appendix samples). 13 appendix samples clustered together (green box). A group of 10 rectal samples (blue box) clustered separately from the appendix samples, suggesting that the microbiome of the rectum differs from the microbiome of the appendix. Only one pair of rectal-appendix samples from the same subject (subject 10; red arrows) clustered together. The appendix cluster (green box) was composed almost entirely (12 out of 13 samples) of appendicitis samples, both non-perforated and perforated, suggesting that the appendix microbiome associated with appendicitis differs from the microbiome of the normal appendix. For the rectal sample cluster, 8 samples out of 10 samples from patients with appendicitis, both non-perforating and perforating, clustered together, suggesting that the microbiome of the rectum in patients with appendicitis is distinct from the microbiome of the rectum from patients without appendicitis. Samples are listed by ID number, SnX/Y, where n is the subject identification number, X describes the body site (A for appendix, R for rectum), and Y describes the patient's diagnosis (N for normal appendix, NP for an appendix with non-perforating appendicitis, and P for an appendix with perforating appendicitis).

Discussion

Appendicitis is the most common surgical emergency. It will affect approximately 8% of persons living in Western countries at

Table 2. Bacterial Genera with Significantly Different Abundance in the Normal Appendix vs. Normal Rectum.

Bacteria	Rectum	Appendix	P-value
Fusibacter	0	0.12%+/−0.07%	**0.009**
Frankineae	0.008%+/−0.008%	0	**0.019**
Dyadobacter	0.008%+/−0.008%	0	**0.019**
Selenomas	0	0.03%+/−0.02%	**0.026**
Actinomycineae	1.66%+/−0.92%	0.065+/−0.025%	**0.033**
Melissococcus	0.007%+/−0.007%	0	**0.042**
Curvibacter	0.007%+/−0.007%	0	**0.042**
Variovorax	0.007%+/−0.007%	0	**0.042**
Larkinella	0.007%+/−0.007%	0	**0.042**
Peptostreptococcus	0.016%+/−0.016%	0.32%+/−0.19%	**0.049**

Relative abundance percentage (+/− standard error) of taxa in the normal rectum and normal appendix. The normal appendix had 3 bacteria with significantly elevated abundance compared to the normal rectum.

Table 3. Bacterial Genera with Significantly Different Abundance in the Normal Appendix vs. the Appendix in Appendicitis Patients.

Bacteria	Normal Appendix	Appendicitis	P-value
Peptostreptococcus	0.32%+/−0.19%	5.07%+/−1.2%	**0.0003**
Bilophila	0.07%+/−0.06%	0.88%+/−0.21%	**0.0003**
Parvimonas	4.38%+/−3.61%	23.9%+/−5.33%	**0.003**
Paenibacillaceae 1	0.03%+/−0.03%	0	**0.005**
Porphyromonas	0.58%+/−0.43%	4.56%+/−1.54	**0.010**
Bulleidia	0.70%+/−0.45%	3.79%+/−1.21%	**0.012**
Mogibacterium	0.003%+/−0.002%	0.04%+/−0.01%	**0.012**
Fusobacterium	1.04%+/−0.67%	3.21%+/−0.69	**0.018**
Acidobacteriaceae Gp4	0.019%+/−0.019%	0	**0.018**
Pseudocardineae	0.026%+/−0.026%	0.00105%+/−0.00105%	**0.019**
Bergeyella	0.0086%+/−0.0086%	0.0019%+/−0.0019%	**0.019**
Aminobacterium	0.004%+/−0.004%	0.13%+/−0.05%	**0.019**
Proteus	0	0.015%+/−0.015%	**0.028**
Actinomycineae	0.060%+/−0.025%	1.42%+/−0.65%	**0.028**
Anaerovorax	0.14%+/−0.08%	0.37%+/−0.08%	**0.042**
Rhizobium	0.026%+/−0.026%	0.0017%+/−0.0017%	**0.045**
Anaerofilum	0.01%+/−0.0044%	0.04%+/−0.013%	**0.045**

Taxa with significant relative abundance percentage differences in the normal vs. diseased appendix. Relative abundance (percent, +/− standard error) of bacteria in the normal appendix and appendicitis. The normal appendix had 5 bacteria with significantly elevated abundance compared to the diseased appendix.

some point in their lifetimes. Despite the frequent occurrence of appendicitis, our understanding of the normal function and physiology of the appendix remains limited. While the findings we present are more extensive than previously published studies that used more limited culture techniques or FISH, our results are consistent with those previous results, which identified *Bilophilia* and *Fusobacterium* in the appendix via culture techniques and FISH respectively [21,23]. Our 16S rRNA gene sequencing-based study results are also are consistent with the identification of *Fusobacterium* and *Parvimonas* as notable genera in the appendix microbiota [22], but the results we present also identified additional bacterial genera, not previously reported, which are found in the microbial community of the appendix, healthy and diseased. The first reported gene sequencing study examined those patients being evaluated for appendicitis while the current study observed those being evaluated for appendicitis as well as those without appendicitis, enabling a comparison to the normal appendix microbiota. It might have been desirable from a purely scientific point of view to study patients who had not been treated with antibiotics, since antibiotics could conceivably distort the composition of the appendiceal microbiota; however this would have been ethically impossible because antibiotics are considered an important element of the standard-of-care treatment of patients with suspected appendicitis, and for any patient undergoing laparotomy or laparoscopy with a surgical resection of the GI tract. While antibiotics could have altered the composition of the microbiota it is important to note that all patients were given antibiotics: patients with suspected appendicitis who were found to have appendicitis by pathologic examination, patients with clinically suspected appendicitis who were found to not have appendicitis by pathologic examination, and patients who underwent incidental appendectomy, since it is standard-of-care to give patients perioperative prophylactic antibiotics. In addition, since our study employed DNA sequence analysis of the relatively short 16S rRNA gene, not living bacterial cells, since DNA is reasonably stable, and since the time between antibiotic administration and surgery was short, it is unlikely that the administration of antibiotics substantially altered our findings. Another possible confounder is the single 5 month old infant who was included in the control group, and who underwent surgery to rule out malrotation. Since the infant GI microbiota changes significantly during development [34], the microbiota of a 5 month old may not be strictly comparable to the microbiota of an older child or an adult, but we do not believe that the inclusion of this single control subject substantially alters the conclusions of the study.

Our results show that the microbial community of the appendix is distinct from the microbial community observed in the rectal samples, suggesting that the appendix and rectum are two quite different environments, and hence support two different microbial communities. Comparing the normal appendix to the normal rectum, the normal appendix exhibits an elevated abundance of *Selenomonas*, *Fusobacterium*, and *Streptococcus*, while the normal rectum has an increased abundance of *Frankineae*, *Dyadobacter*, *Curvibacter*, *Melissococcus*, *Variovorax*, *Larkinella*, and *Actinomycineae* compared to the normal appendix. Interestingly, *Selenomonas*, in the family Veillonellaceae is perhaps best known as a colonizer of the anaerobic environment of the ruminant rumen and guinea pig cecum and while not fibrinolytic itself works in synergy with other fibrinolytic bacteria to promote dietary fiber digestion [35]. *Selenomonas* is also known as a genus that colonizes gingival pockets and is associated with severe periodontitis [36]. If the model that the appendix serves as a reservoir for beneficial microbiota is correct, then given the observation that GI microbial metabolism serves as a source of small, but significant fraction of human nutrition, then *Selenomonas* provided by the appendix may be partially responsible. *Fusobacterium* is a well-known colonizer of mammalian mucous membrane compartments. Some *Fusobacterium sp* can ferment carbohydrates and amino acids to produce butyrate and acetic acids [37]. *Fusobacterium sp* can also, however, cause invasive infections, have been implicated in periodontal

Table 4. Bacterial Genera with Significantly Different Abundance in the Rectum of Patients With and Without Appendicitis.

Bacteria	Rectum w/o Appendicitis	Rectum w/Appendicitis	P-value
Bulleidia	0.0021%+/−0.0021%	0.0238%+/−0.11%	**0.034**
Porphyromonas	0.103%+/−0.091%	0.65%+/−0.23%	**0.026**
Dialister	0.066%+/−0.037%	0.77%+/−0.23%	**0.003**

Relative abundance (percent, +/− standard error) of taxa in the rectal samples from patients without appendicitis and rectal samples with appendicitis.

disease and are an important agent in Lemierre's syndrome [38,39]. *Peptostreptococcus* is an anaerobic, typically commensal species in humans that lives predominantly in the mouth, skin, gastrointestinal, vagina and urinary tracts. This species can become pathogenic under immunosuppressed or traumatic conditions [40,41].

While the microbial species identified as having different abundances in the normal and diseased appendix are interesting and could conceivably be responsible either for the disease itself or sequellae associated with the disease, it is important to note that our study identifies associations only, and cannot definitively assign causality. Another important consideration is that some of the taxa we identified as being differentially present in the different specimen types and/or disease states were of relatively low abundance, which may make it more challenging to determine the exact contribution these low abundant taxa make to the pathogenesis of appendicitis or to the diagnosis of appendicitis. However, it is important to note that presence at low abundance certainly does not rule out the possibility that a microbe plays an important part in disease pathogenesis. For example, in an experimental model of *Shigella* infection, *Shigella* was by far a minority taxon in the GI tract, even though clinical effects were clearly evident [42].

Much work has studied the microbial communities of feces or the lower GI tract for clues to the pathogenesis of disease in more proximal regions of the GI tract [29,43,44]. This is mainly because fecal material can be collected easily, noninvasively and contains a large number of microbial cells. While these studies have yielded important information, our findings that the community observed in the rectum differs substantially from the community observed in the appendix suggests that the rectal microbial community may not be a completely valid window into the microbial physiology of more proximal areas of the GI tract. This may need to be taken into account in designing future, more extensive studies of the lower GI tract microbiota.

Table 5. Bacterial Genera with Significantly Different Abundance in the Appendix of Patients with Perforated Appendicitis vs. Appendicitis Without Perforation.

Bacteria	Perforated Appendicitis	Appendicitis	P-value
Bulleidia	5.72%+/−1.72%	0.88%+/−0.58%	**0.005**
Fusibacter	0.29%+/−008%	0.05%+/−0.04%	**0.005**
Prevotella	7.66%+/−1.82%	2.77%+/−1.53%	**0.022**
Porphyromonas	6.50%+/−2.32%	1.65%+/−0.99%	**0.032**
Dialister	0.97%+/−0.30%	0.26%+/−0.23%	**0.003**

Bacteria with significant relative abundance percentage differences in appendix samples from patients with perforated vs. non perforated appendicitis.

The bacteria in the normal and diseased appendix differ from those isolated in normal rectal samples with the exception of *Actinomycineae*, which was found to be significantly abundant in both appendicitis and normal rectal samples. Interestingly, two of the bacteria identified in non-perforated appendicitis were also identified in significant quantities in corresponding rectal samples (*Bulleidia* and *Porphyromonas*) and three of the five bacteria identified in perforated appendicitis were identified in corresponding rectal samples (*Bulleidia, Porphyromonas and Dialister*). Thus, identification of *Bulleidia*, *Porphyromonas* and *Dialister* in the rectum may be a secondary indicator of appendicitis, an indicator that could conceivably be used to develop diagnostics for appendicitis, although the clinical significance of such indicator bacterial species would have to be confirmed by larger scale prospective clinical studies.

The bacteria identified in the normal and diseased appendix include organisms several of which are found in the healthy human microbiota in many sites, including the gastrointestinal tract, upper respiratory tract, vagina and oral cavity. If the human host is compromised (in this case, secondary to appendiceal obstruction causing bacterial overgrowth), many of these organisms may be involved in bacteremia and septicemia (ie. *Peptostreptococcus, Bilophila, Fusobacterium, Parvimonas, Proteus, Dialister, Prevotella, Porphyromas*) [45,46]. A study by Dharmani et al showed that *Fusobacterium nucleatum* (a normal inhabitant of the human mouth and gut) derived from the inflamed intestines of Crohn's disease patients evoked significantly greater gene expression of mucin and tumor necrosis factor alpha gene than other bacteria isolated from the non-inflamed gut in human colonic epithelial cells [47]. Another study by Qin et al showed that 155 bacterial species of the fecal microbiota were found to be present at significantly different relative abundance between patients with Crohn's disease, ulcerative colitis and healthy control patients [48,49]. While no specific mechanisms have been identified that implicate the bacteria identified in our current study as contributing to the disease characteristics of appendicitis, the studies point to instances in which specific bacteria evoke unique inflammatory responses characteristic of the symptoms in inflammatory bowel disease. It must be noted, however, that our observations only report associations and so cannot definitively establish a causal relationship. More studies will be needed to elucidate the specific bacterial mechanisms that contribute to appendicitis pathogenesis.

It is possible that obstruction from a fecalith or prominent lymphoid tissue leads to alterations in the microbiota of the normal appendix, leading to colonization by organisms associated with appendicitis, which then produce the clinical sequelae of inflammation, compromised perfusion and, ultimately, perforation. Larger scale studies that examine abundance and virulence factor shifts in the normal and diseased appendix are needed to further elucidate the complete process of appendicitis pathogenesis.

Our finding that some of the organisms that have increased abundance in the diseased appendix are also present in increased

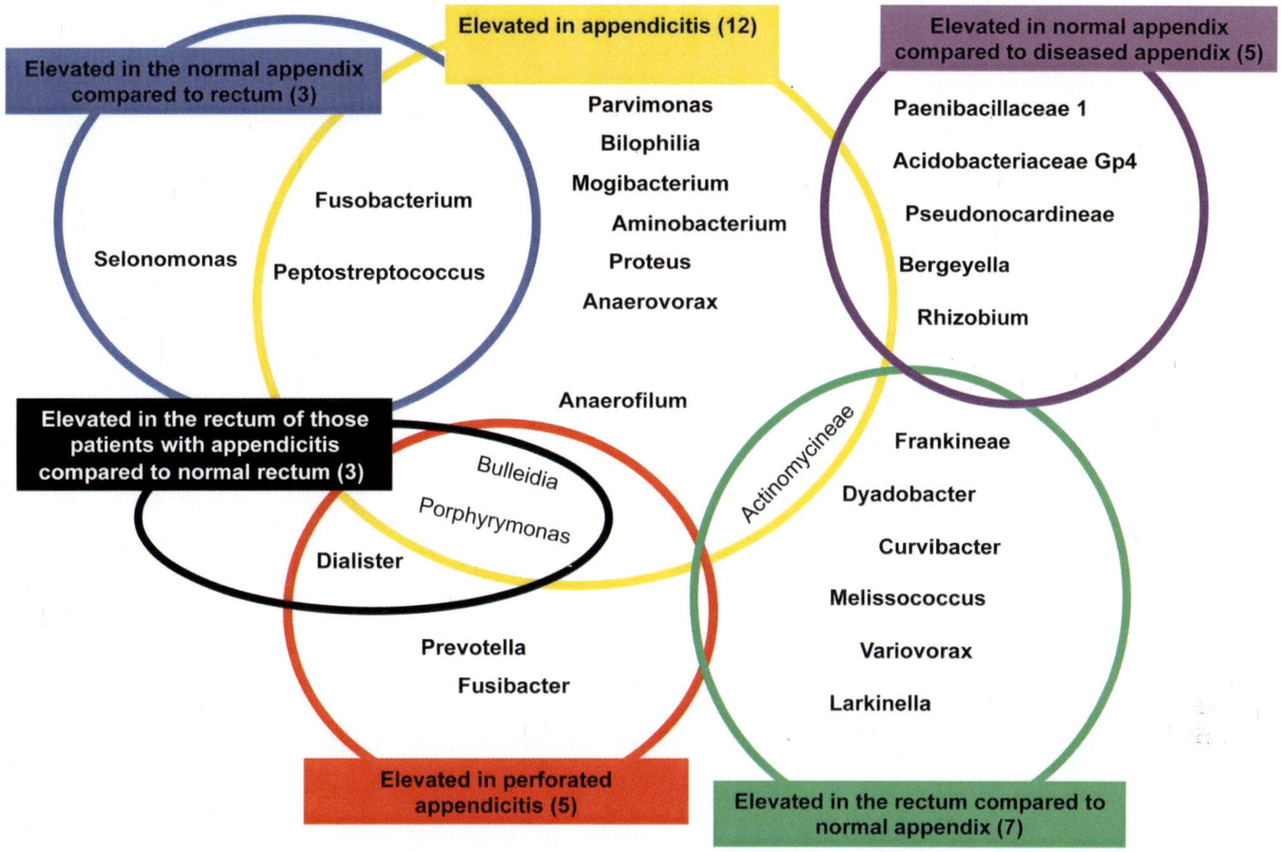

Figure 3. Schematic of Bacterial Genera with Significant Differences in Abundance in Appendix and Rectum, in Patients with and without Appendicitis. Top row, left to right: bacteria with elevated abundance in the normal appendix compared to the rectum, elevated abundance in appendicitis and elevated abundance in the normal appendix compared to the diseased appendix (appendicitis); Bottom row, left to right: Elevated abundance in the rectum of patient's with appendicitis compared to those with normal rectum samples, elevated abundance in perforated appendicitis compared to non perforated appendicitis and elevated abundance in the normal rectum compared to the normal appendix. The figure lists the taxa in each category; the numbers in parentheses for each heading lists the number of genera in that category.

abundance in the rectal samples of those with appendicitis raises some intriguing questions. The data suggest that with appendicitis, organisms linked to appendicitis are not confined to the appendix, perhaps because the normal physiology of the appendix is compromised. The data further suggest that the detection of appendicitis-associated microbes in the rectum may represent a remote microbial signal of appendicitis, a signal that could perhaps be exploited to develop rectal microbe-based diagnostics for appendicitis.

Additional limitations of our study include its sample size and the administration of antibiotics. More samples, particularly more normal samples, are needed in future studies to better characterize the normal microbiome of the appendix. While each participant received antibiotics regardless of surgical indication, (ie. appendicitis vs. appendectomy incidental to surgery for other indications), the impact of these antibiotics on the composition of the appendiceal and rectal microbiota is unclear. It is not ethically possible to withhold antibiotics from a patient with suspected appendicitis about to undergo abdominal surgery, so it will be impossible to definitively assess the microbiota of the appendix in patients who have not received antibiotics.

Looking forward, study of specific pathogens identified through culture-independent 16S rRNA sequence determination and analysis could not only help to further characterize the normal microbiota of the appendix and other gastrointestinal organs, but may lead to enhanced preoperative evaluation, differential diagnosis, and expedited care in the treatment of appendicitis and other medical/surgical conditions.

Supporting Information

File S1 This file contains Figure S1–Figure S3. Figure S1, Bacterial Community Richness and Diversity Estimators by Sample. The figure shows, for each sample, the sample type (appendix or rectum), the diagnosis (normal, appendicitis, perforated appendicitis), the observed number of OTUs, and the Chao1, ACE (richness), Shannon (diversity), and Simpson values. Figure S2, Bacterial community composition at the phylum level. The figure shows the bacterial relative abundance (fraction of total sequence reads assigned to each of the bacteria phyla listed in the legend on the right side) for each of the samples studied. The sample names follow the convention used in Figure 1: Samples are listed by ID number, SnX/Y, where n is the subject identification number, X describes the body site (A for appendix, R for rectum), and Y describes the patient's diagnosis (N for normal appendix, NP for an appendix with non-perforating appendicitis, and P for an appendix with perforating appendicitis). Figure S3, Bacterial community composition at the genus level. The figure shows the bacterial relative abundance (fraction of total sequence reads assigned to each of the bacteria genera listed in the legend on the right side). The sample names follow the convention used in Figure 1: Samples are listed by ID number, SnX/Y, where n is the subject identification number, X describes the body site (A for appendix, R for rectum), and Y describes the patient's diagnosis (N for normal appendix, NP for an appendix with non-perforating appendicitis, and P for an appendix with perforating appendicitis). (DOC)

Author Contributions

Conceived and designed the experiments: SLZ ADS CMF EFM. Performed the experiments: HTJ EFM KPD. Analyzed the data: HTJ EFM SLZ. Contributed reagents/materials/analysis tools: HTJ KPD. Wrote the paper: HTJ EFM SLZ. Patient interactions and consents: KPD HTJ.

References

1. Gebbers JO, Laissue JA (2004) Bacterial translocation in the normal human appendix parallels the development of the local immune system. Ann NY Acad Sci 1029: 337–343.
2. Rhee KJ, Jasper PJ, Sethupathi P, Shanmugam M, Lanning D, et al. (2005) Positive selection of the peripheral B cell repertoire in gut-associated lymphoid tissues. J Exp Med 201: 55–62.
3. Randal Bollinger R, Barbas AS, Bush EL, Lin SS, Parker W (2007) Biofilms in the large bowel suggest an apparent function of the human vermiform appendix. J Theor Biol 249: 826–831.
4. Rhee KJ, Sethupathi P, Driks A, Lanning DK, Knight KL (2004) Role of commensal bacteria in development of gut-associated lymphoid tissues and preimmune antibody repertoire. J Immunol 172: 1118–1124.
5. Fitz R (1886) Perforating inflammation of the vermiform appendix. Philadelphia, PA: Wm. J. Dornan, Printer. 74 p.
6. Kalisova M (1944) Acute appendicitis, treated with penicilin. Brit Med J 2: 1.
7. Guthery S, Hutchings C, Dean J, Hoff C (2004) National estimates of hospital utilization by children with gastrointestinal disorders: analysis of the 1997 kids' inpatient database. J Peds 144: 589–594.
8. Addiss D, Shaffer N, Fowler B, Tauxe R (1990) The epidemiology of appendicitis and appendectomy in the United States. Am J Epidemiol 132: 910–925.
9. Walker A, Segal I (1990) What causes appendicitis? J Clin Gastroenterol 12: 127–129.
10. Primatesta P, Goldacre M (1994) Appendicectomy for acute appendicitis and for other conditions: an epidemiological study. Int J Epidemiol 23: 155–160.
11. Jones B, Demetriades D, Segal I, Burkitt D (1985) The prevalence of appendiceal fecaliths in patients with and without appendicitis. A comparative study from Canada and South Africa. Ann Surgery 202: 80–82.
12. Nitecki S, Karmeli R, Sarr M (1990) Appendiceal calculi and fecaliths as indications for appendectomy. Surgery, Gynecol & Obstet 171: 185–188.
13. Shaw R (1965) Appendix calculi and acute appendicitis. Brit J Surg 52: 451–459.
14. Gearhart S (2008) Acute Appendicitis. In: Fauci A BE, Kasper D, Hauser S, Longo D, Jameson JL, Loscalzo J editor. Harrison's Principles of Internal Medicine. 17 ed. New York: McGraw-Hill. pp. 1914–1917.
15. Humes D (2006) Acute appendicitis. Brit Med J 333: 530.
16. Bundy D, Byerley J, Liles E, Perrin E, Katznelson J, et al. (2007) Does this child have appendicitis? J Am Med Assoc 298: 438–451.
17. Brook I (1980) Bacterial studies of peritoneal cavity and postoperative surgical wound drainage following perforated appendix in children. Ann Surg 192: 208–212.
18. Lau WY, Teoh-Chan CH, Fan ST, Yam WC, Lau KF, et al. (1984) The bacteriology and septic complication of patients with appendicitis. Ann Surg 200: 576–581.
19. Leigh DA, Simmons K, Norman E (1974) Bacterial flora of the appendix fossa in appendicitis and postoperative wound infection. J Clin Pathol 27: 997–1000.
20. Roberts JP (1988) Quantitative bacterial flora of acute appendicitis. Arch Dis Child 63: 536–540.
21. Baron EJ, Summanen P, Downes J, Roberts MC, Wexler H, et al. (1989) Bilophila wadsworthia, gen. nov. and sp. nov., a unique gram-negative anaerobic rod recovered from appendicitis specimens and human faeces. J Gen Microbiol 135: 3405–3411.
22. Guinane CM, Tadrous A, Fouhy F, Ryan CA, Dempsey EM, et al. (2013) Microbial composition of human appendices from patients following appendectomy. MBio 4.
23. Swidsinski A, Dorffel Y, Loening-Baucke V, Theissig F, Ruckert J, et al. (2011) Acute appendicitis is characterised by local invasion with Fusobacterium nucleatum/necrophorum. Gut 60: 34–40.
24. Ebringer A, Rashid T, Wilson C (2003) Rheumatoid arthritis: proposal for the use of anti-microbial therapy in early cases. Scand J Rheumatol 32: 2–11.
25. Syed SA, Svanberg M, Svanberg G (1981) The predominant cultivable dental plaque flora of beagle dogs with periodontitis. J Clin Periodontol 8: 45–56.
26. Hugenholtz P, Goebel BM, Pace NR (1998) Impact of culture-independent studies on the emerging phylogenetic view of bacterial diversity. J Bacteriol 180: 4765–4774.
27. Bik EM, Eckburg PB, Gill SR, Nelson KE, Purdom EA, et al. (2006) Molecular analysis of the bacterial microbiota in the human stomach. Proc Nat Acad Sci USA 103: 732–737.
28. Dekio I, Hayashi H, Sakamoto M, Kitahara M, Nishikawa T, et al. (2005) Detection of potentially novel bacterial components of the human skin microbiota using culture-independent molecular profiling. J Med Microbiol 54: 1231–1238.
29. Eckburg PB, Bik EM, Bernstein CN, Purdom E, Dethlefsen L, et al. (2005) Diversity of the human intestinal microbial flora. Science 308: 1635–1638.
30. Zupancic ML, Cantarel BL, Liu Z, Drabek EF, Ryan KA, et al. (2012) Analysis of the gut microbiota in the old order Amish and its relation to the metabolic syndrome. PLoS One 7: e43052.
31. Angiuoli SV, Matalka M, Gussman A, Galens K, Vangala M, et al. (2011) CloVR: a virtual machine for automated and portable sequence analysis from the desktop using cloud computing. BMC Bioinformatics 12: 356.
32. Bray JR, Curtis JT (1957) An ordination of the upland forest communities of southern Wisconsin. Ecol Monogr 27: 325–349.
33. Field JG, Clarke KR, Warwick RM (1982) A practical strategy for analyzing multispecies distribution patterns. Mar Ecol Prog Ser 8: 37–52.
34. Palmer C, Bik EM, Digiulio DB, Relman DA, Brown PO (2007) Development of the human infant intestinal microbiota. PLoS Biol 5: e177.
35. Sawanon S, Koike S, Kobayashi Y (2011) Evidence for the possible involvement of Selenomonas ruminantium in rumen fiber digestion. FEMS Microbiol Lett 325: 170–179.
36. Goncalves LF, Fermiano D, Feres M, Figueiredo LC, Teles FR, et al. (2012) Levels of Selenomonas species in generalized aggressive periodontitis. J Periodont Res 47: 711–718.
37. Buckel W, Barker HA (1974) Two pathways of glutamate fermentation by anaerobic bacteria. J Bacteriol 117: 1248–1260.
38. Kuppalli K, Livorsi D, Talati NJ, Osborn M (2012) Lemierre's syndrome due to Fusobacterium necrophorum. Lancet Infect Dis 12: 808–815.
39. Sundqvist G (1992) Associations between microbial species in dental root canal infections. Oral Microbiol Immunol 7: 257–262.
40. Finegold SM (1995) Anaerobic infections in humans: an overview. Anaerobe 1: 3–9.
41. Murdoch DA (1998) Gram-positive anaerobic cocci. Clin Microbiol Rev 11: 81–120.
42. Seekatz AM, Panda A, Rasko DA, Toapanta FR, Eloe-Fadrosh EA, et al. (2013) Differential response of the cynomolgus macaque gut microbiota to Shigella infection. PloS One 8: e64212.
43. Zoetendal EG, von Wright A, Vilpponen-Salmela T, Ben-Amor K, Akkermans AD, et al. (2002) Mucosa-associated bacteria in the human gastrointestinal tract are uniformly distributed along the colon and differ from the community recovered from feces. Appl Environ Microbiol 68: 3401–3407.
44. Gerritsen J, Smidt H, Rijkers GT, de Vos WM (2011) Intestinal microbiota in human health and disease: the impact of probiotics. Genes Nutr 6: 209–240.
45. Lau SK, Woo PC, Teng JL, Leung KW, Yuen KY (2002) Identification by 16S ribosomal RNA gene sequencing of Arcobacter butzleri bacteraemia in a patient with acute gangrenous appendicitis. Mol Pathol 55: 182–185.
46. Spiegelman D, Whissell G, Greer CW (2005) A survey of the methods for the characterization of microbial consortia and communities. Canad J Microbiol 51: 355–386.
47. Dharmani P, Strauss J, Ambrose C, Allen-Vercoe E, Chadee K (2011) Fusobacterium nucleatum infection of colonic cells stimulates MUC2 mucin and tumor necrosis factor alpha. Infect Immun 79: 2597–2607.
48. Pflughoeft KJ, Versalovic J (2012) Human microbiome in health and disease. Annu Rev Pathol 7: 99–122.
49. Qin J, Li R, Raes J, Arumugam M, Burgdorf KS, et al. (2010) A human gut microbial gene catalogue established by metagenomic sequencing. Nature 464: 59–65.

13

Use of Liver Stiffness Measurement for Liver Resection Surgery: Correlation with Indocyanine Green Clearance Testing and Post-Operative Outcome

James Fung[1], Ronnie T. P. Poon[2], Wan-Ching Yu[2], See-Ching Chan[2], Albert C. Y. Chan[2], Kenneth S. H. Chok[2], Tan-To Cheung[2], Wai-Kay Seto[1], Chung-Mau Lo[2], Ching-Lung Lai[1], Man-Fung Yuen[1]*

1 Department of Medicine, The University of Hong Kong, Hong Kong, China, **2** Department of Surgery, The University of Hong Kong, Hong Kong, China

Abstract

Background: Liver stiffness measurement (LSM) using transient elastography has recently become available for the assessment of liver fibrosis. Whether LSM can predict the functional liver reserve in patients undergoing liver resection is not certain.

Aim: To correlate liver stiffness measurement (LSM) with indocyanine green (ICG) clearance test and liver biochemistry, and to determine its usefulness in predicting postoperative outcomes in patients undergoing liver resection.

Patients and Methods: Transient elastography and ICG clearance test were performed pre-operatively in 44 patients with hepatocellular carcinoma. The LSM and ICG retention rate at 15 minutes (R15) were correlated with pre-operative factors and post-operative outcomes.

Results: There was significant correlation between ICG R15 and LSM. In patients with LSM $\geq$11 kPa vs $<$11 kPa, there was significantly higher ICG R15 (17.1% vs 10.0% respectively, $p = 0.025$). For patients with ICG R15$\geq$10% compared to those $<$10%, there was significantly higher LSM (12.0 vs 7.6 kPa respectively, $p = 0.015$). Twenty-eight patients proceeded to resection. There was a significant correlation between LSM and the peak INR after liver resection ($r = 0.426$, $p = 0.024$). There was a significant correlation between ICG R15 and the post-operative peak AST level ($r = -0.414$, $p = 0.029$) and peak ALT level ($r = -0.568$, $p = 0.002$). The operative time was a significant independent factor associated with post-operative complications and peak INR.

Conclusion: LSM correlated well with ICG R15 in patients undergoing liver resection, and predicted early post-operative complications. Addition of LSM to ICG R15 testing may provide better prognostic information for patients undergoing resection.

Editor: Kwan Man, The University of Hong Kong, Hong Kong

Funding: There are no current external funding sources for this study.

Competing Interests: The authors have declared that no competing interests exist.

* E-mail: mfyuen@hkucc.hku.hk

Background

Hepatocellular carcinoma (HCC) is the most common primary tumour of the liver, and the fifth commonest malignancy worldwide [1]. Under normal circumstances, hepatic resection is well tolerated as the liver regenerates rapidly. However, in patients with HCC, the remnant liver is often abnormal due to underlying chronic liver disease. For patients with HCC, bridging fibrosis or established cirrhosis is frequently observed in the non-tumour tissue. It is therefore of paramount importance that the underlying liver function is not severely compromised to cause decompensation and death after liver resection. Stringent pre-operative assessment is therefore essential to prevent post- resection morbidity and mortality. Routine liver biochemistry, the Child Pugh classification, and the Model for End-stage Liver Disease (MELD) score provides an estimation of the severity of liver disease, but cannot predict the liver synthetic function reserve, or the ability of the liver to regenerate after resection [2,3,4].

Indocyanine green (ICG) clearance test, a more objective measurement for liver reserve is commonly adopted in many centers because of its high predictive value for postoperative outcome after liver resection [5]. ICG is a synthetic dye which binds completely to albumin and β-lipoprotein and is eliminated by the liver into the bile virtually unchanged without any extrahepatic metabolism or excretion [6]. Excretion of ICG is dependent on hepatic adenosine triphosphate concentration, and decreased levels may reflect reduced ability to regenerate after liver resection. The ICG retention value at 15 minutes (ICG R15) after injection is approximately 10% in normal persons. A cut-off value for a safe major hepatectomy is 14%, although the cut-off may be higher for centres with more operative experience, patients with adequate remnant liver volume and/or with limited resections [7,8]. Infrared digital measurement based on pulse spectrophotometry can be used at bedside to replace repetitive blood taking, and has been shown to be accurate in determining blood ICG concentration [9,10,11].

Recently, liver stiffness measurement (LSM) by transient elastography has become available for the non-invasive assessment of liver fibrosis. LSM has been shown to correlate well with liver biochemistry, liver histology, and predictive of long term outcome in Asian patients with chronic hepatitis B [12,13,14]. In patients with established cirrhosis, higher LSM may also predict complications of cirrhosis including the presence of varices and the development of HCC [15,16]. A pilot study also demonstrated that LSM may be useful in predicting development of postoperative hepatic insufficiency after resection for HCC [17]. Therefore, LSM may be able to predict the functional liver reserve indirectly through the assessment of fibrosis level.

The current study aims to correlate LSM with ICG clearance test and routine liver biochemistry, and to determine its usefulness in predicting postoperative outcomes in patients with HCC undergoing liver resection.

Patients and Methods

Patients with HCC scheduled for potential liver resection from October 2010 to December 2011 at Queen Mary Hospital, Hong Kong, were prospectively recruited. All patients enrolled in the study underwent ICG clearance testing (Pulsion Medical Systems AG, Munich, Germany) and LSM using transient elastography (Echosens, Paris, France) on the same day. Routine liver biochemistry was performed. Basic patient demographics and operation details were recorded. Pre- and post-operative laboratory results and outcome were monitored. Written informed consent was obtained from all subjects. This study was approved by the Ethics Committee/Institutional Review Board of the University of Hong Kong and Hospital Authority Western Cluster. All clinical investigations were conducted according to the principles expressed in the Declaration of Helsinki.

ICG Clearance Test

The ICG clearance test was performed with the patient fasted for 6 hours. ICG was administered intravenously at a dose of 0.5 mg/kg. The ICG Plasma Disappearance Rate (PDR) was measured transcutaneously using a near-infrared finger clip sensor. The ICG retention rate at 15 minutes (R15) was then calculated. The ICG retention value at 15 minutes (ICG R15) after injection is approximately 10% in normal persons, and this value was used for stratification of patients in the current study [18].

Liver Stiffness Measurement

This procedure has been well described previously [12]. The LSM was performed by a single experienced operator (who had performed over 2000 scans). The operator was blinded of the ICG results of the patients. At least 10 valid measurements were obtained for each patient. The median values of the validated measurements for each patient were representative of the liver stiffness and expressed in units of kilopascals (kPa). The results were valid only for the final analysis if the success rate was greater than 50% and the interquartile range (IQR)-to-liver stiffness ratio was below 30%. A cut-off value of 11 kPa has been shown to be predictive of the presence of cirrhosis, and this was used for stratification in the current study [19].

Statistical Analyses

All statistical analyses were performed using SPSS version 17.0 (SPSS Inc, Chicago, IL). Chi-squared test or Fisher's exact test was used for categorical variables when appropriate. Continuous variables with skewed distribution were analyzed using Mann-Whitney test. The comparison of different median values of more than two groups was made by Kruskal-Wallis test. The correlation co-efficient was calculated using Spearman test. Multivariate analysis was performed using linear regression. The area under receiver operating characteristic (AUROC) curve was used to derive an optimal cut-off of liver stiffness measurement for predicting short-term complications after liver resection. A p-value of <0.05 was considered statistically significant.

Results

A total of 68 patients were enrolled during the recruitment period in the current study. Twenty four were excluded from the final analysis due to suboptimal (22 patients had high IQR/LSM ratio) or invalid LSM (2 patients had less than 10 valid measurements). Forty-four patients were included in the final analysis. Thirty six (82%) were male. The median age was 59 years (range, 46–75). The basic patient demographics and laboratory data are summarized in table 1. The correlation between ICG clearance and LSM with age and other routine laboratory parameters are summarized in table 2. There were significant correlations between ICG R15 and LSM, bilirubin, albumin, international normalized ratio (INR), platelet levels, and MELD scores, and between LSM and AST, albumin, INR, and MELD scores. A previous study of CHB patients identified a LSM cut-off value of 11 kPa for the presence of cirrhosis [19]. In our patients with LSM $\geq$11 kPa vs $<$11 kPa, there was significantly higher ICG R15 (17.1% vs 10.0% respectively, $p=0.025$), lower albumin (38 vs 45 g/L respectively, $p<0.001$), higher INR (1.1 vs 1.0 respectively, $p<0.001$), and lower platelet counts (131 vs 170×10^{9}/L respectively, $p=0.043$). The normal ICG R15 is $<$10% [18]. For patients with ICG R15$\geq$10% compared to those $<$10%, there was significantly higher LSM (12.0 vs 7.6 kPa respectively, $p=0.015$), higher bilirubin (12 vs 8 umol/L respectively, $p=0.039$), lower albumin (41 vs 46 g/L respectively, $p<0.001$), higher INR (1.1 vs 1.0 respectively, $p<0.001$), and lower platelet counts (132 vs 178×10^{9}/L respectively, $p=0.027$). The comparison between LSM and ICG R15 is shown in figure 1. Using multivariate analysis, only albumin remained a significant factor associated with both ICG R15 and LSM ($p=0.011$ and $p=0.007$ respectively).

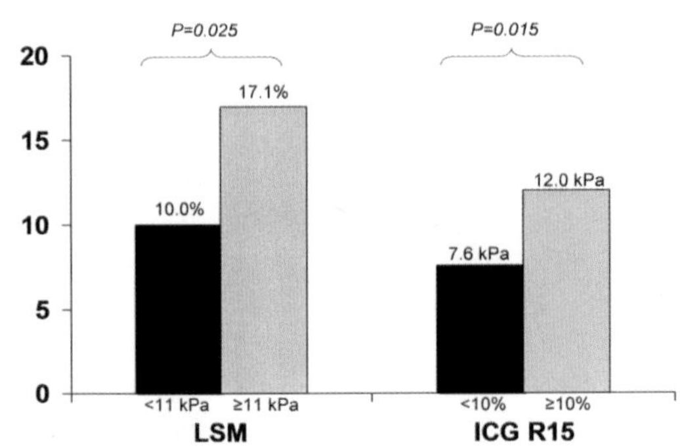

Figure 1. Comparison between LSM and ICG R15.

Table 1. Basic patient demographics and laboratory data.

Parameter	Value
Total patients (N)	68
Invalid fibroscan	24
Numbers in final analysis (n)	44
Male sex, n(%)	36 (82%)
Age (years)	59 (46–75)
Bilirubin (umol/L)	9 (5–29)
ALT (U/L)	39 (16–167)
AST (U/L)	47 (21–263)
Albumin (g/L)	42 (26–52)
Creatinine (umol/L)	80 (57–485)
INR	1.0 (0.9–1.2)
AFP (ng/ml)	37 (3–539700)
Plalelet (x10^9/L)	155 (23–466)
MELD score	7.3 (6.4–13.7)
HCC size (cm)	3.5 (1–14)
Liver stiffness (kPa)	10.2 (3.3–75.0)
ICG R15 (%)	11.8 (5.9–40.7)

Continuous variables are expressed as median values (range).

Post-operative Outcomes

Of the 44 patients with valid LSM, 28 proceeded to liver resection. The remaining 16 patients underwent one of the following treatments: loco-ablative therapy, chemotherapy, or palliation. Of the 28 patients who underwent resection, 10 had segmentectomy, 4 had sectionectomy, 5 had wedge resection, and 9 had lobectomy. The characteristics of the resected patients are shown in table 3. The correlations between operative and post-operative parameters with pre-operative parameters are shown in table 4. There was significant correlation between operative blood loss and HCC size ($r = 0.632$, $p < 0.001$) and operative time ($r = 0.510$, $p = 0.006$), and between operative time and HCC size ($r = 0.573$, $p = 0.001$).

Table 3. Characteristics of patients undergoing liver resection.

Parameters	Value
Number of resected patients	28
Presence of cirrhosis	19 (68%)
Child Pugh Class (A:B:C)	27: 1:0
MELD score	7.2 (6.4–11.7)
Number of tumours	1 (1–6)
Size of largest HCC (cm)	4.2 (2–14)
Hepatitis B	23 (82%)
Hepatitis C	2 (7%)
Cryotpgenic cirrhosis	2 (7%)
Gastrointestinal stromal tumour	1 (4%)
Segmentectomy	18
Sectionectomy	4
Wedge resection	5
Lobectomy	9
Operation time (minutes)	343 (45–1149)
Blood loss (mls)	517 (50–2000)
Bilirubin (umol/L)	33 (18–79)
AST (U/L)	344 (66–3000)
ALT (U/L)	312 (39–3000)
INR	1.4 (1–2.3)
Length of hospital stay (days)	6 (3–21)

Continuous variables are expressed as median values (range).

Correlation with LSM

There was a significant correlation between LSM and the peak INR after liver resection ($r = 0.426$, $p = 0.024$). No significant correlation was observed between LSM and peak levels of bilirubin, AST, and ALT, and length of hospital stay after resection (table 4). In patients with LSM >11.0 kPa, a larger HCC, greater blood loss, and a higher peak INR after resection

Table 2. Correlation between LSM, ICG R15 and other laboratory parameters.

Parameters	Liver stiffness r co-efficient	Liver stiffness P value	ICG R15 r co-efficient	ICG R15 P value
Liver stiffness	–	–	0.342	0.023
ICG R15	0.342	0.023	–	–
Age	−0.032	0.836	0.100	0.517
Bilirubin	0.136	0.378	0.349	**0.020**
ALT	0.228	0.137	−.080	0.605
AST	0.455	**0.002**	0.095	0.541
Albumin	−.0710	**<0.001**	−0.525	**<0.001**
Creatinine	0.071	0.649	0.141	0.361
INR	0.682	**<0.001**	0.548	**<0.001**
AFP	0.140	0.369	0.081	0.605
Platelet count	−0.176	0.253	−0.322	0.033
MELD score	0.431	**0.003**	0.519	**<0.001**
HCC size	0.248	0.108	−0.211	0.174

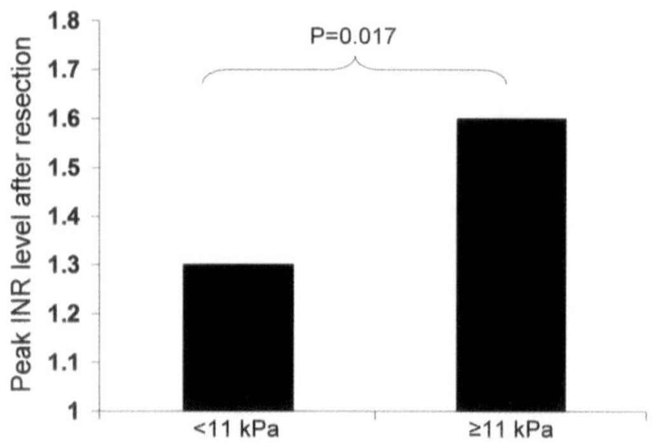

Figure 2. Pre-operative liver stiffness associated with higher post-resection INR.

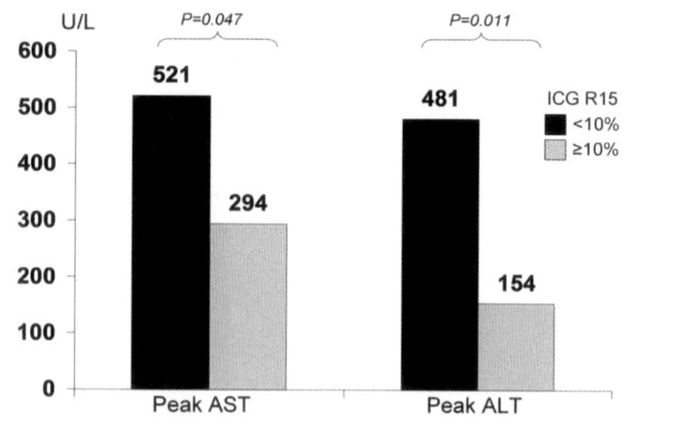

Figure 3. Pre-operative ICG R15 associated with higher post-operative transaminases.

was observed. The comparison between pre-operative LSM and post-resection INR is shown in figure 2. No significant difference was observed with respect to operative time, peak levels of bilirubin, AST, and ALT after resection, and length of hospital stay.

Apart from LSM, other parameters significantly correlated with peak post-operative INR included pre-op AST ($r=0.424$, $p=0.025$), HCC size ($r=0.605$, $p<0.001$), and operative time ($r=0.768$, $p<0.001$). Using multivariate analysis, only the operative time remained significantly associated with the peak INR.

Correlation with ICG R15

There was a significant correlation between ICG R15 and the post-operative peak AST level ($r=-0.414$, $p=0.029$) and peak ALT level ($r=-0.568$, $p=0.002$). There was no correlation between ICG R15 and post-operative peak bilirubin and INR levels, and length of hospital stay (table 4). In patients with ICG R15≥10%, vs <10%, there was a significant lower peak levels of AST (294 vs 521 U/L respectively, $p=0.047$) and ALT (154 vs 481 U/L respectively, $p=0.011$) after resection (as shown in figure 3). There was no significant difference with HCC size, amount of operative blood loss, length of operative time, length of hospital stay, and peak level of bilirubin and INR.

In addition to ICG R15, other factors that was significantly correlated with peak AST included pre-operative platelet levels ($r=0.379$, $p=0.047$) and operative time ($r=0.506$, $p=0.006$). For peak ALT, other factors with significant correlations included pre-operative bilirubin ($r=-0.419$, $p=0.027$), pre-operative albumin (0.479, $p=0.010$), pre-operative INR ($r=-0.426$, $p=0.024$), pre-operative platelet count ($r-0.412$, $p=0.030$), and operative time ($r=0.505$, $p=0.006$). Using multivariate analysis, only the operative time remains significantly associated with both peak AST and ALT levels after resection.

Of the 28 patients, 9 had hepatic inflow occlusion intra-operatively, and there was no significant differences when compared to the 19 patients without occlusion with respect to peak AST (437 vs 284 U/L respectively, $p=0.156$) and ALT (344 vs 154 U/L respectively, $p=0.085$).

Presence of Cirrhosis

In patients who underwent liver resection, the surrounding non-tumour tissue was assessed histologically for the presence of cirrhosis. Of the 28 patients, 19 had evidence of established cirrhosis on histology. In cirrhotic patients versus non-cirrhotic patients, there was significantly higher LSM (9.9 vs 6.3 kPa respectively, $p=0.012$). There was no difference between cirrhotic patients vs non-cirrhotic patients with respect to ICG R15 (14.6 vs 10.0% respectively, $p=0.498$). There were no significant differences between cirrhotic and non-cirrhotic patients with respect to

Table 4. Correlation between pre- and post- operative parameters.

Parameters	Peak Br	P value	Peak ALT	P value	Peak AST	P value	Peak INR	P value	Hospital Stay	P value
Pre-operative										
Age	−0.200	0.308	−0.116	0.556	−0.091	0.646	−0.087	0.659	0.037	0.851
MELD score	0.165	0.402	−0.252	0.196	−0.219	0.264	0.126	0.524	−0.029	0.882
AFP	0.447	**0.019**	−0.161	0.423	0.033	0.871	−0.064	0.753	−0.179	0.372
HCC size	0.176	0.369	0.359	0.060	0.369	0.053	0.605	**0.001**	0.615	**0.001**
ICG R15	−0.015	0.939	−0.568	**0.002**	−0.414	**0.029**	−0.169	0.390	−0.048	0.808
LSM	0.274	0.158	−0.272	0.161	−0.132	0.504	0.426	**0.024**	0.185	0.345
Operative										
Operation time	0.026	0.895	0.505	**0.006**	0.506	**0.006**	0.768	**<0.001**	0.619	**<0.001**
Blood loss	0.169	0.391	0.261	0.179	0.334	0.082	0.659	**<0.001**	0.412	**0.029**

the operative time, amount of blood loss, and peak levels of post-operative bilirubin, AST, ALT, and INR.

Short-term Outcome

Of the 28 patients undergoing resection, all were discharged well with a median hospital stay of 6 days (range, 3–21). We defined post-operative complications as any deviation from the normal recovery course with or without the need for pharmacological treatment or surgical, endoscopic, and radiological interventions. Seven patients had evidence of early (<1 month) post-operative complications, with a median time from operation to development of complication of 11 days (range, 2–17). Ascites developed in 4 patients and was the most common complication. The remaining 3 complications included a combination of wound leakage and pneumonia. The only factor significantly associated with the development of complications was the operative time ($p = 0.008$). Age, ICG, LSM, albumin, platelet, MELD score, the presence of cirrhosis, HCC size and operative blood loss were not significantly associated with the development of complications.The HCC size, LSM, intra-operative blood loss, and operative time were significantly associated with the post-operative peak INR. After multivariate analysis, only the operative time remained the only significant factor ($p = 0.002$), whereas ICG, LSM, albumin, platelet count, MELD score, presence of cirrhosis, HCC size and intra-operative blood loss were not significant factors.

Discussion

For patients undergoing liver resection, assessment of the liver function is essential to ensure that sufficient liver function remains after resection to allow for regeneration of the remnant liver and to prevent decompensation and death. Current methods to assess liver function include using the Child Pugh score, MELD score, and the ICG R15. Routine laboratory, endoscopic and radiological assessment can also be used to determine the presence of underlying portal hypertension. More recently, transient elastography has become available as a non-invasive method for assessing liver fibrosis and cirrhosis. Previous studies have shown good correlation between LSM and the degree of fibrosis [12,13,14]. In patients with established cirrhosis, higher LSM was also correlated with complications of cirrhosis, including the presence of varices [13,15,16].

In contrast to LSM, ICG testing determines the functional capacity rather than the degree of architectural change in the liver. Although ICG is extracted exclusively by the liver with negligible extrahepatic elimination, the clearance rate is dependent on hepatic blood flow and plasma volume. Therefore, it remains an imperfect test for assessing hepatic functional reserve. A previous pilot study has suggested a potential role for LSM to predict post-resection hepatic insufficiency [17]. A more recent study demonstrated that elevated LSM was an independent predictor of postoperative liver failure; those with LSM <14.8 kPa had no liver failure [20]. Another study showed that LSM >12.0 kPa predicted worst outcomes after hepatectomy, and was better than ICG test in predicting major postoperative complications [21].

In the current study, significant correlation between ICG R15 and LSM was demonstrated in patients undergoing liver resection. However, after multivariate analysis, only albumin remained a significant factor that was correlated with either ICG R15 or LSM. This would suggest that the correlation between ICG R15 and LSM is not independent of other more important factors such as the level of serum albumin. This is not surprising given that ICG R15 is a functional test whereas LSM is a structural assessment. In fact, in patients with cirrhosis, the LSM was significantly higher than non-cirrhotic patients, in comparison to ICG R15 where no differences were observed.

There was also significant correlation of LSM and ICG R15 with post-operative outcomes. Interestingly, the post-operative peak INR was correlated with LSM whereas the post-operative peak AST and ALT were inversely correlated with ICG R15. The higher INR observed is consistent with the fact that those patients with higher LSM have more advanced fibrosis/cirrhosis, resulting in a higher INR after resection. This implies that the risk of liver decompensation may be higher in patients with high LSM who undergo liver resection. This may be an important consideration for those who have major liver resection. It will be interesting to define in future studies, the role of LSM to stratify post-operative risks in patients with different extent of liver resection.

Elevation of transaminases is commonly observed after liver resection. The causes are multifactorial, including the duration of operation, transaction surface and any ischemic injury to the liver during operation. In the current study, only the length of operation remains significantly associated with the post-resection peak INR and transaminase after multivariate analysis. However, it should be noted that the results of the multivariate analysis may be affected by the relatively small number of patients ($n = 28$) who eventually underwent liver resection. Further studies are required to examine specifically whether LSM and ICG R15 are important measurement to correlate liver decompensation and hepatocyte damage respectively after liver resection.

There are several limitations to the current study. Firstly, there was an unusually high rate of invalid FS (35%), so the number included in the final analysis was reduced. This is most likely due to the higher IQR that is often observed in patients with established cirrhosis. In fact, only 2 of the patients excluded because of invalid LSM were due to insufficient success rate. Secondly, the patients included in the study have already been selected as potential candidate for resection based on their normal clinical parameters and the absence of overt portal hypertension. To determine a cut-off value of ICG R15 and LSM whereby resection is contra-indicated would require a proportion of patients who decompensated after resection. As all 28 patients were discharged without evidence of severe decompensation, this would suggest that at least in pre-selected patients with compensated cirrhosis and without evidence of portal hypertension, the addition of LSM may not provide further decisional value in addition to ICG R15. However, it is noteworthy that the majority of patients underwent minor resection rather than lobectomy. LSM may still have a role in assessing the risk of decompensation in patients undergoing major hepatectomy and this needs a further study to clarify.

In conclusion, LSM correlated well with ICG R15 in patients undergoing liver resection, and may predict complications in the early post-operative phase. Further studies are required to determine whether the addition of LSM to ICG R15 testing has any added benefit in the pre-operative assessment to select out patients suitable for hepatectomy.

Author Contributions

Conceived and designed the experiments: JF RP SC AC KC TC WS C. Lai C. Lo MY. Performed the experiments: JF RP WY SC AC KC TC C. Lai WS C. Lo MY. Analyzed the data: JF C. Lai MY. Contributed reagents/materials/analysis tools: JF C. Lai MY WY. Wrote the paper: JF RP SC AC KC TC WS C. Lai C. Lo MY.

References

1. Bruix J, Sherman M (2005) Management of hepatocellular carcinoma. Hepatology 42: 1208–1236.
2. Ichikawa T, Uenishi T, Takemura S, Oba K, Ogawa M, et al. (2009) A simple, noninvasively determined index predicting hepatic failure following liver resection for hepatocellular carcinoma. J Hepatobiliary Pancreat Surg 16: 42–48.
3. Kamath PS, Wiesner RH, Malinchoc M, Kremers W, Therneau TM, et al. (2001) A model to predict survival in patients with end-stage liver disease. Hepatology 33: 464–470.
4. Cescon M, Cucchetti A, Grazi GL, Ferrero A, Vigano L, et al. (2009) Indication of the extent of hepatectomy for hepatocellular carcinoma on cirrhosis by a simple algorithm based on preoperative variables. Arch Surg 144: 57–63; discussion 63.
5. Lau H, Man K, Fan ST, Yu WC, Lo CM, et al. (1997) Evaluation of preoperative hepatic function in patients with hepatocellular carcinoma undergoing hepatectomy. Br J Surg 84: 1255–1259.
6. Caesar J, Shaldon S, Chiandussi L, Guevara L, Sherlock S (1961) The use of indocyanine green in the measurement of hepatic blood flow and as a test of hepatic function. Clin Sci 21: 43–57.
7. Fan ST, Lai EC, Lo CM, Ng IO, Wong J (1995) Hospital mortality of major hepatectomy for hepatocellular carcinoma associated with cirrhosis. Arch Surg 130: 198–203.
8. Lam CM, Fan ST, Lo CM, Wong J (1999) Major hepatectomy for hepatocellular carcinoma in patients with an unsatisfactory indocyanine green clearance test. Br J Surg 86: 1012–1017.
9. Ohwada S, Kawate S, Hamada K, Yamada T, Sunose Y, et al. (2006) Perioperative real-time monitoring of indocyanine green clearance by pulse spectrophotometry predicts remnant liver functional reserve in resection of hepatocellular carcinoma. Br J Surg 93: 339–346.
10. Purcell R, Kruger P, Jones M (2006) Indocyanine green elimination: a comparison of the LiMON and serial blood sampling methods. ANZ J Surg 76: 75–77.
11. Hsieh CB, Chen CJ, Chen TW, Yu JC, Shen KL, et al. (2004) Accuracy of indocyanine green pulse spectrophotometry clearance test for liver function prediction in transplanted patients. World J Gastroenterol 10: 2394–2396.
12. Fung J, Lai CL, Fong DY, Yuen JC, Wong DK, et al. (2008) Correlation of liver biochemistry with liver stiffness in chronic hepatitis B and development of a predictive model for liver fibrosis. Liver Int 28: 1408–1416.
13. Fung J, Lai CL, Seto WK, Wong DK, Yuen MF (2010) Prognostic significance of liver stiffness for hepatocellular carcinoma and mortality in HBeAg-negative chronic hepatitis B. J Viral Hepat.
14. Fung J, Lai CL, Chan SC, But D, Seto WK, et al. (2010) Correlation of liver stiffness and histological features in healthy persons and in patients with occult hepatitis B, chronic active hepatitis B, or hepatitis B cirrhosis. Am J Gastroenterol 105: 1116–1122.
15. Castera L, Le Bail B, Roudot-Thoraval F, Bernard PH, Foucher J, et al. (2009) Early detection in routine clinical practice of cirrhosis and oesophageal varices in chronic hepatitis C: comparison of transient elastography (FibroScan) with standard laboratory tests and non-invasive scores. J Hepatol 50: 59–68.
16. Masuzaki R, Tateishi R, Yoshida H, Goto E, Sato T, et al. (2009) Prospective risk assessment for hepatocellular carcinoma development in patients with chronic hepatitis C by transient elastography. Hepatology 49: 1954–1961.
17. Kim SU, Ahn SH, Park JY, Kim do Y, Chon CY, et al. (2008) Prediction of postoperative hepatic insufficiency by liver stiffness measurement (FibroScan((R))) before curative resection of hepatocellular carcinoma: a pilot study. Hepatol Int 2: 471–477.
18. Watanabe Y, Kumon K (1999) Assessment by pulse dye-densitometry indocyanine green (ICG) clearance test of hepatic function of patients before cardiac surgery: its value as a predictor of serious postoperative liver dysfunction. J Cardiothorac Vasc Anesth 13: 299–303.
19. Marcellin P, Ziol M, Bedossa P, Douvin C, Poupon R, et al. (2009) Non-invasive assessment of liver fibrosis by stiffness measurement in patients with chronic hepatitis B. Liver Int 29: 242–247.
20. Cescon M, Colecchia A, Cucchetti A, Peri E, Montrone L, et al. (2012) Value of transient elastography measured with FibroScan in predicting the outcome of hepatic resection for hepatocellular carcinoma. Ann Surg 256: 706–712; discussion 712–703.
21. Wong JS, Wong GL, Chan AW, Wong VW, Cheung YS, et al. (2013) Liver stiffness measurement by transient elastography as a predictor on posthepatectomy outcomes. Ann Surg 257: 922–928.

A Preclinical Evaluation of Alternative Synthetic Biomaterials for Fascial Defect Repair Using a Rat Abdominal Hernia Model

Daniela Ulrich[1,2,4], Sharon L. Edwards[3], Jacinta F. White[3], Tommy Supit[1], John A. M. Ramshaw[3], Camden Lo[1], Anna Rosamilia[4], Jerome A. Werkmeister[3], Caroline E. Gargett[1,4]*

1 Monash Institute of Medical Research, Clayton, Victoria, Australia, 2 Medical University Graz, Graz, Austria, 3 CSIRO Materials Science and Engineering, Clayton, Victoria, Australia, 4 Department of Obstetrics and Gynaecology and Monash Micro Imaging, Monash Medical Centre, Monash University, Clayton, Victoria, Australia

Abstract

Introduction: Fascial defects are a common problem in the abdominal wall and in the vagina leading to hernia or pelvic organ prolapse that requires mesh enhancement to reduce operation failure. However, the long-term outcome of synthetic mesh surgery may be unsatisfactory due to post-surgical complications. We hypothesized that mesh fabricated from alternative synthetic polymers may evoke a different tissue response, and provide more appropriate mechanical properties for hernia repair. Our aim was to compare the in vivo biocompatibility of new synthetic meshes with a commercial mesh.

Methods: We have fabricated 3 new warp-knitted synthetic meshes from different polymers with different tensile properties polyetheretherketone (PEEK), polyamide (PA) and a composite, gelatin coated PA (PA+G). The rat abdominal hernia model was used to implant the meshes (25×35 mm, n = 24/ group). After 7, 30, 60, 90 days tissues were explanted for immunohistochemical assessment of foreign body reaction and tissue integration, using CD31, CD45, CD68, alpha-SMA antibodies. The images were analysed using an image analysis software program. Biomechanical properties were uniaxially evaluated using an Instron Tensile® Tester.

Results: This study showed that the new meshes induced complex differences in the type of foreign body reaction over the time course of implantation. The PA, and particularly the composite PA+G meshes, evoked a milder early inflammatory response, and macrophages were apparent throughout the time course. Our meshes led to better tissue integration and new collagen deposition, particularly with the PA+G meshes, as well as greater and sustained neovascularisation compared with the PP meshes.

Conclusion: PA, PA+G and PEEK appear to be well tolerated and are biocompatible, evoking an overlapping and different host tissue response with time that might convey mechanical variations in the healing tissue. These new meshes comprising different polymers may provide an alternative option for future treatment of fascial defects.

Editor: Nuno M. Neves, University of Minho, Portugal

Funding: Supported by Australian National Health and Medical Research Council grants (1021126) (CEG, JW, AR) and R.D Wright Career Development Award 465121 (CEG), the Australian Stem Cell Centre (SDF5) and South East Melbourne Alliance for Regenerative Therapies (SMART)grants (CEG, JW, AR, SE) the Victorian Government's Operational Infrastructure Support Program and a Monash Postgraduate Award (DU). In kind support as a gift of Polypropylene meshes were kindly provided by Boston Scientific, USA. The funders had no role in study design, data collection and analysis, decision to publish, or preparation of the manuscript.

Competing Interests: Polypropylene meshes were kindly provided to Dr. Anna Rosamilia by Boston Scientific, USA for use in this study.

* E-mail: Caroline.Gargett@med.monash.edu.au

Introduction

Incisional ventral hernias occur in up to 49% of patients after abdominal surgery for trauma, infection, herniation or surgical resection [1–3]. Similarly, hernias in the female lower urogenital tract known as pelvic organ prolapse (POP) occur in up to 25% of women with childbirth, ageing and obesity being the most common causes [4]. Recurrence rates with tissue approximation procedures occur in up to 17% for abdominal hernias [5] and 30% for POP repair [6], respectively, which has led to the implantation of synthetic meshes to improve surgical outcomes.

Polypropylene (PP) mesh is the most commonly used mesh, and is knitted from monofilament yarn to a relatively large pore size, in order to allow tissue ingrowth [7]. Synthetic non-degradable meshes are used to provide a permanent solution and are believed to work by inducing an inflammatory foreign body reaction, resulting in fibrosis that provides strength, albeit not necessarily mechanically optimal, to the weakened support structures [8,9]. However, the presence of an inflammatory response may reflect poor tissue biocompatibility, depending on the extent and type of response. It is also primarily responsible for the significant complications arising from the use of synthetic meshes reported in up to 42%, including mesh contraction, infection, pain, and exposure of mesh [10,11].

With PP mesh dominating the market, we believe that mesh manufactured from alternative synthetic polymers may evoke a different biological response, and provide more appropriate mechanical properties for hernia repair. PA and PEEK polymers were chosen as alternative polymers to PP, due to differences in yarn tensile properties. Gelatin coating was also used to further improve tissue integration [12,13].Gelatin works as a carrier for delivering large number of cells and can be adapted as a basis for cell based therapies in the future [14].

The aim of this study was to compare the *in vivo* host tissue response of synthetic meshes fabricated from alternative polymers and a composite mesh coated with gelatin, with a clinical PP mesh, using a rat abdominal hernia model as a preclinical model for hernia repair surgery.

Materials and Methods

Polyetheretherketone (PEEK) and polyamide (PA) meshes were warp knitted to the same pattern using 100 μm PEEK (Invibio; UK) and PA (Ri-Thai International; Taiwan) monofilament yarns. Meshes were knitted to possess pore sizes ranging 1310 to 1487 μm and weights ranging 69 to 85 g/m^2. A clinical PP mesh (Polyform TM; Boston Scientific; USA), of similar knit pattern, filament diameter and pore size, with a weight of 42 g/m^2 [15], was also used in the study. Additionally, fabricated PA mesh was coated with gelatin (PA+G). Briefly, PA mesh was immersed in a 0.2 μm filter sterilised solution of 12% porcine gelatin (Type A, 300 bloom; Sigma; USA), in water. Once fully wetted the mesh was placed onto ice-cold 2% glutaraldehyde (Sigma) in PBS for 8 minutes on either side. All the subsequent steps were for 15 minutes duration and at room temperature. The mesh was washed, placed into 2% w/v glycine (Merck; Australia) in water, washed, placed in 2% v/v H_2O_2 (Merck) in water, washed, then 4% w/v glycerol (Merck) in water. Finally, the mesh was air-dried overnight. All mesh samples were gamma ray irradiated at 25 kGy prior to implantation.

Animals

The experimental procedures and rat husbandry were approved by the Monash Medical Centre Animal Ethics Committee A (2009/50). Sprague Dawley rats were housed in the animal house of Monash Animal Service facilities in compliance with the National Health and Medical Research guidelines for the care and use of laboratory animals. The rats were provided with food and water *ad libitum* and were kept under controlled environmental conditions at 20°C and a 12 h day/night cycle.

Surgical Procedure

125 female rats were divided into 5 experimental groups (24 rats/group) and were implanted with one of 4 mesh types; PA, PA+G, PEEK, or PP. A sham operation was used as a negative control as described below. The rats were anaesthetised with 2.5% Isoflurane® and analgesia was provided with Carprofen (5 mg/kg bodyweight). The abdomen was shaved and disinfected and covered with sterile drapes. A longitudinal 3 cm skin incision was performed in the lower abdomen and a full thickness fascial defect of the abdominal wall, 20×30 mm, was created [16] (Fig. S1A) . Before implantation, mesh thickness was measured with a calliper. Each mesh (25 mm×35 mm) was implanted using the overlay technique (Fig. S1A) and sutured with PP sutures as previously described [16,17] (Fig. S1C). Rats in the control group were sham-operated without mesh implantation. A 25×35 mm full-thickness abdominal wall defect was created on the right lateral side of the midline. A muscle flap with preserved vascularisation from the contralateral side was created, rotated 45° clockwise and sutured with 3/0 Surgipro^{TM} II (polypropylene thread) to cover the initial defect (Fig. S1B). Skin closure in all groups was performed by intracutaneous continuous suture with 3/0 Vicryl* Plus (polyglactin thread).

Following recovery, the animals were monitored daily until they were sacrificed at 7, 30, 60 and 90 days (n = 6/ group/ timepoint). Each rat was euthanized in a CO_2 chamber. The adhesion area of the mesh on the intestinal side was recorded and calculated as a percentage of total mesh area. Adhesion tenacity to the intestinal wall was also recorded as previously described [18]. Adhesion scores were graded from 1–4 with 4 being the most adhesive. The mesh was dissected with a 5 mm border of adjacent tissue and divided into three parts; for biomechanical analysis, histology and immunohistochemistry, using the same pattern of dissection for each mesh. Adhesive organs to the mesh were peeled off manually. The meshes used for biomechanical analysis were stored at −20 degrees prior to testing. Additionally, explant dimensions (length, width and thickness) were measured with a calliper at 3 random regions and the mean recorded. Mesh contraction was calculated by dividing the mesh size after explantation by the original mesh size.

Biomechanical Analysis

The frozen samples were thawed overnight at 4 degrees and kept moist during testing. Day 7 and day 90 explants and tissue from the control rats were uniaxially tensile tested using an Instron® Tensile Tester (Instron Corp; USA) and a 5 kN load cell. Samples (typically n = 10), with dimensions of 4×25 mm, were cut in the explant cross direction and tested using a 14 mm gauge length (noted as the initial length). Samples were pre-loaded to 100 mN at an elongation rate of 14 mm/min to remove any sample slack. Subsequent testing was conducted at an elongation rate of 30 mm/min to break. Average load-elongation curves were plotted for each mesh type and the control (failure region not included in curve) from the data obtained. Tensile strain (%) was calculated by dividing mesh elongation by the initial mesh length and multiplying by 100. Mesh stiffness is represented by the slope of the curve, with a steeper curve indicating a stiffer mesh.

Histology

The explanted tissue for histological analysis was fixed in 4% w/v paraformaldehyde (PFA) for 24 h, then embedded in paraffin and sectioned into 5 μm thick sections. After dewaxing and rehydrating in graded alcohols, sections were stained with haematoxylin and eosin (H+E) or Sirius red F3B (0.1 g/100 ml saturated aqueous picric acid) (Sigma Aldrich®, St. Louis, MO USA) for one hour at room temperature (RT).

Immunohistochemistry (IHC)

To examine for tissue macrophages, a monoclonal anti rat CD68 antibody (details in Table 1) was used. Sections underwent dewaxing, rehydrating in graded alcohols. Antigen retrieval using citric acid buffer (0.1 M, pH 6.0) was done by microwaving for 5 minutes on high power. After cooling to RT and washes in PBS, endogenous peroxidase was quenched with 3% v/v H_2O_2 followed by protein blocking (Protein Block serum free, Dako®, Glostrup, Denmark) for 30 minutes at RT. The primary CD68 antibody and isotype controls (mouse IgG_1) were incubated overnight at 4°C, sections washed and the secondary Streptavidin HRP-conjugated antibody was applied for 30 minutes at RT, respectively (Table 1). 3,3′-Diaminoben-

Table 1. Details of antibodies used for immunohistochemistry.

Primary antibody	Clone	Dilution	Isotype	supplier	Secondary antibody	Dilution	supplier
α smooth muscle actin	1A4	1:400	Mouse IgG2a	Dako®, Glostrup. Denmark	Alexa fluor 488 goat anti-mouse IgG	1:200	Invitrogen®, Mulgrave, VIC, Australia
CD 31 PECAM-1	TLD-3A12	1:200	Mouse IgG1	BD Pharmingen® NJ, USA	Alexa fluor 568 donkey anti-mouse IgG (H+L)	1:200	Invitrogen® Mulgrave, VIC, Australia
CD 45 Leukocyte common antigen	OX-1	1:200	Mouse IgG1	BD Pharmingen® NJ, USA	Alexa fluor 568 donkey anti-mouse IgG (H+L)	1:200	Invitrogen® Mulgrave, VIC, Australia
CD 68/ MCA341R	ED 1	1:500	Mouse IgG1	AbD Serotec®, Oxford, UK	EnVison+System- HRP Labelled Polymer (anti-mouse)	Ready to use	Dako®, CA, USA

zidine (Sigma-Aldrich®, St. Louis, MO, USA) was used as a chromogen, counterstaining was with haematoxylin. The slides were dehydrated in graded alcohols and mounted with DPX mounting medium.

Immunofluorescence

4% w/v PFA fixed, paraffin embedded tissues were used for immunofluorescence analysis and 5 μm sections dewaxed, dehydrated, blocked and washed as above. Sections were incubated with the primary monoclonal anti-alpha smooth muscle actin (αSMA) antibody for one hour at 37°C (Table 1) to label smooth muscle cells, myofibroblasts and myoepithelial cells. Mouse IgG_{2a} isotype was used for the negative control and applied at the same concentration. Bound antibodies were detected with Alexa-Fluor-488- conjugated secondary antibody (Table 1) for 30 minutes at RT after 3 washes in PBS. Nuclei were stained with Hoechst 33258. The slides were mounted with fluorescent mounting medium (Dako®, Glostrup, Denmark).

CD31 and CD45 immunofluorescence was used to visualise endothelial cells and leukocytes, respectively (Table 1). Tissue for frozen sections was snap frozen in optimal compound tissue solution (OCT, Tissue-Tek, Miles, IN, USA). The frozen sections cut (5 μm) were thawed at RT, fixed in ice cold acetone for 10 minutes followed by protein block (Dako®, Glostrup, Denmark) for 30 minutes at RT. After three washes in PBS, primary antibodies were incubated for 1hr at 37°C and with Alexa-Fluor-568- conjugated secondary antibody (Table 1) for 30 minutes at RT, respectively. The slides were mounted as above.

Histomorphometric Analysis

Four images were taken per section stained with Sirius red or immunostained with CD68, αSMA, CD31 or CD45 for each explant at each timepoint using a Leica® DMR Fluorescence Microscope at 20X 0.6NA magnification and at 10X 0.3NA for H+E. Images of the 4 most central mesh filaments were captured (Fig. S2A, B, Fig. 1A), to achieve consistency and overcome bias, and to avoid any foreign body reaction associated with anchoring sutures. The images were analysed using the image analysis software, Metamorph® (v7.7 Molecular Devices, LLC, CA, USA). The software was programmed to identify individual mesh filaments (Fig. 1B) and trace contoured concentric area bands around filament bundles in 50 μm increments (Fig. 1C, D). The positive signal area (pixels) for each shape was recorded and divided by the total tissue area examined (Fig. 1B). Neotissue formation (as indicated by Sirius, αSMA and CD31) was analyzed using the whole image, assessing the entire surrounding tissue. Foreign body cells were assessed close to the mesh filaments.

Statistics

GraphPad Prism 5 was used for statistical analysis. Results are reported as mean ± SEM for each experimental group ($n = 6$ animals/ group/ timepoint). Since the data was not normally distributed (D'Agostino & Pearson omnibus normality test), non-parametric analysis using Kruskal – Wallis ANOVA, were undertaken to assess differences between timepoints for the various meshes, followed by Bonferroni correction for pairwise comparisons. P values <0.05 were considered as statistically significant. For statistical analysis of load-elongation curves, 95% confidence intervals were plotted as error bars to determine whether the differences were significant at the $p < 0.05$ level of significance.

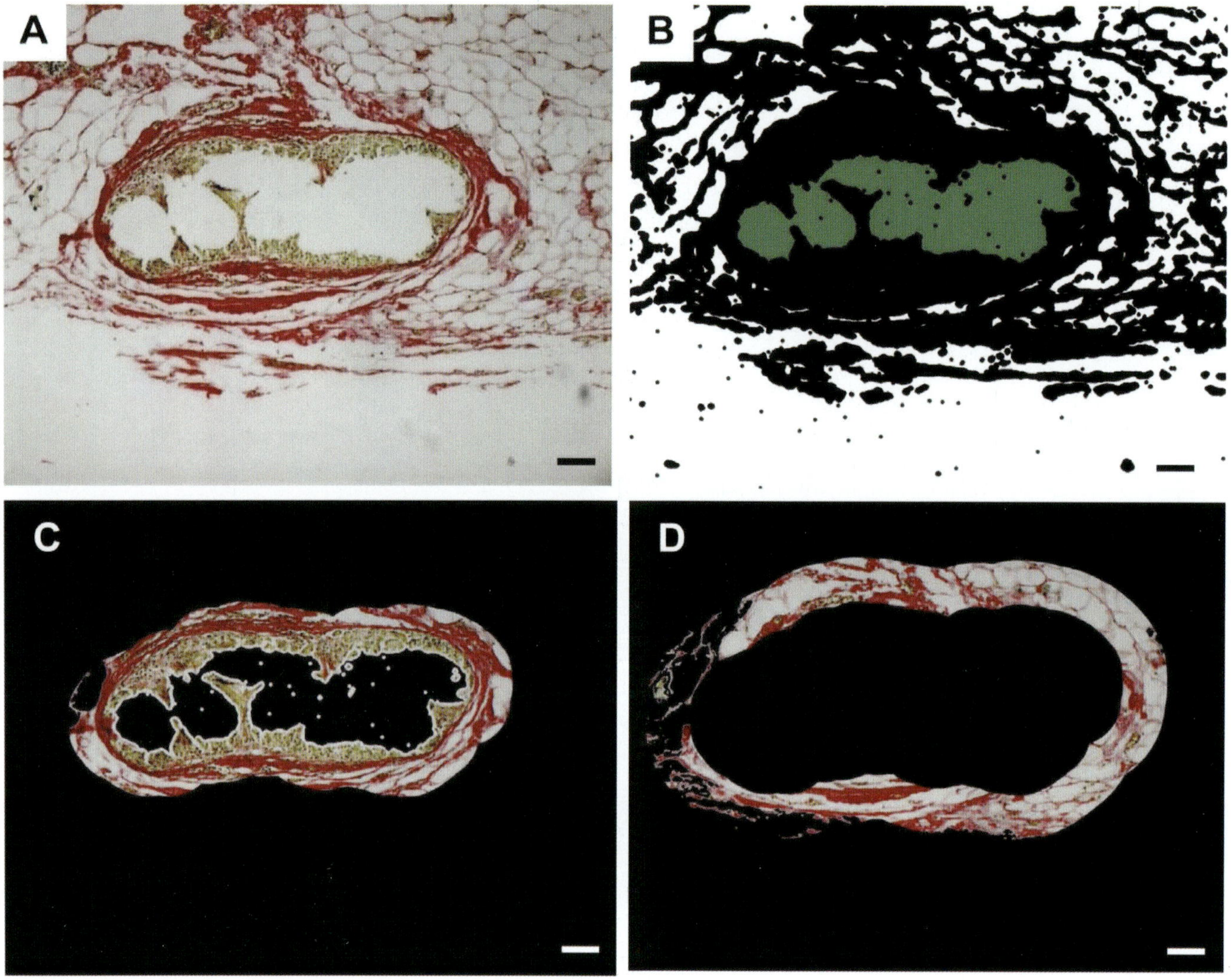

Figure 1. Image analysis using Metamorph®. Software. A. Original image showing Sirius red staining of tissue around a central filament bundle, scale bar — 100 μm. B. binarized image with mesh recognition. C. First 50 μm increment surrounding filament bundle. D. Second 50 μm increment (50–100 μm) surrounding filament bundle.

Results

Macroscopic Tissue Compatibility of New Meshes

Two new meshes, warp-knitted from PA and PEEK monofilaments in a similar pattern as commercially available PP mesh, were examined for tissue biocompatibility using a standard rat abdominal hernia model. In addition, a gelatin-coated PA mesh was studied, since this composite could be adapted for delivering cells in future experiments. Of the 125 animals operated, all had a normal post-operative recovery. Five rats developed wound infection or wound dehiscence with no differences between the mesh groups, necessitating killing these animals according to local ethics committee regulations. Therefore a total number of 120 animals (6 per group at each timepoint) were included for analysis.

All mesh types were well tolerated. Rats gained weight 30 days after operation and weight gain increased significantly in rats implanted with PA, PEEK and PP meshes at 60 days ($p<0.05$) (Fig. 2). At 90 days, rats implanted with PA and PA+G meshes showed significantly greater weight gain compared to control rats, and rats implanted with PEEK and PP meshes ($p<0.001$). Ninety days after surgery, weight gain was significantly higher in all groups compared to 7 days (pairwise comparisons $p<0.0001$).

At the time of necropsy (Fig. S1D, E), intraperitoneal adhesions were noted mainly with the ileum and the omentum over the whole implant surface for all materials as well as to the sutures in all mesh groups. The adhesion scores are shown in Table 2. No differences were observed at 7 and 30 days between the mesh groups. PA meshes showed a significantly lower adhesion score compared to PA+G ($p<0.05$), PEEK and PP ($p<0.001$) at 90 days. Adhesion scores for PA+G, PEEK and PP meshes were significantly increased at 60 and 90 days compared to the earlier timepoints for the same mesh type ($p<0.05$).

While all meshes displayed the greatest adhesion area at 7 days (range 73 to 88%, Table 3), the strength of adhesion was low (adhesion score of 1.0, Table 2). The extent of adhesion was lowest with the PA+G mesh at day 7 without statistically significant differences (Table 3). At 30 days, the extent of adhesion with the PA+G and PEEK meshes was significantly less than observed with PA and PP ($p<0.05$), with no significant difference by 60 and 90 days. All meshes reached the lowest adhesion area at 60 days, with

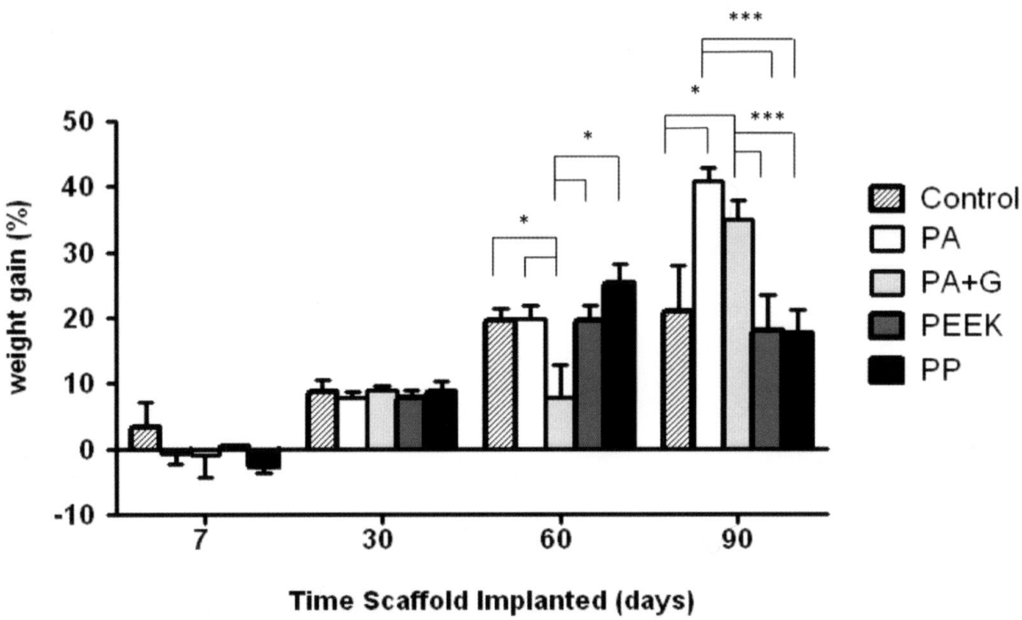

Figure 2. Body weight gain of rats implanted with different synthetic meshes: PA, PA+G, PEEK or PP and controls. Data are mean ± SEM of n=6 animals/ group, * $p<0.05$, *** $p<0.001$. PA, polyamide; PA+G, polyamide gelatin composite; PEEK, polyetheretherketone; PP, polypropylene.

no further reduction at 90 days, although none of these differences were significant.

Folding of the meshes, which contributes to apparent mesh shrinkage, was occasionally observed, with the highest incidence seen in the PA and PP groups. Folding may have arisen from poor suturing but could also be due to extensive tissue ingrowth. These meshes were included in the analysis of mesh contraction. Contraction was significantly greater at 30 days compared to 7 days for PA+G and PP meshes; no significant differences in mesh contraction for PA and PEEK meshes were observed between these timepoints (Table 4). PEEK meshes shrank significantly less than PA and PP meshes at 30 days; however no significant difference was observed at 60 or 90 days (range at 90 days 9 to 19.4%, Table 4).

Biomechanical Properties

The load-elongation curves for the day 7 and day 90 explants are shown in Figure 3 and in Fig. S3. The mechanical properties of meshes prior to implantation were not significantly different to those measured after 7 days implantation. Comparable load-elongation curves, with similar levels of stiffness, were observed for explanted mesh types and the control tissue on day 7; error bars suggest that curves were not significantly different from each other ($p>0.05$). The curves of day 7 meshes suggest some bilinearality, with a linear region from 1.7 mm elongation (Fig. 3 inset), however this is less obvious than for the day 90 meshes (which have distinct toe and linear regions). The load-elongation curves of all meshes explanted at day 90 were significantly ($p<0.05$) different to their day 7 counterparts exceeding 0.9 mm elongation (6.4% strain), and generally had increased stiffness (with steeper slopes) in the linear region of the curves (generally exceeding 0.6 mm elongation: 4.2% strain) (Fig. 3). At day 90, the PA+G explanted meshes were the stiffest of all the explanted meshes, and comparable to the control tissue explants, although this was only significant ($p<0.05$) at elongations exceeding 2.0 mm (14% strain).

Tissue Biocompatibility of Meshes

We examined the microscopic changes induced by the implanted mesh materials using histological stains and immunohistochemistry. As shown in Fig. S2A and B there was substantial cell and tissue formation around the mesh filaments at 7 days. At

Table 2. Adhesion scores of rats implanted with meshes.

Time (days)	PA	PA+G	PEEK	PP
7	1.0±0.0	1.0±0.0	1.0±0.0	1.0±0.0
30	1.0±0.0	1.0±0.0	1.0±0.0	1.0±0.0
60	2.0±0.3	2.0±0.0	1.8±0.2	2.3±0.2
90	1.3±0.2[a,b]	1.8±0.2	2.0±0.0	2.0±0.0

Data are mean ± SEM.
[a]$p<0.05$ compared to PA+G.
[b]$p<0.001$ compared to PEEK and PP.

Table 3. Percentage adhesion area of meshes implanted into abdominal fascial wound in rats.

Time (days)	PA	PA+G	PEEK	PP
7	88±4	73±14	86±5	80±9
30	72±10[a]	40±4	40±8	73±8[b]
60	48±8	42±8	43±8	63±7
90	52±8	53±4	55±6	72±4

Data are mean ± SEM.
[a]$p<0.05$ compared to PA+G and PEEK.
[b]$p<0.05$ compared to PA+G and PEEK.

Table 4. Percentage mesh contraction in rats implanted with meshes.

Timepoints	PA	PA+G	PEEK	PP
7	17.8±2.0	7.1±1.9	19.7±5.1	8.7±2.5
30	29.9±7.0[a]	21.1±5.0	10.9±4.3	26.7±3.0[b]
60	13.0±5.0	9.2±2.4	11.2±2.4	14.6±2.0
90	14.7±5.4	9.0±4.3	19.4±3.0	15.1±2.8

Data are presented as percentage reduction in size from original implanted mesh as mean ± SEM.
[a]$p<0.01$ compared to PEEK.
[b]$p<0.05$ compared to PEEK.
*denotes gelatin around PA filaments.

90 days some encapsulation tissue was still apparent around all filament bundles. PA+G meshes had a greater tissue and cell response around the mesh filaments at 90 days compared to the other mesh types. No microscopic differences were apparent in the control group between 7 and 90 days.

To quantify this tissue response, image analysis was undertaken to examine the gradient of positive staining in 50 µm increments from the central mesh filaments. A diminishing gradient, with a significant decrease, in CD45 and CD68 immunostaining was observed with increasing distance from the filaments (Fig. S4A). We therefore studied the immediate area surrounding the mesh (within 50 µm). No continuous gradient was observed for the other stains (Sirius red, αSMA and CD31) (Fig. S4B), which were analysed using the entire micrograph.

Inflammatory Foreign Body Reaction

The inflammatory response to the implanted meshes was evaluated by examining the extent of $CD45^+$ leukocyte distribution in and around the meshes. CD45 is expressed on all hematopoietic cells except erythrocytes. Larger numbers of leukocytes (red fluorescence) were observed around the meshes (Fig. 4A) at all time points (Fig. 4C), compared to controls where no meshes were present (Fig. 4C). There were significantly fewer CD45 positive cells at 7 and 30 days in the control and PA+G groups compared to PA, PEEK and PP ($p<0.001$) (Fig. 4C). At 60 days PA, PA+G and PEEK attracted significantly more leukocytes than the control ($p<0.05$), with higher positive staining for PEEK, compared to PP ($p<0.05$). At 90 days, the new meshes showed greater leukocyte infiltration than the control and PP groups ($p<0.001$) (Fig. 4C).

To assess macrophage involvement we used the CD68 antibody (Fig. 5). The kinetics of macrophage infiltration varied between mesh types. For example, for the PA mesh, macrophages significantly increased over time from day 7 (Fig. 5A) to day 90 (Fig. 5C) ($p<0.001$). Significantly more macrophages were observed around the filaments for all mesh types than in the control group ($p<0.001$), at all timepoints (Fig. 5C). At 90 days PA meshes were surrounded by significantly more macrophages than PP ($p<0.05$) (Fig. 5C).

Collagen Deposition

Collagen deposition was assessed using Sirius red staining which shows the collagen as red stained material in bright-field microscopy (Figure 6A, B). On day 7 PEEK meshes showed pronounced Sirius red staining loosely distributed around a dense cellular infiltrate (Fig. 6A). At day 90, the cellular infiltrate was less and collagen levels were reduced but more localised around the filaments of the porous mesh (Fig. 6B). At 7 days, a significantly lower collagen content was observed in the control and PP groups

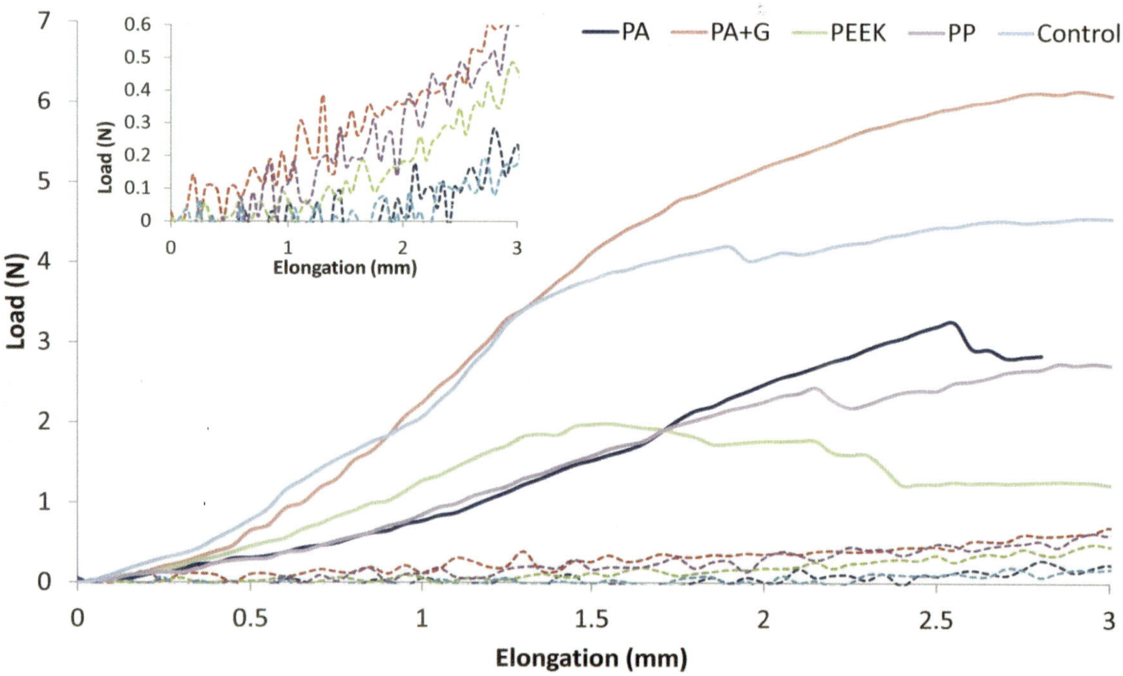

Figure 3. Biomechanical properties of explanted mesh types and control on day 7 (- - -) and day 90 (—). Failure region of graph has not been included. Average explant stiffness is indicated by the slope of the curve, with stiffer materials possessing a steeper gradient. Inset is an enlargement of day 7 meshes.

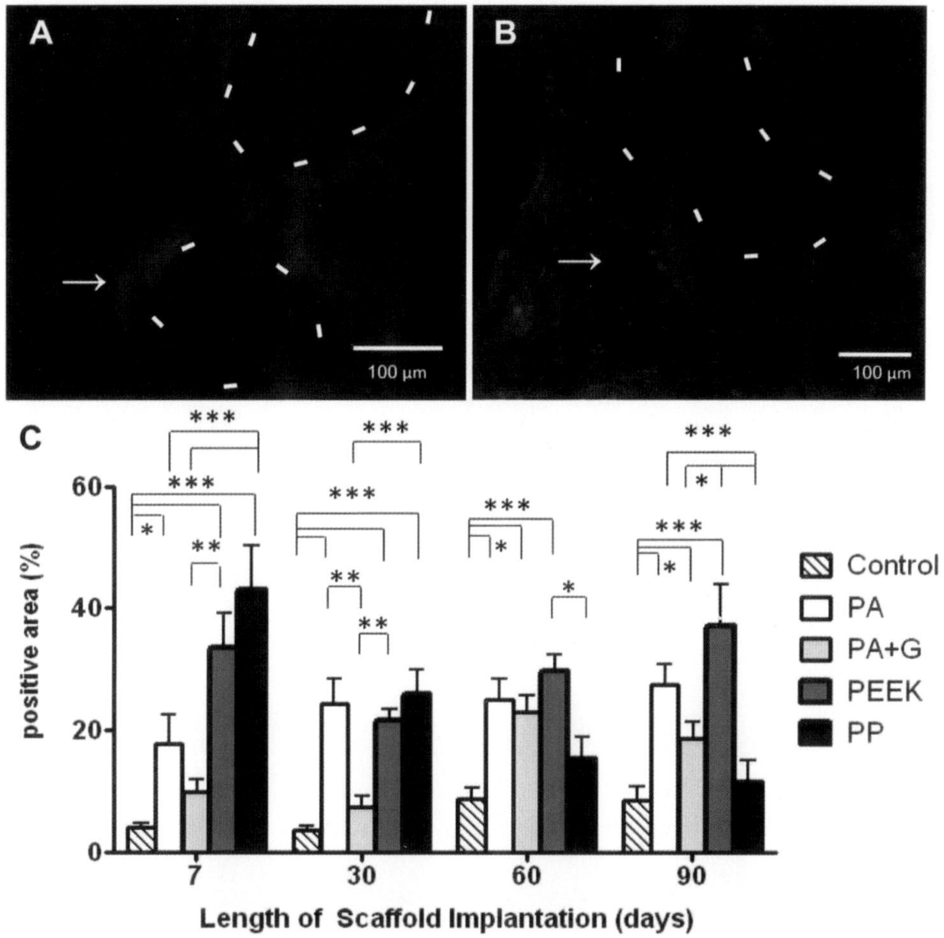

Figure 4. CD45 immunostaining in rats implanted with synthetic mesh. A. PA after 7 days (- - - line indicates mesh filament) and B. After 90 days implantation (arrow indicates a representative CD45 positive cell). C. Percentage CD45 positive area within the 50 μm radius of central mesh filament bundles. Data are mean ± SEM of n=6 animals/ group *: $p<0.05$, **: $p<0.01$ Scale bar, 100 μm.

compared to PA, PA+G and PEEK meshes ($p<0.001$) (Fig. 6C). At 30 days, PA+G mesh induced the highest collagen deposition which was significantly greater than PA, PEEK and PP meshes ($p<0.001$), and comparable to control animals. At 90 days PA, PEEK and PP meshes were all significantly lower in collagen content ($p<0.001$) than the control, whilst the PA+G mesh was significantly higher, and comparable to the control (Fig. 6C). Compared to 7 days, collagen content decreased significantly in both PA and PEEK meshes ($p<0.05$) at 90 days, whereas collagen increased significantly in PP meshes ($p<0.05$).

Vascularisation

The development of vascular structures in the explanted meshes was assessed using the marker CD31 which is expressed on endothelial cells, platelets and subsets of leukocytes. It predominantly stains endothelial cells on small and large blood vessels. Similar to all mesh types, the PA +G meshes were vascularised by day 7 (Fig. 7A), with vessels present at each time point, until day 90 (Fig. 7B). The positive area for CD31 (Fig. 7C) was similar between all mesh groups, and comparable with control animals, on day 7. On day 30 the control group and PEEK meshes showed significantly more positive staining than the PP meshes ($p<0.01$, $p<0.05$ respectively) (Fig. 7C). Vascularisation of PA and PEEK mesh types, and control animals was significantly higher than in PP meshes, at 60 and 90 days ($p<0.01$) (Fig. 7C). The extent of vascularisation increased with time for the PA meshes, and was significantly greater at 60 and 90 days compared to day 7 and day 30 ($p<0.05$). Vascularisation in the PEEK and PA+G meshes was similar at the different timepoints, as were the PP meshes, which had the least CD31 staining overall. To assess larger (stabilized) vessels having a smooth muscle cell coat, αSMA staining was performed. Figure 8A shows a large number of immunostained myofibroblasts in the PEEK meshes on day 7, which were similarly observed in all mesh types at 7 and 30 days. Larger vessels were seen at 90 days, for example in PEEK meshes (Fig. 8B). All meshes induced similar levels of myofibroblast differentiation and smooth muscle cells at 7 and 30 days (Fig. 8C). At 60 days, PA, PA+G and PEEK meshes had significantly more αSMA staining compared to PP meshes ($P<0.01$). At 90 days, all mesh types had a significantly lower positive signal compared to the other time points with no differences between the mesh groups.

Discussion

In this study we compared the *in vivo* biocompatibility of alternative synthetic meshes with a clinical PP mesh, and a tissue control, by investigating biomechanics, collagen deposition, vascularisation and foreign body tissue reaction. Synthetic mesh, manufactured from alternative polymers to a clinical PP mesh,

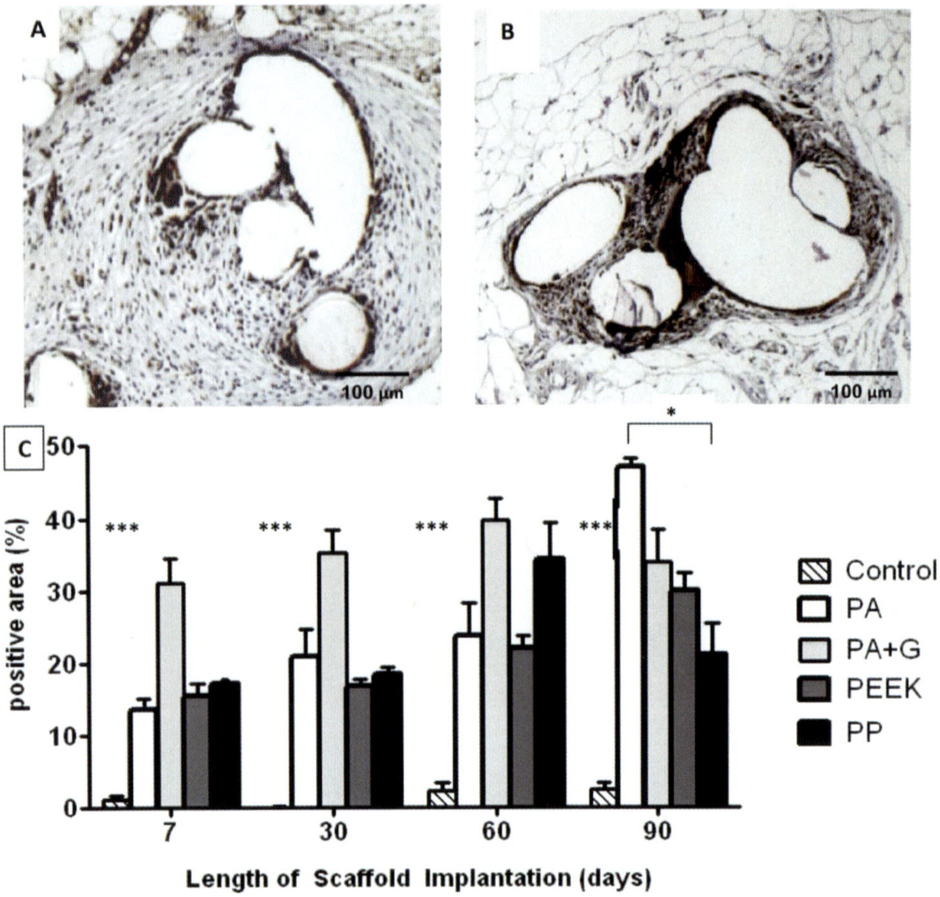

Figure 5. CD68 immunostaining in rats implanted with synthetic mesh. A. PA after 7 days and B. after 90 days implantation (- - - line around mesh filament). Brown staining indicates $CD68^+$ macrophages. C. Percentage CD68 positive area within 50 µm radius of central mesh filament bundle. Data are mean ± SEM of n=6 animals/ group, * $p<0.05$; *** $p<0.001$. Scale bar, 100 µm.

were warp knitted to a similar pattern, using yarn of the same diameter. This ensured that mesh pores were similar in size. Any differences in the host biological response were, therefore, a result of the polymer alone or of the coating. We studied the effect of gelatin coating only in the PA mesh as the tissue response to this composite mesh deemed to be representative for all polymers. This study showed that our new meshes induced a typical foreign body reaction over the time course, largely comparable with the PP meshes, but that there were differences with the extent and type of responses associated with inflammation, macrophage infiltration, collagen deposition and neovascularisation over the 90 day period.

In general, the PA+G meshes showed the least early CD45+ve inflammatory response at 7 and 30 days suggesting that the coating acts like a biofilm, while the PEEK and PP meshes were associated with a more acute inflammation that persisted with the PEEK meshes and subsided with the PP meshes over time. Nonetheless, the macrophage CD68 response depicted a general acute response to all implants. Generally, after implantation of a mesh an acute inflammatory reaction occurs, with macrophages dominating the acute phase at 7 days [16]. In our study, the inflammatory response to the foreign materials showed typical temporal differences. The PA+G meshes had notably more macrophages than the other mesh types at Day 7. Given that these mesh types had the lowest CD45 response at the same time point, it is likely that the major acute response here is due to macrophages. The PP response is similar to that described by Spelzini et al who also showed a lower foreign body reaction at 90 days around the PP implant compared to silk implants [19]. Apart from its role in acute inflammation and early vascularisation, macrophages also have a critical role in the subsequent chronic phase of the host response. In particular, macrophages can potentially differentiate towards two pathways, one leading to an immediate and/or persistent inflammation, the other leading to a constructive remodelling and new tissue generation [20]. This M1/M2 macrophage polarisation has not been studied in this current study. In the case with the PA+G meshes, the gelatin was found to be degrading at the later stages of implantation, associated with more available porous openings allowing fibroblast infiltration and new collagen deposition. It is likely, although speculative, that in these meshes immunoregulatory M2 macrophages are the major type of cell.

Consistent with this, our meshes led to better tissue integration (collagen deposition for PA+G on day 90) and neovascularisation at day 60 compared with the PP meshes. All mesh types were generally well tolerated, with significant weight gain in all rats by 90 days. PA and PA+G implanted rats gained significantly more weight at 90 days compared to the other mesh types and the control, suggesting that these were better tolerated by the animals.

In line with previous studies examining several commercially available mesh types [21,22], both our new meshes and the PP meshes showed contraction at all time points. In general, a correlation can be drawn between collagen deposition and mesh

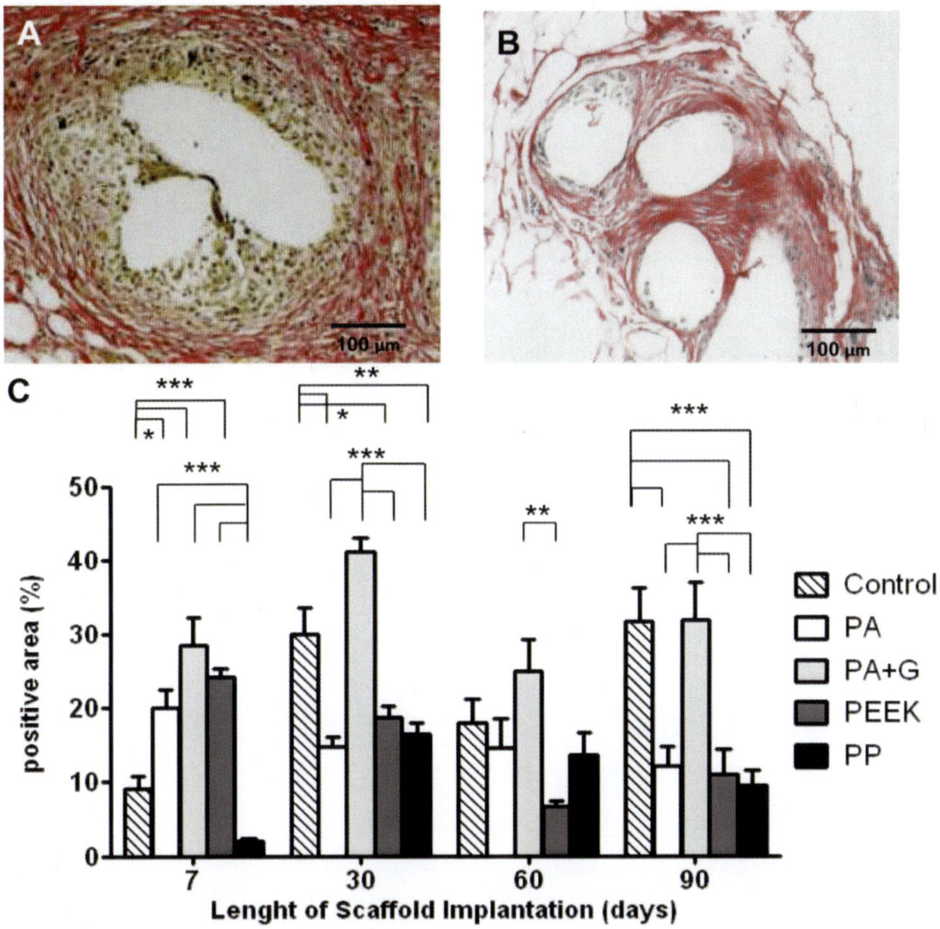

Figure 6. Sirius red staining of collagen fibres in rats implanted with synthetic mesh. A. PEEK after 7 days and B. After 90 days implantation. C. Percentage Sirius red stained area within 50 µm radius of central mesh filament bundle. Data are mean ± SEM of n = 6 animals/ group *: $p<0.05$; **: $p<0.01$, ***: $p<0.001$, Scale bar, 100 µm.

contraction for the PA+G, PEEK and PP mesh types, with an increase in collagen deposition leading to an increase in mesh contraction. It has been reported that both folding and contraction after implantation are responsible for side effects such as pain and tissue erosion [8]. No major differences in adhesion scores were determined between the mesh types assessed using the Lorenz adhesion scores [18]. PA had a significantly smaller adhesion area at 90 days compared to PEEK and PP, indicating that PA might produce fewer adhesions in the long term. No significant differences were found between the other mesh groups. Similar to our findings Boehm et al. compared Ultrapro® (combined PP and absorbable Monocryl®) and Prolene® (polypropylene) with no significant differences in terms of adhesions between the groups [21].

Uniaxial tensile testing was used to assess the biomechanical properties of explanted meshes, with stiffness represented by the slope of the load-elongation curve. Curves for the day 90 explants were found to be bilinear, with a region of initial low stiffness (toe region), followed by a region of higher stiffness (linear stiffness), as found by Afonso et al [23]. Biomechanical testing found all mesh types to be stiffer on day 90 compared to their day 7 counterparts, when loaded beyond strains of 4.2%. Collagen levels decreased between days 7 and 90 for some mesh types, suggesting that collagen alone did not contribute to increased explant stiffness; nor did mesh contraction since contraction was similar for all mesh types except PP. The present results are likely due to a combination of innate mesh mechanical properties and the amount, type and orientation of collagen formed, as suggested by the relative differences in stiffness between the 90 day explanted meshes and collagen levels. Separate tensile studies conducted on these meshes gave no indication of mesh creep, and without a necrotic response, it seems unlikely that any plasticizing material in the polymer was released. The large quantity of collagen present on the PA+G meshes at all time points, except day 60 (for which low rat weights were recorded), suggests that the gelatin coating promoted collagen deposition, or was associated with a cellular response that promoted an environment for fibroblast infiltration, collagen secretion and tissue remodelling. When the gelatin coating had almost fully degraded by day 90 (Fig. S2C), mesh pores became accessible to cells (Fig. S2B h), and permitted collagen synthesis, particularly within the large pores, between the filament bundles. Generally, the level of collagen decreased between 30 and 90 days for all mesh types. This outcome could be related to the fact that the meshes themselves do not promote tissue integration in the long term, or the type of tissue response is too rapid and does not allow for gradual cell infiltration, collagen synthesis and tissue remodelling that may be occurring with the PA+G meshes. We have addressed the need for a more objective analysis of collagen in mesh explants as identified in previous studies [17]. However it is difficult to make comparisons with these

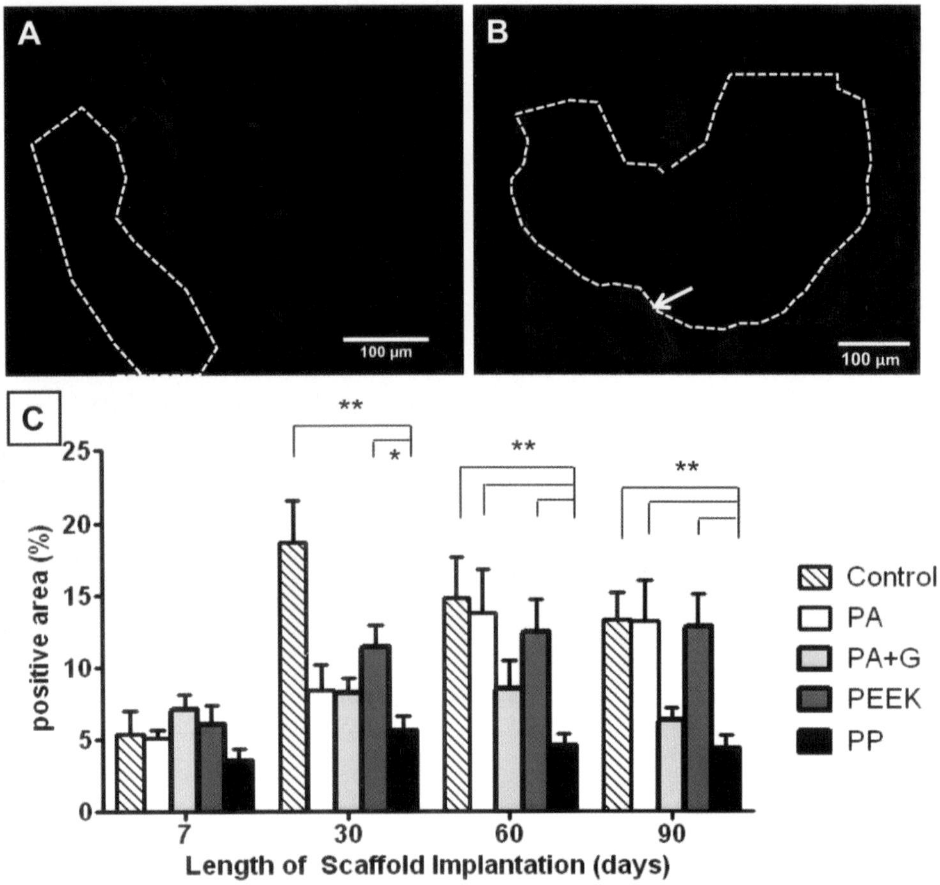

Figure 7. CD31 immunostaining in rats implanted with synthetic mesh. A. PA+G after 7 days and B. After 90 days implantation (- - - line around mesh filament). C: Percentage positive CD31 area within 50 µm radius of mesh. Data are mean ± SEM of n=6 animals/ group, *p<0.05, **p<0.01.

studies and the current quantitative evaluation. Our novel image analysis enables quantification of the amount of collagen and its relationship to the mesh filaments, whereas other studies have scored the organisation of collagen fibres which is also important for mechanical strength [16,24]. Irrespective of this, collagen levels diminish, where in fact, collagen remained more closely associated with mesh filaments, rather than encapsulating the entire implant. In addition, the Sirius red stain does not take into account packing density of collagen fibrils or type of collagen around the mesh filaments, both of which will impact on the mechanical behaviour of the tissue.

Neovascularisation as measured by CD31 immunostaining reached highest levels at 60 and 90 days which is in agreement with previous studies for PP meshes [7,17]. In the current study, PP meshes were consistently less vascularised over the entire time period compared with all new mesh types. In particular, PA and PEEK meshes were superior to PP meshes at 60 and 90 days, perhaps indicating these materials are intrinsically more permissive for angiogenic processes, or are simply comparable to vascularisation in control tissues, and the PP meshes actually inhibit the process. Vascularisation could be further improved by incorporating angiogenic factors onto the mesh filaments during fabrication [25].

Smooth muscle cells and myofibroblasts are cells implicated in wound healing where strengthening wound tissue is important. Our studies show a steady increase in alpha smooth muscle actin until 60 days. At this time point, all 3 new meshes were associated with significantly elevated smooth muscle cells compared with the PP meshes. These cells are finally lost through apoptosis after healing is complete explaining the significant decrease at 90 days. Acquisition of a smooth muscle cell coat by neovessels increases their stability, a desirable feature in the repair of tissues, including those that have herniated, by providing a stable blood supply to nourish neotissue and maintain its integrity in the long term.

In addition to the novelty of the new types of polymer meshes and biological coating used in this study, the strength of the current study is reflected in the use of computer-based analysis of the immunohistochemically stained slides using image analysis software. Histological analysis is the most commonly used technique in assessing new meshes [9]. Qualitative and semi-quantitative analysis of tissue by histology/immunohistochemistry has its limitations. Apart from the fact that different parts of the meshes are studied for histology making comparisons difficult [26,27] more relevant is the problem of subjectivity during the scoring process. In the current study, subjective bias during the scoring process is excluded as the software detects the positive signal in each immunostained image on the same set of 4 centrally placed mesh filaments and calculates the percentage stained area. Also, for the first time, we report a significant gradient for inflammatory cells surrounding mesh filaments, by using the software to examine staining and cell numbers within 50 µm increments from the surface of the filament bundles. Using the

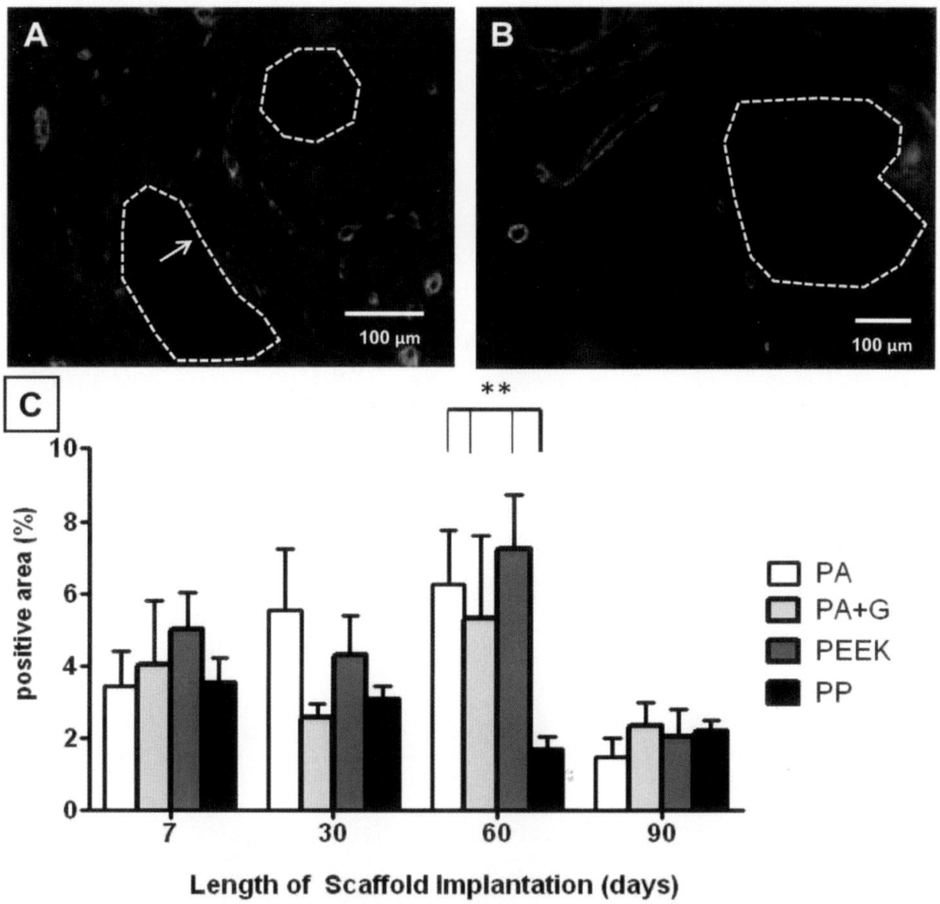

Figure 8. αSMA staining in rats implanted with synthetic mesh. A. PEEK after 7 days and B. after 90 days after implantation (dotted line around mesh filament, arrow indicates vessel). C. Percentage of positive αSMA staining. Data are mean ± SEM of n = 6 animals/ group, **: $p<0.01$. Scale bar, 100 µm.

image analysis software allowed us to investigate the same area of stained tissue for every image and precisely focus on the area of interest.

A limitation of this study is the choice of model for assessing *in vivo* biocompatibility of mesh to be used for fascial defect repair. The rat abdominal wall hernia model does not mimic the clinical environment. However, this model is well accepted for initial testing of newly designed meshes for both synthetic and biological materials in hernia repair, including pelvic organ prolapse [28]. The clinical interpretation needs to be carefully considered in animals lacking any pathological conditions.

The optimal mesh for hernia or POP repair has not been developed yet [8]. Our ongoing studies indicate that PA+G meshes promote good cell attachment and proliferation for mesenchymal stem cell growth and may be suitable as meshes, (data not published). In conclusion, the new mesh types investigated in this study might form the basis of a new option for the future treatment of fascial defects.

Supporting Information

Figure S1 Schematic of overlay technique. A: Ventral full-thickness abdominal defect involving the transversalis fascia, rectus abdominis muscle, and peritoneum. Meshes (dotted green line), in direct contact with the viscera and skin were sutured with slight overlay to the abdominal wall, B: Rat incisional hernia model in control groups. The defect (dotted red lines) was repaired by manipulating the contralateral full-thickness abdominal wall (blue line). Photographs of rat abdominal wall C. At time of mesh implantation (PA) B. At 7 days of mesh implantation (PA+G) C. At 90 days of mesh implantation (PA+G) representative for all mesh groups.

Figure S2 H+E stained sections from rats implanted with synthetic mesh. A. Composite picture showing typical distribution of mesh filament bundles of PA at 7 days. B. Composite picture with several mesh filaments of PA at 90 days. C. Single filament bundles at higher power for control, PA, PA+G, PEEK and PP mesh after 7 days and. 90 days implantation. * denotes gelatin around PA filaments.

Figure S3 Biomechanical properties of explanted mesh types and control on day 7 (- - - lines) and day 90 (— lines). Explant stiffness is indicated by the slope of the curve, with stiffer materials possessing a steeper gradient. This is the same data shown in Figure 3 (means) and in addition includes 95% CI error bars.

Figure S4 Gradient analysis around the mesh filaments in 50 µm increments in PEEK meshes (representative

example for all meshes). A. CD68 positive staining at 7, 30, 60 and 90 days. *: $p<0.05$, ***: $p<0.001$. B. αSMA staining at 7, 30, 60 and 90 days. *: $p<0.05$, ***: $p<0.001$

Acknowledgments

We thank Dr Keith McLean for advice and Dr Vincent Letouzey for critical reading of the manuscript.

Author Contributions

Conceived and designed the experiments: SLE JAW JAMR AR CEG. Performed the experiments: DU SLE JFW TS. Analyzed the data: DU SLE TS CL. Contributed reagents/materials/analysis tools: CL AR. Wrote the paper: DU SLE AR JAW CEG.

References

1. Mudge M, Hughes LE (1985) Incisional Hernia - A 10 year prospective -study of incidence and attitudes. Br J Surg 72: 70–71.
2. Sailes FC, Walls J, Guelig D, Mirzabeigi M, Long WD, et al. (2011) Ventral Hernia Repairs: 10-Year Single-Institution Review at Thomas Jefferson University Hospital. J Am Coll Surg 212: 119–123.
3. Cassar K, Munro A (2002) Surgical treatment of incisional hernia. Br J Surg 89: 534–545.
4. Hunskaar S, Burgio K, Clark A, Lapitan MC, Nelson R, et al. (2005) Epidemiology of urinary (UI) and faecal (FI) incontinence and pelvic organ prolapse (POP); Abrams P, Cardozo L, Khoury S, Wien A, editors. Available: http://www.icsoffice.org/Publications/ICI_3/v1.pdf/chap5.pdf. 255–312 p. Accessed 22.10.2012.
5. Butters M, Redecke J, Koninger J (2007) Long-term results of a randomized clinical trial of Shouldice, Lichtenstein and transabdominal preperitoneal hernia repairs. Br J Surg 94: 562–565.
6. Stanford EJ, Cassidenti A, Moen MD (2012) Traditional native tissue versus mesh-augmented pelvic organ prolapse repairs: providing an accurate interpretation of current literature. Int Urogynecol J 23: 19–28.
7. Konstantinovic ML, Pille E, Malinowska M, Verbeken E, De Ridder D, et al. (2007) Tensile strength and host response towards different polypropylene implant materials used for augmentation of fascial repair in a rat model. Int Urogynecol J Pelvic Floor Dysfunct 18: 619–626.
8. Deprest J, Zheng F, Konstantinovic M, Spelzini F, Claerhout F, et al. (2006) The biology behind fascial defects and the use of implants in pelvic organ prolapse repair. Int Urogynecol J Pelvic Floor Dysfunct 17 Suppl 1: S16–25.
9. de Tayrac R, Alves A, Therin M (2007) Collagen-coated vs noncoated low-weight polypropylene meshes in a sheep model for vaginal surgery. A pilot study. Int Urogynecol J Pelvic Floor Dysfunct 18: 513–520.
10. Lim YN, Muller R, Corstiaans A, Hitchins S, Barry C, et al. (2007) A long-term review of posterior colporrhaphy with Vypro 2 mesh. Int Urogynecol J Pelvic Floor Dysfunct 18: 1053–1057.
11. Robinson TN, Clarke JH, Schoen J, Walsh MD (2005) Major mesh-related complications following hernia repair - Events reported to the Food and Drug Administration. Surgical Endoscopy and Other Interventional Techniques 19: 1556–1560.
12. Pereira-Lucena CG, Artigiani-Neto R, Lopes GJ, Frazao CVG, Goldenberg A, et al. (2010) Experimental study comparing meshes made of polypropylene, polypropylene plus polyglactin and polypropylene plus titanium: inflammatory cytokines, histological changes and morphometric analysis of collagen. Hernia 14: 299–304.
13. Felemovicius I, Bonsack ME, Hagerman G, Delaney JP (2004) Prevention of adhesions to polypropylene mesh. J Am Coll Surg 198: 543–548.
14. Tadokoro M, Matsushima A, Kotobuki N, Hirose M, Kimura Y, et al. (2012) Bone morphogenetic protein-2 in biodegradable gelatin and ss-tricalcium phosphate sponges enhances the in vivo bone-forming capability of bone marrow mesenchymal stem cells. J Tissue Eng Regen Med 6: 253–260.
15. Bostonscientific website. Available: http://www.bostonscientific.com/templatedata/imports/collateral/Gynecology/broc_Polyform_01_ug_us.pdf. Accessed 22.10.2012.
16. Zheng F, Lin Y, Verbeken E, Claerhout F, Fastrez M, et al. (2004) Host response after reconstruction of abdominal wall defects with porcine dermal collagen in a rat model. Am J Obstet Gynecol 191: 1961–1970.
17. Ozog Y, Konstantinovic ML, Verschueren S, Spelzini F, De Ridder D, et al. (2009) Experimental comparison of abdominal wall repair using different methods of enhancement by small intestinal submucosa graft. Int Urogynecol J Pelvic Floor Dysfunct 20: 435–441.
18. Zuhlke HV, Lorenz EMP, Straub EM, Savvas V (1990) PATHOPHYSIOLOGY AND CLASSIFICATION OF ADHESIONS. Langenbecks Arch Chir: 1009–1016.
19. Spelzini F, Konstantinovic ML, Guelinckx I, Verbist G, Verbeken E, et al. (2007) Tensile strength and host response towards silk and type i polypropylene implants used for augmentation of fascial repair in a rat model. Gynecol Obstet Invest 63: 155–162.
20. Mantovani A, Sica A, Sozzani S, Allavena P, Vecchi A, et al. (2004) The chemokine system in diverse forms of macrophage activation and polarization. Trends in Immunology 25: 677–686.
21. Bohm G, Steinau G, Krahling E, Schumpelick V, Hermanns-Sachweh B, et al. (2011) Is Biocompatibility Affected by Constant Shear Stress? - Comparison of Three Commercially Available Meshes in a Rabbit Model. J Biomater Appl 25: 721–741.
22. Garcia-Urena MA, Ruiz VV, Godoy AD, Perea JMB, Gomez LMM, et al. (2007) Differences in polypropylene shrinkage depending on mesh position in an experimental study. Am J Surg 193: 538–542.
23. Afonso JS, Martins P, Girao M, Jorge RMN, Ferreira AJM, et al. (2008) Mechanical properties of polypropylene mesh used in pelvic floor repair. Int Urogynecol J 19: 375–380.
24. Konstantinovic ML, Lagae P, Zheng F, Verbeken EK, De Ridder D, et al. (2005) Comparison of host response to polypropylene and non-cross-linked porcine small intestine serosal-derived collagen implants in a rat model. Bjog 112: 1554–1560.
25. Oh HH, Lu HX, Kawazoe N, Chen GP (2012) Micropatterned angiogenesis induced by poly(D,L-lactic-co-glycolic acid) mesh-structured scaffolds. J Bioact Compat Polym 27: 97–106.
26. Bellows CF, Wheatley BM, Moroz K, Rosales SC, Morici LA (2011) The Effect of Bacterial Infection on the Biomechanical Properties of Biological Mesh in a Rat Model. Plos One 6(6): e21228.
27. Boennelycke M, Christensen L, Nielsen LF, Everland H, Lose G (2011) Tissue response to a new type of biomaterial implanted subcutaneously in rats. Int Urogynecol J 22: 191–196.
28. Abramowitch SD, Feola A, Jallah Z, Moalli PA (2009) Tissue mechanics, animal models, and pelvic organ prolapse: A review. EJOG 144: S146–S158.

15

Insulin-Like Growth Factor 1 Predicts Post-Load Hypoglycemia following Bariatric Surgery

Bianca K. Itariu[1,2], Maximilian Zeyda[1,2], Gerhard Prager[3], Thomas M. Stulnig[1,2]*

1 Division of Endocrinology and Metabolism, Department of Medicine III, Medical University Vienna, Vienna, Austria, **2** Christian Doppler Laboratory for Cardio-Metabolic Immunotherapy, Medical University Vienna, Vienna, Austria, **3** Department of Surgery, Medical University of Vienna, Vienna, Austria

Abstract

Postprandial hypoglycemia is a complication following gastric bypass surgery, which frequently remains undetected. Severe hypoglycemic episodes, however, put patients at risk, e.g., for syncope. A major cause of hypoglycemia following gastric bypass is hyperinsulinemic nesidioblastosis. Since pancreatic islets in nesidioblastosis overexpress insulin-like growth factor 1 (IGF-1) receptor α and administration of recombinant IGF-1 provokes hypoglycemia, our main objective was to investigate the occurrence of post-load hypoglycemia one year after bariatric surgery and its relation to pre- and post-operative IGF-1 serum concentrations. We evaluated metabolic parameters including 2 h 75 g oral glucose tolerance test (OGTT) and measured IGF-1 serum concentration in thirty-six non-diabetic patients (29 f/7 m), aged 41.3±2.0 y with a median (IQR) BMI of 30.9 kg/m^2 (27.5–34.3 kg/m^2), who underwent elective bariatric surgery (predominantly gastric bypass, 83%) at our hospital. Post-load hypoglycemia as defined by a 2 h glucose concentration <60 mg/dl was detected in 50% of patients. Serum insulin and C-peptide concentration during the OGTT and HOMA-IR (homeostatic model assessment–insulin resistance) were similar in hypoglycemic and euglycemic patients. Strikingly, pre- and post-operative serum IGF-1 concentrations were significantly higher in hypoglycemic patients ($p = 0.012$ and $p = 0.007$ respectively). IGF-1 serum concentration before surgery negatively correlated with 2 h glucose concentration during the OGTT (rho = −0.58, $p = 0.0003$). Finally, IGF-1 serum concentrations before and after surgery significantly predicted post-load hypoglycemia with odds ratios of 1.28 (95%CI:1.03–1.55, $p = 0.029$) and 1.18 (95%CI:1.03–1.33, $p = 0.015$), respectively, for each 10 ng/ml increment. IGF-1 serum concentration could be a valuable biomarker to identify patients at risk for hypoglycemia following bariatric surgery independently of a diagnostic OGTT. Thus, IGF-1 testing could help to prevent a significant complication of gastric bypass surgery.

Editor: Alan Stitt, Queen's University Belfast, United Kingdom

Funding: This work was supported by the Austrian National Bank Project no. 12735; the European Community's 7th Framework Programme (FP7/2007-2013) under grant agreement no. 201608 and the Federal Ministry of Economy, Family and Youth; and the National Foundation for Research, Technology and Development (all to T.M.S). The funders had no role in study design, data collection and analysis, decision to publish, or preparation of the manuscript.

Competing Interests: This work was partly supported by the Austrian National Bank Project. There are no patents, products in development or marketed products to declare.

* E-mail: thomas.stulnig@meduniwien.ac.at

Introduction

Bariatric surgery is currently the most effective treatment to achieve and maintain clinically significant long-term weight-loss in severely obese subjects [1]. The mortality rate from disease-related causes decreases in surgically treated patients, but the rate of non-disease deaths, caused by accidents, poisoning of undetermined intent or suicide is twice as high in postoperative patients compared to matched controls [2]. Postprandial, severe and recurrent hypoglycemia is a late complication of Roux-en-Y gastric bypass surgery (RYGB) [3] and could contribute to the post-operative increase in mortality unrelated to disease. Its occurrence is increasingly reported in recent bariatric surgery literature, with symptomatic or asymptomatic forms prevailing to a similar extent [4–6]. The published prevalence of hypoglycemia following bariatric surgery varies greatly depending on the applied definition with a range of 0.2% for patients requiring hospitalisation for severe hypoglycemia to 72% for reactive hypoglycemia in a glucose tolerance test [7,8]. Postoperative hypoglycemia seems to be caused by post-prandial hyperinsulinemia, accompanied or not by pancreatic nesidioblastosis [9–11], or altered incretin release [12–14], even though other causes cannot be ruled out [9]. Hyperinsulinemic hypoglycemia has been described decades ago as a complication of gastrectomy and can lead to life-threatening neuroglycopenia [15]. Therapeutic approaches to prevent hypoglycemia following RYGB are not standardized and comprise dietary interventions, drugs, such as acarbose, diazoxide or verapamil as well as invasive procedures such as subtotal or total pancreatectomy [16,17]. In order to prevent post-prandial hypoglycemia, pre-operative individual risk assessment would be imperative. However, factors predicting the onset of post-load hypoglycemia following bariatric surgery are widely unknown.

Insulin-like growth factor-1 (IGF-1) is a hormone with structural and functional similarities to insulin, whose main functions are regulation of somatic growth, proliferation and apoptosis. IGF-1 enhances insulin sensitivity and lowers glycaemia by stimulating glucose transport in muscle and adipose tissue via signalling mechanisms linked to insulin receptor activation [18]. It also enhances glucose uptake into several cells including osteoblasts by binding to the IGF-1 receptor [19]. Some glucose-related effects may be mediated through the IGF-2 and insulin receptors, although the binding occurs with low affinity. Furthermore IGF-1 promotes bone formation, protein synthesis, neuronal survival and also myelin synthesis [20]. During periods of food deprivation IGF-1 can reverse the negative nitrogen balance and inhibit protein catabolism in muscle [20]. Higher IGF-1 serum concentrations are associated with a higher risk of breast cancer in women and prostate cancer in men [21,22]. IGF-1 concentration is directly related to insulin sensitivity, irrespective of confounders such as age, BMI, WHR or glucose tolerance status, but its association to insulin resistance seems U shaped [23,24]. Bariatric surgery seems to have little effect on circulating IGF-1 concentrations [25,26]. Recombinant IGF-1 is used as a long-term therapy in patients suffering from Laron Syndrome. Due to its insulin-like action, the most common side-effect to exogenous IGF-1 is hypoglycemia, which occurs in a dose-dependent manner [27].

Insulin-like growth factor 1 (IGF-1) receptor α is overexpressed in pancreatic islets in nesidioblastosis and administration of recombinant IGF-1 causes hypoglycemia [27,28]. Given the direct effect of IGF-1 on glucose metabolism we hypothesised that IGF-1 is an indicator for the occurrence of post-prandial hypoglycemia in patients who underwent bariatric surgery. Consequently, high IGF-1 serum levels would be associated with hypoglycemia before and after bariatric surgery independent of insulin secretion. Therefore, we aimed to investigate the occurrence of post-load hypoglycemia by a 2 h OGTT and to assess the utility of IGF-1 serum levels before and after bariatric surgery as a biomarker for post-load hypoglycemia. Our data identified IGF-1 as a novel predicting factor for the occurrence of post-prandial hypoglycemia following bariatric surgery.

Subjects and Methods

Ethics statement

The study was conducted in compliance with the Declaration of Helsinki and Good Clinical Practice guidelines at the Department of Medicine III, Medical University of Vienna, and has been previously approved by the Ethics Committee of the Medical University of Vienna (EK Nr. 963/2009). All subjects provided written informed consent.

Subjects

In this prospective study, we performed longitudinal measurements of metabolic and routine parameters in non-diabetic patients shortly before and approximately one year after the patients underwent elective bariatric surgery (mean follow up time 14±1.9 months). Surgeries were performed at the Department of Surgery of the Medical University of Vienna. We invited patients >18 years of age, who participated in our previous studies [29,30] and from which we collected preoperative anthropometric and metabolic data (n = 55) to participate in this study. Patients were excluded in case of acute illness within the last two weeks, diagnosed type 2 diabetes, acquired immunodeficiency (HIV infection, AIDS), significant liver disease, severe or untreated cardiovascular, renal, pulmonary disease, active malignant disease, etc. Pregnancy or breast feeding were also among the exclusion criteria. Of the 55 patients we aimed to recruit, six patients did not respond to our invitation, five patients refused to participate or did not show up at the scheduled visit, one patient underwent surgery due to complications related to the initial procedure, one patient had died, and four patients were pregnant. We thus recruited 36 patients. Of these, 30 patients underwent RYGB, 3 patients underwent gastric banding and 3 patients underwent sleeve gastrectomy. None of the subjects were on oral antidiabetics of any kind, insulin, or corticosteroids. Before surgery 6 patients were on diuretics but treatment discontinued after surgery. One patient was on antipsychotic mediation before and after surgery. Antipsychotics can influence blood glucose concentration but the medication was continuously administered at both time points, before and after surgery. All samples and data were collected at the Clinical Research Unit of the Division of Endocrinology and Metabolism of the Medical University of Vienna. We advised patients to fast overnight before the examination. Preoperatively and at the follow-up visit, we performed anthropometric and hemodynamic measurements (body mass index (BMI), waist and hip circumference, systolic and diastolic blood pressure), blood sampling for routine laboratory analyses and a standardized 75 g 2 h oral glucose tolerance test (OGTT). Due to technical reasons we failed to perform the OGTT in one patient. After short venous stasis and venipuncture, blood was collected into evacuated vials and the samples were transferred to the Department of Laboratory Medicine of the Medical University of Vienna, where serum concentrations of triglycerides, total-, HDL- and LDL-cholesterol, ALT, GGT, HbA1c, glucose, insulin and C-peptide were determined by routine laboratory analyses.

Metabolic assessment

Fasting serum concentrations of blood lipids (triglycerides, cholesterol, high-density lipoprotein (HDL) cholesterol, low-density lipoprotein (LDL) cholesterol), glucose, liver enzymes [alanine transaminase (ALT), gamma-glutamyl-transferase (GGT)] as well as hemoglobin A_{1c} (HbA_{1c}) were determined by routine laboratory methods at the Department of Laboratory Medicine, Medical University of Vienna; insulin and C-peptide were measured by chemiluminescence immunoassays (Roche Diagnostics GmBH).

Insulin resistance was assessed by the homeostatic model assessment index of insulin resistance (HOMA-IR) calculated as the product of the fasting serum insulin concentration (in milliunits per liter) and fasting plasma glucose concentration (in millimoles per liter) divided by 22.5 [31] and incremental area under the curve (AUC) was calculated for the time course of glucose, insulin and C-peptide concentration during the OGTT. Post-load hypoglycemia was defined by a blood glucose concentration<60 mg/dl (3.3 mmol/l) in the 2nd hour of the OGTT. We calculated beta cell function during the entire OGTT by calculating the dynamic area under the curve of serum C-peptide concentrations as total AUC-(180× basal concentration) [32]. Established OGTT-derived indexes such as the Matsuda Index, the insulinogenic index and the disposition index were calculated in order to assess insulin sensitivity and beta cell function [33]. Disposition index was calculated as insulinogenic index * Matsuda index. Insulinogenic index was calculated as [ΔInsulin30-0(microU/ml)/ΔGlucose30–0(mmol/l)*18]. The C-peptide AUC to insulin AUC ratio was calculated as a measure of hepatic insulin extraction.

Metabolic syndrome was assessed according to the of International Diabetes Federation (IDF) consensus criteria published in 2006 [34], i.e. central obesity (waist >80 cm in women and > 94 cm in men), plus any two of the following criteria: raised triglycerides (≥150 mg/dl), reduced HDL-cholesterol (<50 mg/dl in women and <40 mg/dl in men), raised blood pressure (systolic ≥130 mmHg or diastolic ≥85 mmHg or treatment for previous diagnosed hypertension) or raised fasting plasma glucose (≥100 mg/dl or previously diagnosed diabetes mellitus type 2).

Table 1. Characteristics of obese patients before and one year after bariatric surgery.

	pre-operative	post-operative	P
Sex (f/m)	29/7		
Age (y)	39.9±2.0	41.3±2.0	
Metabolic syndrome (IDF)[a]	19/36	2/36	<0.0001
Anthropometric measurements			
BMI (kg/m^2)	45.4 (41.0–50.7)	30.9 (27.5–34.3)	**<0.0001**
Weight (kg)	130.2±3.7	87.3±2.9	**<0.0001**
Waist (cm)	131.0±2.2	102.2±2.5	<0.0001
WHR	0.92±0.01	0.88±0.01	**0.003**
Systolic BP (mmHg)	128±3	112±2	**0.0002**
Diastolic BP (mmHg)	83±2	71±2,	**0.0001**
Metabolic Parameters			
Triglycerides (mg/dl)	154±9	98.8±5.8	**<0.0001**
Total cholesterol (mg/dl)	205±5	165.5±5.3	**<0.0001**
HDL-C (mg/dl)	47±2	50.7±1.4	**0.002**
LDL-C (mg/dl)	127.8±4.9	95.0±4.2	**<0.0001**
ALT (U/l)	32±3	21.0±1.5	**0.003**
GGT (U/l)	39±4	19.7±1.8	**<0.0001**
FLI	96.9±0.5	51.9±5.7	**<0.0001**
HbA1c%	5.5±0.1	5.2±0.1	**<0.0001**
Fasting Glucose (mg/dl)	94±2	78±1	**<0.0001**
Insulin (µU/ml)	17.3 (7.4–28.8)	2.0 (2.0–5.4)	**<0.0001**
C-peptide (ng/ml)	4.0±0.3	1.8±0.1	**<0.0001**
AUC glucose (mg/dl*2 h)	140.6±4.1	77.4±6.6	**<0.0001**
AUC insulin (µU/ml*2 h)	117.8±21.8	79.2±10.3	**0.019**
AUC C-peptide (ng/ml*2 h)	11.5±0.8	10.8±0.7	0.31
HOMA-IR	3.9 (1.6–6.8)	0.4 (0.4–1.0)	**<0.0001**
IGF-1 (ng/ml)	125.1±8.2	145.6±11.5	0.053

[a]Metabolic syndrome was defined according to IDF criteria;
ALT, alanine transaminase; BP, blood pressure; FLI, fatty liver index; GGT, gamma-glutamyl-transferase; HDL-C, high density lipoprotein cholesterol; LDL-C, low density lipoprotein cholesterol, WHR, waist to hip ratio.

Serum IGF-1 concentration pre- and one year post surgery was determined by chemiluminescent immunoassay on a Siemens Immulite analyzer (Siemens Healthcare Medical Diagnostics, Bad Nauheim, Germany). The assays were performed according to the manufacturer's recommendations by skilled technical laboratory personal methods at the Department of Laboratory Medicine, Medical University of Vienna. Interassay coefficients of variation varied between 2.0–8.5% and the lowest detection limit was 15 ng/ml.

The presence of fatty liver was calculated by an algorithm based on BMI (in kg/m^2), waist circumference (cm), serum triglycerides (mg/dl) and GGT (U/l), called the "fatty liver index" (FLI), with an accuracy in detecting fatty liver of 0.84 (95%CI: 0.81–0.87) [35]. FLI is calculated as $(e^{(0.953\times \mathrm{loge}\ (\mathrm{triglycerides})+0.139\times \mathrm{BMI}+0.718\times \mathrm{loge}(\mathrm{GGT})+0.053\times \mathrm{waist}-15.745)}/(1+e^{(0.953\times \mathrm{loge}\ (\mathrm{triglycerides})+0.139\times \mathrm{BMI}+0.718\times \mathrm{loge}(\mathrm{GGT})+0.053\times \mathrm{waist}-15.745)})*100$ [35].

Statistical analysis

Statistical analysis included all patients. Continuous variables are presented as mean ± SEM if normally distributed, otherwise as median (IQR). Differences between continuous variables before and one year after bariatric surgery were analyzed by paired t-test or the non-parametric Wilcoxon signed rank test, as necessary. Categorical variables were compared by chi-square test. Differences between continuous variables in patients experiencing or not post-load hypoglycemia were calculated by unpaired student's t-test for normally distributed variables otherwise by Mann Whitney U-Test. Correlations were explored by Spearman's rank method. Odds ratios were computed by logistic regression to estimate the predictive value of IGF-1 on post-load hypoglycemia. The risk estimation model for post-load hypoglycemia was calculated for each participant using receiver operating characteristic (ROC) curves. The ROC-AUC and 95% CIs were estimated by non-parametric methods. All analyses were performed with IBM SPSS Statistics 20.0 (IBM Corporation, New York, USA). Differences were considered statistically significant with two sided $p<0.05$ and there were no considerations to adjust for multiplicity.

Results

Patients one year after bariatric surgery are at risk for post-load hypoglycemia

Post-operative changes in anthropometric and laboratory parameters were dramatic (Table 1). Patients on average lost

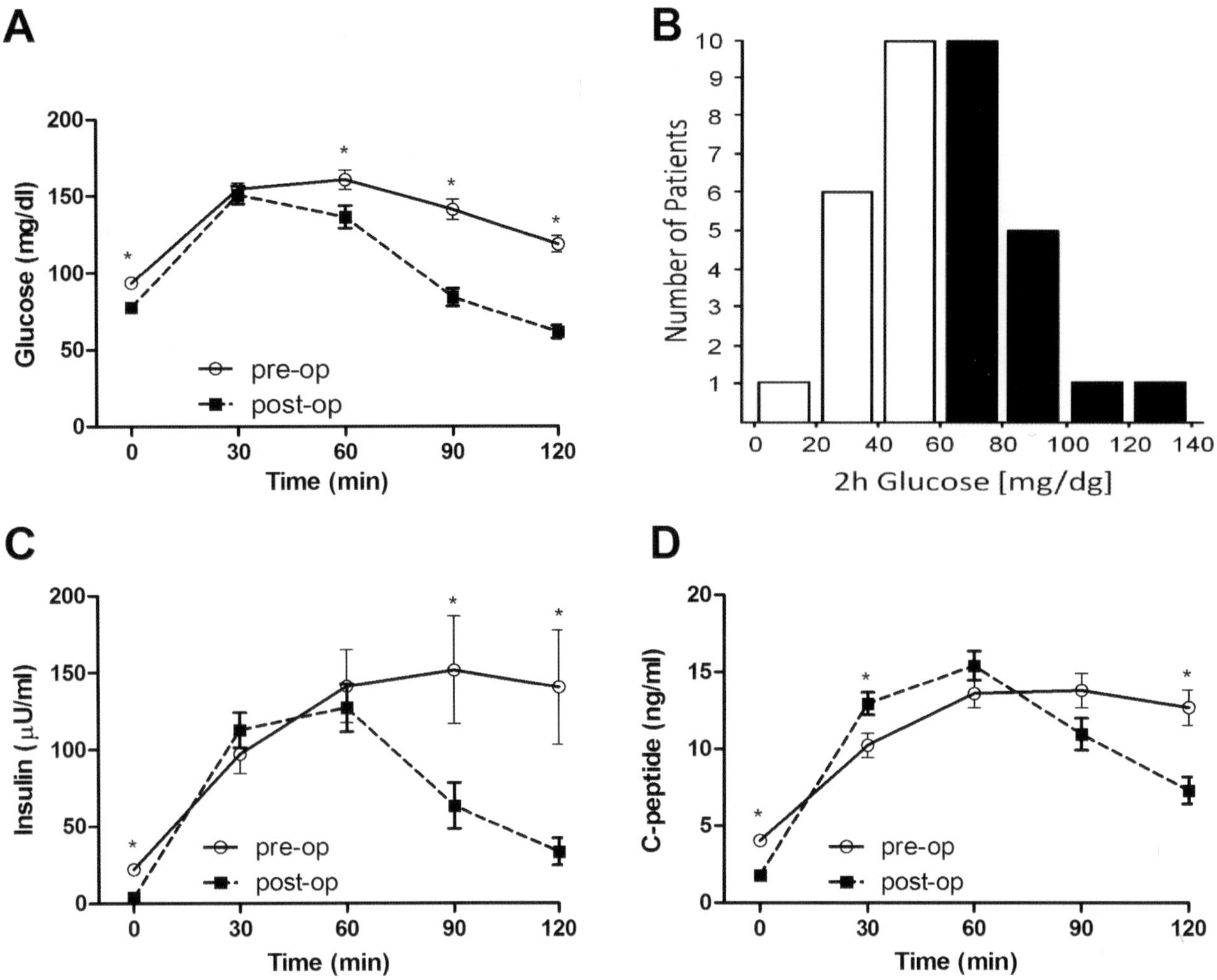

Figure 1. Glucose, insulin and C-peptide concentration during pre-operative and post-operative OGTT. (A) Glucose concentrations during the course of the pre-operative 2 h OGTT (n = 35, full lines) compared to the post-operative OGTT (n = 35, dashed lines). (B) Histogram of post-operative 2 h glucose concentrations during the OGTT (n = 35). Post-load hypoglycemia was defined by a 2 h glucose concentration<60 mg/dl. (C) Insulin and (D) C-peptide concentrations during the course of the pre-operative 2 h OGTT (n = 35, full lines) compared to the post-operative OGTT (n = 35, dashed lines).

15.1±0.8 BMI units, corresponding to a mean weight loss of 43.2±2.5 kg. Parallel to the weight loss, we observed a significant reduction in the number of patients with metabolic syndrome, from 19 before surgery to 2 one year after ($p<0.0001$). Accordingly, we detected a significant improvement in patients' lipid profiles (triglycerides, total, LDL- and HDL-cholesterol, all $p<0.01$). Circulating concentration of liver enzymes ALT and GGT was also reduced, as was the fatty liver index (FLI) (all $p<0.01$), indicating a reduction of obesity-associated fatty liver disease.

Plasma HbA_{1c} concentration after surgery was lower than before surgery and in the normal range at both time-points. Fasting plasma glucose and fasting serum insulin concentrations were significantly reduced after the surgery, as was HOMA-IR (all $p<0.0001$). Glucose concentration during the course of the 2 h-OGTT was drastically changed in the postoperative setting, with significantly lower concentrations after the first hour, which is also reflected by the reduced area under the curve (AUC) - Figure 1A, Table 1. Moreover, post-load hypoglycemia as defined by blood plasma glucose concentration <60 mg/dl at 2 h of the OGTT was detected in half (50%) of all patients (n = 18, Figure 1B). These were mainly patients who underwent RYGB (n = 16). Surprisingly, most patients who experienced post-load hypoglycemia reported no complaints at all, including one patient whose blood glucose concentration reached 14 mg/dl (0.78 mmol/l). First phase insulin response to glucose load (calculated as the insulinogenic index) remained similar to the response observed before surgery, but insulin levels were significantly reduced during the second hour of the OGTT (Figure 1C). The post-operative AUC for insulin concentration was significantly lower than before surgery ($p = 0.019$; Table 1). Interestingly, the C-peptide concentration at 30 minutes of the test was higher after compared to before the operation (Figure 1D; $p = 0.001$), but the AUC for C-peptide concentration was not significantly different (Table 1). Serum IGF-1 concentration increased after surgery by a mean of 20.5±10.2 ng/dl and the increase was significant in trend ($p = 0.053$).

Characteristics of patients with post-load hypoglycemia

We split patients into two groups according to their glycaemic condition at 2 h during the post-operative OGTT (post-load hypoglycemia/euglycemia) and compared the changes in glucose,

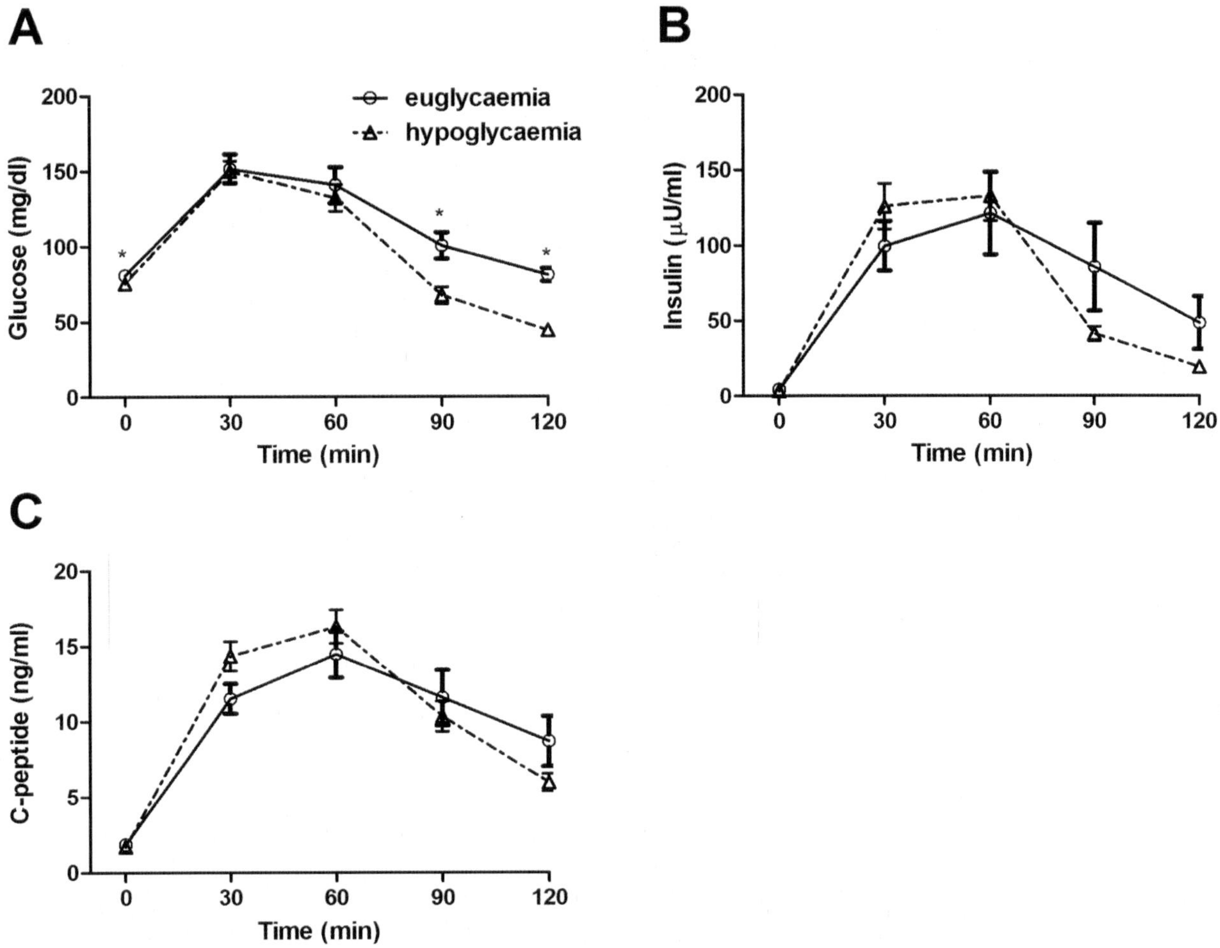

Figure 2. Post-operative OGTT glucose, insulin and C-peptide concentration in patients with euglycemia and hypoglycemia. (A) Glucose, (B) insulin and (C) C-peptide concentrations during the course of the post-operative 2 h OGTT in patients with euglycemia (n = 17, full lines) and patients with post-load hypoglycemia (n = 18, dashed lines). Differences between pre and post-operative values were calculated with paired t-test. Differences between patients with euglycemia and hypoglycemia were calculated by unpaired student's t-test.*p<0.05.

insulin and C-peptide concentrations and respective AUC. We detected significant differences in glucose concentration at time point 0′, 90′ and 120′ during the OGTT (p = 0.020, p = 0.003 and p<0.0001 respectively, Figure 2A), but insulin or C-peptide concentrations during the course of the OGTT were not altered (Figure 2B,C) except for a slight elevation of C-peptide concentration at 30 minutes (p = 0.06). The calculated AUC for glucose, insulin and C-peptide were similar in both groups (Table 2). Beta cell function as assessed by the dynamic AUC of serum C-peptide was not significantly different between the two groups (p = 0.47). There was no difference in the established OGTT-derived indices: Matsuda index, insulinogenic index and disposition index between the two groups (data not shown). Hepatic insulin extraction as calculated by the C-peptide AUC to insulin AUC ratio was not different between the groups (p = 0.24) and was not related to IGF-1 levels before or after surgery.

By comparing anthropometric and laboratory parameters of patients with post-load hypoglycemia and patients with euglycemia, we found that age, WHR, serum triglyceride, fasting plasma glucose and IGF-1 serum concentrations were lower in patients with post-load hypoglycemia - Table 2. Glucose concentration at 2 h during the OGTT correlated with post-operative WHR (rho = 0.48, p = 0.004) and serum triglyceride concentration (rho = 0.50; p = 0.002). Other parameters, including BMI, serum lipids other than triglycerides, liver enzymes and FLI, did not differ between the groups.

Differences between the two groups in baseline anthropometric and laboratory parameters before surgery are presented in Table S1.

IGF-1 serum concentration before and after surgery

We hypothesised that increased IGF-1 concentration could contribute to the susceptibility to develop post-load hypoglycemia. As shown in Table 2, mean post-operative IGF-1 serum concentration for all patients increased in trend, compared to IGF-1 concentration measured before the operation (146±12 vs. 125±8 ng/ml; p = 0.0535). Notably, post-operative IGF-1 concentration was significantly higher in patients with post-load hypoglycemia (n = 18) compared to patients with euglycemia (n = 17, Figure 3A). Interestingly, patients with post-load hypoglycemia had significantly higher serum IGF-1 concentrations compared to patients with euglycemia, already before surgery (145±12 ng/dl vs. 105±9 ng/dl respectively, p = 0.0122). When we analysed other differences in other pre-operative parameters with respect to post-load hypoglycemia, we found that only IGF-1 and age were significantly different between patients with hypoglycemia and euglycemia. Pre-operative IGF-1 serum con-

Table 2. Characteristics of patients with post-load hypoglycemia and euglycemia at 2 h during the post-operative OGTT.

	post-load hypoglycemia	euglycemia	P
Age	36.3±2.6	44.7±2.8	**0.037**
Anthropometric measurements			
BMI (kg/m^2)	31.1 (27.0–35.9)	30.8 (28.0–34.7)	0.88
Weight (kg)	87.0±4.8	88.0±3.6	0.87
Waist (cm)	99.3±3.5	105.6±3.6	0.22
WHR	0.85±0.01	0.91±0.02	**0.018**
Metabolic Parameters			
Triglycerides (mg/dl)	84.1±5.0	114.6±9.7	**0.010**
Total cholesterol (mg/dl)	160.4±6.2	171.2±9.0	0.33
HDL-C (mg/dl)	51.1±2.3	49.9±1.8	0.69
LDL-C (mg/dl)	92.5±5.1	98.4±7.2	0.51
ALT (U/l)	20.4±2.3	20.7±1.9	0.93
GGT (U/l)	17.1±2.3	23.1±2.8	0.10
FLI	46.2±7.8	61.3±8.7	0.21
HbA1c %	5.2±0.1	5.3±0.1	0.34
Fasting Glucose (mg/dl)	75±2	81±1	**0.019**
Insulin (µU/ml)	2.0 (2.0–5.2)	2.0 (2.0–5.4)	0.88
C-peptide (ng/ml)	1.7±0.1	1.9±0.2	0.49
AUC glucose (mg/dl*2 h)	78.8±7.2	75.9±11.4	0.84
AUC insulin (µU/ml*2 h)	75.5±8.4	83.2±19.6	0.72
AUC C-peptide (ng/ml*2 h)	10.9±0.8	10.7±1.2	0.92
HOMA-IR	0.4 (0.4–1.0)	0.4 (0.4–1.1)	0.37
IGF-1 (ng/ml)	168.3±17.1	112.8±8.9	**0.007**

ALT, alanine transaminase; FLI, fatty liver index; GGT, gamma-glutamyl-transferase; HDL-C, high density lipoprotein cholesterol; LDL-C, low density lipoprotein cholesterol; WHR, waist to hip ratio.

centration correlated negatively with glucose concentration at 2 h during the OGTT (rho = −0.58, p = 0.0003), whereas post-operative IGF-1 concentration correlated only in trend (rho = −0.30, p = 0.08; Figure 3B,C). The risk of post-load hypoglycemia one year after bariatric surgery increased by 28% with every 10 ng/ml increment of pre-operative IGF-1 serum concentration (OR 1.28; 95%CI: 1.03–1.55; p = 0.0297) and by 18% with post-operative IGF-1 concentrations (OR 1.18; 95%CI: 1.03–1.33; p = 0.0155). Moreover, patients with a pre-operative serum IGF-1 concentration above the calculated median of the whole cohort of 111 ng/ml had a significantly higher risk of post-load hypoglycemia (OR 4.8; 95%CI: 1.15–20.1; p = 0.0275) while the median cut-off value for post-operative IGF-1 concentration was not significantly associated with a higher risk. Multiple logistic regression for post-operative parameters including IGF-1, age, triglycerides and WHR revealed that only IGF-1 significantly predicted the occurrence of post-load hypoglycemia (OR 1.22; 95%CI: 1.02–1.42, p = 0.0300). The ROC analysis of the risk estimation by pre-operative IGF-1 revealed an AUC of 0.79 (95%CI: 0.64–0.94, p = 0.0033) and hence showed a good accuracy to detect hypoglycemia one year after bariatric surgery (Figure 3D; ROC-AUC of 1.00 represents a perfect test and 0.50 an insignificant test).

Discussion

The main finding of our study was that post-load hypoglycemia approximately one year after bariatric surgery was closely associated with increased circulating IGF-1 concentrations before and after surgery. This could indicate that IGF-1 plays an important role in glucose homeostasis following RYBG.

We noticed a trend increase in post-operative IGF-1 serum concentration compared to pre-operative values. This increase could be attributed to an improvement in liver function following weight loss. Indeed obesity-associated fatty liver disease is likely to improve after weight loss, as reflected by a reduction of BMI, WHR, serum triglycerides and GGT, i.e. the most relevant variables for determining the fatty liver index. However, the reduction of hepatic steatosis, reflected by a reduced fatty liver index, does not seem to affect the risk of hypoglycemia, since both hypoglycemic as well as euglycemic patients had similar fatty liver indices. Therefore, we believe that IGF-1 is in itself a good predictor of post-load hypoglycemia, irrespective of improvements in liver function.

Here we identified increased IGF-1 concentrations before and after surgery as a major risk factor for post-load hypoglycemia. IGF-1 is synthesized in the liver, has structural similarities to proinsulin [36] and augments insulin actions such as stimulating glucose uptake, via phosphorylation of IRS-1, and suppresses hepatic gluconeogenesis [37,38]. Thus, IGF-1 is known to enhance insulin sensitivity in humans and recombinant IGF-1 induces hypoglycemia as does its ectopic secretion [30,39,40]. Interestingly, both pre- and post-operative IGF-1 serum concentrations were significantly higher in subjects with post-load hypoglycemia and the pre-operative levels correlated negatively with 2 h glucose concentration. Thus, IGF-1 concentration was related to hypo-

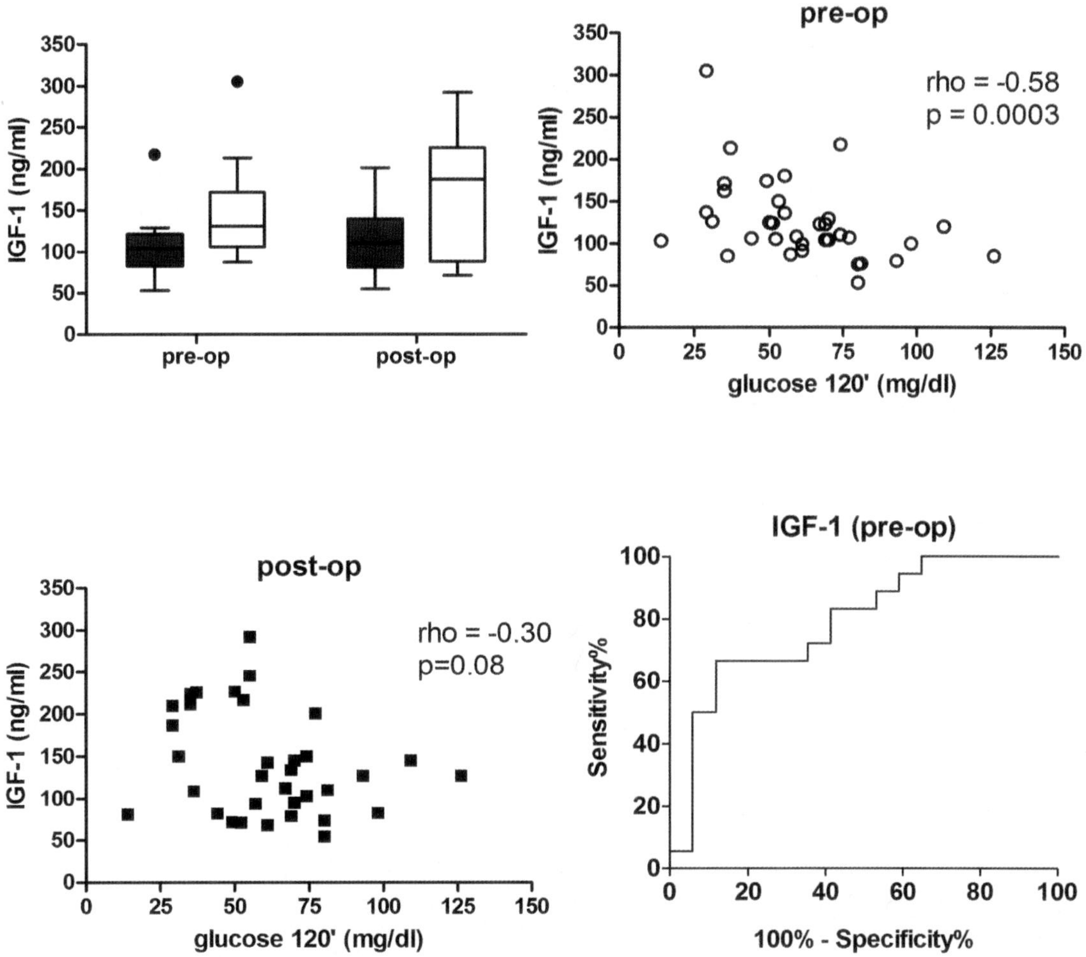

Figure 3. IGF-1 in patients with euglycemia and post-load hypoglycemia at 2 h during the post-operative OGTT. (A) Box-plots of pre- and post-operative serum IGF-1 concentrations in patients with euglycemia (n = 17, black bars) and post-load hypoglycemia (n = 18, white bars). Outliers are represented by dots. (B) Pre-operative serum IGF-1 concentration plotted against 2 h glucose concentration during the post-operative OGTT (n = 35). (C) Post-operative serum IGF-1 concentration plotted against 2 h glucose concentration during the post-operative OGTT (n = 35). (D) ROC-AUC curve for detecting post-load hypoglycemia according to pre-operative IGF-1 concentration (n = 35). Differences between IGF-1 concentrations between the two groups were calculated by unpaired student's t-test. The association between pre- and post-operative serum IGF-1 concentration and post-operative 2 h glucose concentration during the OGTT was analyzed using Spearman's rank correlation,*$p<0.05$.

glycemia risk. Moreover pre-operative IGF-1 serum concentration was the only parameter to be detected before surgery that predicted post-load hypoglycemia. Post-operative IGF-1 serum concentration was also predictive for the risk of hypoglycemia, alone and even after adjustment for other potential risk factors such as age, WHR and triglycerides. Higher IGF-1 concentrations can be detected under physiologic conditions in the young and pathologically in patients with growth hormone secreting pituitary adenomas (acromegaly or gigantism), but these patients present with hyperglycemia. IGF-1 secretion decreases with increasing age and we also observed a negative correlation between pre and post-operative IGF-1 concentration and age ($r = -0.53$, $p = 0.0008$ and $r = -0.41$, $p = 0.013$, respectively). We found no association between IGF-1 and serum triglycerides or IGF-1 and WHR, similar to the findings of Gram et *al* [41]. Furthermore, triglycerides and WHR were no longer significant when added to a multiple logistic regression for hypoglycemia risk, indicating the independent relation of IGF-1 to hypoglycemia.

Patients suffering from hypoglycemia during the OGTT had a similar BMI, but patients with hypoglycemia were younger, had lower WHR, and lower serum triglyceride concentrations than patients with euglycemia. This is partly consistent with work suggesting that diabetes remission is more common in younger, leaner, more insulin sensitive patients with adequate beta-cell function at baseline [42]. These latter correlations suggest that reductions in abdominal fat may be important for decreasing blood lipids and alleviating lipotoxicity effects on post-prandial blood glucose regulation. A possible explanation for post-load hypoglycemia may have been differences in insulin concentrations [9], but we noticed similar insulin and C-peptide responses to the oral glucose load in patients with hypoglycemia and patients with euglycemia. Furthermore both groups were comparable with respect to circulating serum total-, LDL- and HDL-cholesterol, liver enzymes, hepatic insulin extraction and fatty liver index.

Since clinical predictors for post-operative hypoglycemia are missing, we aimed to identify potential risk factors for post-load hypoglycemia occurring one year after bariatric surgery, in a cohort of non-diabetic patients. Strikingly, in an unexpectedly high percentage, namely half of all patients, we detected moderate to severe post-load hypoglycemia at 2 h during an OGTT. This finding was surprising, as the frequency for hypoglycemia following RYGB described in the literature is much lower [1,4,7–9]. Emerging evidence of an increased susceptibility to postprandial hypoglycemia following gastric bypass surgery [43] points to the fact that hypoglycemia might contribute to the increased risk of death from non-disease related causes, such as accidental deaths and suicide [2,44], as hypoglycemia is known to determine an increase in depressive symptoms [45]. Similar to patients under insulin treatment for type 1 or type 2 diabetes, most of the patients we evaluated were completely unaware of hypoglycemia during the test. Hence these patients could suffer from hypoglycemia-related impairments of cognitive and motor functions [46] without being aware of it. Therefore, we believe it is crucial to identify patients at risk for post-prandial hypoglycemia following bariatric surgery. We detected a clinically applicable "threshold" of 111 ng/ml in pre-operative IGF-1 concentration which can be somewhat useful in assessing the risk of hypoglycemia. The association of insulin resistance with IGF-1 concentrations seems to be U shaped [23,24] in patients who did not undergo bariatric surgery and there is not enough data to make such an assumption for bariatric surgery patients. Nevertheless, higher values are predictive of post-load hypoglycaemia following bariatric surgery. Of note, serum IGF-1 concentration can be determined independent of an elaborate and time-consuming oral tolerance test, which further requires patient compliance. As an additional advantage, IGF-1 concentration as a predictive marker can be determined even before the operation and may hence contribute to patient selection for gastric bypass surgery, while all other parameters relating to post-operative hypoglycemia – except from age – need to be determined in the post-operative setting, thus demanding a strict follow-up of patients.

We are aware of some limitation to our study, including the small sample size and the fact that we could not compare the incidence of post-load hypoglycemia across a wider spectrum of surgical techniques, since the most prevalent surgical procedure performed in this cohort, was RYGB. Although the sample size was modest, the differences we observed were consistent enough to encourage further researcher. As for the operating technique, RYGB is most representative, since it is the most commonly performed bariatric procedure worldwide [47]. Moreover, 80% of the patients were women, which is a common finding in bariatric surgery literature and we cannot make the assumption our findings would be identical in men. Further work should be performed including more men and also type two diabetics, since we included only non-diabetic patients.

In conclusion, post- and particularly pre-operative IGF-1 serum concentrations help in identifying patients at risk for developing post-load hypoglycemia. Identification of patients at hypoglycemia risk based on IGF-1 may improve patient selection for gastric bypass surgery, help to tailor dietary recommendations, promote awareness of patients and health-care professionals for this complication, and may hence further improve the prognosis of these patients.

Acknowledgments

We thank the patients for participating in our study. We thank Dr. Christian S. Göbl, from the Department of Gynecology and Obstetrics, Medical University of Vienna, for helpful discussions regarding the statistical analysis.

Author Contributions

Conceived and designed the experiments: TMS BKI. Performed the experiments: BKI GP. Analyzed the data: BKI MZ TMS. Contributed reagents/materials/analysis tools: TMS MZ GP. Wrote the paper: BKI. Critically reviewed the manuscript: TMS MZ GP.

References

1. Karlsson J, Taft C, Ryden A, Sjostrom L, Sullivan M (2007) Ten-year trends in health-related quality of life after surgical and conventional treatment for severe obesity: the SOS intervention study. International journal of obesity 31: 1248–1261.
2. Adams TD, Gress RE, Smith SC, Halverson RC, Simper SC, et al. (2007) Long-term mortality after gastric bypass surgery. The New England journal of medicine 357: 753–761.
3. Neff KJ, Olbers T, le Roux CW (2013) Bariatric surgery: the challenges with candidate selection, individualizing treatment and clinical outcomes. BMC medicine 11: 8.
4. Service GJ, Thompson GB, Service FJ, Andrews JC, Collazo-Clavell ML, et al. (2005) Hyperinsulinemic hypoglycemia with nesidioblastosis after gastric-bypass surgery. The New England journal of medicine 353: 249–254.
5. Kim SH, Liu TC, Abbasi F, Lamendola C, Morton JM, et al. (2009) Plasma glucose and insulin regulation is abnormal following gastric bypass surgery with or without neuroglycopenia. Obesity surgery 19: 1550–1556.
6. Parsaik AK, Carter RE, Myers LA, Dong M, Basu A, et al. (2012) Outcomes of community-dwelling adults without diabetes mellitus who require ambulance services for hypoglycemia. Journal of diabetes science and technology 6: 1107–1113.
7. Marsk R, Jonas E, Rasmussen F, Naslund E (2010) Nationwide cohort study of post-gastric bypass hypoglycaemia including 5,040 patients undergoing surgery for obesity in 1986–2006 in Sweden. Diabetologia 53: 2307–2311.
8. Roslin M, Damani T, Oren J, Andrews R, Yatco E, et al. (2011) Abnormal glucose tolerance testing following gastric bypass demonstrates reactive hypoglycemia. Surgical endoscopy 25: 1926–1932.
9. Patti ME, Goldfine AB (2010) Hypoglycaemia following gastric bypass surgery--diabetes remission in the extreme? Diabetologia 53: 2276–2279.
10. Clancy TE, Moore FD Jr, Zinner MJ (2006) Post-gastric bypass hyperinsulinism with nesidioblastosis: subtotal or total pancreatectomy may be needed to prevent recurrent hypoglycemia. Journal of gastrointestinal surgery: official journal of the Society for Surgery of the Alimentary Tract 10: 1116–1119.
11. Patti ME, McMahon G, Mun EC, Bitton A, Holst JJ, et al. (2005) Severe hypoglycaemia post-gastric bypass requiring partial pancreatectomy: evidence for inappropriate insulin secretion and pancreatic islet hyperplasia. Diabetologia 48: 2236–2240.
12. Anderwald CH, Tura A, Promintzer-Schifferl M, Prager G, Stadler M, et al. (2012) Alterations in gastrointestinal, endocrine, and metabolic processes after bariatric Roux-en-Y gastric bypass surgery. Diabetes care 35: 2580–2587.
13. Holdstock C, Zethelius B, Sundbom M, Karlsson FA, Eden Engstrom B (2008) Postprandial changes in gut regulatory peptides in gastric bypass patients. International journal of obesity 32: 1640–1646.
14. Goldfine AB, Mun EC, Devine E, Bernier R, Baz-Hecht M, et al. (2007) Patients with neuroglycopenia after gastric bypass surgery have exaggerated incretin and insulin secretory responses to a mixed meal. The Journal of clinical endocrinology and metabolism 92: 4678–4685.
15. Roth DA, Meade RC (1965) Hyperinsulinism-Hypoglycemia in the Postgastrectomy Patient. Diabetes 14: 526–528.
16. Moreira RO, Moreira RB, Machado NA, Goncalves TB, Coutinho WF (2008) Post-prandial hypoglycemia after bariatric surgery: pharmacological treatment with verapamil and acarbose. Obesity surgery 18: 1618–1621.
17. Cui Y, Elahi D, Andersen DK (2011) Advances in the etiology and management of hyperinsulinemic hypoglycemia after Roux-en-Y gastric bypass. Journal of gastrointestinal surgery: official journal of the Society for Surgery of the Alimentary Tract 15: 1879–1888.
18. Clemmons DR (2004) Role of insulin-like growth factor iin maintaining normal glucose homeostasis. Hormone research 62 Suppl 1: 77–82.
19. Zoidis E, Ghirlanda-Keller C, Schmid C (2011) Stimulation of glucose transport in osteoblastic cells by parathyroid hormone and insulin-like growth factor I. Molecular and cellular biochemistry 348: 33–42.
20. Laron Z (2001) Insulin-like growth factor 1 (IGF-1): a growth hormone. Molecular pathology: MP 54: 311–316.
21. Key TJ, Appleby PN, Reeves GK, Roddam AW (2010) Insulin-like growth factor 1 (IGF1), IGF binding protein 3 (IGFBP3), and breast cancer risk: pooled

individual data analysis of 17 prospective studies. The lancet oncology 11: 530–542.
22. Roddam AW, Allen NE, Appleby P, Key TJ, Ferrucci L, et al. (2008) Insulin-like growth factors, their binding proteins, and prostate cancer risk: analysis of individual patient data from 12 prospective studies. Annals of internal medicine 149: 461–471, W483–468.
23. Sesti G, Sciacqua A, Cardellini M, Marini MA, Maio R, et al. (2005) Plasma concentration of IGF-I is independently associated with insulin sensitivity in subjects with different degrees of glucose tolerance. Diabetes care 28: 120–125.
24. Friedrich N, Thuesen B, Jorgensen T, Juul A, Spielhagen C, et al. (2012) The association between IGF-I and insulin resistance: a general population study in Danish adults. Diabetes care 35: 768–773.
25. Pellitero S, Granada ML, Martinez E, Balibrea JM, Guanyabens E, et al. (2013) IGF1 modifications after bariatric surgery in morbidly obese patients: potential implications of nutritional status according to specific surgical technique. European journal of endocrinology / European Federation of Endocrine Societies 169: 695–703.
26. Mittempergher F, Pata G, Crea N, Di Betta E, Vilardi A, et al. (2013) Preoperative prediction of growth hormone (GH)/insulin-like growth factor-1 (IGF-1) axis modification and postoperative changes in candidates for bariatric surgery. Obes Surg 23: 594–601.
27. Chernausek SD, Backeljauw PF, Frane J, Kuntze J, Underwood LE (2007) Long-term treatment with recombinant insulin-like growth factor (IGF)-I in children with severe IGF-I deficiency due to growth hormone insensitivity. The Journal of clinical endocrinology and metabolism 92: 902–910.
28. Rumilla KM, Erickson LA, Service FJ, Vella A, Thompson GB, et al. (2009) Hyperinsulinemic hypoglycemia with nesidioblastosis: histologic features and growth factor expression. Modern pathology: an official journal of the United States and Canadian Academy of Pathology, Inc 22: 239–245.
29. Itariu BK, Zeyda M, Hochbrugger EE, Neuhofer A, Prager G, et al. (2012) Long-chain n-3 PUFAs reduce adipose tissue and systemic inflammation in severely obese nondiabetic patients: a randomized controlled trial. The American journal of clinical nutrition 96: 1137–1149.
30. Itariu BK, Zeyda M, Leitner L, Marculescu R, Stulnig TM (2013) Treatment with n-3 polyunsaturated fatty acids overcomes the inverse association of vitamin D deficiency with inflammation in severely obese patients: a randomized controlled trial. PloS one 8: e54634.
31. Matthews DR, Hosker JP, Rudenski AS, Naylor BA, Treacher DF, et al. (1985) Homeostasis model assessment: insulin resistance and beta-cell function from fasting plasma glucose and insulin concentrations in man. Diabetologia 28: 412–419.
32. Anderwald CH, Tura A, Gessl A, Luger A, Pacini G, et al. (2013) Adequately adapted insulin secretion and decreased hepatic insulin extraction cause elevated insulin concentrations in insulin resistant non-diabetic adrenal incidentaloma patients. PloS one 8: e77326.
33. Matsuda M, DeFronzo RA (1999) Insulin sensitivity indices obtained from oral glucose tolerance testing: comparison with the euglycemic insulin clamp. Diabetes care 22: 1462–1470.
34. Alberti KG, Zimmet P, Shaw J (2006) Metabolic syndrome—a new world-wide definition. A Consensus Statement from the International Diabetes Federation. Diabetic medicine: a journal of the British Diabetic Association 23: 469–480.
35. Bedogni G, Bellentani S, Miglioli L, Masutti F, Passalacqua M, et al. (2006) The Fatty Liver Index: a simple and accurate predictor of hepatic steatosis in the general population. BMC gastroenterology 6: 33.
36. Rinderknecht E, Humbel RE (1978) The amino acid sequence of human insulin-like growth factor I and its structural homology with proinsulin. The Journal of biological chemistry 253: 2769–2776.
37. Yakar S, Liu JL, Fernandez AM, Wu Y, Schally AV, et al. (2001) Liver-specific igf-1 gene deletion leads to muscle insulin insensitivity. Diabetes 50: 1110–1118.
38. Ogiwara Y, Mori S, Iwama M, Sawabe M, Takemoto M, et al. (2010) Hypoglycemia due to ectopic secretion of insulin-like growth factor-I in a patient with an isolated sarcoidosis of the spleen. Endocrine journal 57: 325–330.
39. Li JB, Wang CY, Chen JW, Feng ZQ, Ma HT (2004) Expression of liver insulin-like growth factor 1 gene and its serum level in patients with diabetes. World journal of gastroenterology: WJG 10: 255–259.
40. Laron Z (1999) The essential role of IGF-I: lessons from the long-term study and treatment of children and adults with Laron syndrome. The Journal of clinical endocrinology and metabolism 84: 4397–4404.
41. Gram IT, Norat T, Rinaldi S, Dossus L, Lukanova A, et al. (2006) Body mass index, waist circumference and waist-hip ratio and serum levels of IGF-I and IGFBP-3 in European women. International journal of obesity 30: 1623–1631.
42. Hirsch FF, Pareja JC, Geloneze SR, Chaim E, Cazzo E, et al. (2012) Comparison of metabolic effects of surgical-induced massive weight loss in patients with long-term remission versus non-remission of type 2 diabetes. Obes Surg 22: 910–917.
43. Khoo CM, Muehlbauer MJ, Stevens RD, Pamuklar Z, Chen J, et al. (2013) Postprandial Metabolite Profiles Reveal Differential Nutrient Handling After Bariatric Surgery Compared With Matched Caloric Restriction. Annals of surgery.
44. Mitchell JE, Crosby R, de Zwaan M, Engel S, Roerig J, et al. (2013) Possible risk factors for increased suicide following bariatric surgery. Obesity 21: 665–672.
45. Chaput JP, Tremblay A (2009) The glucostatic theory of appetite control and the risk of obesity and diabetes. International journal of obesity 33: 46–53.
46. Cox DJ, Gonder-Frederick LA, Kovatchev BP, Julian DM, Clarke WL (2000) Progressive hypoglycemia's impact on driving simulation performance. Occurrence, awareness and correction. Diabetes care 23: 163–170.
47. Buchwald H, Oien DM (2013) Metabolic/bariatric surgery worldwide 2011. Obesity surgery 23: 427–436.

Volume-Outcome Relation for Acute Appendicitis: Evidence from a Nationwide Population-Based Study

Po-Li Wei[1,2], Shih-Ping Liu[3], Joseph J. Keller[4], Herng-Ching Lin[5]*

1 Division of General Surgery, Department of Surgery, Taipei Medical University Hospital, Taipei, Taiwan, **2** Department of Surgery, School of Medicine, College of Medicine, Taipei Medical University, Taipei, Taiwan, **3** Department of Urology, National Taiwan University Hospital and College of Medicine, Taipei, Taiwan, **4** School of Public Health, Taipei Medical University, Taipei, Taiwan, **5** School of Health Care Administration, Taipei Medical University, Taipei, Taiwan

Abstract

Background: Although procedures like appendectomy have been studied extensively, the relative importance of each surgeon's surgical volume-to-ruptured appendicitis has not been explored. The purpose of this study was to investigate the rate of ruptured appendicitis by surgeon-volume groups as a measure of quality of care for appendicitis by using a nationwide population-based dataset.

Methods: We identified 65,339 first-time hospitalizations with a discharge diagnosis of acute appendicitis (International Classification of Disease, Ninth Revision, Clinical Modification (ICD-9-CM) codes 540, 540.0, 540.1 and 540.9) between January 2007 and December 2009. We used "whether or not a patient had a perforated appendicitis" as the outcome measure. A conditional (fixed-effect) logistic regression model was performed to explore the odds of perforated appendicitis among surgeon case volume groups.

Results: Patients treated by low-volume surgeons had significantly higher morbidity rates than those treated by high-volume (28.1% vs. 26.15, $p<0.001$) and very-high-volume surgeons (28.1% vs. 21.4%, $p<0.001$). After adjusting for surgeon practice location, and teaching status of practice hospital, and patient age, gender, and Charlson Comorbidity Index, and hospital acute appendicitis volume, patients treated by low-volume surgeons had significantly higher rates of perforated appendicitis than those treated by medium-volume surgeons ($OR=1.09$, $p<0.001$), high-volume surgeons ($OR=1.16$, $p<0.001$), or very-high-volume surgeons ($OR=1.54$, $p<0.001$).

Conclusion: Our study suggested that surgeon volume is an important factor with regard to the rate of ruptured appendicitis.

Editor: Jorge I F Salluh, D'or Institute of Research and Education, Brazil

Funding: The authors have no support or funding to report.

Competing Interests: The authors have declared that no competing interests exist.

* E-mail: henry11111@tmu.edu.tw

Introduction

Acute appendicitis is the most common surgical emergency. Although the exact mechanism is still obscure, it is likely that luminal obstruction plays a key pathogenic role [1–3]. Luminal obstruction leads to increased mucus production and bacterial overgrowth, which increases the intra-luminal pressure and decreases blood ow to the appendiceal wall. Subsequently, necrosis and perforation of the appendix occur. The primary adverse outcome of appendicitis is appendiceal rupture. In comparison with simple appendicitis, patients with an appendiceal rupture at the time of surgical exploration have been shown to have a higher risk of post-operative complication, such as intra-abdominal abscess, wound infection, and postoperative paralytic ileus (39% vs 8%) [4,5]. It has been assumed that the natural history of appendiceal rupture is within the control of the hospital and attending physician, and that a high rate of rupture reflects a failure of medical care [6]. As a result, appendiceal rupture rates have been proposed as a measure of intrinsic hospital quality, and early surgical exploration has been encouraged to decrease the rupture rate [7,8].

The impact of hospital volume on operative mortality with surgical procedures has been previously studied [9]. One recent review suggested that thousands of preventable surgical morbidities and mortalities occur each year in the United States, and that patients can significantly reduce their risk of operative death by selecting a high-volume hospital [10]. Despite recent interest in surgical volume, many question the applicability of previous research to the volume and outcomes of current practice.

First, due to recent decreases in surgical mortality associated with many procedures [11], it is possible that the relative importance of the volume of procedures performed may be declining. Second, most published studies on volume and outcome have used state-level databases or regional populations that are served by a small number of high-volume centers [12,13].

Although procedures like appendectomy have been studied extensively, the relative importance of each surgeon's surgical volume to ruptured appendicitis has either not been explored or

Table 1. Perforated appendicitis rate and patient and physician characteristics across physician pulmonary embolism caseload volume groups (n = 65,339).

Variable	All	Physician acute appendicitis case volume				*p* value
		Low (≤65)	Medium (66~120)	High (121~190)	Very High (≥191)	
Perforated appendicitis rate (%)	25.8	28.1	27.0	26.1	21.4	<0.001
Patient characteristics						
No. (%) of patients	65,339	16,094 (24.6)	16,614 (25.4)	18,055 (27.7)	14,576 (22.3)	
Age, mean (SD), years	36.7 (19.3)	36.5 (21.0)	37.5 (19.4)	37.2 (18.3)	35.5 (18.4)	<0.001
Charlson Comorbidity Index score						<0.001
0	60,381 (92.4)	14,489 (90.0)	15,382 (92.6)	16,813 (93.1)	13,697 (94.0)	
1	3,639 (5.6)	1,067 (6.6)	932 (5.6)	967 (5.4)	673 (4.6)	
2	610 (0.9)	202 (1.3)	157 (0.9)	141 (0.8)	110 (0.7)	
3 or more	709 (1.1)	336 (2.1)	143 (0.9)	134 (0.7)	96 (0.7)	
Surgeon characteristics						
No. (%) of surgeons	2,536	2,178 (85.9)	182 (7.2)	118 (4.7)	58 (2.3)	
Age, mean (SD), years	43.7 (8.7)	43.9 (8.8)	43.9 (7.9)	42.3 (7.8)	41.4 (6.1)	0.201
No. (%) of Practice location						0.100
Urban	1,849 (72.9)	1,582 (72.6)	126 (69.2)	93 (78.8)	48 (82.8)	
Rural	687 (27.1)	596 (27.4)	56 (30.8)	25 (21.2)	10 (17.2)	

has been studied in samples that were too small to permit assessment of performance at meaningful surgical volumes. The purpose of this study was to investigate the rate of ruptured appendicitis with surgeon volume groups as a measure of quality of care for appendicitis by using a nationwide, population-based dataset (from 2007 through 2009). Since some previous studies have suggested that volume-outcome relationships may exist for surgeons but not for hospitals in Taiwan [14,15], the present study focused on the volume-outcome relationship for surgeons. However, we took hospital volume into consideration in the regression model.

Methods

Database

We used data sourced between 2007 and 2009 from the National Health Insurance Research Database (NHIRD). The NHIRD, published by the Taiwan National Health Research Institute, includes all the original claims data and registration files for beneficiaries enrolled under the National Health Insurance (NHI) program. As the end of 2009, about 22.60 of Taiwan's 22.96 million residents (over 98% coverage rate) were enrolled under the NHI program. Taiwan's NHI program is a single plan with generous benefits, very low co-payments, and free choice of a widely-dispersed network of healthcare providers. Furthermore, the NHI Bureau implements routine sample cross-checks between each hospital's claims and medical charts, followed by punitive measures for coding infractions to deter diagnosis upcoding. Therefore, although there are no documented sensitivity and specificity studies for coding accuracy, it is generally believed that the NHI's checks and balances foster accurate coding.

This study was exempted from full review by an Institutional Review Board (IRB) after consulting with the director of the Taipei Medical University IRB since the NHIRD consists of de-identified secondary data released to the public for research purposes.

Study Sample

We identified 65,339 first-time hospitalizations with a discharge diagnosis of acute appendicitis (International Classification of Disease, Ninth Revision, Clinical Modification (ICD-9-CM) codes 540, 540.0, 540.1 and 540.9) between January 2007 and December 2009. If a patient had ≥2 hospitalizations within a 30-day period, they were regarded as the same episode and we only included the first hospitalization. The mean age for these 65,339 patients was 36.7 (±19.3 years) years, with a range between 2 and 97 years.

Surgeon Acute Appendicitis Volume Groups

The NHIRD included unique physician identifiers for each medical claim submitted, which enabled us to identify the same physician who performed one or more appendectomies during the three-year study period. Surgeons were sorted in ascending order of appendectomy volume, with volume cutoff points being determined in accordance with prior studies so that the sampled patients were classified into four, approximately equally-sized groups [6,7]. We divided the sample of 65,339 patients into four surgeon volume groups: ≤65 cases (hereafter referred to as low volume), 66–120 cases (medium volume), 121–190 (high volume), and ≥191 cases (very-high volume).

Key Variables of Interest

The key independent variable of interest was surgeon appendectomy caseload volume. Prior studies have used the proportion of cases of perforated appendicitis as a measure of quality of care for appendicitis [16,17]. Therefore, in this study, we used "whether or not a patient had a perforated appendicitis" as the outcome measure. Patients were regarded as having perforated appendicitis if they had an ICD-9-CM code of 540.0 (acute appendicitis with generalized peritonitis) or 540.1 (acute appendicitis with peritoneal abscess).

Table 2. Distributions of perforated appendicitis by surgeon and patient characteristics and comorbidities (n = 65,339).

Variable	Perforated appendicitis		*p* value
	Yes, *n* (row %)	**No, *n* (row %)**	
Surgeon characteristics			
Surgeon age (years)			0.217
<41	711 (42.2)	20,794 (42.9)	
41~50	6,758 (40.1)	19,326 (39.9)	
>50	2,984 (17.7)	8,366 (17.2)	
Surgeon gender			0.989
Male	16,284 (96.6)	46,848 (96.6)	
Female	569 (3.4)	1,638 (3.4)	
Practice location			<0.001
Urban	13,323 (79.1)	36,874 (76.1)	
Rural	3,530 (20.9)	11,612 (23.9)	
Teaching status			<0.001
Yes	15,660 (92.9)	43,162 (89.0)	
No	1,193 (7.1)	5,324 (11.0)	
Patient characteristics			
Patient age (years)			<0.001
≤19	3,452 (20.5)	10,320 (21.3)	
20~39	4,443 (26.4)	20,877 (43.1)	
40~59	5,024 (29.8)	12,477 (25.7)	
≥60	3,934 (23.3)	4,812 (9.9)	
Patient gender			<0.001
Male	9,883 (58.6)	25,526 (52.7)	
Female	6,970 (41.4)	22,960 (47.3)	
Charlson Comorbidity Index score			<0.001
0	14,612 (86.7)	45,769 (94.4)	
1	1,564 (9.3)	2,075 (4.3)	
2	307 (1.8)	303 (0.6)	
3 or more	370 (2.2)	339 (0.7)	

Statistical Analysis

We used the SAS package (Version 9.1) for statistical analysis in this study. Chi-squared tests were used to examine differences among surgeon volume groups in terms of both surgeon and patient characteristics. Surgeon characteristics included age, gender, practice location (urban vs. rural), and teaching status of practice hospital, while patient characteristics included age, gender, and Charlson Comorbidity Index (CCI). CCI was used to quantify pre-existing co-morbidities as a means of adjusting for the higher mortality risks associated with co-morbidities (the higher the score, the greater the number of co-morbidities). We then performed a conditional (fixed-effect) logistic regression model (conditional on hospitals in order to partition out systematic hospital-specific variation) to explore the odds of perforated appendicitis among surgeon case volume groups. This conditional model also uses a clustered method for variance estimation to account for the possibility that the patients of each physician have more similar outcomes than patients viewed across physicians. A two-sided p value of less than, or equal to, 0.05 was considered to be statistically significant.

Results

Table 1 presents the distribution of the rate of perforated appendicitis and patient and surgeon characteristics across surgeon acute appendicitis case volume groups. Of the 65,339 patients admitted for the treatment of acute appendicitis between January 2007 and December 2009, 16,857 (25.8%) had perforated appendicitis; the rate of perforated appendicitis consistently decreased with increasing surgeon acute appendicitis caseload volume. Patients treated by low-volume surgeons had significantly higher morbidity rates than those treated by high-volume (28.1% vs. 26.15, $p<0.001$) or very-high-volume surgeons (28.1% vs. 21.4%, $p<0.001$). In addition, patients in the low surgeon volume quartile were more likely to have a greater number of co-morbidities ($p<0.001$).

Table 1 also shows that patients with acute appendicitis were treated by 2,536 surgeons between 2007 and 2009, at a mean volume per surgeon of 25.8 (±53.2) cases. The χ^2 analyses indicate that the surgeons in the low-volume group were more likely to be female ($p<0.001$) and practice in non-teaching hospitals ($p<0.001$) than their counterparts in other volume groups. No significant relationships were found in the surgeon distributions in terms of mean age ($p=0.201$) and practice location ($p=0.100$) across caseload volume groups.

Table 2 presents the distributions of the rates of perforated appendicitis according to surgeon and patient characteristics. Global χ^2 analyses revealed that there were significant differences in the rate of perforated appendicitis associated with surgeon practice location ($p<0.001$), teaching status of practice hospital ($p<0.001$), patient age ($p<0.001$), patients gender ($p<0.001$), and CCI ($p<0.001$).

Table 3 provides the crude and covariate-adjusted odds ratio (OR) estimates of the likelihood of perforated appendicitis by surgeon acute appendicitis case volume and surgeon and patient characteristics. The ORs of perforated appendicitis for those patients treated by medium-volume, high-volume, and very-high-volume surgeons were 0.95 (95% CI = 0.90–0.99), 0.91 (95% CI = 0.86–0.95), and 0.70 (95% CI = 0.66–0.73), respectively, compared to patients treated by low-volume surgeons. After adjusting for surgeon practice location, and teaching status of practice hospital, and patient age, gender, CCI, and hospital acute appendicitis case volume, patients treated by low-volume surgeons had significantly higher rates of perforated appendicitis than those treated by medium-volume surgeons (OR = 1.09, reciprocal of 0.92, $p<0.001$), high-volume surgeons (OR = 1.16, $p<0.001$), or very-high-volume surgeons (OR = 1.54, $p<0.001$). In addition, it is also worth noting that higher rates of perforated appendicitis were detected among patients treated by surgeon practicing in the urban areas (adjusted OR = 1.09) and teaching hospitals (OR = 1.61).

Discussion

To the best of our knowledge, this is the first study to use nationwide data to investigate the relationship between surgeon volume and the perforation rate of appendicitis. Our study demonstrated that low volume surgeons were more likely to have a greater number of perforated appendicitis.

Earlier studies have suggested that higher hospital volumes are associated with better outcomes for several surgical procedures [18,19]. The proposed explanation for this inverse volume-outcome relationship is commonly known as the 'practice makes perfect' hypothesis. This hypothesis is based upon the rationale that a larger volume of patients provides clinicians with the opportunity to better hone their surgical skills and accumulate

Table 3. Crude and adjusted odds ratios for perforated appendicitis, by surgeon acute appendicitis case volume.

Variables	Crude odds ratio		Adjusted odds ratio	
	95% CI	P value	95% CI	P value
Surgeon acute appendicitis case volume				
≤65	1.00		1.00	
66~120	0.95 (0.90–0.99)	0.031	0.92 (0.87–0.96)	<0.001
121~190	0.91 (0.86–0.95)	<0.001	0.86 (0.82–0.91)	<0.001
≥191	0.70 (0.66–0.73)	<0.001	0.66 (0.62–0.70)	<0.001
Surgeon characteristics				
Practice location				
Urban	1.19 (1.14–1.24)	<0.001	1.09 (1.03–1.14)	<0.001
Rural	1.00		1.00	
Hospital teaching status				
Yes	1.62 (1.52–1.73)	<0.001	1.61 (1.49–1.73)	<0.001
No	1.00		1.00	
Patient characteristics				
Patient age (years)				
≤19	1.00		1.00	
20~39	0.64 (0.61–0.67)	<0.001	0.65 (0.62–0.68)	<0.001
40~59	1.20 (1.14–1.27)	<0.001	1.18 (1.12–1.24)	<0.001
≥60	2.44 (2.31–2.59)	<0.001	2.19 (2.06–2.33)	<0.001
Patient gender				
Male	1.28 (1.23–1.32)	<0.001	1.33 (1.28–1.38)	<0.001
Female	1.00		1.00	
Charlson Comorbidity Index score				
0	1.00		1.00	
1	2.36 (2.21–2.53)	<0.001	1.54 (1.43–1.66)	<0.001
2	3.17 (2.71–3.72)	<0.001	1.81 (1.53–2.13)	<0.001
3 or more	3.42 (2.95–3.95)	<0.001	2.01 (1.73–2.35)	<0.001
Hospital appendicitis case volume	1.00 (1.00–1.00)	<0.001	1.00 (1.00–1.00)	<0.001

experience in operation management. Therefore, high-volume providers are more likely to achieve superior clinical performance on account of their greater experience, improved skills, and operational judgment.

In the case of acute appendicitis, the severity and complication rate are closely associated with the time interval between symptom onset and treatment [20], and the rupture rate is generally not the result of surgical technique related error but rather pre- and in-hospital delay. Therefore, high-volume surgeons who have more experience in dealing with patients with acute appendicitis may reduce unnecessary in-hospital delays and lead to better outcomes. A corollary to the "practice makes perfect" hypothesis then, is that low-volume surgeons with poor outcomes would be able to substantially reduce the rate of ruptured appendicitis by simply increasing their patient volumes or having the opportunity to practice under the guidance of more experienced high-volume surgeons.

A second hypothesis used to explain volume-outcome relationships involves 'selective-referral'. This hypothesis suggests that patients are selectively referred to providers with superior outcomes. Thus, the best providers have the highest volumes on account of their prior record of superior outcomes. However, this hypothesis is unlikely to offer a valid explanation for this study. The progression of appendicitis is rapid, and most patients promptly receive treatment at nearby hospitals. Therefore, 'selective-referral' may not be a major factor contributing to the inverse relationship between the patient outcome sand surgeon volumes observed in this study.

The main strength of this study was its use of a nation-wide population-based dataset from Taiwan. Taiwan is a country with more than 23 million people on a 35.8 thousand square kilometer island, which launched a universal national health insurance (NHI) program in the end of 1995. Under a single-payer system operated by the Taiwanese government, the NHI program covered 98% of Taiwan's population by 2009. The population-based dataset associated with this program offered the statistical power necessary to detect real differences. Furthermore, Taiwan is over 98% Han Chinese, and this study could therefore exclude the influence of race and insurance status from our analysis, both of which were previously demonstrated to be important factors influencing the rate of ruptured appendicitis [21,22].

There are some limitations to this study. First, as pathologic confirmation was unavailable in this study, the definition of perforated appendicitis was dependent on ICD-9 codes sourced from an administrative database. These codes may be less accurate than data collected prospectively. For example, while ICD-9-CM code 540 is theoretically reserved exclusively for uncomplicated appendicitis, we cannot rule out the possibility that miscoding occurred. Furthermore, as coding is a skill itself, it is possible that lower volume surgeons would have been more likely to miscode more specific codes referring to complicated appendicitis (ICD-9-CM codes 540.0 and 540.1) as ICD-9-CM code 540. If this were the case, our results would be biased toward an underestimation of the effect size. Secondly, although this study has controlled for patient co-morbidities, the administrative database used by this study is extremely limited in its ability to account for the differences in the severity of appendicitis among patients. Therefore it is possible that the associations detected in this study were biased by the residual confounding of severity. Third, this study also lacked any data describing the rate of negative appendectomies which may have biased our results, as higher rates of negative appendectomies would have decreased the rate of perforated appendicitis [23]. Fourth, the dataset used in this study did not have any data on pre-hospital care (the time from the onset of symptoms to first seeking medical attention), advanced diagnostic testing, or the use of antibiotics. Therefore, these potentially confounding factors could not be considered in our analysis. Finally, the very small appendectomy caseloads seen among some surgeons in the very low-volume group may have prohibited their meaningful statistical comparison.

In conclusion, our study suggested that surgeon volume is an important factor with regard to the rate of ruptured appendicitis. Future investigations will need to be undertaken to determine a threshold of surgeon volume for best practice, and to identify the differences in clinical approach between high-volume surgeons with superior outcomes, and low-volume surgeons with inferior outcomes. The identification of such differences may be useful toward aiding low-volume surgeons with inferior outcomes to reduce the incidence of perforated appendicitis.

Author Contributions

Conceived and designed the experiments: HCL PLW. Analyzed the data: HCL SPL. Contributed reagents/materials/analysis tools: HCL. Wrote the paper: HCL PLW SPL JJK. Critical revision: HCL PLW SPL JJK.

References

1. Addiss DG, Shaffer N, Fowler BS, Tauxe RV (1990) The epidemiology of appendicitis and appendectomy in the United States. Am J Epidemiol 132: 910–925.
2. Williams GR (1983) Presidential Address: a history of appendicitis. With anecdotes illustrating its importance. Ann Surg 197: 495–506.
3. Nitecki S, Karmeli R, Sarr MG (1990) Appendiceal calculi and fecaliths as indications for appendectomy. Surg Gynecol Obstet171: 185–188.
4. Williams NM, Jackson D, Everson NW, Johnstone JM (1998) Is the incidence of acute appendicitis really falling? Ann R Coll Surg Engl 80: 122–124.
5. Al-Omran M, Mamdani M, McLeod RS (2003) Epidemiologic features of acute appendicitis in Ontario, Canada. Can J Surg 46: 263–268.
6. Andersson RE (2007) The natural history and traditional management of appendicitis revisited: spontaneous resolution and predominance of prehospital perforations imply that a correct diagnosis is more important than an early diagnosis. World J Surg 31: 86–92.
7. Balthazar EJ, Rofsky NM, Zucker R (1998) Appendicitis: the impact of computed tomography imaging on negative appendectomy and perforation rates. Am J Gastroenterol 93: 768–771.
8. Fuchs JR, Schlamberg JS, Shortsleeve MJ, Schuler JG (2002) Impact of abdominal CT imaging on the management of appendicitis: an update. J Surg Res 106: 131–136.
9. Hannan EL, O'Donnell JF, Kilburn H Jr, Bernard HR, Yazici A (1989) Investigation of the relationship between volume and mortality for surgical procedures performed in New York State hospitals. JAMA 262: 503–510.
10. Birkmeyer JD, Siewers AE, Finlayson EV, Stukel TA, Lucas FL, et al. (2002) Hospital volume and surgical mortality in the United States. N Engl J Med 346: 1128–1137.
11. Welke KF, Diggs BS, Karamlou T, Ungerleider RM (2009) Comparison of pediatric cardiac surgical mortality rates from national administrative data to contemporary clinical standards. Ann Thorac Surg 87: 216–222.
12. Lien WC, Lee WC, Wang HP, Chen YC, Liu KL, et al. (2011) Male gender is a risk factor for recurrent appendicitis following nonoperative treatment. World J Surg 35: 1636–1642.
13. Paquette IM, Zuckerman R, Finlayson SR (2011) Perforated appendicitis among rural and urban patients: implications of access to care. Ann Surg 253: 534–538.
14. Lien YC, Huang MT, Lin HC (2007) Association between surgeon and hospital volume and in-hospital fatalities after lung cancer resections: the experience of an Asian country. Ann Thorac Surg 83: 1837–1843.
15. Wen HC, Tang CH, Lin HC, Tsai CS, Chen CS, et al. (2006) Association between surgeon and hospital volume in coronary artery bypass graft surgery outcomes: a population-based study. Ann Thorac Surg 81: 835–842.
16. Ponsky TA, Huang ZJ, Kittle K, Eichelberger MR, Gilbert JC, et al. (2004) Hospital- and patient-level characteristics and the risk of appendiceal rupture and negative appendectomy in children. JAMA 292: 1977–1982.
17. Ditillo MF, Dziura JD, Rabinovici R (2006) Is it safe to delay appendectomy in adults with acute appendicitis? Ann Surg 244: 656–660.
18. Lin HC, Xirasagar S, Lee HC, Chai CY (2006) Hospital volume and inpatient mortality after cancer-related gastrointestinal resections: the experience of an Asian country. Ann Surg Oncol 13: 1182–1188.
19. Nallamothu BK, Saint S, Hofer TP, Vijan S, Eagle KA, et al. (2005) Impact of patient risk on the hospital volume-outcome relationship in coronary artery bypass grafting. Arch Intern Med 165: 333–337.
20. Pittman-Waller VA, Myers JG, Stewart RM, Dent DL, Page CP, et al. (2000) Appendicitis: why so complicated? Analysis of 5755 consecutive appendectomies. Am Surg 66: 548–554.
21. Smink DS, Fishman SJ, Kleinman K, Finkelstein JA (2005) Effects of race, insurance status, and hospital volume on perforated appendicitis in children. Pediatrics 115: 920–925.
22. Camp M, Chang DC, Zhang Y, Arnold M, Sharpe L, et al. (2010) Provider density and health system facility factors and their relationship to rates of pediatric perforated appendicitis in US counties. Arch Surg 145: 1139–1144.
23. Hale DA, Molloy M, Pearl RH, Schutt DC, Jaques DP (1997) Appendectomy: a contemporary appraisal. Ann Surg 225: 252–261.

Bacteriology and Changes in Antibiotic Susceptibility in Adults with Community-Acquired Perforated Appendicitis

Hong Gil Jeon[1], Hyeong Uk Ju[1], Gyu Yeol Kim[2], Joseph Jeong[3], Min-Ho Kim[4], Jae-Bum Jun[1]*

1 Department of Internal Medicine, Ulsan University Hospital, University of Ulsan College of Medicine, Ulsan, Republic of Korea, **2** Department of Surgery, Ulsan University Hospital, University of Ulsan College of Medicine, Ulsan, Republic of Korea, **3** Department of Laboratory Medicine, Ulsan University Hospital, University of Ulsan College of Medicine, Ulsan, Republic of Korea, **4** Biomedical Research Center, Ulsan University Hospital, University of Ulsan College of Medicine, Ulsan, Republic of Korea

Abstract

This study evaluated bacterial etiology and antibiotic susceptibility in patients diagnosed with community-acquired perforated appendicitis over a 12-year-period. We retrospectively reviewed records of adult patients diagnosed with perforated appendicitis at an 800-bed teaching hospital between January 2000 and December 2011. In total, 415 culture-positive perforated appendicitis cases were analyzed. *Escherichia coli* was the most common pathogen (277/415, 66.7%), followed by *Streptococcus* species (61/415, 14.7%). The susceptibility of *E. coli* to ampicillin, piperacillin/tazobactam, ceftriaxone, cefepime, amikacin, gentamicin, and imipenem was 35.1%, 97.1%, 97.0%, 98.2%, 98.9%, 81.8%, and 100%, respectively. The overall susceptibility of *E. coli* to quinolones (ciprofloxacin or levofloxacin) was 78.7%. During the study period, univariate logistic regression analysis showed a significant decrease in *E. coli* susceptibility to quinolones (OR = 0.91, 95% CI 0.84–0.99, $P = 0.040$). We therefore do not recommend quinolones as empirical therapy for community-acquired perforated appendicitis.

Editor: D William Cameron, University of Ottawa, Canada

Funding: The authors have no support or funding to report.

Competing Interests: The authors have declared that no competing interests exist.

* Email: uvgotletter@hanmail.net

Introduction

Acute appendicitis is one of the most common abdominal surgical emergencies; it is also typically a community-acquired infection. Despite the generally favorable outcome, complicated appendicitis, such as perforated appendicitis, is associated with increased morbidity compared with simple acute appendicitis [1,2]. Because *Escherichia coli* and *Bacteroides fragilis* are most commonly associated with appendicitis, antibiotic therapies are generally selected to target these bacteria [3,4].

For adult patients with community-acquired complicated intra-abdominal infections of mild-to moderate severity, the use of ticarcillin-clavulanate, cefoxitin, ertapenem, moxifloxacin, or tigecycline as single-agent therapy or combinations of metronidazole with cefazolin, cefuroxime, ceftriaxone, cefotaxime, levofloxacin, or ciprofloxacin are recommended by Infectious Diseases Society of America (IDSA) guidelines [5]. However, with increased *E. coli* resistance to quinolones, investigation of local microbiologic findings had been proposed when selecting empirical therapies [5].

Because previous literature has reported a proportionally greater ratio of extended-spectrum β-lactamase (ESBL) and quinolone-resistant *E. coli* among bacteria responsible for community-acquired abdominal infections in Asia compared to other regions, careful selection of empirical antibiotics is particularly important in Asia [6–8]. We therefore conducted a study of the local microbiological profile and changes in antibiotic resistance in community-acquired perforated appendicitis over the past 12 years. These results may help us to inform selection of empirical antibiotic treatments for community-acquired complicated appendicitis.

Materials and Methods

Patient selection and data collection

We retrospectively reviewed the records of adult patients (age ≥ 18 years) who were diagnosed to have perforated appendicitis at Ulsan University Hospital, an 800-bed teaching hospital, between January 2000 to December 2011. Hospital charts and follow-up records were reviewed.

Definitions

Perforated appendicitis was defined as either gross or microscopic evidence of appendiceal perforation. The appendix was not considered to be ruptured by the mere presence of suppurative peritoneal fluid or gangrenous appendicitis without microscopic evidence of perforation.

Community-acquired appendicitis was defined as appendicitis that occurred within 48 hours of hospital admission. Patients were excluded from the study if they had at least 1 of the following health care risk factors: 1) presence of an invasive device at time of admission, 2) history of MRSA infection or colonization, 3) history of surgery, hospitalization, dialysis, or residence in a long-term care facility in the 12 months preceding the culture date [5].

Systemic inflammatory response syndrome (SIRS), sepsis, severe sepsis, and septic shock were defined as described elsewhere [9].

Specimen culture, species identification, and susceptibility testing

Specimens were obtained by swabbing the suppurative peritoneal fluid or periappendiceal abscess. In some cases, specimens were obtained by swabbing the lumen of appendix or by retrieving the suppurative peritoneal fluid via syringe aspiration. The swab specimens were transported to the laboratory in a transport medium (Amies transport medium without Charcoal; Asan Pharmaceuticals Co., Ltd., Hwasung, Korea). The specimens were either dispatched to the microbiology laboratory directly or stored in the operating room until the next day if collected after the working hours. The specimens were inoculated on blood agar, chocolate agar, and MacConkey agar plates. Samples were not inoculated into anaerobic culture. An automated VITEK 2 system (bioMerieux, Inc. Durham, NC, USA) was used to identify pathogens and perform ESBL susceptibility testing. The Vitek 2 ESBL test has 6 wells containing cefepime at 1 µg/mL, cefotaxime at 0.5 µg/mL, and ceftazidime at 0.5 µg/mL alone and in combination with clavulanic acid (10 µg/mL, 4 µg/mL, and 4 µg/mL, respectively); growth rate in each well is quantitatively assessed with an optical scanner. The proportional growth reduction (over 50%) in wells containing cephalosporin plus clavulanic acid compared with those containing cephalosporin alone was considered evidence of ESBL production. Susceptibility testing results were interpreted according to the National Committee for Clinical Laboratory Standards (CLSI) guidelines published in 2009 [10]. However, cephalosporin susceptibility results of ESBL-positive strains were interpreted on the basis of the strains' respective minimal inhibitory concentration (MIC) breakpoints.

Ethics statement

This retrospective study was approved by the Institutional Review Board (IRB) committee of Ulsan University Hospital. Written consent given by the patients was waived by the approving IRB.

Statistical analysis

Statistical analyses were performed by using IBM SPSS Statistics for Windows, version 21 (IBM Corp., Armonk, NY, USA). The Chi-squared test was used to compare frequencies. A univariate logistic regression model was used to calculate odds ratios (OR), 95% confidence intervals, and p-values. The significance level was set at 0.05.

Results

Study population and clinical characteristics

Of 3,379 patients, 567 (16.7%) who received appendectomies during the study period were diagnosed with perforated appendicitis. Of these, we discarded 4 cases of health care-associated infection, 6 without confirmatory cultures, and 142 culture-negative cases; in total, we analyzed 415 culture-positive perforated appendicitis cases. The average length of hospitalization was 9.1±5.1 days. Patient ages ranged between 20 years and 94 years (mean 48.6±17.0 years), with 51.1% (212/415) men (Table 1). A majority of patients (404, 97.3%) underwent open appendectomy via a McBurney incision; laparotomy with a low midline incision was performed in 9 patients (2.2%) and laparoscopic appendectomy was performed in 2 patients (0.5%). The most common underlying disease was hypertension, reported in 56 patients (13.5%). Severe sepsis or septic shock was observed in 70 patients (16.8%), while 1 patient (0.2%) died of sepsis after mechanical ileus. Post-operative complications included wound infection in 18 patients (4.3%), abdominal abscesses or peritonitis in 7 patients (1.6%), and mechanical ileus in 6 patients (1.4%). A combination therapy comprising cephalosporin and metronidazole was the most frequent empirical antibiotic treatment.

Microbiological features

The most commonly isolated bacteria was *E. coli* (277 isolates, 66.7%), followed by *Streptococcus* spp. (61, 14.7%), *Enterococcus* spp. (32, 7.7%), *Klebsiella* spp. (25, 6.0%), and *Pseudomonas aeruginosa* (24, 5.8%) (Table 2). More than 2 organisms were isolated in 75 cases (18.0%).

Antibiotic susceptibilities of isolated organisms

Data on antibiotic susceptibilities of isolated organisms showed that *E. coli* had 78.7% susceptibility to quinolones (ciprofloxacin or levofloxacin). Susceptibilities to ampicillin, aztreonam, ampicillin/sulbactam, amoxicillin/clavulanic acid, piperacillin/tazobactam, cefazolin, cefoxitin, ceftriaxone, cefepime, trimethoprim/sulfamethoxazole, amikacin, gentamicin, tobramycin, and imipenem were 35.1%, 95.2%, 41.4%, 83.5%, 97.1%, 89.8%, 97.7%, 97.0%, 98.2%, 65.6%, 98.9%, 81.8%, 83.4%, and 100%, respectively (Table 3). ESBL-producing strains accounted for 3.9% of *E. coli* species. *Streptococcus* species showed 68.9% susceptibility to penicillin, and 100% susceptibility to ceftriaxone. *Enterococcus* species were 71.9% susceptible to penicillin. The susceptibilities of *P. aeruginosa* to piperacillin/tazobactam, cefepime, quinolones, amikacin, and imipenem were 95.2%, 100%, 87.5%, 100%, and 95.8%, respectively.

Comparisons of bacterial species and *E. coli* isolate antibiotic susceptibilities by clinical severity

We compared the bacterial species and antibiotic susceptibilities of *E. coli* isolates according to the clinically indicated severity (Table 4). The cases were redistributed into two major groups: "sepsis" and "severe sepsis." Infected patients without SIRS and the patients with sepsis were grouped together in the "sepsis" group, whereas the patients with severe sepsis and septic shock were grouped together in the "severe sepsis" group. A total of 345 patients (83.1%) were included in the sepsis group and 70 (16.9%) were included in the severe sepsis group. *E. coli* isolates were found more frequently in the severe sepsis group (74.3%) than in the sepsis group (65.2%), but the difference was not statistically significant. The isolation rates of the other species were also not significantly different between groups. There were no statistically significant differences in *E. coli* susceptibility to all antibiotics between groups.

Changes in *E. coli* antimicrobial susceptibility according to the year

Yearly changes in *E. coli* antimicrobial susceptibility during the study period were examined (Fig. 1). Univariate logistic regression analysis showed that *E. coli* susceptibility to quinolones significantly decreased, with annual susceptibility rates of 89.4%, 83.3%, 89.2%, 84.2%, 66.6%, 74.0%, 82.6%, 69.2%, 80.0%, 61.9%, 65.0%, and 85.0%, during the period of 2000 to 2011 (OR = 0.91, 95% CI 0.84–0.99, $P = 0.040$). In particular, *E. coli* susceptibility to cefoxitin ($P = 0.052$) and ceftriaxone ($P = 0.054$) decreased during the study period, but the change was not statistically

Table 1. Baseline characteristics of patients with perforated appendicitis.

Characteristics	Number (%)
Number of culture positive patients	415
Hospital day (Mean ± SD)	9.1±5.1
Age (Mean ± SD)	48.6±17.0
Sex	
male	212 (51.1)
female	203 (48.9)
Operation method	
laparoscopic	2 (0.5)
McBurney	404 (97.3)
laparotomy	9 (2.2)
Underlying disease	
hypertension	56 (13.5)
diabetes mellitus	26 (6.3)
hepatitis B virus	16 (3.9)
solid cancer	12 (2.9)
Initial manifestation	
infection without SIRS	73 (17.6)
sepsis	272 (65.7)
severe sepsis	67 (16.1)
septic shock	3 (0.7)
In-hospital mortality	
alive	414 (99.8)
death	1 (0.2)
Infectious complication	
wound infection	18 (4.3)
intra-abdominal abscess or peritonitis	7 (1.6)
mechanical ileus	6 (1.4)
Antibiotics	
1st (or 2nd) generation cephalosporin + metronidazole	215 (51.8)
3rd generation cephalosporin + metronidazole	193 (46.5)
ciprofloxacin + metronidazole	4 (1.0)
piperacillin/tazobactam	3 (0.7)

SIRS = systemic inflammatory response syndrome.

significant. Nor were any statistically significant changes observed in *E. coli* susceptibility to other antibiotics such as ampicillin ($P=0.235$), aztreonam ($P=0.168$), piperacillin/tazobactam ($P=0.645$), cefazolin ($P=0.126$), cefepime ($P=0.393$), trimethoprim/sulfamethoxazole ($P=0.732$), amikacin ($P=0.835$), gentamicin ($P=0.389$), and tobramycin ($P=0.645$).

Discussion

This study evaluated microbiological profiles and antibiotic susceptibilities of pathogens isolated from cases of perforated appendicitis. The flora detected in complicated intra-abdominal infection differs between community-acquired and nosocomial infections. We considered appendicitis suitable for studying community-acquired bacterial infections since this illness is largely community-acquired. In fact, only 4 patients discarded from analysis owing to health care-associated infections. *P. aeruginosa* isolates in this study showed overall high levels of antibiotic susceptibility with no multidrug-resistant strains, supporting the idea that appendicitis is more commonly a community-acquired rather than nosocomial infection [11].

E. coli was the most common pathogen identified in this study (66.7% of all isolates), similar to findings in previous appendicitis literature [3,12]. Similarly, *Streptococcus* and *Enterococcus* species were the most frequently isolated gram-positive organisms [12,13]. The ratio of ESBL-producing *E. coli* was 3.9%, within previously reported ranges of 3.5–15.4% [8,14]. The isolation rate of *E. coli* was greater in the severe sepsis group, although this difference was not statistically significant. Some studies have reported that *P. aeruginosa* is a commonly isolated strain in appendicitis, with an isolation rate of 19–32%; however, this was not the case in the current study [12,15].

Although *E. coli* showed a high susceptibility rate of 97% to second- and third-generation cephalosporins that are most

Table 2. Distribution of bacterial species.

	Species	Number (%)[f]
Gram negative organism	*Escherichia coli*	277 (66.7)
	Klebsiella species[a]	25 (6.0)
	Pseudomonas aeruginosa	24 (5.8)
	Other gram negative organism[b]	45 (10.8)
Gram positive organism	*Streptococcus* species[c]	61 (14.7)
	Enterococcus species[d]	32 (7.7)
	Staphylococcus aureus	6 (1.4)
	Other gram positive organism[e]	23 (5.5)

[a]Includes: *K. pneumoniae, K. oxytoca.*
[b]Includes: *Achromobacter xylosoxidans, Acinetobacter lwoffii, Aeromonas hydrophila, Comamonas testosteroni, Hafnia alvei, Proteus mirabilis, Raoultella planticola, Serratia* species, *Enterobacter cloacae.*
[c]Includes: *S. alactolyticus, S. anginosus, S. cristatus, S. constellatus, S. gordonii, S. intermedius, S. mitis, S. salivarius, S. sanguinis*, Viridans Streptococci.
[d]Includes: *E. avium, E. faecalis, E. faecium, E. gallinarum, E. hirae, E. raffinosus.*
[e]Includes: *Gemella morbillorum, Lactococcus garvieae, Leuconostoc mesenteroides, Pediococcus pentosaceus.*
[f]Polymicrobial infection: 75 cases (18.0%).

Table 3. Antibiotic susceptibilities of isolated organisms that caused perforated appendicitis.

	E. coli **(total)**	*E. coli* **(non-ESBL)**	*E. coli* **(ESBL)**	*Streptococcus* **species**	*Enterococcus* **species**	*P. aeruginosa*
Antibiotic	**(n = 277)**	**(n = 266)**	**(n = 11)**	**(n = 61)**	**(n = 32)**	**(n = 24)**
Penicillin				42/61 (68.9)	23/32 (71.9)	
Ampicillin	97/276 (35.1)	97/265 (36.6)	0/11 (0)		24/27 (88.8)	
Aztreonam	220/231 (95.2)	217/220 (98.6)	3/11 (27.2)			
Ampicillin/sulbactam	84/203 (41.4)	84/200 (42.0)	0/3 (0)			
Amoxicillin/clavulanic acid	61/73 (83.5)	55/65 (84.6)	6/8 (75.0)			
Piperacillin/tazobactam	240/247 (97.1)	229/236 (97.0)	11/11 (100)			20/21 (95.2)
Cefazolin	248/276 (89.8)	248/265 (93.5)	0/11 (0)			
Cefoxitin	264/270 (97.7)	254/259 (98.0)	10/11 (90.9)			
Ceftriaxone	267/275 (97.0)	262/264 (99.2)	5/11 (45.4)	39/39 (100)		2/24 (8.3)
Cefepime	227/231 (98.2)	220/220 (100)	7/11 (63.6)			22/22 (100)
Quinolone	218/277 (78.7)	215/266 (80.8)	3/11 (27.2)		25/28 (89.2)	21/24 (87.5)
Trimethoprim/sulfamethoxazole	181/276 (65.6)	177/265 (66.7)	4/11 (36.3)	34/47 (72.3)	11/17 (64.7)	1/24 (4.1)
Amikacin	274/277 (98.9)	264/266 (99.2)	10/11 (90.9)			24/24 (100)
Gentamicin	226/276 (81.8)	221/265 (83.4)	5/11 (45.4)			24/24 (100)
Tobramycin	231/277 (83.4)	227/266 (85.3)	4/11 (36.3)			24/24 (100)
Vancomycin				60/61 (98.3)	30/32 (93.7)	
Imipenem	276/276 (100)	265/265 (100)	11/11 (100)	11/11 (100)	23/26 (88.5)	23/24 (95.8)

Table 4. Comparisons of bacterial species and antibiotic susceptibilities of *E. coli* between the sepsis group and the severe sepsis group.

	Sepsis[a] (%)	Severe sepsis[b] (%)	*P*-value
Species			
E. coli	225/345 (65.2)	52/70 (74.3)	0.142
P. aeruginosa	20/345 (5.8)	4/70 (5.7)	0.978
Streptococcus species	52/345 (15.1)	9/70 (12.9)	0.633
Enterococcus species	25/345 (7.3)	7/70 (10.0)	0.431
Antibiotics susceptibilities of *E. coli*			
Piperacillin/tazobactam	197/202 (97.5)	43/45 (95.6)	0.472
Cefoxitin	214/220 (97.3)	50/50 (100)	0.238
Ceftriaxone	215/223 (96.4)	52/52 (100)	0.166
Cefepime	184/187 (98.4)	43/44 (97.7)	0.760
Ciprofloxacin or levofloxacin	176/225 (78.2)	42/52 (80.8)	0.686

[a]Infection without SIRS (systemic inflammatory response syndrome) & sepsis.
[b]Severe sepsis & septic shock.

commonly used for empirical antibiotic treatment, the susceptibility decreased during the study period, albeit without statistical significance ($P = 0.052$ and $P = 0.054$, respectively). The susceptibility to quinolones was 78.7%, with a statistically significant ($P = 0.040$) decrease during the study period. Previous studies by Bochicchio et al (2006) and Rob et al (2013) reported that the susceptibility rate of *E. coli*, isolated from appendicitis samples, to quinolones was 71.4–85.6% [6,8]. The *E. coli* susceptibility to quinolones and cephalosporins reported by Rob et al (2013) was lower than that reported by Bochicchio et al (2006). This may be attributable to *E. coli*'s increased resistance to the antibiotics or the lowered MIC breakpoint for cephalosporins set by the CLSI guidelines. For most antibiotics, *E. coli* susceptibility rates observed in this study were similar to those reported by Bochicchio et al (2006), with the susceptibility rate to quinolones being slightly lower. Both previous studies found high susceptibilities to carbapenem, amikacin, and piperacillin/tazobactam; in this study, ESBL-producing organisms were particularly sensitive to piperacillin/tazobactam (12/12, 100%). The susceptibility of *Streptococcus* species to penicillin was 68.9%, and all strains were susceptible to ceftriaxone. *P. aeruginosa* isolated in this study was highly susceptible to amikacin, cefepime, piperacillin/tazobactam, and carbapenem, but was slightly less susceptible to quinolones (87.5%).

All patients undergoing operation for appendicitis should receive antimicrobial therapy [16]. Appropriate antimicrobial therapy includes agents effective against facultative and aerobic gram-negative organisms and anaerobic organisms. There are

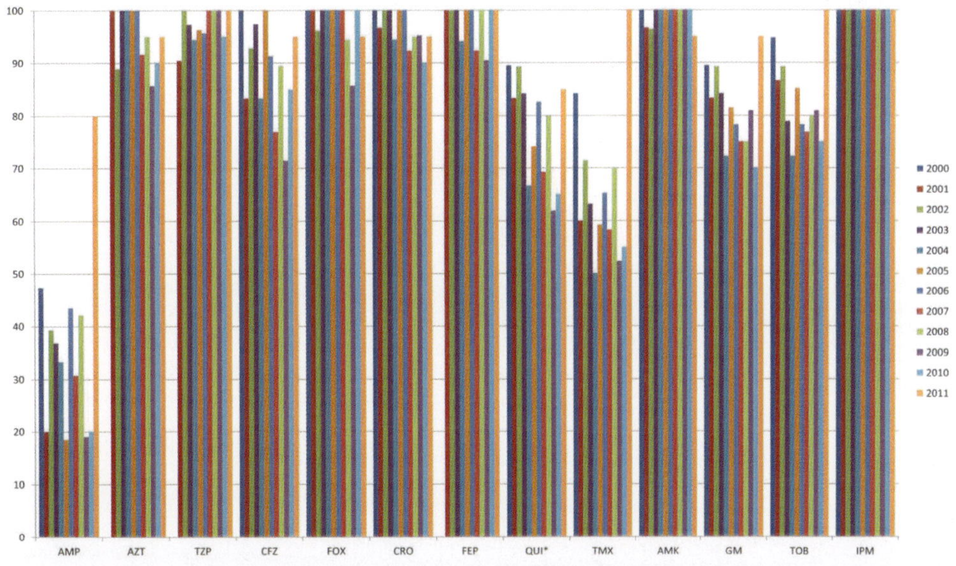

Figure 1. Change of antimicrobial susceptibility among *E. coli* during the 12-year-period. AMP, ampicillin; AZT, aztreonam; TZP, piperacillin/tazobactam; CFZ, cefazolin; FOX, cefoxitin; CRO, ceftriaxone; FEP, cefepime; QUI, quinolone; TMX, trimethoprim/sulfamethoxazole; AMK, amikacin; GM, gentamicin; TOB, tobramycin; IPM, imipenem. * During the study period, there was a significant decrease in antimicrobial susceptibility on univariate logistic regression analysis ($P = 0.040$).

data that inadequate empiric antibiotic therapy results in increased morbidity or treatment failure in complicated appendicitis [17,18]. If resistance to a given antibiotic is present in 10%–20% or more of isolates of a common intra-abdominal pathogen in the community, use of that agent should be avoided [5]. A report in Taiwan proposed that a quinolone be used to treat community-acquired complicated intra-abdominal infections, as *E. coli* was found to be 82–85% susceptible to ciprofloxacin and levofloxacin [19]. In this study, however, the resistance rate of *E. coli* to quinolones is >20%; therefore, its use as an empirical antibiotic is not advisable in Korea. Second- and third-generation cephalosporins appeared to be an appropriate treatment for this application according to our results. Although third-generation cephalosporins might be a better treatment choice because that *Streptococcus* species showed 100% susceptibility to ceftriaxone, further studies are needed to thoroughly trace variations in susceptibility, given that the decrease in *E. coli* susceptibility, observed during the study period, was not statistically significant. Piperacillin/tazobactam and carbapenem might be considered to treat *P. aeruginosa* or ESBL-producing organisms in patients with signs of severe sepsis such as organ dysfunction. However, these species were not frequently isolated in all patient groups including the severe sepsis group of the current study, and spectrum of these antibiotics may be too broad. *E. coli* also showed high susceptibility to amikacin, but concerns remain regarding use of aminoglycoside antibiotics owing to their nephrotoxicity and ototoxicity. Considering the high resistance of *E. coli* to ampicillin and ampicillin/sulbactam–and the questionable significance of enterococci as pathogens in complicated intra-abdominal infections–these antibiotics are not recommended for treating perforated appendicitis.

On the basis of evidence that culture testing of intraoperative specimens does not affect the prognosis of patients with perforated appendicitis, many institutions may not perform routine culture testing [20,21]. However, considering the current reality of increasing antibiotic resistance, routine culture testing might be useful to identify changes in susceptibility and to select appropriate antibiotics [5]. Anaerobic cultures are not necessary for patients with community-acquired intra-abdominal infection if empiric antimicrobial therapy active against common anaerobic pathogens is provide [5]. Although anaerobic bacteria culturing was not performed in this study, previous reports on anaerobic culture showed that *Bacteroides fragilis*, along with *E. coli*, was the most commonly isolated pathogen in appendicitis [14,20]. In past studies of appendicitis that conducted anaerobic susceptibility testing, *B. fragilis* was found to be more than 95% susceptible to metronidazole [4,14,22]. Anaerobic bacteria culturing could be considered for future studies if an increase in anaerobic bacterial resistance to metronidazole is observed.

The retrospective nature of the present study might have resulted in intrinsic bias and the data may not represent the entire population because data was collected from a single institution. However, considering that the quinolone resistance rate we observed was similar to that reported in previous studies conducted in Korea [23,24]–which involved community-acquired *E. coli* bacteremia originated from various infections including intra-abdominal infection–we speculated that quinolone resistance rate among *E. coli* causing intra-abdominal infection in Korea should be similar to the one determined in this study.

In conclusion, *E. coli* was the most commonly identified pathogen in patients with perforated appendicitis. The quinolone resistance rate was >20% in *E. coli* isolated from community-acquired perforated appendicitis. The isolates were decreasingly susceptible to quinolones during the study period. We advise against the use of quinolones as a first line antibiotic therapy in community-acquired perforated appendicitis in Korea.

Author Contributions

Conceived and designed the experiments: J-BJ. Performed the experiments: HGJ HUJ. Analyzed the data: GYK JJ M-HK. Contributed to the writing of the manuscript: J-BJ.

References

1. Lau WY, Wong SH (1981) Randomized, prospective trial of topical hydrogen peroxide in appendectomy wound infection. High risk factors. Am J Surg 142: 393–397.
2. Schmit PJ, Hiyama DT, Swisher SG, Bennion RS, Thompson JE Jr (1994) Analysis of risk factors of postappendectomy intra-abdominal abscess. J Am Coll Surg 179: 721–726.
3. Bennion RS, Baron EJ, Thompson JE Jr, Downes J, Summanen P, et al. (1990) The bacteriology of gangrenous and perforated appendicitis–revisited. Ann Surg 211: 165–171.
4. Lau WY, Teoh-Chan CH, Fan ST, Yam WC, Lau KF, et al. (1984) The bacteriology and septic complication of patients with appendicitis. Ann Surg 200: 576–581.
5. Solomkin JS, Mazuski JE, Bradley JS, Rodvold KA, Goldstein EJ, et al. (2010) Diagnosis and management of complicated intra-abdominal infection in adults and children: guidelines by the Surgical Infection Society and the Infectious Diseases Society of America. Clin Infect Dis 50: 133–164.
6. Bochicchio GV, Baquero F, Hsueh PR, Paterson DL, Rossi F, et al. (2006) In vitro susceptibilities of Escherichia coli isolated from patients with intra-abdominal infections worldwide in 2002–2004: results from SMART (Study for Monitoring Antimicrobial Resistance Trends). Surg Infect (Larchmt) 7: 537–545.
7. Paterson DL, Rossi F, Baquero F, Hsueh PR, Woods GL, et al. (2005) In vitro susceptibilities of aerobic and facultative Gram-negative bacilli isolated from patients with intra-abdominal infections worldwide: the 2003 Study for Monitoring Antimicrobial Resistance Trends (SMART). J Antimicrob Chemother 55: 965–973.
8. Lob SH, Badal RE, Bouchillon SK, Hawser SP, Hackel MA, et al. (2013) Epidemiology and susceptibility of Gram-negative appendicitis pathogens: SMART 2008–2010. Surg Infect (Larchmt) 14: 203–208.
9. Bone RC, Sibbald WJ, Sprung CL (1992) The ACCP-SCCM consensus conference on sepsis and organ failure. Chest 101: 1481–1483.
10. Clinical and Laboratory Standards Institute (2009) Performance standards for antimicrobial susceptibility testing. Nineteenth informational supplement. Document M100–S19. Wayne, PA: CLSI.
11. Montravers P, Lepape A, Dubreuil L, Gauzit R, Pean Y, et al. (2009) Clinical and microbiological profiles of community-acquired and nosocomial intra-abdominal infections: results of the French prospective, observational EBIIA study. J Antimicrob Chemother 63: 785–794.
12. Guillet-Caruba C, Cheikhelard A, Guillet M, Bille E, Descamps P, et al. (2011) Bacteriologic epidemiology and empirical treatment of pediatric complicated appendicitis. Diagn Microbiol Infect Dis 69: 376–381.
13. Chen CY, Chen YC, Pu HN, Tsai CH, Chen WT, et al. (2012) Bacteriology of acute appendicitis and its implication for the use of prophylactic antibiotics. Surg Infect (Larchmt) 13: 383–390.
14. Chan KW, Lee KH, Mou JW, Cheung ST, Sihoe JD, et al. (2010) Evidence-based adjustment of antibiotic in pediatric complicated appendicitis in the era of antibiotic resistance. Pediatr Surg Int 26: 157–160.
15. Fallon SC, Hassan SF, Larimer EL, Rodriguez JR, Brandt ML, et al. (2013) Modification of an evidence-based protocol for advanced appendicitis in children. J Surg Res 185: 273–277.
16. Andersen BR, Kallehave FL, Andersen HK (2001) Antibiotics versus placebo for prevention of postoperative infection after appendectomy. Cochrane Database Syst Rev: CD001439.
17. Yellin AE, Heseltine PN, Berne TV, Appleman MD, Gill MA, et al. (1985) The role of Pseudomonas species in patients treated with ampicillin and Sulbactam for gangrenous and perforated appendicitis. Surg Gynecol Obstet 161: 303–307.
18. Berne TV, Yellin AW, Appleman MD, Heseltine PN (1982) Antibiotic management of surgically treated gangrenous or perforated appendicitis. Comparison of gentamicin and clindamycin versus cefamandole versus cefoperazone. Am J Surg 144: 8–13.
19. Lau YJ, Chen YH, Huang CT, Lee WS, Liu CY, et al. (2012) Role of moxifloxacin for the treatment of community-acquired [corrected] complicated intra-abdominal infections in Taiwan. J Microbiol Immunol Infect 45: 1–6.

20. Kokoska ER, Silen ML, Tracy TF Jr, Dillon PA, Kennedy DJ, et al. (1999) The impact of intraoperative culture on treatment and outcome in children with perforated appendicitis. J Pediatr Surg 34: 749–753.
21. Foo FJ, Beckingham IJ, Ahmed I (2008) Intra-operative culture swabs in acute appendicitis: a waste of resources. Surgeon 6: 278–281.
22. Wojcik-Stojek B, Bulanda M, Martirosian G, Heczko P, Meisel-Mikolajczyk F (2000) In vitro antibiotic susceptibility of Bacteroides fragilis strains isolated from excised appendix of patients with phlegmonous or gangrenous appendicitis. Acta Microbiol Pol 49: 171–175.
23. Lee S, Han SW, Kim KW, Song do Y, Kwon KT (2014) Third-generation cephalosporin resistance of community-onset Escherichia coli and Klebsiella pneumoniae bacteremia in a secondary hospital. Korean J Intern Med 29: 49–56.
24. Park S, Park J, Lee S (2005) Analysis on the etiology and prognostic factors of community-acquired bacteremia in a community-based tertiary hospital. Infect Chemother 37: 255–264.

18

Peripheral Surgical Wounding and Age-Dependent Neuroinflammation in Mice

Zhipeng Xu[1]¶, Yuanlin Dong[1]¶, Hui Wang[1,2], Deborah J. Culley[3], Edward R. Marcantonio[4], Gregory Crosby[3], Rudolph E. Tanzi[5], Yiying Zhang[1], Zhongcong Xie[1]*

1 Geriatric Anesthesia Research Unit, Department of Anesthesia, Critical Care and Pain Medicine, Massachusetts General Hospital and Harvard Medical School, Charlestown, Massachusetts, **2** Department of Anesthesia, Beijing Chaoyang Hospital, Capital Medical University, Beijing, P. R. China, **3** Department of Anesthesia, Brigham & Women's Hospital and Harvard Medical School, Boston, Massachusetts, **4** Divisions of General Medicine and Primary Care and Gerontology, Department of Medicine, Beth Israel Deaconess Medical Center and Harvard Medical School, Boston, Massachusetts, **5** Genetics and Aging Research Unit, MassGeneral Institute for Neurodegenerative Disease, Department of Neurology, Massachusetts General Hospital and Harvard Medical School, Charlestown, Massachusetts

Abstract

Post-operative cognitive dysfunction is associated with morbidity and mortality. However, its neuropathogenesis remains largely to be determined. Neuroinflammation and accumulation of β-amyloid (Aβ) have been reported to contribute to cognitive dysfunction in humans and cognitive impairment in animals. Our recent studies have established a pre-clinical model in mice, and have found that the peripheral surgical wounding without the influence of general anesthesia induces an age-dependent Aβ accumulation and cognitive impairment in mice. We therefore set out to assess the effects of peripheral surgical wounding, in the absence of general anesthesia, on neuroinflammation in mice with different ages. Abdominal surgery under local anesthesia was established in 9 and 18 month-old mice. The levels of tumor necrosis factor-α (TNF-α), interleukin-6 (IL-6), Iba1 positive cells (the marker of microglia activation), CD33, and cognitive function in mice were determined. The peripheral surgical wounding increased the levels of TNF-α, IL-6, and Iba1 positive cells in the hippocampus of both 9 and 18 month-old mice, and age potentiated these effects. The peripheral surgical wounding increased the levels of CD33 in the hippocampus of 18, but not 9, month-old mice. Finally, anti-inflammatory drug ibuprofen ameliorated the peripheral surgical wounding-induced cognitive impairment in 18 month-old mice. These data suggested that the peripheral surgical wounding could induce an age-dependent neuroinflammation and elevation of CD33 levels in the hippocampus of mice, which could lead to cognitive impairment in aged mice. Pending further studies, anti-inflammatory therapies may reduce the risk of postoperative cognitive dysfunction in elderly patients.

Editor: Zhiyi Zuo, University of Virginia, United States of America

Funding: This study was supported by National Institutes of Health grants (Bethesda, Maryland) (R21 AG029856, R21 AG038994, R01 GM088801 and R01 AG041274); American Geriatrics Society Jahnigen Award (New York, NY); Investigator-Initiated Research Grant from Alzheimer's Association (Chicago, IL) and Cure Alzheimer's Fund to ZX. EM is supported by a Midcareer Investigator Award in Patient-Oriented Research from the National Institute on Aging [K24 AG035075]. The funders had no role in study design, data collection and analysis, decision to publish, or preparation of the manuscript.

* E-mail: zxie@mgh.harvard.edu

¶ These authors contributed equally to this work.

Introduction

Post-operative cognitive dysfunction (POCD) is one of the most common post-operative complications in senior patients [1], and is associated with increased cost, morbidity, and mortality [2,3,4]. However, the neuropathogenesis of POCD remains largely to be determined and this gap in knowledge impedes the further research of POCD.

In our previous studies, we have established a pre-clinical model of open abdominal surgery under local anesthesia in mice to determine the effects of peripheral surgical wounding without the influence of general anesthesia on Aβ accumulation and cognitive impairment [5]. We have found that the peripheral surgical wounding without the influence of general anesthesia can induce an age dependent Aβ accumulation and cognitive impairment [5].

Neuroinflammation, including increases in levels of pro-inflammatory cytokine tumor necrosis factor-α (TNF-α) and interleukin-6 (IL-6), as well as microglia activation, has been reported to contribute to the cognitive impairment induced by surgery under anesthesia ([6,7,8,9], reviewed in [10]). However, whether the peripheral surgical wounding without the influence of general anesthesia can induce an age dependent neuroinflammation has not been investigated.

Therefore, we studied the neuropathogenesis of POCD by assessing whether the peripheral surgical wounding without the influence of general anesthesia could induce an age-dependent neuroinflammation in mice. Finally, ibuprofen is a non-steroidal anti-inflammatory drug (NSAIDs). We therefore assessed whether ibuprofen could attenuate the peripheral surgical wounding-induced cognitive impairment in the 18 month-old mice.

We chose TNF-α and IL-6 in the current studies because these two pre-inflammatory cytokines have been shown to be associated with the neuroinflammation associated with surgery under anesthesia ([6,7,8,9,11], reviewed in [10]). Finally, *CD33* is a newly suggested AD associated gene [12]. Protein CD33 is a member of the SIGLEC family of lectins can bind to sialic acid and regulate the innate immune system [13]. Moreover, a recent study has shown that the reduction in the protein levels of *CD33* can ameliorate Aβ pathology [14]. Both Aβ accumulation (reviewed in [15]) and neuroinflammation (reviewed in [10]) have been shown to be associated with cognitive impairment. Taken together, we assessed the effects of the peripheral surgical wounding, in the absence of general anesthesia, on the levels of TNF-α, IL-6, microglia activation, and CD33 in the hippocampus of mice, as well as the cognitive function in the mice.

Results

The Peripheral Surgical Wounding Increased TNF-α Levels in the Hippocampus of Mice at Three and Six Hours after the Procedure

Neuroinflammation may be associated with cognitive impairment in animals [6,8] and in patients [16]. Therefore, we assessed the effects of the peripheral surgical wounding without the influence of general anesthesia on neuroinflammation. ELISA of TNF-α showed that the peripheral surgical wounding increased the TNF-α levels in the hippocampus of both 9 (6.9 pg/ml±1.07 versus 4.2 pg/ml±0.57, P = 0.047) and 18 (9.0 pg/ml±2.51 versus 3.1 pg/ml±0.6, P = 0.048) month-old mice at three hours after the peripheral surgical wounding (Figure 1A). Two-way ANOVA indicated that age potentiated the peripheral surgical wounding-induced increases in TNF-α levels (Figure 1A, P = 0.003). The peripheral surgical wounding also increased the TNF-α levels in the hippocampus of both 9 (8.9 pg/ml±1.53 versus 4.2 pg/ml±0.57, P = 0.040) and 18 (11.1 pg/ml±2.50 versus 3.1 pg/ml±0.6, P = 0.040) month-old mice at six hours after the peripheral surgical wounding (Figure 1B). Two-way ANOVA indicated that age potentiated the peripheral surgical wounding-induced increases in TNF-α levels (Figure 1B, P = 0.04). The peripheral surgical wounding did not significantly alter the TNF-α levels in the hippocampus of mice of 9 and 18 month-old mice at 12 hours after the peripheral surgical wounding (data not shown). These data suggested that the peripheral surgical wounding without the influence of general anesthesia induced a time- and age-dependent increase in the pro-inflammatory cytokine TNF-α levels in the hippocampus of mice.

The Peripheral Surgical Wounding Increased IL-6 Levels in the Hippocampus of Mice at 12 Hours after the Procedure

ELISA studies showed that the levels of pro-inflammatory cytokine IL-6 increased at 12 hours post-surgery in the hippocampus of both 9 month-old mice: 7.1 pg/ml±0.40 versus 3.1 pg/ml±0.26, **P = 0.009; and 18 month-old mice: 9.9 pg/ml±1.06 versus 4.3 pg/ml±0.44, **P = 0.0001 (Figure 2). Two-way ANOVA indicated that age potentiated the peripheral surgical wounding-induced increases in the levels of IL-6 (Figure 2, ^^P = 0.003) in the mouse hippocampus. The peripheral surgical wounding did not increase the IL-6 levels at three or six hours after the procedure (data not shown). These data suggested that the peripheral surgical wounding induced a time- and age-dependent increase in the pro-inflammatory cytokine IL-6 levels in the hippocampus of mice.

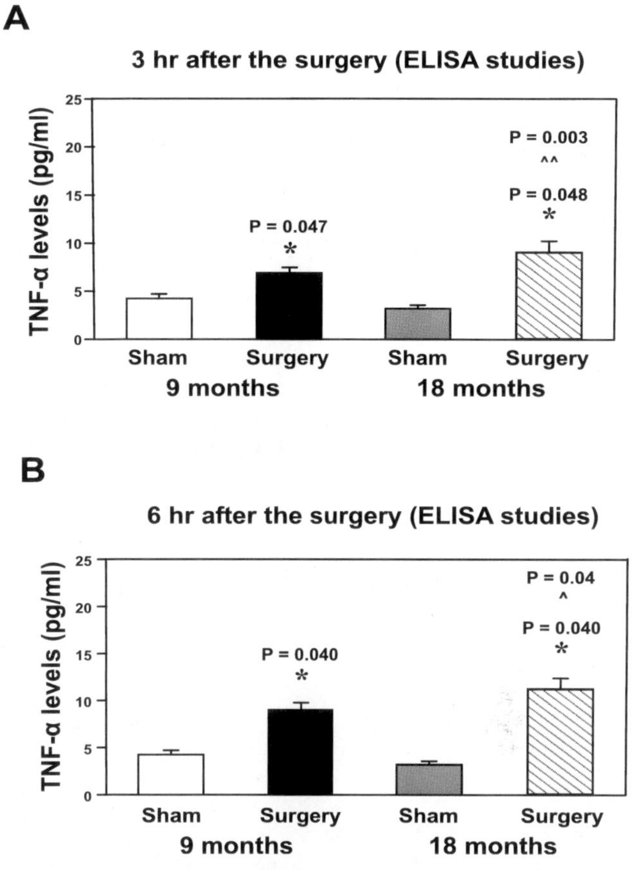

Figure 1. Peripheral surgical wounding increases TNF-α levels in the mouse hippocampus. A. Peripheral surgical wounding increases the levels of TNF-α in the hippocampus of both 9 and 18 month-old mice at three hours after the peripheral surgical wounding. Age potentiates the peripheral surgical wounding-induced elevation of TNF-α levels. **B.** Peripheral surgical wounding increases the levels of TNF-α in the hippocampus of both 9 and 18 month-old mice at six hours after the peripheral surgical wounding. Age potentiates the peripheral surgical wounding-induced elevation of TNF-α levels. (*: the difference between sham and peripheral surgical wounding; ^ or ^^: the interaction between the group and the treatment). TNF-α, tumor necrosis factor-α. N = 6.

The Peripheral Surgical Wounding Increased Iba1 Positive Cells in the Hippocampus of Mice at 12 Hours after the Procedure

Immunostaining of Iba1, a marker of microglia cell activation [17], illustrated that the peripheral surgical wounding increased the number of Iba1 positive cells in the hippocampus of both 9 month-old mice: 75, 62.3–123.3 (median, interquartile range) versus 66, 38.8–89.8 (median, interquartile range), **P = 0.003; and 18 month-old mice: 136, 102.0–149.0 (median, interquartile range) versus 62, 56.0–77.0 (median, interquartile range), ##P = 0.0001 at 12 hours post-surgery (Figure 3A and 3B). Two-way ANOVA indicated that age potentiated the peripheral surgical wounding-induced increases in the levels of microglia cell activation, as evidenced by the increase in the number of Iba1 positive cells, in the hippocampus of mice (Figure 3B, ^^P = 0.002). These data suggested that the peripheral surgical wounding was able to induce microglia activation and age potentiated it.

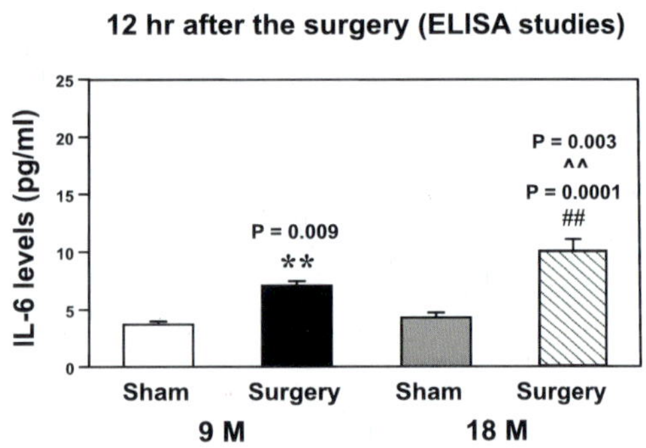

Figure 2. Peripheral surgical wounding increases IL-6 levels in the mouse hippocampus. Peripheral surgical wounding increases the levels of IL-6 in the hippocampus of both 9 and 18 month-old mice at 12 hours after the peripheral surgical wounding. Age potentiates the peripheral surgical wounding-induced elevation of TNF-α levels. (** or ##: the difference between sham and peripheral surgical wounding; ^^: the interaction between the group and the treatment). IL, interleukin. N = 6.

Peripheral Surgical Wounding Increased Protein Levels of Gene *CD33* in the Hippocampus of Aged Mice

CD33 is a newly suggested AD associated gene [12]. As a member of the SIGLEC family of lectins, protein CD33 binds sialic acid and regulates the innate immune system [13]. We therefore assessed the effects of the peripheral surgical wounding without the influence of general anesthesia on the levels of CD33. Immunoblotting of CD33 showed that the peripheral surgical wounding increased the protein levels of *CD33* (CD33) (Figure 4A and 4B): 141% ± 15 versus 100% ± 16, *P = 0.030 in the hippocampus of 18 month-old mice at 12 hours after the procedure. However, the quantitative western blot showed that the peripheral surgical wounding did not significantly alter the CD33 levels in the hippocampus of 9 month-old mice at 12 hours after the procedure (Figure 4C and 4D). These data suggested that the peripheral surgical wounding induced an age-dependent enhancement of CD33 levels in the hippocampus of mice.

Ibuprofen Ameliorated the Peripheral Surgical Wounding-induced Cognitive Impairment in Aged Mice

Given that the peripheral surgical wounding without the influence of general anesthesia could induce neuroinflammation (Figure 1, 2 and 3), and Aβ accumulation and cognitive impairment in aged mice [5], we assessed the cause-effect relationship by employing ibuprofen, a nonsteroidal anti-inflammatory drug (NSAID), which has been shown to attenuate neuroinflammation [18] and reduce Aβ levels [19]. We found that a treatment with ibuprofen for 7 days post-surgery ameliorated the peripheral surgical wounding-induced cognitive impairments in aged mice (Figure 5A: context test, ^^P = 0.002, two-way ANOVA) and (Figure 5B: tone text, ^^P = 0.0001, two-way ANOVA). These findings provided additional information to suggest that the peripheral surgical wounding could induce cognitive impairment in aged mice via neuroinflammation, and curbing neuroinflammation, e.g. with NSAIDs, might reduce the risk of POCD.

Discussion

The neuropathogenesis of POCD remains largely to be determined. Neuroinflammation has been reported to be associated with POCD in humans and cognitive impairment in animals ([6,7,8,9], reviewed in [10]). Our recent studies have shown that peripheral surgical wounding without the influence of general anesthesia can induce an age-dependent Aβ accumulation and cognitive impairment in mice [5]. We therefore assessed whether the peripheral surgical wounding without the influence of general anesthesia could cause an age-dependent neuroinflammation.

We found that the peripheral surgical wounding increased the levels of TNF-α (Figure 1), IL-6 (Figure 2) and Iba1 positive cells

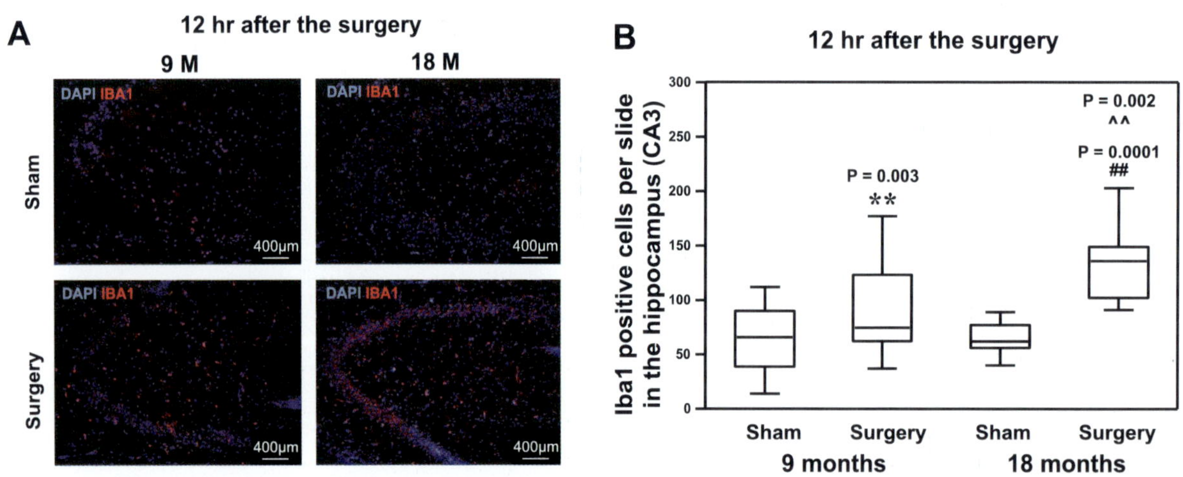

Figure 3. Peripheral surgical wounding increases the levels of Iba1 positive cells in the mouse hippocampus. A. The immunohistochemistry staining showed that peripheral surgical wounding increases the levels of Iba1 positive cells in the hippocampus of both 9 and 18 month-old mice at 12 hours after the peripheral surgical wounding as compared to sham. There are more Iba1 positive cells in the hippocampus of 18 month-old mice than that of 9 month-old mice following the peripheral surgical wounding. **B.** The quantification of the images shows that the peripheral surgical wounding increases the number of Ibal positive cells in the hippocampus of both 9 and 18 month-old mice at 12 hours after the peripheral surgical wounding as compared to sham. Age potentiates the peripheral surgical wounding-induced increases in the levels of Iba1 cells. (** or ##: the difference between sham and peripheral surgical wounding group; ^^: the interaction between the group and the treatment). Iba1, ionized calcium-binding adapter molecule 1. N = 6.

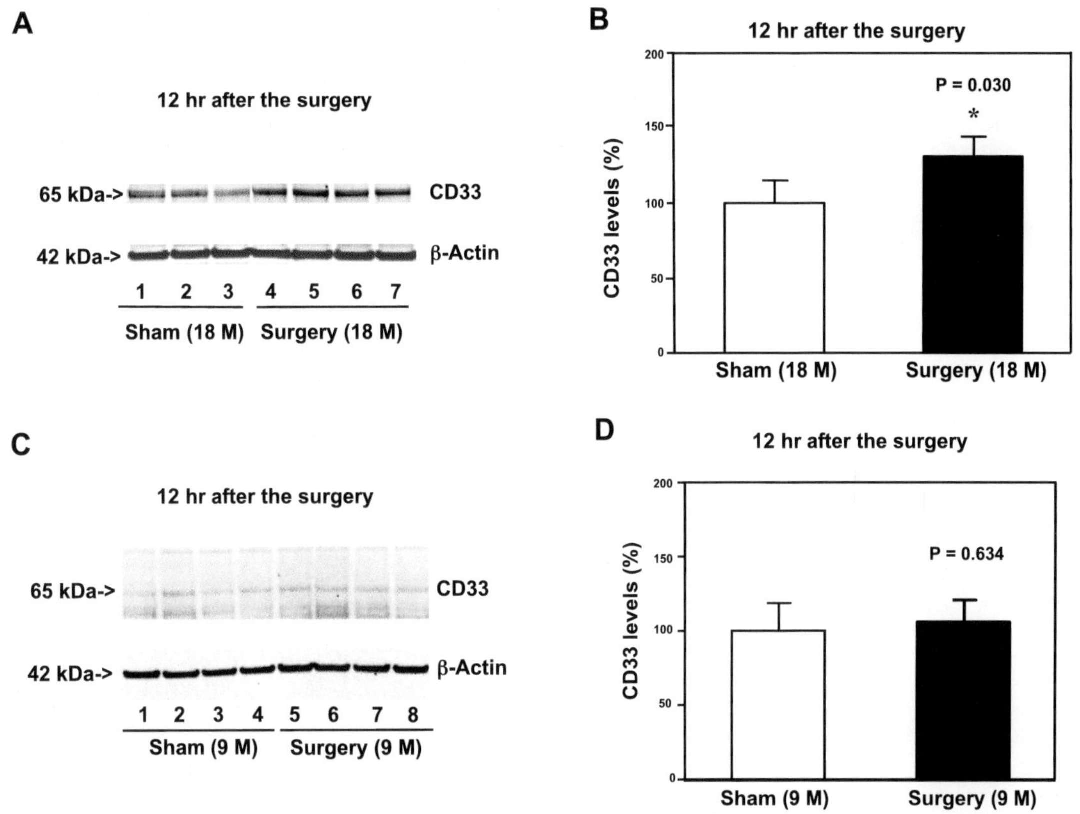

Figure 4. Peripheral surgical wounding only increases the levels of Iba1 positive cells in the hippocampus of 18 month-old mice. A. Peripheral surgical wounding increases the CD33 levels in the hippocampus of 18 month-old mice as compared to sham. There is no significant difference in β-actin levels between the peripheral surgical wounding mice and sham mice. **B.** The quantification of the Western blot shows that the peripheral surgical wounding increases the CD33 levels in the hippocampus of 18 month-old mice as compared to sham. **C.** Peripheral surgical wounding does not increase the CD33 levels in the hippocampus of 9 month-old mice as compared to sham. There is no significant difference in β-actin levels between the peripheral surgical wounding mice and sham mice. **D.** The quantification of the Western blot shows that the peripheral surgical wounding does not increase the CD33 levels in the hippocampus of 18 month-old mice as compared to sham. (*: the difference between sham and peripheral surgical wounding). N = 6.

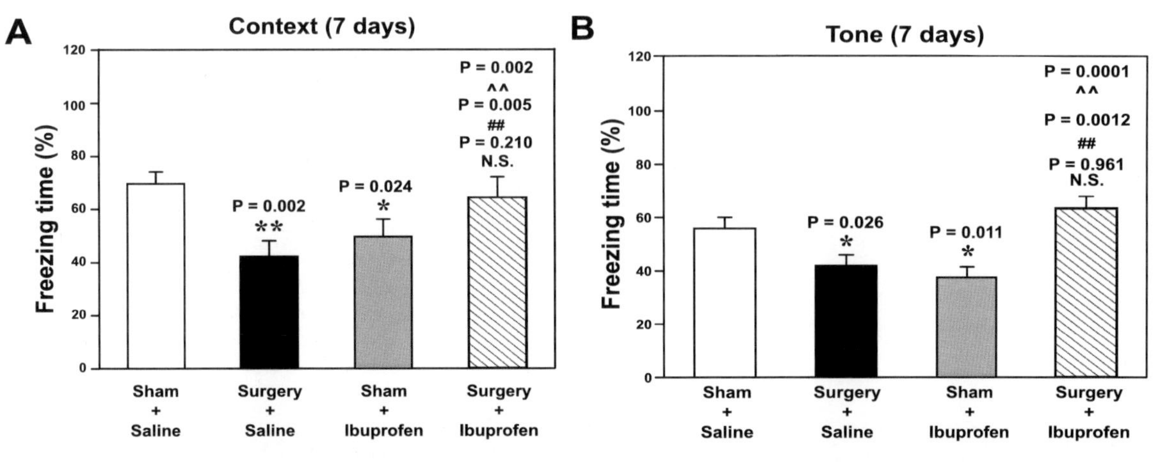

Figure 5. Ibuprofen attenuates the peripheral surgical wounding-induced cognitive impairment in aged mice. Peripheral surgical wounding without the influence of general anesthesia induces cognitive impairment in the context test (*A*) and tone test (*B*) of the FCS at 7 days post-surgery in 18 month-old mice. Ibuprofen attenuates the peripheral surgical wounding-induced reduction in freezing time of the context test (*A*) and the tone test (*B*) of the FCS at 7 days post-surgery (* or **: the difference between sham and peripheral surgical wounding group; ##: the difference between saline and ibuprofen treatment; ^^: the interaction between the group and the treatment). FCT, fear conditioning system. N = 10.

(Figure 3) in the hippocampus of both 9 and 18 month-old mice. More importantly, age potentiated the peripheral surgical wounding-induced elevations in the levels of TNF-α, IL-6 and Iba1 positive cells. These data suggested that the peripheral surgical wounding without the influence of general anesthesia could induce an age-dependent neuroinflammation (increases in pro-inflammatory cytokine levels and microglia activation), and that aged mice might be more vulnerable to the development of neuroinflammation following the insult of peripheral surgical wounding.

Note that the increases in TNF-α levels occurred at 3 and 6, but not 12 hours, after the peripheral surgical wounding, but the peripheral surgical wounding-induced increases in IL-6 levels only occurred at 12 hours after the procedure. These data suggested that the peripheral surgical wounding-induced increases in TNF-α levels could be precedent of the peripheral surgical wounding-induced increases in IL-6 levels. Terrando et al. has shown that TNF-α is upstream of IL-1 following a surgery under anesthesia in mice [6]. It is conceivable that increases in TNF-α levels following the peripheral surgical wounding could also lead to the increase in IL-6 levels. The future studies to test this hypothesis were warranted.

CD33 is a newly suggested AD associated gene [12] and *CD33* is involved in both innate immunity and Aβ pathology [14]. A recent study has shown that the reduction in the protein levels of *CD33* (CD33) can ameliorate Aβ pathology [14]. Consistently, we found that the peripheral surgical wounding increased CD33 levels in the hippocampus of 18 month-old mice, but not in the hippocampus of the 9 month-old mice (Figure 4). These findings suggested that there was also an age-dependent changes in CD33 levels in the hippocampus of mice following the peripheral surgical wounding. Whether the difference in the CD33 levels in the hippocampus of 9 and 18 month-old mice following the peripheral surgical wounding is responsible for the difference in the neuroinflammation observed in the 9 and 18 month-old mice following the peripheral surgical wounding is not known at the present time, but warrants further investigation in the future.

Finally, non-steroidal anti-inflammatory drug ibuprofen, which has anti-inflammatory and lowers Aβ level effects [18,19], mitigated the peripheral surgical wounding-induced cognitive impairment in the 18 month-old mice (Figure 5). These results demonstrated the cause-effect relationship of the peripheral surgical wounding-induced neuroinflammation and the peripheral surgical wounding-induced cognitive impairment. Moreover, these findings showed the potential application of anti-inflammatory treatment in preventing and treating POCD, pending further studies.

The aged TNF-α, IL-6, or CD33 knockout mice (e.g., 18 month-old mice) were not available at the time of the experiments. We therefore could not investigate the mechanism (s) underlying the effects of TNF-α, IL-6, or CD33 knockout. However, the main objective of the current studies was to determine whether there was an age-dependent change in neuroinflammation in mice following the peripheral surgical wounding without the influence of general anesthesia. We will determine whether the peripheral surgical wounding without the influence of general anesthesia can still induce cognitive impairment in aged TNF-α, IL-6, or CD33 knockout mice in our future studies.

Interestingly, there is no significant difference in the baseline levels of TNF-α, IL-6, and microglia activation (Iba1 positive cells) in the hippocampus between the 9 (adult) and 18 (aged) month-old mice in the current experiments. The exact reasons of these findings are unknown at the present time. However, it remains possible that there is still a significant difference in the baseline levels of TNF-α, IL-6, and microglia activation (Iba1 positive cells) in other brain regions of the mice, e.g., cortex, between the 9 (adult) and 18 (aged) month-old mice. The experiments to illustrate such differences may be included in future studies.

The studies have several limitations. First, we did not measure the effects of ibuprofen on the levels of TNF-α, IL-6, and microglia activation in the studies. However, the objective of the ibuprofen studies was to demonstrate the general cause-effect relationship of the peripheral surgical wounding-induced neuroinflammation and the peripheral surgical wounding-induced cognitive impairment. Second, levobupivacaine has been reported to suppress inflammation [20,21], therefore, we cannot totally rule out the influence of local anesthetics on the levels of TNF-α, IL-6, and microglia activation, as well as the cognitive function observed in the current studies. However, our previous studies showed that local anesthetic bupivacaine (0.5% and 0.1 ml) did not affect the cognitive function in the mice [5]. Moreover, the sham mice also received the bupivacaine injection in the current studies. Finally, employment of EMLA might cause side effects. A case report showed that a 7-month-old girl with pulmonary dysplasia receiving inhaled nitric oxide developed cyanosis caused by methemoglobinemia after prolonged use of EMLA. We did not observe such side effects in mice after the use of EMLA in our previous experiments [5,22].

In conclusion, we have shown that open abdominal surgery, in the absence of general anesthesia (under local anesthesia), induced an age-dependent neuroinflammation (e.g., increases in TNF-α and IL-6 levels, and microglia activation) and changes in CD33 levels in the hippocampus of mice. The aged mice are more vulnerable to the peripheral surgical wounding-induced neuroinflammation and increases in CD33 levels. Ibuprofen, an anti-inflammatory drug, ameliorated the peripheral surgical wounding-induced cognitive impairment in aged mice. Taken together, these findings carry insightful implications for the surgical care of elderly patients and suggest that the aging brain could be more susceptible to the development of neuroinflammation following peripheral surgical wounding. Pending further studies, it may be useful to consider anti-inflammatory to reduce the risk of POCD in elderly patients.

Methods

Mice Surgery and Treatment

All experiments followed the National Institutes of Health guidelines and the animal protocol was approved by the Massachusetts General Hospital (Boston, Massachusetts) Standing Committee on the Use of Animals in Research and Teaching. Efforts were made to minimize the number of animals used. Since it is technically difficult to perform an epidural or spinal anesthesia in mice, we have established an animal model of open abdominal surgery under local anesthesia in mice [5]. Specifically, wild type C57BL/6J female mice (9 month-old, The Jackson Laboratory, Bar Harbor, ME; and 18 month-old, National Institute of Aging, Bethesda, MD) were used in the studies. The mice were randomly assigned to a surgery or sham group by weight. The mice were gently restrained to a heating pad (37°C) using paper tape. A local anesthetic bupivacine (0.5% and 0.1 ml) was injected into the skin and subcutaneous tissue of the abdominal area. A 2.5 cm incision was made in the middle of the abdomen to open and then close the abdominal cavity in the mouse. The procedure lasted about five minutes. We did not use sedative medicine in an effort to reveal the effects of surgery alone and to minimize all other variables. EMLA cream (2.5% lidocaine and 2.5% prilocaine) was used every 8 hours for the first and second post-operative days to treat the surgery-associated pain. We did not use antibiotics because the procedure was aseptic. The non-surgery (sham) mice underwent the same procedure, only without the incision. For the interaction studies, each of the mice received ibuprofen (30 mg/kg, PO, CVS Pharmacy, Inc., Woonsocket, RI) or saline once per day for 7 days post-surgery [18,23]. We chose abdominal surgery because it is associated with POCD in humans [24]. In addition, the surgery is easy to perform, and behavioral tests can be run without difficulty post-surgery. There was no significant difference in blood pressure, blood gas, levels of blood glucose and epinephrine, locomotor activity, or pain threshold between the surgery and sham mice, as demonstrated in our previous studies [5]. Local anesthetic induced neither neuroinflammation nor cognitive impairment in the aged mice (18 month-old mice) [5].

Brain Tissue Lysis, Protein Amount Quantification

The harvested hippocampus tissues were homogenized on ice using immunoprecipitation buffer (10 mM Tris-HCl, pH 7.4, 150 mM NaCl, 2 mM EDTA, 0.5% Nonidet P-40) plus protease inhibitors (1 μg/ml aprotinin, 1 μg/ml leupeptin, 1 μg/ml pepstatin A). The lysates were collected, centrifuged at 12,000 rpm for 15 minutes, and quantified for total proteins by bicinchoninic acid protein assay kit (Pierce, Iselin, NJ). The hippocampus tissues were then subjected to Western blot analysis as described by Xie et al. [25].

Western Blot Analysis

Antibody C33 (1:200, Santa Cruz, Santa Cruz, CA, Cat. Number: sc-53199) was used to recognize protein CD33 (67 kDa). Western blot quantification was performed as described by Xie et al. [25]. Briefly, signal intensity was analyzed using a Bio-Rad (Hercules, CA) image program (Quantity One). We quantified Western blots in two steps. First, we used β-Actin levels to normalize (e.g., determining ratio of CD33 to β-Actin amount) protein levels and control for loading differences in total protein amount. Second, we presented protein level changes in the mice receiving the surgery as a percentage of those in the sham group mice. 100% of protein level changes refer to control levels for the purpose of comparison to experimental conditions.

Immunohistochemistry

Mice were anesthetized with isoflurane briefly (1.4% isoflurane for five minutes) and perfused transcardially with heparinized saline followed by 4% paraformaldehyde in 0.1 M phosphate buffer at pH 7.4. Mouse hippocampus tissues were removed and kept at 4 degrees C in paraformaldehyde. Five μm frozen sections from mouse brain hemispheres were used for the immunohistochemistry staining. The sections were incubated with ionized calcium binding adaptor molecule 1 (Iba1) antibody (1:500, Wako, Cat. Number: 019-19741) and secondary antibody (Alexa Fluor594, 1:500, Invitrogen, Cat. Number: A11037). Finally, the sections were analyzed in mounting medium under a 20 × objective lens fluorescence microscope and photos of the sections were taken. An investigator who was blind to the experimental design counted the number of the Iba1 positive cells using Image J Version 1.38 (National Institutes of Health, Bethesda, MD).

Enzyme-Linked Immunosorbent Assay (ELISA) Determination of TNF-α and IL-6

The mouse TNF-α Immunoassay kit (R&D Systems, Minneapolis, MN, Catalog number: MTA00B) and IL-6 Immunoassay kit (R&D Systems, Catalog number: M6000B) was used to determine the levels of TNF-α and IL-6 in the hippocampus tissues of the mice. Briefly, a monoclonal antibody specific for mouse TNF-α or IL-6 has been coated onto microplates. We added 50 ul of standard or samples, and then added 50 μL of assay diluent RD1-14 to the center of each well. Wells were incubated for two hours at room temperature, and washed five times. Then 100 μL of mouse TNF-α or IL-6 conjugate was added to each well and incubated for another two hours and repeated the washing. At last, wells were incubated in 100 μL of substrate solution for 30 minutes and stopped with stop solution. Determination of the optical density of each well was set at 450 nm, and corrected at 570 nm.

Fear Conditioning System (FCS)

The FCS studies were performed as described in our previous studies with modifications [5]. Specifically, the pairing in the FCS (Stoelting Co., Wood Dale, IL) was performed at 24 hours post-surgery, mimicking the condition that patients may have difficulty learning new things after surgery. The pairing was performed twice with two minutes in between. For pairing, each mouse was allowed to explore the FCS chamber for 180 seconds before presentation of a 2-Hz pulsating tone (80 dB, 3,600 Hz) that persisted for 60 seconds. The tone was immediately followed by a mild foot shock (0.8 mA for 0.5 second). The mice were tested in FCS at 7 days after the procedure. Each mouse was allowed to stay in the same chamber for a total of 390 seconds. Cognitive functions (e.g., learning and memory) in the context and tone test were assessed by measuring the amount of time the mouse demonstrated "freezing behavior", which is defined as a completely immobile posture except for respiratory efforts during the second 180 seconds. "Freezing behavior" was analyzed by Any-Maze (freezing on threshold: 10; freezing off threshold: 20; minimum freezing duration: one second) (Stoelting Co.). The percentage of freezing time was calculated by dividing the actual freezing time with the observed time (180 seconds).

Statistics

The nature of the hypothesis testing was two-tailed. Data were expressed as mean ± Standard Error of the Mean (SEM). The data for the number of Iba1 positive cells were not normally distributed, thus were expressed as median and interquartile range (IQR). The number of samples varied from 6 (biochemistry studies) to 10 (behavioral studies). Two-way ANOVA was used to determine the interaction between group (9 and 18 month-old mice) and treatment (sham and peripheral surgical wounding) in FCS studies, and in the levels of TNF-α and IL-6. Student t-test was used to determine the difference in CD33 levels between the peripheral surgical wounding and sham. P values less than 0.05 (*, # and ^) and 0.01 (**, ## and ^^) were considered statistically significant. Prism 6 software (La Jolla, CA, USA) software was used for all statistical analyses.

Acknowledgments

The authors would like to thank Dr. Mark Baxter from Mount Sinai School of Medicine for constructive discussion, Dr. Hui Zheng from Massachusetts General Hospital for the help of statistical analysis of the data, and Joshua J. Busscher from Massachusetts General Hospital for technical help.

Author Contributions

Conceived and designed the experiments: Z. Xie GC DC EM RT YZ. Performed the experiments: Z. Xu YD HW YZ. Analyzed the data: Z. Xie Z. Xu YD YZ. Contributed reagents/materials/analysis tools: RT GC. Contributed to the writing of the manuscript: Z. Xie RT EM.

References

1. Liu LL, Leung JM (2000) Predicting adverse postoperative outcomes in patients aged 80 years or older. J Am Geriatr Soc 48: 405–412.
2. Monk TG, Weldon BC, Garvan CW, Dede DE, van der Aa MT, et al. (2008) Predictors of cognitive dysfunction after major noncardiac surgery. Anesthesiology 108: 18–30.
3. Deiner S, Silverstein JH (2009) Postoperative delirium and cognitive dysfunction. Br J Anaesth 103 Suppl 1: i41–46.
4. Steinmetz J, Christensen KB, Lund T, Lohse N, Rasmussen LS (2009) Long-term consequences of postoperative cognitive dysfunction. Anesthesiology 110: 548–555.
5. Xu Z, Dong Y, Wang H, Culley DJ, Marcantonio ER, et al. (2014) Age-dependent postoperative cognitive impairment and Alzheimer-related neuropathology in mice. Scientific reports 4: 3766.
6. Terrando N, Monaco C, Ma D, Foxwell BM, Feldmann M, et al. (2010) Tumor necrosis factor-alpha triggers a cytokine cascade yielding postoperative cognitive decline. Proc Natl Acad Sci U S A 107: 20518–20522.
7. Wan Y, Xu J, Ma D, Zeng Y, Cibelli M, et al. (2007) Postoperative impairment of cognitive function in rats: a possible role for cytokine-mediated inflammation in the hippocampus. Anesthesiology 106: 436–443.
8. Wan Y, Xu J, Meng F, Bao Y, Ge Y, et al. (2010) Cognitive decline following major surgery is associated with gliosis, beta-amyloid accumulation, and tau phosphorylation in old mice. Crit Care Med.
9. Cibelli M, Fidalgo AR, Terrando N, Ma D, Monaco C, et al. (2010) Role of interleukin-1beta in postoperative cognitive dysfunction. Ann Neurol 68: 360–368.
10. Terrando N, Brzezinski M, Degos V, Eriksson LI, Kramer JH, et al. (2011) Perioperative cognitive decline in the aging population. Mayo Clin Proc 86: 885–893.
11. Shen X, Dong Y, Xu Z, Wang H, Miao C, et al. (2013) Selective Anesthesia-induced Neuroinflammation in Developing Mouse Brain and Cognitive Impairment. Anesthesiology 118: 502–515.
12. Bertram L, Lange C, Mullin K, Parkinson M, Hsiao M, et al. (2008) Genome-wide association analysis reveals putative Alzheimer's disease susceptibility loci in addition to APOE. Am J Hum Genet 83: 623–632.
13. von Gunten S, Simon HU (2006) Sialic acid binding immunoglobulin-like lectins may regulate innate immune responses by modulating the life span of granulocytes. FASEB J 20: 601–605.
14. Griciuc A, Serrano-Pozo A, Parrado AR, Lesinski AN, Asselin CN, et al. (2013) Alzheimer's Disease Risk Gene CD33 Inhibits Microglial Uptake of Amyloid Beta. Neuron.
15. Querfurth HW, LaFerla FM (2010) Alzheimer's disease. N Engl J Med 362: 329–344.
16. Teeling JL, Perry VH (2009) Systemic infection and inflammation in acute CNS injury and chronic neurodegeneration: underlying mechanisms. Neuroscience 158: 1062–1073.
17. Willuweit A, Velden J, Godemann R, Manook A, Jetzek F, et al. (2009) Early-onset and robust amyloid pathology in a new homozygous mouse model of Alzheimer's disease. PLoS One 4: e7931.
18. Sliva J, Dolezal T, Sykora D, Vosmanska M, Krsiak M (2009) Guaifenesin enhances the analgesic potency of ibuprofen, nimesulide and celecoxib in mice. Neuro Endocrinol Lett 30: 352–356.
19. Weggen S, Eriksen JL, Das P, Sagi SA, Wang R, et al. (2001) A subset of NSAIDs lower amyloidogenic Abeta42 independently of cyclooxygenase activity. Nature 414: 212–216.
20. Huang YH, Yen JC, Lee JJ, Liao JF, Liaw WJ, et al. (2013) Suppressive effects of levobupivacaine on endotoxin-induced microglial activation. The Journal of surgical research 184: 989–996.
21. Duman U, Yilmazlar A, Ozturk E, Aker S, Sarandol E, et al. (2010) Anti-inflammatory efficiency of levobupivacaine in an experimental colitis model. World journal of gastroenterology: WJG 16: 2537–2541.
22. Zhang X, Xin X, Dong Y, Zhang Y, Yu B, et al. (2013) Surgical Incision-Induced Nociception Causes Cognitive Impairment and Reduction in Synaptic NMDA Receptor 2B in Mice. The Journal of neuroscience: the official journal of the Society for Neuroscience 33: 17737–17748.
23. Cauli O, Rodrigo R, Piedrafita B, Llansola M, Mansouri MT, et al. (2009) Neuroinflammation contributes to hypokinesia in rats with hepatic encephalopathy: ibuprofen restores its motor activity. J Neurosci Res 87: 1369–1374.
24. Hocker J, Stapelfeldt C, Leiendecker J, Meybohm P, Hanss R, et al. (2009) Postoperative neurocognitive dysfunction in elderly patients after xenon versus propofol anesthesia for major noncardiac surgery: a double-blinded randomized controlled pilot study. Anesthesiology 110: 1068–1076.
25. Xie Z, Culley DJ, Dong Y, Zhang G, Zhang B, et al. (2008) The common inhalation anesthetic isoflurane induces caspase activation and increases amyloid beta-protein level in vivo. Ann Neurol 64: 618–627.

Comparison of Hemodynamic and Inflammatory Changes between Transoral and Transthoracic Thoracoscopic Surgery

Yen Chu[1]¶, Chien-Ying Liu[2]¶, Yi-Cheng Wu[1], Ming-Ju Hsieh[1], Tzu-Ping Chen[1], Ying-Kai Chao[1], Ching-Yang Wu[1], Hsu-Chia Yuan[3], Po-Jen Ko[1], Yun-Hen Liu[1]*, Hui-Ping Liu[1]*

1 Department of Thoracic Surgery, Chang Gung Memorial Hospital, Chang Gung University, Taoyuan, Taiwan, **2** Department of Thoracic Medicine, Chang Gung Memorial Hospital, Chang Gung University, Taoyuan, Taiwan, **3** Laboratory Animal Center, Chang Gung Memorial Hospital, Chang Gung University, Taoyuan, Taiwan

Abstract

Background: Natural orifice transluminal endoscopy has been developed for abdominal surgical procedures. The aim of this study was to compare the surgical outcome between a novel transoral approach and a standard transthoracic approach for the thoracic cavity in a canine model.

Methods: Twenty-eight dogs were assigned to transoral (n = 14) or standard thoracoscopy (n = 14). Each group underwent thoracic exploration, pre-determined surgical lung biopsy, and pericardial window creation. Blood draws were obtained before surgery and at postoperative days 1, 3, 7, and 14. Operative time, complications, laboratory parameters, hemodynamic parameters, and inflammatory parameters were compared between the two procedures. The animals were monitored for two weeks and necropsy were performed for surgical outcome evaluation.

Results: The thoracic procedures were successfully performed in all of the dogs, with the exception of one animal in the transoral group. There were no serious acute or delayed complications related to surgery. There was no difference between the two surgical groups for each of the hemodynamic parameters that were evaluated. Regarding the immunological impact of the surgeries, transoral thoracoscopy was associated with significant elevations in interleukin 6 and c-reactive protein levels on postoperative days 1 and 3, respectively, when compared with the standard thoracoscopy. All dogs recovered well, without signs of mediastinitis or thoracic infection. Necropsy revealed absence of infection, no injury to vital organs, and confirmed the success of the novel procedure.

Conclusions: This study suggests that both techniques were comparable with respect to procedure success rate, hemodynamic impact, and inflammatory changes. Furthermore, there was no difference in the incidence of postoperative discomfort between groups.

Editor: Sai Yendamuri, Roswell Park Cancer Institute, United States of America

Funding: This work was supported by Chang-Gung Memorial Hospital (CMRPG-391912 for YHL, and CMRPG-28028 and CMRPG-3A0371 for CYL, Taiwan) and by the National Science Council of Taiwan (NSC 100-2314-B-182A-052 for CYL). The funders had no role in study design, data collection and analysis, decision to publish, or preparation of the manuscript.

Competing Interests: The authors have declared that no competing interests exist.

* E-mail: foreverairmail@gmail.com (Y-HL); zebraairmail@gmail.com (H-PL)

¶ These authors contributed equally to this work.

Introduction

Natural orifice transluminal endoscopic surgery (NOTES) has been used as a diagnostic and therapeutic platform to perform a wide variety of abdominal surgical procedures, including peritoneoscopy, cancer staging, appendectomy, cholecystectomy, and nephrectomy [1]–[4]. By eliminating conventional abdominal incisions, several potential advantages have been proposed, including faster recovery, shorter hospital stay, less postoperative pain, better post-surgery pulmonary function, and improved cosmetic outcome. Recent reports have also confirmed the safety and benefits of NOTES in abdominal surgery in human studies [5]–[7].

The feasibility of NOTES thoracoscopy has been demonstrated in various access methods (transvesical, transesophageal, transtracheal, and transoral) in porcine and canine models [8]–[10]. However, there have been no large, randomized, controlled trials of NOTES in thoracic surgery. We previously reported the use of a transoral technique to perform thoracoscopy, pericardial window creation, and surgical lung biopsy without complications in a survival canine model [11]–[13]. To further evaluate the potential benefits of transoral thoracoscopy, we aimed to compare the surgical outcome of minor thoracic intervention using the recently developed transoral method compared with the standard transthoracic thoracoscopy in a randomized study. The experiment focused on surgical outcomes and evaluated relevant safety issues, including operative complications, cardiopulmonary impact, and inflammatory changes. Oxidative activity of neutrophils, inducible nitric oxide synthase (iNOS) expression of monocytes, and cytokine interleukin 6 (IL-6) are good guides in the assessment of the activation of the systemic inflammation to tissue injury. The expression of these mediators as well as c-reactive protein (CRP) play a major role in the acute-phase response against surgical stress [14]–[15]. They are objective and quantitative parameters in the assessment of inflammatory system activation in response to operative trauma. Therefore, these mediators were measured to clarify the surgical stress of thoracoscopy via different approaches.

Methods

Ethics Statement

The study was conducted in accordance with the Guide for the Care and Use of Laboratory Animals as promulgated by Institutional of Laboratory Animal Resources, National Research Council, U.S.A. The protocol of the animal experiment was approved by the Institutional Animal Care and Use Committee (IACUC) of Chang Gung Memorial Hospital in Taiwan (No. 2009121003).

Dogs and surgical procedures

Twenty-eight dogs with a mean body weight of 8.5 kg (7.2–10.6 kg) were obtained from BioVet Beagle Farm, Pingtung, Taiwan. They were housed under standard lighting (12 hours light/dark cycle) and temperature conditions, and received humane care for the animal research at laboratory animal center of Chang Gung Memorial Hospital in Taouyan, Taiwan. All animals were fed with regular diet, and then fast overnight with unrestricted to water prior to surgery. The procedures were performed with the animals under general anesthesia using intramuscular injection of ketamine (5 mg/kg, Pfizer Inc, Taipei, Taiwan) and xylazine hydrochloric acid (HCL, 10 mg/kg). The animals were then placed in the supine position and intubated with a homemade endotracheal tube into a mainstem bronchus to provide single lung ventilation during surgery. The general anesthesia was maintained with 2% isoflurane. Before performing the thoracoscopy, an antibiotic (cefazolin, 20 mg/kg, Standard Chem & Pharm, Tainan, Taiwan) was administered for prevention of postoperative infection.

A 9 mm homemade metal tube was introduced through the vestibular incision and advanced down to the mandibular periosteum. The metal tube was advanced carefully from the premandibular space, through the pretracheal space, and into the submanubrial space. The mediastinal incision was carefully performed according to a previously reported procedure [11]–[13]. Briefly, the blunt tip of the metal tube was used to make a linear incision over the upper anterior mediastinal pleura by blunt dilation. Once the incision was complete, the metal tube was advanced into the thoracic cavity. The bronchoscope was then advanced through the metal tube for thoracic cavity exploration. For pericardial window creation, a needle knife (KD-10Q-1, Olympus Optical Co. Ltd., Tokyo, Japan) was introduced through the working channel of the flexible bronchoscope. The pericardium was incised anterior to the phrenic nerve with the tip of needle knife. The endoscope was then advanced through this window into the pericardial cavity using the needle knife as a guide, and was used to explore the pericardial cavity. For surgical lung biopsy, the predetermined lung region was resected with the electrocautery loop (Olympus Optical Co. Ltd., Tokyo, Japan) and endoscopic grasper through a 1.9 mm bronchoscopic working channel. The resected lung margin was reinforced with a homemade (Ethicon, Somerville, NJ, USA) endoloop ligature to prevent air leakage. The vestibular incision was then closed with a running 3-0 Vicryl suture (Ethicon, San Angelo, TX, USA) as previously described [11]–[13]. Soon after completion of wound closure, postoperative local anesthesia with xylocaine 20 mg was administrated over the incision. The animal was then recovered from anesthesia and returned to their cages. The arterial blood gases were analyzed immediately before and after surgery and on the 14th day.

Care after surgery

Regular oral feeding was restarted after the animals were recovered from anesthesia. The animals were closely monitored daily for general status, eating status, social behavior, and signs of mediastinitis, sepsis, clinical signs of postoperative discomfort (decreased food intake, weight reduction, or inappropriate social behavior), and survival for 2 weeks after experiment. The animals were euthanized with xylocaine 200 mg intravenously after sedation with the ketamine and xylazine hydrochloric acid combination described above. The necropsy was performed via medial sternotomy incision and evaluated for evidence of infection, bleeding, or signs of injury to adjacent organs.

Hemodynamic study

Immediately following intubation and then at 5 min intervals until the animal completely recovered from anesthesia, in addition to respiratory rate (breaths per minute, bpm), the values of mean arterial pressure (MAP, mmHg), heart rate (HR, beats per minute, bpm), cardiac index (CI, $L/[min \cdot m^2]$), systemic vascular resistance (SVRI, $[dyn \cdot s]/[cm^{-5} \cdot m^2]$), and global end-diastolic volume index (GEDVI, mL/m^2) were recorded by transpulmonary thermodilution technique operated by the pulse contour cardiac output (PiCCO®) system (Pulsion Medical Systems, Munich, Germany)

Leukocyte subset analysis and isolation of neutrophils and mononuclear cells

Total leukocyte count was measured preoperatively and postoperatively at day 1, day 3, day 7, and day 14. Specific mouse anti-canine CD3, CD4, CD8, CD14, or CD45 monoclonal antibodies (BD PharMingen™, BD Biosciences, Franklin Lakes, NJ, USA) were used to define the subpopulations of leukocytes ($CD4^+$ and $CD8^+$ lymphocytes, monocytes and neutrophils) by flow cytometry (Becton Dickinson, Mountain View, CA, USA).

Intracellular oxidative activity of neutrophils

The neutrophils (2×10^5 cells in 200 µL of supplemented RPMI medium) were supplemented with cell-permeable, fluorogenic 2′,7′-dichlorohydrofluorescein-diacetate (DCFH-DA, 5 µM; Sigma, St. Louis, MO, USA) for 30 min. Upon intracellular hydrolysis and subsequent oxidization, fluorescent DCFH was generated and analyzed quantitatively by flow cytometry.

iNOS expression of monocytes

After cytospin preparation of peripheral blood mononuclear cells and fixation in methanol, the slides were prepared as previously described [16]. A rabbit polyclonal antibody to canine iNOS (Abcam Biochemicals, Cambridge, UK) was used for immunological staining. Antibody labeling was visualized by an avidin-biotin complex method (LSAB 2 kit, Dako, Carpenteria and Vector Laboratories, Burlingame, CA, USA). An image analyzer was used to determine the intensity of iNOS expression of monocytes.

Enzyme-linked immunosorbent assay for IL- 6 and CRP

Serum for IL-6 and CRP analysis was stored at −80°C, and the levels of IL-6 and CRP were determined using a commercially available enzyme-linked immunosorbent assay (ELISA) kit with monoclonal antibodies specific for IL-6 (Quantikine, R & D Systems Inc., Minneapolis, Minnesota, USA) and CRP (PharMingen, BD Biosciences, San Diego, California, USA), according to the manufacturers' instructions.

Statistical analysis

Data are presented as mean and 95% confidence interval (C.I.) except otherwise mentioned. Since the data did not approximate a Gaussian distribution (for example, the mean value did not approximate the median value), nonparametric statistical analyses were used. The Mann–Whitney *U* test was performed to assess the significance of differences between 2 groups. The frequency distributions between 2 groups were tested by using a Fisher exact probability test. GraphPad Prism (version 4.0, GraphPad Software, San Diego, CA, USA) was used for all statistical analyses. Statistical significance was defined as $P<0.05$.

Results

All animals survived the follow-up period of 14 days. Thoracoscopy with surgical biopsy and pericardial window creation was successfully performed in 27 animals, with the exception of 1 animal in the transoral group. There was no different in the mean procedure time and mean weight gain between groups. None of the animals in either group had intraoperative or perioperative complications related to surgery. No postoperative complications such as infection or mediastinitis were found during the 2-week postoperative period (Table 1).

Temperature

Six animals showed rectal temperature elevation after surgery. In 2 dogs from the transoral group, the temperature rose above normal on day 1–3 and returned to normal 7 days after surgery. In the transthoracic group, 4 animals had elevated temperatures at 3–7 days after surgery, which returned to baseline at 2 weeks in 3 of the animals (Table 1).

Hemodynamic study

Comprehensive hemodynamic changes were recorded in 24 animals. We observed a significant decline in HR and a moderate variation in CI during surgery. We also observed a minor decrease in GEDI and MAP compared to baseline. However, the change in the cardiopulmonary parameters between the groups was not statistically significant, and no clinically relevant immediate or late complications were identified after surgery (Fig. 1).

White blood cells

Among the 28 animals, 25 animals showed an increased white blood cell count above baseline 1 day after surgery, which included 15 animals from the transthoracic group and 10 from the transoral group. The white blood cell (WBC) count returned to baseline in 24 of the 28 animals at 2 weeks. The WBC count of transthoracic group was significantly higher on day 1 after surgery relative to the transoral group, but there was no significant difference in WBC count between the groups thereafter (Fig. 2).

Neutrophils and oxidative activity

The number of neutrophils was elevated on postoperative day 1, 3, and 7 in both groups. This variation was significantly increased in the transthoracic group relative to the transoral group on the first postoperative day. Neutrophil activation was revealed by expression of DCFH, which increased significantly in both groups on postoperative day 1 and returned to preoperative levels at 1 week. However, DCFH expression was not significantly different between the groups (Fig. 3A and 3B).

Monocytes and the intensity of iNOS expression

During the postoperative period, the number of monocytes increased significantly in both groups following surgery, and remained elevated above the baseline until 7 days post-surgery.

Table 1. Characteristics of the Experimental Animals.

Characteristics	Total	Thoracic Surgery		P value
		Transoral	Transthoracic	
Dogs (No.)	28	14	14	
Body weight (kg, mean ± SD)	8.5±1.2	8.8±1.1	8.3±1.3	0.2229
Surgical time (min, mean ± SD)	55.8±14.4	55.4±13.1	56.3±16.1	0.9632
Successful procedure	27	13	14	
Weight gain (after 14 days, kg, mean ± SD)	0.33±0.53	0.20±0.59	0.46±0.13	0.1956
Postoperative complications (No.)				
Fever	6	2	4	0.6483
Infection or mediastinitis	0	0	0	
Pain	4	2 (1 mild, 1 severe)	2 (severe)	1.0
Necropsy after 14 days (No.)				
Infection	0	0	0	
Organ injury	0	0	0	
Correct lung biopsy	27	13	14	1.0
Good healing of pericardial window	17	8	9	1.0
Local adhesion	25	12	13	1.0

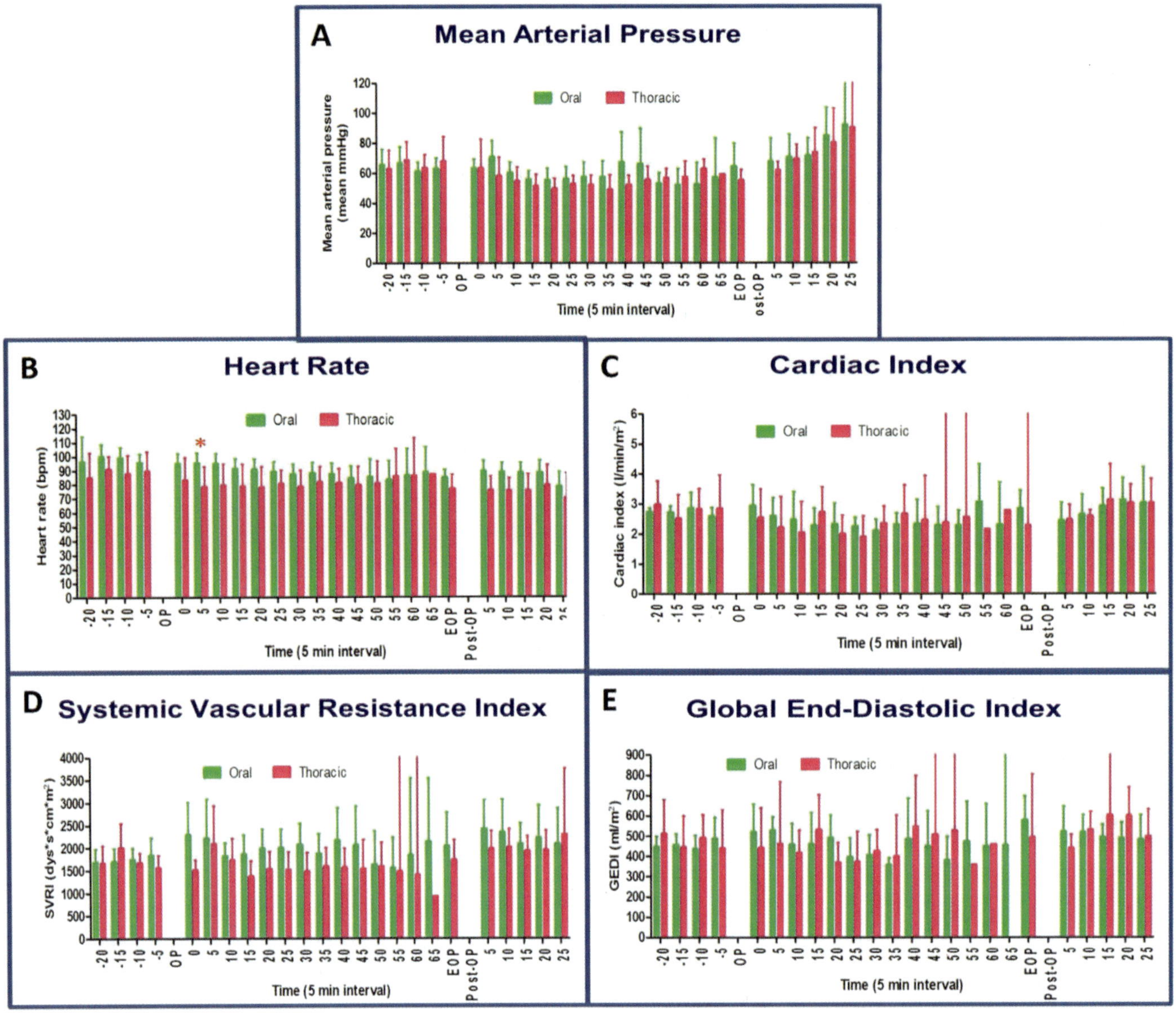

Figure 1. Hemodynamic analyses, including mean arterial pressure (A), heart rate (B), cardiac index (C), systemic vascular resistance index (D), and global end-diastolic index (E). N = 12 for the transoral approach and n = 12 for the transthoracic approach. *$P<0.05$, transoral vs. transthoracic approach for the same time interval, by Mann–Whitney *U* test.

Significantly increased iNOS levels were observed in both groups during the postoperative period; however, there were no statistically significant differences between the transoral and transthoracic groups with regard to monocyte cell counts and iNOS expression (Fig. 3C and 3D).

Lymphocytes and CD4/CD8 T lymphocyte subset analysis

There was a significant decrease in the total lymphocyte count on postoperative day 1 in both groups. Thereafter, the total lymphocyte count increased significantly above the baseline on postoperative day 3. With regard to T lymphocyte subsets, the number of $CD4^{+}$ T cells increased on postoperative days 3 and 7, the number of $CD8^{+}$ T cells did not differ significantly from preoperative levels at any of the time points throughout the study, and a significant elevation in the CD4:CD8 ratio was also noted on postoperative day 3 in both groups. However, there were no significant differences in total lymphocyte count, T lymphocyte subsets, or CD4:CD8 ratio between the groups at any of the study time points (Fig. 4).

Interleukin 6 and C-reactive protein levels

Plasma levels of CRP increased significantly 1 day after surgery in both groups. The CRP levels were significantly higher in the transoral group compared with the transthoracic group at day 3. However, there was no group difference in the plasma levels of CRP on day 7 and day 14. The serum concentration of IL-6 was increased over preoperative levels in early postoperative period in both groups. This elevation in IL-6 levels was greater in the transoral group than in the transthoracic group at day 1 after surgery. However, no differences were observed between the groups 3 days after surgery (Fig. 5).

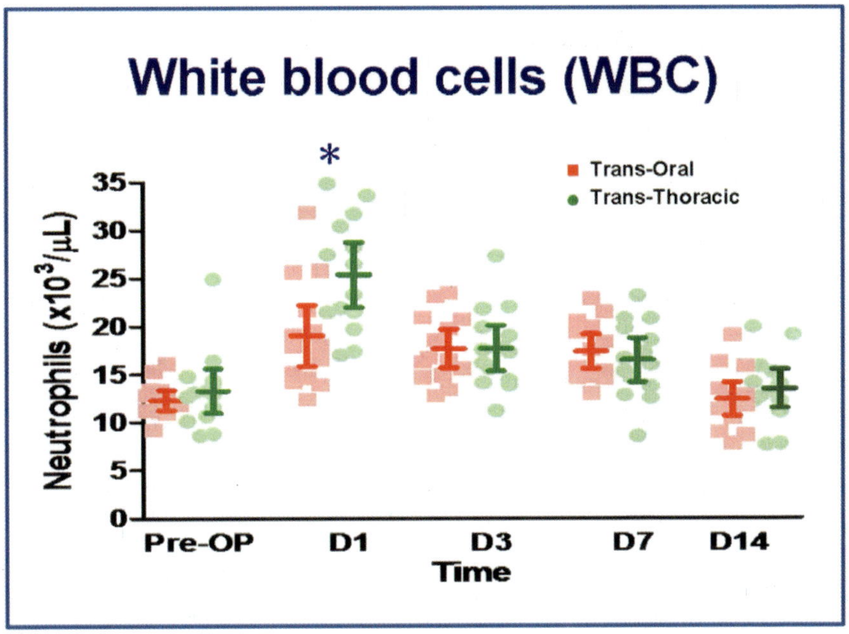

Figure 2. White blood cell counts. N = 14 for the transoral approach and n = 14 for the transthoracic approach. *P<0.05, transoral vs. transthoracic approach for the same time point, by Mann–Whitney *U* test.

Arterial blood gas

There was no significant change in PaO2 values before and after the procedure. The pH value was decreased and PaCO2 level was elevated immediately after the procedure. Both values returned to the pre-operative levels before day 14 post-operatively. There was no difference in the values of pH, PaO2, and PaCO2 between the two approaches at the same time point (Fig. 6).

Postoperative pain

In the study animals, postoperative discomfort manifested as decreased food intake, weight reduction, or inappropriate social behavior after surgery; 4 of 28 dogs presented with moderate to severe postoperative wound pain. There was no significant difference in the severity of pain between the groups (1 animal with mild pain and 1 animal with severe pain in the transoral group vs. 2 animals with severe pain in the transthoracic group; Table 1).

Necropsy

At the time of necropsy, there were no signs of infection or evidence of organ injury in either the thoracic cavity or the mediastinum. The lung biopsy was correctly performed in 27 out of the 28 animals (n = 13 in the transoral group, n = 14 in the transthoracic group, P = 1.0). The pericardial window had obliterated and the surgical wounds were difficult to identify in 17 out of the 28 animals (n = 8 in the transoral group, n = 9 in the transthoracic group, P = 1.0). Twenty-five animals revealed adhesions either on the pleural or mediastinum at the surgical lung biopsy region (n = 12 in the transoral group, n = 13 in the transthoracic group, P = 1.0; Table 1).

Discussion

We recently published a study demonstrating the successful performance of a minor thoracic procedure via a transoral approach in a canine model [11]–[13]. In line with these findings, our present study further demonstrated the safety and efficacy of the transoral approach in hemodynamic, inflammatory conditions. These findings are clinically relevant, as our study included thoracic exploration, surgical lung biopsy, and pericardial window creation in a survival canine model, and each of these procedures is commonly performed in daily practice.

Since Kallo et al. reported the first transgastric peritoneoscopy in 2004, NOTES has been increasingly used in the diagnosis and therapy of both benign and malignant disease of the abdomen [17] Natural orifice surgery (NOS) has potential advantages over conventional laparoscopic surgery; however, the development of NOTES in thoracic surgery was delayed. The critical problem that hindered the implementation of NOTES in thoracic disease was the lack of a reliable platform for approaching the thoracic cavity via a natural orifice. Furthermore, potential complications during the procedure, including incision leakage, mediastinal organ injury, and infection were important concerns.

Several studies have investigated the feasibility of using the natural orifice as a novel platform for thoracic intervention and emphasized that an optimal approach was key to successful natural orifice thoracic surgery. Lima et al. reported their experience with 6 pigs that underwent transvesical lung biopsy. Their overall success rate was 100%. The authors found that a major disadvantage of this intervention is difficulty in performing the procedure over the upper mediastinum and pleural region [8]. Palma et al. reported another study of 4 pigs that underwent transgastric lung biopsy. Their success rate was 100%; however, results from a few of the experimental animals failed to effectively assure the safety of a transgastric approach [18]. Sumiyama and colleagues performed transesophageal thoracoscopy in 9 pigs and demonstrated an increased risk of tension pneumothorax and massive bleeding [19]. Our group previously described the utilization of transtracheal thoracoscopy in 12 dogs; we encountered 3 cases of tension pneumothorax due to inadvertent injury to the lung during creation of a tracheal access site [20]. Recently, we have made significant progress in using a transoral route for

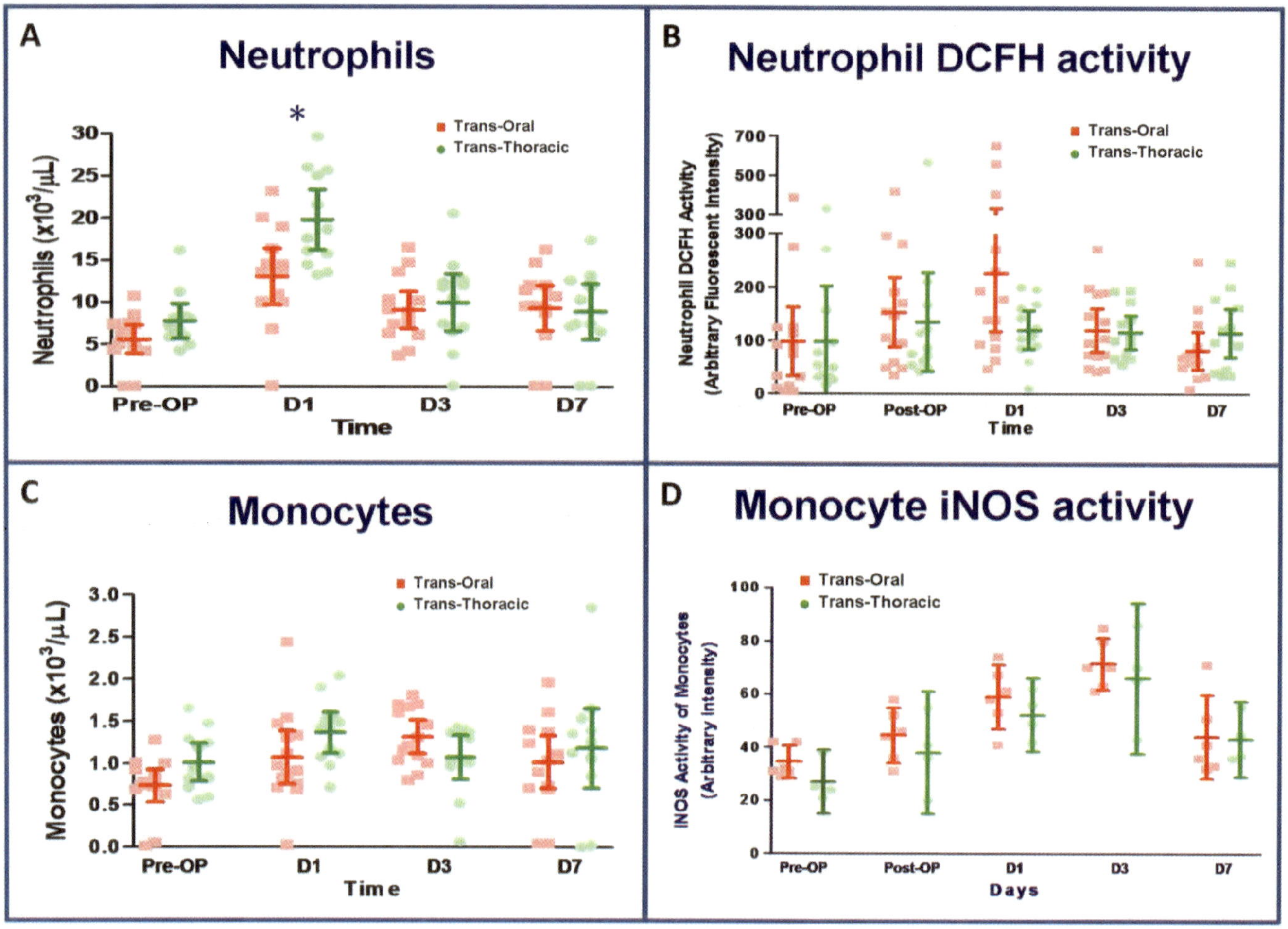

Figure 3. Neutrophil cell counts (A) and dichlorodihydrofluorescein (DCFH) activity (B) as well as monocyte cell counts (C) and iNOS activity (D). N = 14 for the transoral approach and n = 14 for the transthoracic approach. *$P<0.05$, transoral vs. transthoracic approach for the same time point, by Mann–Whitney *U* test.

surgical lung biopsy and pericardial window creation, without major intraoperative or postoperative complications [10]–[13]. Our findings suggest that a transoral approach can be used as a novel platform for studies of NOTES for intrathoracic surgery. However, its clinical application has yet to be implemented, as there is uncertainty regarding the impact of hemodynamic and inflammatory status during the procedure.

In 2011, our research group showed that identification of the anterior medial aspect of the thoracic cavity is possible with the transoral approach, and creation of a pericardial window and surgical lung biopsy is technically feasible in a canine model [11]–[13]. In this comparative study, 93% of the target lung regions were successfully accessed by the present approach. We expect that the present transoral method will play a central role in the development of NOTES in intrathoracic surgery. The safety of novel surgical procedures is one of the most critical barriers to gaining acceptance in clinical practice. Our previous study demonstrated that 90% to 95% of surgical lung biopsies could be completed by using the transoral route without major complications. The present study also demonstrates that using the transoral route for thoracic intervention is safe and practical in a canine model. This method did not cause infection or injury to the vital organs in all 14 animals, suggesting that the use of transoral thoracoscopy is a potential alternative to the current transthoracic endoscopic method, especially in young adults that are concerned about postoperative cosmesis.

Many recent reports in the literature regarding the hemodynamic impact of NOTES during surgery have been studied in a porcine model. In 2011, Suzuki et al. evaluated the cardiopulmonary effect of transvaginal NOTES cholecystectomy in 10 pigs [21]. This study demonstrated that there was similar cardiopulmonary stability in both the transvaginal NOTES and the laparoscopic cholecystectomy groups. With regard to cardiopulmonary safety of NOTES in intrathoracic surgery, Von Delius et al. studied hemodynamic impact in 8 pigs that underwent transesophageal mediastinostomy [22]. They observed hemodynamic instability in 3 animals, due to an injury in the parietal pleura, which resulted in tension pneumothorax and mortality in 1 pig. These results highlight the importance of using a safe and effective surgical platform and monitoring the hemodynamic status during NOTES. Our current study revealed a similar impact of hemodynamic status in the transoral and standard transthoracic approaches in a comparative animal study, which suggests that transoral access to the thoracic cavity is a safe platform compared with the standard transthoracic approach.

When the clinical application of the novel platform is considered, the invasiveness of the procedure is another major concern that must be addressed. Several researchers have

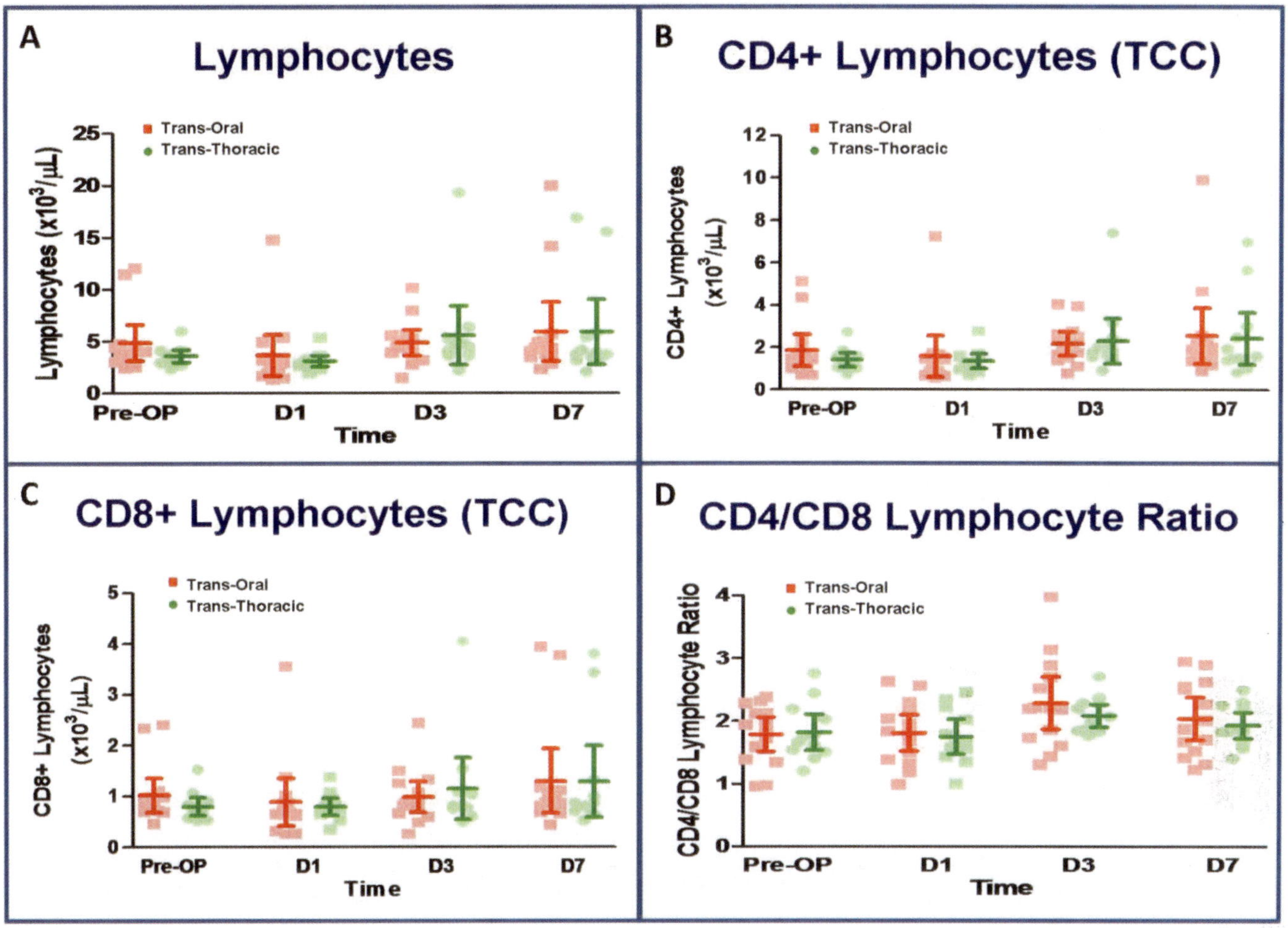

Figure 4. Lymphocyte cell counts (A), the CD4 (B) and CD8 (B) subsets, and CD4/CD8 lymphocyte ratio (D). N = 14 for the transoral approach and n = 12 for the transthoracic approach. *$P < 0.05$, transoral vs. transthoracic approach for the same time point, by Mann–Whitney *U* test.

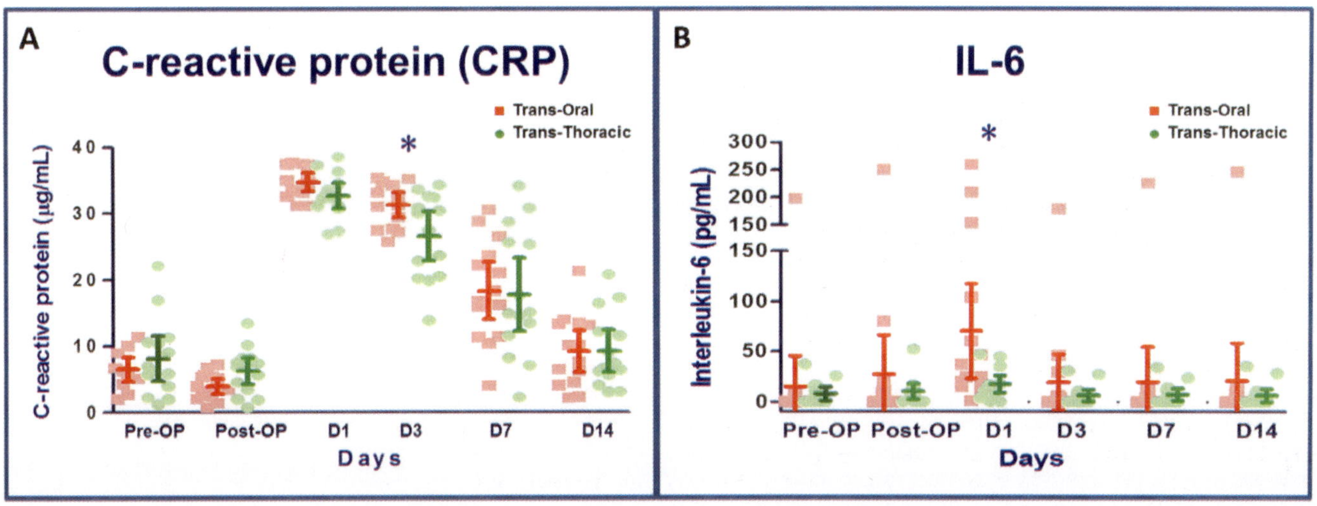

Figure 5. Serum levels of c-reactive protein (A) and interleukin 6 (B). N = 14 for the transoral approach and n = 14 for the transthoracic approach. *$P < 0.05$, transoral vs. transthoracic approach for the same time point, by Mann–Whitney *U* test.

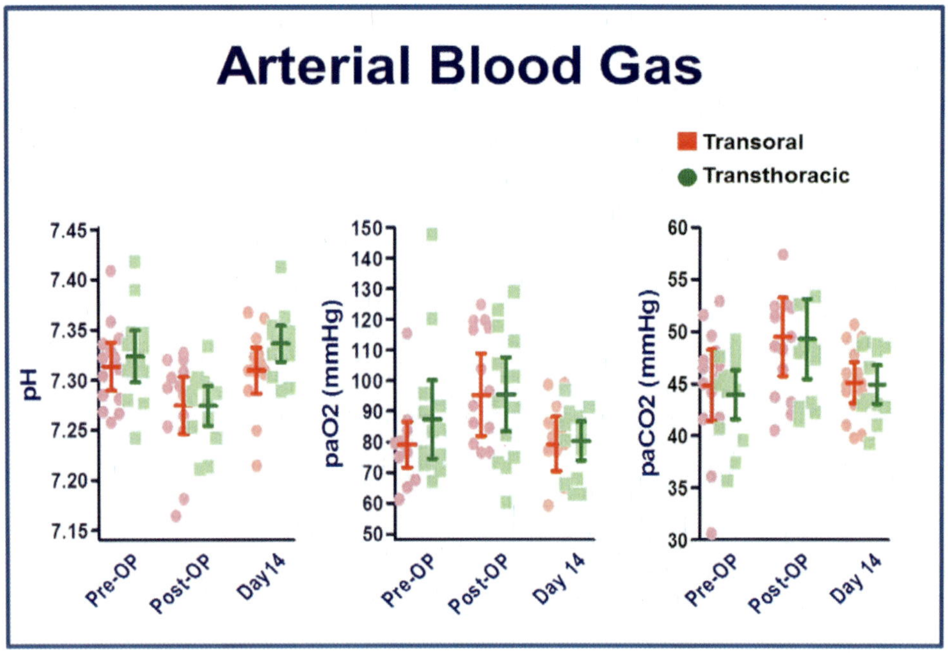

Figure 6. Arterial blood gas analysis. N = 14 for the transoral approach and n = 14 for the transthoracic approach. *$P<0.05$, transoral vs. transthoracic approach for the same time point, by Mann–Whitney *U* test.

evaluated inflammatory and immunologic responses in both animal and human studies following endoscopic and open surgery, and suggest that endoscopic surgery is associated with less surgical stress than the open surgical approach [14]–[15]. In the current study, the transthoracic group showed higher IL-6 and CRP levels than the transoral group. However, only 1 of 6 IL-6 and CRP measurements was found to be significantly different. Furthermore, there were no clinically apparent complications in both groups. Regarding the cellular responses to the surgical procedure, we found a similar change in iNOS, DCFH, and CD4/CD8 indicators in the transoral group compared with those that underwent conventional thoracoscopy. Based on these results, our study suggests that transoral thoracoscopy results in similar surgical stress as the current transthoracic approach. Additionally, the arterial blood gas analysis revealed no difference between groups, suggesting that transoral thoracoscopy did not increase pulmonary dysfunction, compared to the transthoracic approach.

The present transoral method offers several potential advantages over the transthoracic technique that is currently in use. First, the technique demonstrated good cosmetic outcomes, as the surgery was completed without any external thoracic incision. Second, the transoral group experienced similar acute postoperative pain compared with the animals undergoing transthoracic surgery. However, many studies reported that thoracic incisions may result in post-thoracotomy discomfort and intercostal neuralgia, which can be avoided by using the transoral approach.

The present study has some limitations. First, our transoral approach for thoracic cavity techniques in a canine model may face difficulty in clinical practice, particularly in obese patients with a thick or short neck. Second, a relatively small sample size was obtained for the cellular immunity study, which may contribute to the non-significant difference observed in the cellular immune reactions between the groups. Third, we were unable to measure the complete cardiopulmonary data that were influenced by arterial line dysfunction. Fourth, since the IL-6 and CRP assays were performed 1 day after surgery in our study, we could not explore the change in inflammatory cytokine secretion immediately after surgery. Finally, we only performed the surgical lung biopsy over the anterior aspect of thorax. Thus, we cannot determine whether approaching the posterior thorax under the decubital position would be successful. Nevertheless, we designed the present experiment to be as relevant to surgical practice as possible, and in clinical daily practice surgical lung biopsy is one of the most commonly performed endoscopic procedures in thoracic surgery.

In summary, this study revealed that utilizing a transoral approach for thoracic cavity procedures was feasible, efficacious, and safe in a canine survival study. We also found that the immunologic, inflammatory, and hemodynamic responses to the transoral approach were similar to those of the conventional thoracoscopic approach, with the exception of minimal differences in inflammatory reactions. We conclude that clinical trials are needed to further clarify the clinical role of NOTES in thoracic disease.

Author Contributions

Conceived and designed the experiments: YC CYL YCW YHL HPL. Performed the experiments: YC HCY CYW MJH TPC PJK YHL. Analyzed the data: CYL MJH YKC. Contributed reagents/materials/analysis tools: CYL MJH YKC. Wrote the paper: YC CYL YHL. Supervision and coordination of project: YC YHL HPL.

References

1. Hazey JW, Narula VK, Renton DB, Renton DB, Reavis KM, et al. (2008) Natural orifice transgastric endoscopic peritoneoscopy in humans: initial clinical trial. Surg Endosc 22: 16–20.

2. Dallemagne B, Perretta S, Allemann P, Asakuma M, Marescaux J (2009) Transgastric hybrid cholecystectomy. Br J Surg 96: 1162–1166.

3. Palanivelu C, Rajan PS, Rangarajan M, Parthasarathi R, Senthilnathan P, et al. (2008) Transvaginal endoscopic appendectomy in humans: a unique approach to NOTES - world's first report. Surg Endosc 22: 1343–1347.
4. Alcaraz A, Musquera M, Peri L, Izquierdo L, García-Cruz E, et al. (2011) Feasibility of transvaginal natural orifice transluminal endoscopic surgery-assisted living donor nephrectomy: is kidney vaginal delivery the approach of the future? Eur Urol 59: 1019–1025.
5. Chukwumah C, Zorron R, Marks JM, Ponsky JL (2010) Current status of natural orifice translumenal endoscopic surgery (NOTES). Curr Probl Surg 47: 630–668.
6. Lehmann KS, Ritz JP, Wibmer A, Gellert K, Zornig C, et al. (2010) The German registry for natural orifice translumenal endoscopic surgery: report of the first 551 patients. Ann Surg 252: 263–270.
7. Coomber RS, Sodergren MH, Clark J, Teare J, Yang GZ, et al. (2012) Natural orifice translumenal endoscopic surgery applications in clinical practice. World J Gastrointest Endosc 16: 65–74.
8. Lima E, Henriques-Coelho T, Rolanda C, Pêgo JM, Silva D, et al. (2007) Transvesical thoracoscopy: a natural orifice translumenal endoscopic approach for thoracic surgery. Surg Endosc 21: 854–858.
9. Fritscher-Ravens A, Cuming T, Eisenberger CF, Ghadimi M, Nilges A, et al. (2010) Randomized comparative long-term survival study of endoscopic and thoracoscopic esophageal wall repair after NOTES mediastinoscopy in healthy and compromised animals. Endoscopy 42: 468–474.
10. Liu YH, Chu Y, Liu CY, Liu HP, Wu YC, et al. (2011) Feasibility of the transtracheal approach for the thoracic cavity in a large animal model. Surg Endosc 25: 1652–1658.
11. Liu YH, Chu Y, Wu YC, Chen TP, Lu MS, et al. (2012) Feasibility of endoscopic transoral surgical lung biopsy in a live canine model. Surg Innov 19: 162–170.
12. Ko PJ, Chu Y, Wu YC, Liu CY, Hsieh MJ, et al. (2012) Feasibility of endoscopic transoral thoracic surgical lung biopsy and pericardial window creation. J Surg Res 175: 207–214.
13. Liu YH, Chu Y, Wu YC, Yeh CJ, Liu CY, et al. (2011) Single-dose antimicrobial prophylaxis in transoral surgical lung biopsy: a preliminary experience. Surg Endosc 25: 3912–3917.
14. Wichmann MW, Hüttl TP, Winter H, Spelsberg F, Angele MK, et al. (2005) Immunological effects of laparoscopic vs open colorectal surgery. Arch Surg 140: 692–697.
15. Romeo C, Cruccetti A, Turiaco A, Impellizzeri P, Turiaco N, et al. (2002) Monocytes and neutrophils activity after minor surgical stress. J Pediatr Surg 37: 741–744.
16. Liu CY, Wang CH, Chen TC, Lin HC, Yu CT, et al. (1998) Increased level of exhaled nitric oxide and upregulation of nitric oxide synthase in alveolar macrophages in patients with primary lung cancer. Br J Cancer 78: 534–541.
17. Kalloo AN, Singh VK, Jagannath SB, Niiyama H, Hill SL, et al. (2004) Flexible transgastric peritoneoscopy: a novel approach to diagnostic and therapeutic interventions in the peritoneal cavity. Gastrointest Endosc 60: 114–117.
18. De Palma GD, Siciliano S, Addeo P, Salvatori F, Persico M, et al. (2010) A NOTES approach for thoracic surgery: transgastric thoracoscopy via a diaphragmatic incision in a survival porcine model. Minerva Chir 65: 11–15.
19. Sumiyama K, Gostout CJ, Rajan E, Bakken TA, Knipschield MA (2007) Transesophageal mediastinoscopy by submucosal endoscopy with mucosal flap safety valve technique. Gastrointest Endos 65: 679–683.
20. Sumiyama K, Gostout CJ, Rajan E, Bakken TA, Knipschield MA, et al. (2008) Pilot study of transesophageal endoscopic epicardial coagulation by submucosal endoscopy with the mucosal flap safety valve technique (with videos). Gastrointest Endosc 67: 497–501.
21. Suzuki K, Yasuda K, Kawaguchi K, Yoshizumi F, Inomata M, et al. (2010) Cardiopulmonary and immunologic effects of transvaginal natural-orifice transluminal endoscopic surgery cholecystectomy compared with laparoscopic cholecystectomy in a porcine survival model. Gastrointest Endosc 72: 1241–1248.
22. von Delius S, Wilhelm D, Feussner H, Sager J, Becker V, et al. (2010) Natural orifice transluminal endoscopic surgery: cardiopulmonary safety of transesophageal mediastinoscopy. Endoscopy 42: 405–412.

20

Comparisons of Prediction Models of Quality of Life after Laparoscopic Cholecystectomy: A Longitudinal Prospective Study

Hon-Yi Shi[1], Hao-Hsien Lee[2], Jinn-Tsong Tsai[3], Wen-Hsien Ho[1], Chieh-Fan Chen[4,5], King-Teh Lee[1,6], Chong-Chi Chiu[2,7,8,9]*

1 Department of Healthcare Administration and Medical Informatics, Kaohsiung Medical University, Kaohsiung, Taiwan, **2** Department of Surgery, Chi Mei Medical Center, Liouying, Taiwan, **3** Department of Computer Science, National Pingtung University of Education, Pingtung, Taiwan, **4** Emergency Department, Kaohsiung Municipal United Hospital, Kaohsiung, Taiwan, **5** Department of Health Business Administration, Meiho University, Pigntung, Taiwan, **6** Division of Hepatobiliary Surgery, Department of Surgery, Kaohsiung Medical University Hospital, Kaohsiung, Taiwan, **7** Department of General Surgery, Chi Mei Medical Center, Tainan, Taiwan, **8** Taipei Medical University, Taipei, Taiwan, **9** Chia Nan University of Pharmacy and Science, Tainan, Taiwan

Abstract

Background: Few studies of laparoscopic cholecystectomy (LC) outcome have used longitudinal data for more than two years. Moreover, no studies have considered group differences in factors other than outcome such as age and nonsurgical treatment. Additionally, almost all published articles agree that the essential issue of the internal validity (reproducibility) of the artificial neural network (ANN), support vector machine (SVM), Gaussian process regression (GPR) and multiple linear regression (MLR) models has not been adequately addressed. This study proposed to validate the use of these models for predicting quality of life (QOL) after LC and to compare the predictive capability of ANNs with that of SVM, GPR and MLR.

Methodology/Principal Findings: A total of 400 LC patients completed the SF-36 and the Gastrointestinal Quality of Life Index at baseline and at 2 years postoperatively. The criteria for evaluating the accuracy of the system models were mean square error (MSE) and mean absolute percentage error (MAPE). A global sensitivity analysis was also performed to assess the relative significance of input parameters in the system model and to rank the variables in order of importance. Compared to SVM, GPR and MLR models, the ANN model generally had smaller MSE and MAPE values in the training data set and test data set. Most ANN models had MAPE values ranging from 4.20% to 8.60%, and most had high prediction accuracy. The global sensitivity analysis also showed that preoperative functional status was the best parameter for predicting QOL after LC.

Conclusions/Significance: Compared with SVM, GPR and MLR models, the ANN model in this study was more accurate in predicting patient-reported QOL and had higher overall performance indices. Further studies of this model may consider the effect of a more detailed database that includes complications and clinical examination findings as well as more detailed outcome data.

Editor: Frank Emmert-Streib, Queen's University Belfast, United Kingdom

Funding: This work was in part supported by the National Science Council, Taiwan, Republic of China, under grant numbers NSC99-2314-B-037-069-MY3. The funders had no role in study design, data collection and analysis, decision to publish, or preparation of the manuscript. No additional external funding received for this study.

Competing Interests: The authors have declared that no competing interests exist.

* E-mail: chiuchongchi@yahoo.com.tw

These authors contributed equally to this work.

Introduction

Laparoscopic cholecystectomy (LC) is among the most common operations performed by general surgeons. Accurately predicting quality of life (QOL), a standard outcome measure after LC, is important when selecting treatment modality and when allocating scarce medical resources [1–3].

Regression analysis, one of the most widely used multivariate analysis methods, assumes linear relationships between independent and dependent variables. However, studies show that changes in biomedical variables are often non-linear [4–11]. The major classifier methods use support vector machines (SVMs) to solve classification problems by constructing hyperplanes in a multidimensional space that separates cases of different class labels. However, SVMs have also proven effective for solving regression problems because they can handle multiple continuous variables [4–6]. Gaussian process regression (GPR) is a kernel-based nonlinear regression technique for using either a kernel or a covariance function for implicitly transforming the data into a high-dimensional reproduction of kernel Hilbert space. The method has proven effective for solving various regression problems [7,8]. Artificial neural networks (ANNs) are complex and flexible nonlinear systems with properties not found in other modeling systems. These properties include robust performance in dealing with noisy or incomplete input patterns, high fault tolerance, and the capability to generalize from the input data [9–11]. The computational power of an ANN is derived from the distributed nature of its connections. The ANN model is a well established data mining algorithm that is widely used in various fields, from engineering to biomedical science [9–11].

Although many outcome-predicting models have been developed using conventional statistical procedures, their application at the individual level is hampered by the high interdependence of the clinical variables involved, which potentially may interact with each other and have reciprocal enhancing effects [12,13]. Three major limitations of this algorithm are (1) the inability to capture interactions of the disease, (2) the inability to capture the process dynamics, and (3) the very large confidence interval in individual risk assessment. Hence, conventional statistical approaches have intrinsic limitations in handling this complex nonlinear information [14–16].

Gholipour et al compared ANNs with linear discrimination analysis in terms of their accuracy in predicting conversion of LC to open surgery [14]. They concluded that ANNs that consider the preoperative health characteristics of patients have superior prediction performance compared to discriminant analysis models. Another retrospective analysis of the prevalence of gallbladder disease and its risk factors by Liew et al compared logistic regression and ANN in terms of their accuracy in predicting conversion of LC to open surgery in obese patients [15]. Again, ANN models significantly outperformed the LR models in predicting the risk factors and prevalence of gallbladder disease and gallstone development in obese patients on the basis of multiple variables related to laboratory and pathological features. In Eldar et al, a comparison of logistic regression, linear discriminant analysis and ANN models in predicting conversion of LC to open surgery again showed that ANN-based models are relatively more effective and practical for predicting successful LCs and their conversion [16].

$$^{\#} = |[(B - A)/A]| \times 100\%.$$

Despite their contribution to the growing understanding of LC surgery outcomes, previous studies of LC outcome have had major shortcomings [12,17,18]. Few studies of LC outcome have used longitudinal data for more than two years. Moreover, no studies have considered group differences in factors other than outcome such as age and nonsurgical treatment. Additionally, almost all published articles agree that the essential issue of the internal validity (reproducibility) of ANN, SVM, GPR and multiple linear regression (MLR) models has not been adequately addressed. Therefore, the primary aim of this study was to validate the use of ANN models in predicting patient-reported QOL after LC surgery, and the secondary aim was to compare the predictive capability of ANNs with that of SVM, GPR and MLR models.

Table 1. Demographic and clinical characteristics of analyzed subjects (N = 400).*

Variables		N (%)
Age, years		55.9±14.6
Body mass index, kg/m^2		24.8±3.8
Duration of symptoms, months		11.8±27.9
Charlson co-morbidity index score		0.9±1.1
Gender	Male	171 (42.7%)
	Female	229 (57.3%)
Education	No formal education/ Primary school	138 (34.5%)
	Junior high school	57 (14.3%)
	Senior high school	121 (30.2%)
	College	84 (21.0%)
Marital status	Single	37 (9.3%)
	Married	363 (90.7%)
Previous abdominal surgery	Yes	129 (32.3%)
	No	271 (67.7%)
Surgical factors	Symptomatic gallstones	252 (63.0%)
	Acute cholecystitis with gallstones	148 (37.0%)
Patient referral source	Outpatient department	303 (75.8%)
	Emergency department	97 (24.2%)
Current drinker	Yes	49 (12.3%)
	No	351 (87.7%)
Current smoker	Yes	68 (17.0%)
	No	332 (83.0%)
Length of stay, days		2.7±2.6
Re-hospitalization within 30 days	Yes	12 (3.0%)
	No	388 (97.0%)
Current complications	Yes	27 (6.7%)
	No	373 (93.3%)
Operation time, minutes		85.8±44.1
American Society of Anesthesiologists score		2.1±0.4
Preoperative physical component summary score		48.6±9.3
Preoperative mental component summary score		36.2±20.8
Preoperative total gastrointestinal quality of life index score		102.8±22.5

*Values are means ± standard deviations.

Materials and Methods

Ethics statement

All patients who had undergone LC performed between May, 2007 and June, 2009 by any surgeons practicing at two tertiary academic hospitals in southern Taiwan were surveyed by the SF-36 and the Gastrointestinal Quality of Life (GIQLI) instruments. Ethical approval was provided by Institutional Review Board of the Kaohsiung Medical University Hospital (KMUH-IRB-960169).

Study population

Patients provided written informed consent. Patients with cognitive impairment (n = 1), severe organ disease (n = 4) or

Table 2. Coefficients of significant variables for total gastrointestinal quality of life index (GIQLI) score, physical component summary (PCS) score and mental component summary (MCS) score in linear regression model after surgery.

	Total GIQLI score		PCS score		MCS score	
Variables	**Coefficients**	**P value**	**Coefficients**	**P value**	**Coefficients**	**P value**
Age	−0.028	<0.001	−0.018	0.005	−0.027	0.004
Charlson co-morbidity index	−0.714	<0.001	−0.174	<0.001	−0.283	<0.001
Gender (female vs. male)	0.748	0.004	0.694	0.002	0.249	<0.001
Previous abdominal surgery (no vs. yes)	3.766	0.008	1.764	<0.001	0.188	0.002
Current complications (yes vs. no)	5.559	<0.001	1.601	<0.001	−2.020	<0.001
Operation time	−0.031	0.007	−0.014	0.008	−0.004	0.018
Pre-operative functional status	0.084	<0.001	0.034	<0.001	0.069	<0.001

psychiatric disease (n = 1) were excluded. Of the 518 eligible subjects who gave written consent and were enrolled in the study at baseline, twelve were excluded due to conversion of LC to open cholecystectomy (OC), and 106 were excluded because they did not undergo postoperative assessments. All 400 of the remaining LC subjects completed the preoperative and 2-year postoperative assessments.

Instruments and measurements

The SF-36 (Chinese version) was administered to measure QOL outcomes, and the score was used as a dependent variable. As described in the literature, the physical component summary scale (PCS) and mental component summary scale (MCS) were calculated using norm-based scoring methods to compare QOL in the study population with that of the general Taiwan population [19]. A PCS or MCS value of 50 was considered average for the general Taiwan population. Both PCS and MCS have been widely adopted and were used in the present study to provide an overall QOL index and for further study of longitudinal changes in generic measures as a whole [20].

The GIQLI is recognized as a valid and reliable instrument for measuring functional status, especially in patients undergoing cholecystectomy [13]. Each of its thirty-six items is scored from 0 to 4 with a higher score indicating better health status, and the total GIQLI score ranges from 0 to 144. A Chinese version of the GIQLI has demonstrated validity [2,13].

The following patient data obtained by records review and questionnaire interview were tested as independent variables in this study: age, gender, body mass index (BMI), education, Charlson co-morbidity index (CCI) score, marital status, previous abdominal surgery, surgical factors, patient referral source, current alcohol or tobacco use, preoperative functional status, operating time, American Society of Anesthesiologist (ASA) score, current complications, operation time, length of stay (LOS) and re-hospitalization within 30 days.

System model development

The factors used in the MLR model to predict long-term QOL of LC patients included both demographic and clinical characteristics. The MLR model can be formulated as the following linear equation:

$$\hat{Y} = \beta_0 + \beta_i X_i + \varepsilon_i,\ i = 1, 2, \ldots, m.$$

where $\hat{Y}$ is the actual output value, β_0 is the intercept, β_i is the model coefficient parameter, X_i is the independent or input variable, ε_i is the random error, and m is the number of variables.

The SVM model employs non-linear mapping to transform the original training data into higher-dimensional data and searches for the linear optima that define a hyperplane within the new dimension [4]. With appropriate non-linear mapping to a sufficiently high dimension, a decision boundary can separate data into two classes [4]. In the SVM model, this decision boundary is defined by support vectors and margins.

The GPR applies a Bayesian approach to nonlinear regression. The Bayesian paradigm provides probabilistic modeling of nonlinear regression. The Bayesian approach to regression

Table 3. The mean and standard deviation (SD) of total gastrointestinal quality of life index (GIQLI) score, physical component summary (PCS) score and mental component summary (MCS) score after surgery in forty runs of the data with an 80%–20% random split.

	Training set (320 cases)	Testing set (80 cases)	
Subscales	**Mean ± SD**	**Mean ± SD**	**P value**
Total GIQLI score	122.7±4.9	119.9±4.7	0.171
PCS score	50.5±4.8	50.3±4.9	0.660
MCS score	53.2±6.0	55.0±6.6	0.069

Table 4. Three-layer networks and number of support vectors for total gastrointestinal quality of life index (GIQLI) score, physical component summary (PCS) score and mental component summary (MCS) score in artificial neural network (ANN) and support vector machine (SVM) models.

Subscales	ANN-based model*	SVM-based model#
Total GIQLI score	7-4-1	134
PCS score	7-5-1	88
MCS score	7-4-1	140

*Values are for input layer-hidden layer-output layer.
#Values are numbers of support vectors.

specifies a priori probabilities of the parameters to be estimated, and it computes the maximum a posteriori probabilities given the observed data samples. Unlike non-Bayesian schemes, which typically choose a single parameter based on a specified criterion, the Bayesian probabilistic model obtains both the optimal estimated function and the covariance associated with the estimation. Therefore, the Bayesian paradigm provides more information about the estimated parameters compared to non-Bayesian methodology. The GPR is a memory-based method of storing some or all of the training data for use in testing. Therefore, GPR can be quickly trained, which improves the efficiency of the massive-training methodology [7].

The ANN model used in this study was a standard feed-forward, back-propagation neural network with three layers: an input layer, a hidden layer and an output layer. The multilayer perceptron (MLP) network is an emerging tool for designing special classes of layered feed-forward networks [21]. Its input layer consists of source nodes, and its output layer consists of neurons; these layers connect the network to the outside world. In addition to these two layers, the MLP usually has one or more layers of neurons referred to as hidden neurons because they are not directly accessible. The hidden neurons extract important features contained in the input data.

Statistical analysis

The dataset was divided randomly into two sets, one set of 320 cases (80% of the overall dataset) for training the model and another set of eighty cases for testing the model. The model was built using the training set. Demographic and clinical characteristics were the independent variables, and the outcome (QOL) was the dependent variable. The SVM, GPR, MLR and ANN models were then tested using the eighty cases in the testing dataset.

The model fit and prediction accuracy of the system models were measured in terms of mean square error (MSE) and mean absolute percentage error (MAPE), respectively. The MSE, which is computed between the desired and predicted values and then averaged across all data, is used as an indicator of goodness of fit. The MAPE indicates the average deviation from the desired value and is usually expressed as a percentage [22]. The prediction accuracy of a model is considered excellent if its MAPE value is lower than 10%. Values between 10% and 20%, between 20% and 50%, and higher than 50% are considered indicators of high, average, and low prediction accuracy, respectively [22]. The formulas for calculating MSE and MAPE are

Table 5. Comparison of multiple linear regression (MLR), support vector machine (SVM), Gaussian process regression (GPR) and artificial neural network (ANN) models in predicting total gastrointestinal quality of life index (GIQLI) score, physical component summary (PCS) score and mental component summary (MCS) score.

Indices	Models	Training set (A)	Testing set (B)	Change rate#
Total GIQLI score				
MSE	MLR	82.14	74.73	9.0%
	SVM	76.50	74.52	2.6%
	GPR	1.3×10^{-23}	1038	7.9×10^{27}%
	ANN	65.55	54.42	16.9%
MAPE	MLR	4.7%	6.1%	-
	SVM	5.3%	5.3%	-
	GPR	1.5×10^{-12}%	20.2%	
	ANN	4.2%	4.7%	-
PCS score				
MSE	MLR	19.91	17.48	12.2%
	SVM	23.39	22.68	3.1%
	GPR	14.94	46.66	212.3%
	ANN	18.62	15.65	15.9%
MAPE	MLR	6.3%	6.0%	-
	SVM	6.8%	6.2%	-
	GPR	4.4%	10.7%	
	ANN	5.8%	5.1%	-
MCS score				
MSE	LR	86.68	80.82	6.7%
	SVM	62.60	60.01	4.1%
	GPR	30.42	87.82	188.7%
	ANN	66.31	58.61	11.6%
MAPE	LR	13.9%	10.9%	-
	SVM	9.7%	10.0%	-
	GPR	8.3%	15.8%	
	ANN	8.6%	6.4%	-

MSE = mean square error, MAPE = mean absolute percentage error.

$$\mathrm{MSE} = \frac{1}{n}\sum_{i=1}^{n}(Y_i - \hat{Y}_i)^2,$$

and

$$\mathrm{MAPE} = \frac{1}{n}\sum_{i=1}^{n}\frac{|Y_i - \hat{Y}_i|}{Y_i}\times 100\%,$$

where n is the number of observations, Y_i is the desired (target) value of the ith observation, and $\hat{Y}_i$ is the actual output value of the ith observation.

The change rates are also given. The optimal number of neurons in the hidden layer and the activation functions are iteratively determined by comparing the MSE index of the output error among several neural networks. The network training process continues as long as training and test errors decrease. That

Table 6. Global sensitivity analysis of artificial neural network (ANN) model in predicting total gastrointestinal quality of life index (GIQLI) score, physical component summary (PCS) score and mental component summary (MCS) score.*

	Rank 1st	Rank 2nd	Rank 3rd
ANN model	**Variable sensitivity ratios**	**Variable sensitivity ratios**	**Variable sensitivity ratios**
Total GIQLI score	X_7	X_2	X_4
	1.38	1.24	1.14
PCS score	X_7	X_4	X_3
	1.15	1.06	1.02
MCS score	X_7	X_5	X_4
	1.07	1.02	1.02

*Age (X_1), Charlson co-morbidity index score (X_2), gender (X_3), previous abdominal surgery (X_4), current complications (X_5), operation time (X_6), preoperative functional status (X_7).

is, training stops when the training error rate and test error rate no longer change or when they begin increasing. The prediction accuracy of the model is then judged by computing the MAPE value. The change rate is also used to compare model performance between the training and test sets. This criterion is used to calculate the difference in MSE index between the test and the training sets so that the better model can be identified. Absolute value was defined as [(the MSE value from test set – the MSE value from training set)/(the MSE value from training set)] ×100%. The lower the change rate and the lower the MSE value are, the better the model performs.

The unit of analysis in this study was the individual LC surgery patient. The data analysis was performed in several stages. Firstly, continuous variables were tested for statistical significance by one-way analysis of variance (ANOVA), and categorical variables were tested by Fisher exact analysis. Univariate analyses were applied to identify significant predictors ($P<0.05$). Secondly, STATISTICA 10.0 (StatSoft, Tulsa, OK) software was used to construct the MLP network model, the SVM model, the GPR model and the MLR model of the relationship between the identified predictors and QOL. Finally, sensitivity analysis was performed to assess the importance of variables in the fitted models. To simplify the training process, key variables were introduced, and unnecessary variables were excluded. A global sensitivity analysis was also performed to assess the relative significance of input parameters in the system model and to rank the variables in order of importance. The global sensitivity of the input variables against the output variable was expressed as the ratio of the network error (variable sensitivity ratios, VSR) with a given input omitted to the network error with the input included. A ratio of 1 or lower indicates that the variable degrades network performance and should be removed.

Table 7. Comparison of mean absolute percentage error (MAPE) in total gastrointestinal quality of life index (GIQLI) score, physical component summary (PCS) score and mental component summary (MCS) score predicted by multiple linear regression (MLR), support vector machine (SVM), Gaussian process regression (GPR), and artificial neural network (ANN) models in forty new data sets.

Models	**MAPE**
Total GIQLI score	
MLR model	6.2%
SVM model	6.0%
GPR model	20.8%
ANN model	4.7%
PCS score	
MLR model	7.7%
SVM model	7.8%
GPR model	12.3%
ANN model	6.4%
MCS score	
MLR model	14.7%
SVM model	11.8%
GPR model	20.6%
ANN model	10.6%

Results

Table 1 shows the patient characteristics in this study. The mean age of the study population was (55.9 ± 14.6) years. The average CCI was 0.9 ± 1.1, and 57.3% of the patients were female. Furthermore, Table 2 shows the coefficients for total GIQLI score, PCS score, and MCS score obtained by the training set in the MLR model. The selected variables included in the MLR models were age (X_1), CCI (X_2), gender (X_3), previous abdominal surgery (X_4), current complications (X_5), operation time (X_6), and preoperative functional status (X_7). All selected variables were statistically significant ($P<0.05$) (Table 3). Additionally, in forty runs of the data using an 80%–20% random split, total GIQLI score (Appendix S1), PCS score (Appendix S2) and MCS score (Appendix S3) after surgery did not significantly differ between the training set and testing set.

Table 4 shows the three-layer networks and number of support vectors of total GIQLI score, PCS score and MCS score in ANN and SVM models. The ANN-based approaches provided the 3-layer networks and the relative weights of neurons used for predicting QOL. The activation functions of logistic sigmoid and hyperbolic tangent were used in each neuron of the hidden layer and output layer, respectively.

Table 5 compares the QOL predictions obtained by the ANN, the SVM, the GPR and the MLR models for the training set and the test set. For predicting QOL, the ANN model had relatively larger change rates and MSE values in the test set with the exception of MSE for the testing set at year 2. That is, the ANN model had better QOL prediction capability. Compared to the other three models, the GPR model had smaller MSE and MAPE values in the training set. In the testing set, however, the GPR model had relatively larger MSE and MAPE values and relatively larger change rates for predicting QOL. The poor predictive performance of the GPR in the testing set may have resulted from overfitting to the training data. Apparently, the ANN model also outperformed the SVM model, the GPR model and the MLR model in terms of predictive accuracy. Most MAPE values obtained by the ANN model were lower than 10%, which indicated the excellent accuracy of the ANN in predicting QOL.

The training set was also used to calculate the variable sensitivity ratios (VSR) for the ANN model. Table 6 presents the VSR values for the outcome variable (QOL) in relation to the three most influential variables. In the ANN model, preoperative functional status (VSR 1.38) was the most influential (sensitive) parameter in terms of its effects on total GIQLI score, PCS score, and MCS score (VSR 1.38, 1.15, and 1.07, respectively). All VSR values exceeded one, indicating that the network performs better when all variables are considered.

Table 7 compares the MAPE values obtained by ANN, SVM, GPR and MLR models. Compared to the SVM model, GPR model and the MLR model, the ANN model consistently obtained lower MAPE values for total GIQLI score (4.7% versus 20.8%), PCS score (6.4% versus 12.3%), and MCS score (10.6% versus 20.6%).

Discussion

This study confirmed that, compared to the SVM model, the GPR model and the MLR model, the ANN model is significantly more accurate in predicting QOL ($P<0.001$). To the best of our knowledge, this study is the first to use ANNs for analyzing predictors of QOL after LC surgery. This model was tested against actual outcomes obtained by a neural network model, a support vector machine model and a linear regression model constructed using identical inputs. We also showed that, given the same number of demographic and clinical inputs and the same two outcome measures, the predictive accuracy of ANN is superior to that of SVM, GPR and MLR.

Recently, SVM, GPR and ANN models have been used for non-linear modeling in many fields, particularly bioinformatics [4–11]. Although the efficacy of SVM and GPR models is well established in the field of machine learning, its performance in surgical outcome prediction and prognosis has not been measured. The ANNs are adaptive models that use a dynamic approach to analyzing the risk of outcomes. That is, they perform bottom-up computation by modifying their internal structures in relation to a functional objective (i.e., the model is generated by the data it analyzes). Despite their incapability to deal with missing data, ANNs can simultaneously process numerous variables and can consider outliers and nonlinear interactions among variables. Unlike standard statistical tests, ANNs effectively manage complexity even when samples sizes are small and when ratios between variables and records are unbalanced. In this respect, ANNs avoid the dimensionality problem and can achieve a predictive accuracy superior to those of SVM, GPR and MLR. To ensure a sufficiently robust basis for network training, the present study used a large and homogeneous dataset comprising all demographic and clinical variables shown to affect patient-reported QOL in previous linear regression models [10,11].

Piaggi and colleagues demonstrated that ANN models can accurately predict weight loss in obese women treated by laparoscopic adjustable gastric banding. Their integrated multidisciplinary approach showed that ANN may be a valuable tool for selecting the best candidates for surgery [23]. Segal and colleagues compared ANN with a multiple linear regression model in terms of accuracy in predicting several different functional outcome scores at 1 year after traumatic brain injury [24]. The predictive accuracy of their sophisticated linear models was comparable to that of ANNs. Recently, Salvatore and colleagues combined multiple linear regressions with artificial neural networks to predict how relationships among lower urinary tract symptoms, anatomical findings, and baseline characteristics affect outcome in women with pelvic organ prolapse. They also found that ANNs are valuable instruments for improving understanding of complex biological models [25].

The ANN approach developed in this study extends the predictive range of the linear regression model by replacing identity functions with nonlinear activation functions. The approach is apparently superior to linear regression for describing systems. The ANNs may be trained with data acquired in various clinical contexts and can consider local expertise, racial differences, and other variables with uncertain effects on clinical outcome. The analysis need not be limited to clinical parameters. Other potentially useful variables could be tested to improve the predictive value of the model. The proposed ANN architecture with MLP can also include more than one dependent variable and can perform a non-linear transformation between dependent variables. Future studies may evaluate how other demographic or clinical characteristics affect the proposed architecture.

In ANNs, overfitting occurs when a model describes random error instead of the underlying relationship. Data overfitting is indicated by an increasing testing error concurrent with a steadily decreasing training error. The model with the best predictive performance and the best data fit is that in which testing error is at the global minimum [26]. Based on the above rule for obtaining a fitted model while avoiding overfitting, this study used the testing set as the controlling criterion for determining when to stop training. Additionally, the testing data were not included in the training data.

Throughout this two-year follow-up study, the best single predictor of QOL subscale scores was preoperative functional status, which is consistent with reports that preoperative functional scores are the best predictors of postoperative QOL [2,13]. Therefore, effective counseling is essential for apprising patients of expected post-surgery impairments. If QOL outcomes are considered benchmarks, then preoperative functional status, which is a major predictor of postoperative outcome, is crucial. Patients should also be advised that their postoperative QOL might depend not only on the success of their operations, but also on their preoperative functional status.

Post-surgery QOL may be related to surgical risk. For example, Quintana et al. [27] suggested that men with low surgical risks are more likely to be diagnosed with complicated cholelithiasis compared to men with high surgical risks. Since men with low surgical risks are more likely to experience complicated cholelithiasis, they have greater potential for improvement in QOL. This suggests that gender differences in QOL outcomes may result from gender differences in the treatment of complicated presentations, i.e., in terms of QOL, men may derive a greater benefit compared to women because they have a greater potential for complications and thus a greater potential for improvement. Another possible but untested explanation is gender differences in health care received. Some authors also suggest that patient values and the reporting of health status also differ by gender [18,27]. Another factor is age. This study confirmed previous findings that QOL improvement after LC surgery is inversely related to age [18,27].

Additionally, a recent study indicates that, compared to patients in early stages of a disease, patients in advanced stages not only tend to have more co-morbidities, they also tend to have less social support [2]. Notably, the CCI score in the current study was inversely related to QOL, which is consistent with the reported association between increased comorbidity and poor postcholecystectomy QOL [28–30].

Although all research questions were satisfactorily addressed, several limitations are noted. First, this study collected data for LC surgery patients who had been under the supervision of four surgeons in four different medical centers, each of whom had performed the highest volume of LC surgery procedures in his respective hospital during the previous years. This sample selection procedure ensured that patient outcome data would not be affected by surgeons with limited experience. By focusing the analysis on procedures performed by these four surgeons, the results of this study are more representative of all LC patients compared to one analyzing those performed by a single surgeon. However, a notable limitation is that the first patient in the prospective patient cohort was enrolled in 2007. Therefore, depending on their inclusion date, some surveyed patients had a longer follow-up than others did, which may have caused selection bias. Nonetheless, in most QOL subscales, the characteristics of subjects who continuously participated throughout this 2-year study did not significantly differ from those of subjects who died or dropped out during the study (data not shown).

Conclusions

Compared with the SVM model, the GPR model and the MLR model, the ANN model in the study was more accurate in predicting patient-reported QOL and had higher overall performance indices. The global sensitivity analysis also showed that preoperative functional status is the most important predictor of total GIQLI score, PCS score and MCS score after LC surgery. The predictors analyzed in this study could be addressed in preoperative and postoperative health care consultations to educate candidates for LC surgery in the expected course of recovery and expected functional outcomes. Further studies of this model with differential evolution [31] may consider the effect of a more detailed database that includes complications and clinical examination findings as well as more detailed outcome data. Hopefully, the model will evolve into an effective adjunctive clinical decision making tool.

Supporting Information

Appendix S1 Forty data sets used for comparing predictions of total gastrointestinal quality of life index (GIQLI) score.

Appendix S2 Forty new data sets used for comparing predictions of physical component summary (PCS) score.

Appendix S3 Forty new data sets used for comparing predictions of mental component summary (MCS) score.

Author Contributions

Conceived and designed the experiments: HYS CCC. Performed the experiments: HYS HHL JTT WHH CFC KTL CCC. Analyzed the data: HYS. Contributed reagents/materials/analysis tools: HYS HHL JTT WHH CFC KTL CCC. Wrote the paper: HYS HHL JTT WHH CFC KTL CCC. Administrative, technical, and material support: HYS HHL JTT WHH CFC KTL CCC. Study supervision: HHL KTL CCC.

References

1. Lugtenberg M, Burgers JS, Clancy C, Westert GP, Schneider EC (2011) Current guidelines have limited applicability to patients with comorbid conditions: a systematic analysis of evidence-based guidelines. PLoS One 6: e25987.
2. Shi HY, Lee HH, Tsai MH, Chiu CC, Uen YH, et al. (2011) Long-term outcomes of laparoscopic cholecystectomy: a prospective piecewise linear regression analysis. Surg Endosc 25: 2132–2140.
3. Tao M, Teng Y, Shao H, Wu P, Mills EJ (2011) Knowledge, perceptions and information about hormone therapy (HT) among menopausal women: a systematic review and meta-synthesis. PLoS One 6: e24661.
4. Cortes C, Vapnik V (1995) Support-vector networks. Mach Learn 20: 273–297.
5. Sampson DL, Parker TJ, Upton Z, Hurst CP (2011) A comparison of methods for classifying clinical samples based on proteomics data: a case study for statistical and machine learning approaches. PLoS One 6: e24973.
6. Furey TS, Cristianini N, Duffy N, Bednarski DW, Schummer M, et al. (2000) Support vector machine classification and validation of cancer tissue samples using microarray expression data. Bioinformatics 16: 906–914.
7. Rasmussen CE, Williams CKI (2006) Gaussian Processes for Machine Learning. MIT Press, Cambridge, MA.
8. Kapoor A, Grauman K, Urtasun R, Darrell T (2010) Gaussian processes for object categorization. Int J Comput Vis 88: 169–188.
9. Lancichinetti A, Radicchi F, Ramasco JJ, Fortunato S (2011) Finding statistically significant communities in networks. PLoS One 6: e18961.
10. Zou J, Han Y, So SS (2008) Overview of artificial neural networks. Methods Mol Biol 458: 15–23.
11. Das A, Ben-Menachem T, Cooper GS, Chak A, Sivak MV Jr, et al. (2003) Prediction of outcome in acute lower gastrointestinal haemorrhage based on an artificial neural network: internal and external validation of a predictive model. Lancet 362: 1261–1266.
12. Thakur V, Schlachta CM, Jayaraman S (2011) Minilaparoscopic versus conventional laparoscopic cholecystectomy a systematic review and meta-analysis. Ann Surg 253: 244–258.
13. Shi HY, Lee KT, Lee HH, Uen YH, Tsai JT, et al. (2009) Post-cholecystectomy quality of life: a prospective multicenter cohort study of its associations with preoperative functional status and patient demographics. J Gastrointest Surg 13: 1651–1658.
14. Gholipour C, Fakhree MB, Shalchi RA, Abbasi M (2009) Prediction of conversion of laparoscopic cholecystectomy to open surgery with artificial neural networks. BMC Surg 9: 13.
15. Liew PL, Lee YC, Lin YC, Lee TS, Lee WJ, et al. (2007) Comparison of artificial neural networks with logistic regression in prediction of gallbladder disease among obese patients. Dig Liver Dis 39: 356–362.
16. Eldar S, Siegelmann HT, Buzaglo D, Matter I, Cohen A, et al. (2002) Conversion of laparoscopic cholecystectomy to open cholecystectomy in acute cholecystitis: artificial neural networks improve the prediction of conversion. World J Surg 26: 79–85.
17. Hsu CE, Lee KT, Chang CS, Chiu HC, Chao FT, et al. (2010) Cholecystectomy prevalence and treatment cost: an 8-year study in Taiwan. Surg Endosc 24: 3127–3133.
18. Shi HY, Lee KT, Lee HH, Uen YH, Chiu CC (2011) Response shift effect on gastrointestinal quality of life index after laparoscopic cholecystectomy. Qual Life Res 20: 335–341.
19. Shi HY, Chang JK, Wong CY, Wang JW, Tu YK, et al. (2010) Responsiveness and minimal important differences after revision total hip arthroplasty. BMC Musculoskelet Disord 11: 261.
20. Ware JE, Kosinski M, Bayliss MS, McHorney CA, Rogers WH, et al. (1995) Comparison of methods for the scoring and statistical analysis of SF-36 health profile and summary measures: summary of results from the Medical Outcomes Study. Med Care 33: AS264–279.
21. Rumelhart DE, Hinton GE, Williams RJ (1986) Learning internal representations by error propagation. In Rumelhart, D. E. & McCleland, J. L. (Ed.) Cambridge, MA: MIT Press, pp. 318–362.
22. Chen CF, Ho WH, Chou HY, Yang SM, Chen IT, et al. (2011) Long-term prediction of emergency department revenue and visitor volume using autoregressive integrated moving average model. Comput Math Methods Med 2011: 395690.
23. Piaggi P, Lippi C, Fierabracci P, Maffei M, Calderone A, et al. (2010) Artificial neural networks in the outcome prediction of adjustable gastric banding in obese women. PLoS One 5: e13624.

24. Segal ME, Goodman PH, Goldstein R, Hauck W, Whyte J, et al. (2006) The accuracy of artificial neural networks in predicting long-term outcome after traumatic brain injury. J Head Trauma Rehabil 21: 298–314.
25. Salvatore S, Serati M, Siesto G, Cattoni E, Zanirato M, et al. (2011) Correlation between anatomical findings and symptoms in women with pelvic organ prolapse using an artificial neural network analysis. Int Urogynecol J 22: 453–459.
26. Tetko IV, Livingstone DJ, Luik AI (1995) Neural network studies. 1. Comparison of Overfitting and Overtraining. J Chem Inf Comput Sci 35,826–833.
27. Quintana JM, Arostegui I, Oribe V, López de Tejada I, Barrios B, et al. (2005) Influence of age and gender on quality-of-life outcomes after cholecystectomy. Qual Life Res 14: 815–825.
28. Buddingh KT, Nieuwenhuijs VB (2011) The critical view of safety and routine intraoperative cholangiography complement each other as safety measures during cholecystectomy. J Gastrointest Surg 15: 1069–1070.
29. Noble H, Whitley E, Norton S, Thompson M (2011) A study of preoperative factors associated with a poor outcome following laparoscopic bile duct exploration. Surg Endosc 25: 130–139.
30. Joseph S, Moore BT, Sorensen GB, Earley JW, Tang F, et al. (2011) Single-incision laparoscopic cholecystectomy: a comparison with the gold standard. Surg Endosc 25: 3008–3015.
31. Ho WH, Chou JH, Guo CY (2010) Parameter identification of chaotic systems using improved differential evolution algorithm. Nonlinear Dynamics 61, 29–41.

The Cost-Effectiveness of Wound-Edge Protection Devices Compared to Standard Care in Reducing Surgical Site Infection after Laparotomy: An Economic Evaluation alongside the ROSSINI Trial

Adrian Gheorghe[1], Tracy E. Roberts[2], Thomas D. Pinkney[3,4], David C. Bartlett[4], Dion Morton[3,4], Melanie Calvert[1,4]*, on behalf of the West Midlands Research Collaborative and the ROSSINI Trial Investigators

1 Primary Care Clinical Sciences, University of Birmingham, Birmingham, United Kingdom, **2** Health Economics Unit, University of Birmingham, Birmingham, United Kingdom, **3** Academic Department of Surgery, University of Birmingham, Birmingham, United Kingdom, **4** West Midlands Research Collaborative, Birmingham, United Kingdom

Abstract

Background: Wound-edge protection devices (WEPDs) have been used in surgery for more than 40 years to reduce surgical site infection (SSI). No economic evaluation of WEPDs against any comparator has ever been conducted. The aim of the paper was to assess whether WEPDs are cost-effective in reducing SSI compared to standard care alone in the United Kingdom.

Methods and Findings: An economic evaluation was conducted alongside the ROSSINI trial. The study perspective was that of the UK National Health Service and the time horizon was 30 days post-operatively. The study was conducted in 21 UK hospitals. 760 patients undergoing laparotomy were randomised to either WEPD or standard care and 735 were included in the primary analysis. The main economic outcome was cost-effectiveness based on incremental cost (£) per quality adjusted life year (QALY) gained. Patients in the WEPD arm accessed health care worth £5,420 on average and gained 0.02131 QALYs, compared to £5,130 and 0.02133 QALYs gained in the standard care arm. The WEPD strategy was more costly and equally effective compared to standard care, but there was significant uncertainty around incremental costs and QALYs. The findings were robust to a range of sensitivity analyses.

Conclusions: There is no evidence to suggest that WEPDs can be considered a cost effective device to reduce SSI. Their continued use is a waste of limited health care resources.

Editor: Talitha L. Feenstra, National Institute for Public Health and the Environment, Netherlands

Funding: This study was funded by the National Institute for Health Research; Research for Patient Benefit programme (PB-PG-1208-18234). Wound edge protection devices were provided free of charge by 3M (Bracknell, UK). Representatives from 3M did not sit on the trial management group and had no input in trial design, data collection, data analysis, or manuscript synthesis. AG was supported by a National Institute for Health Research (NIHR) Research Support Facility PhD studentship. The funders had no role in study design, data collection and analysis, decision to publish, or preparation of the manuscript.

Competing Interests: The authors have declared that no competing interests exist.

* E-mail: m.calvert@bham.ac.uk

Introduction

Surgical site infection (SSI) is a common postoperative complication, occurring in up to five percent (5%) of all patients undergoing surgery and 30–40% of patients undergoing abdominal surgery depending on the level of contamination [1,2]. Development of an SSI significantly impacts upon patient mortality and morbidity as well as healthcare costs [3]. In the United Kingdom (UK), hospital length of stay is typically doubled and additional per-patient costs of up to £10,000 have been estimated, the variability depending upon the type and site of surgery and the severity of the infection [4,5].

Wound-edge protection devices (WEPDs) have been used for more than forty years to reduce SSI by creating a physical barrier between the abdominal wound edges and viscera, visceral contents, contaminated instruments and gloves, thereby reducing accumulation of endogenous and exogenous bacteria on the wound edges. Evidence on the clinical effectiveness of WEPDs has been unclear: two systematic reviews of randomised controlled trials (RCTs) suggested that WEPD may be effective in the reduction of SSI [6,7], although the quality of the including RCTs was low. To date there is no published evidence on the cost effectiveness of WEPDs.

The objective of the ROSSINI (Reduction of Surgical Site Infection using a Novel Intervention) trial was to explore the effectiveness and cost-effectiveness of WEPD in reducing SSI after laparotomy. In this paper we report the results of the economic

Table 1. ROSSINI trial: unit costs at 2011 value.

Resource	Unit cost (£)	Source
WEPD (intervention)	15	Manufacturer [13]
HOSPITAL CARE		
Day on general ward	311	NHS Reference Costs 2010/2011 [14]
Day in ITU	1515	NHS Reference Costs 2007/2008* [15]
Day in HDU	856	NHS Reference Costs 2007/2008* [15]
PRIMARY CARE		
GP visit	36	Curtis 2011 [16]
Practice nurse visit	13	Curtis 2011 [16]
District nurse visit	73	Curtis 2011 [16]
Outpatient clinic visit	101	NHS Reference Costs 2010/2011 [14]
Medication	as appropriate	British National Formulary 2011 [17]

*The costs for a day in Intensive Therapy Unit (ITU) and a day in High Dependency Unit (HDU) were not available in NHS Reference Costs 2010/2011. The last available document where they were given explicitly was the 2007/2008 edition. For the purpose of this analysis, the 2007/2008 unit costs were updated to their 2011 value using the appropriate Hospital and community health services (HCHS) pay and price inflation (Curtis 2011).

evaluation conducted alongside ROSSINI which compared the relative cost-effectiveness of WEPD compared to standard care from the perspective of the UK National Health Service (NHS). The economic evaluation is reported in accordance with the CHEERS Statement (Appendix S1).

Methods

The trial protocol (Protocol S1) and recruitment flow chart are presented as supplementary information.

Ethics Statement

The trial protocol [8] was approved before the study began by the National Research Ethics Service (09/H1204/91; North Staffordshire Committee) and the research and development team at each hospital. Written informed consent was obtained from all patients before enrolment on paper forms approved by the aforementioned ethics body. ROSSINI was registered with controlled-trials.com (ISRCTN 40402832).

Study Design

The full report on the trial has been reported elsewhere [9]. Briefly, the trial was a prospective, multicentre, observer blinded, randomised controlled trial with stratification according to baseline infection risk. Randomisation was performed when the patient was in the anaesthetic room immediately before surgery using a centralised secure web system provided by the University of Birmingham. Randomisation was stratified according to the urgency of surgery, likelihood of opening a viscus, and likelihood of creating a stoma, with the use of a minimisation procedure. The trial was conducted between February 2010 and January 2012 at 21 NHS hospitals across the UK. The cost-effectiveness analysis was pre-specified in the trial protocol [8]. The objective of the economic evaluation was to explore the relative cost-effectiveness of WEPD compared to standard care. Cost, resource use and outcome data in terms of QALYs were collected prospectively for both arms of the trial. Costs and QALYs for the WEPD intervention are compared to results of the standard care arm and incremental costs and incremental QALYs are calculated as the difference in costs and QALYs, respectively, between the WEPD arm and the standard care arm. When appropriate, the incremental cost-effectiveness ratio (ICER) was calculated as the ratio of incremental costs (£) to incremental effects (QALY). In this case, the ICER (£/QALY) represents the cost of obtaining an additional QALY when switching from standard care to WEPDs.

Setting and Perspective

The trial-based evaluation took a health care provider perspective and thus considered only cost centres relevant for the NHS and Personal Social Services. The intervention under scrutiny was the use of a WEPD during surgery in addition to standard care. The comparator was no WEPD use, i.e. standard care alone. In order to enhance the generalisability of the trial, the surgical teams were given the liberty to use retraction and SSI prophylactic procedures of their choice. The time horizon was 30 days post-operatively, in accordance with SSI monitoring in the English NHS [10]. Given the short time horizon, no discounting was applied to either costs or outcomes.

Data Collection

Health outcomes, preference-based outcomes and resource use data were collected from the participating sites using custom designed paper-based case report forms (CRFs), which were completed by patients or trial staff, as appropriate, at each site then managed centrally at the Centre for Clinical Trials at the University of Birmingham.

Health Utility

We recorded health-related quality of life using the EuroQol EQ-5D questionnaire (the English three-level response version and validated for use in the UK, Appendix S2), a standardised generic preference based instrument that describes a patient's health status using a single index value [11]. We used EQ-5D in this study because of its relevance for the UK policy makers, particularly the National Institute for Health and Clinical Excellence (NICE) [12]. We administered the EQ-5D instrument to patients in ROSSINI at baseline (prior to surgery) and on two occasions post-operatively. We conducted the first assessment in clinic, after the patient provided informed consent and before randomisation. We performed the second assessment (5 to 7 days) on the hospital ward if still inpatient or at discharge, as applicable. We performed the third assessment (30 to 33 days) on the hospital ward if still

Table 2. ROSSINI trial: summary of resource use by treatment group, detailed.

Resource use item	WEPD (n = 369)	Standard care (n = 366)	p-value
HOSPITAL CARE			
Inpatient days			
N	359	358	
Mean (SD)	12.55 (15.46)	11.56 (11.68)	0.3350
SE	0.82	0.62	
Median	9	9	
Days in ITU	369	366	
N	0.93 (3.12)	1.06 (5.46)	0.6913
Mean (SD)	0.16	0.28	
SE	0	0	
Median			
Days in HDU			
N	369	366	
Mean (SD)	0.60 (1.67)	0.51 (1.03)	0.6396
SE	0.09	0.08	
Median	0	0	
PRIMARY CARE			
GP visits			
N	364	358	
Mean (SD)	0.43 (0.81)	0.51 (1.03)	0.2474
SE	0.04	0.05	
Median	0	0	
District nurse visits			
N	360	355	
Mean (SD)	3.43 (7.24)	3.52 (6.94)	0.8644
SE	0.38	0.37	
Median	0	0	
Practice nurse visits			
N	366	361	
Mean (SD)	0.16 (0.70)	0.32 (1.21)	0.0355
SE	0.04	0.06	
Median	0	0	
Outpatient clinic visits			
N	364	363	
Mean (SD)	0.42 (1.09)	0.31 (0.71)	0.1205
SE	0.06	0.04	
Median	0	0	

inpatient or, more often, in the outpatient clinic on the occasion of the scheduled follow-up visit. Only the baseline and third assessment (30 to 33 days) were used to calculate QALYs; the 5–7 days assessment was employed in the multiple imputation algorithms for missing EQ-5D scores at the final assessment.

Resource Utilisation

We collected data on resource utilisation of health care resources prospectively in both secondary and primary care settings using the custom designed CRFs (Appendix S2). Hospital utilisation items were completed by health care staff and primary care utilisation items were completed by patients in clinic at the 30-day visit.

Unit Costs

Unit costs were valued in £ (2011 value). The cost of the intervention (WEPD) was obtained from the manufacturer [13]. Inpatient care resource items were sourced from the NHS Reference Costs data [14,15]. Primary care resource items were sourced from the Personal Social Services Resource Unit (PSSRU) Unit Costs and Social Care 2010–2011 [16]. Medication unit costs were taken from the British National Formulary 2011 [17]. All unit costs were average national costs. Consistent with the NHS

Table 3. ROSSINI trial: summary of missing data, by treatment group.

Missing data item	Missing observations (% of trial arm)		
	WEPD (n = 369)	Standard care (n = 366)	Trial arm differences (p-value)
HOSPITAL CARE			
Inpatient days	10 (2.7%)	8 (2.2%)	0.64
PRIMARY CARE			
GP visits	5 (1.4%)	8 (2.2%)	0.39
Practice nurse visits	3 (0.8%)	5 (1.4%)	0.47
District nurse visits	9 (2.4%)	11 (3%)	0.63
Outpatient clinic visits	5 (1.4%)	3 (0.8%)	0.48
HEALTH UTILITY			
EQ-5D data, any time point	51 (13.8%)	53 (14.5%)	0.79

perspective, only resource use affecting the NHS budget were considered. Total resource costs were obtained by summation of the individual resource costs for each category of resource item accessed by trial patients. Individual resource costs were obtained by multiplying the resource use by the corresponding unit costs.

Data Analysis

In the base-case analysis we included all the patients with complete primary outcome data. Any missing cost and health utility data, as well as patient-level characteristics, were imputed using the multiple imputations using chained equations method (MICE) (Appendix S3). The analysis included descriptive statistics for the resource use items, resource costs (both at aggregate and individual level) and EQ-5D scores. QALYs were calculated by multiplying the utility weight associated with each individual health state and the time spent in that health state. QALYs were calculated based on the baseline and 30-day EQ-5D assessments and were adjusted for baseline utility [18].

The average differences in costs and outcomes, as well as the 95% confidence intervals around the point estimates, were calculated using bias-corrected and accelerated (BCa) non-parametric bootstrap with 1,000 replications [19]. The resulting incremental costs and effects were plotted on the cost-effectiveness plane, a visual decision-aiding tool representing the incremental costs and effects of the intervention under evaluation relative to the next best option [20]. Cost-effectiveness acceptability curves (CEACs) were plotted, indicating the probability of each of the two alternatives to be cost-effective at varying thresholds of the decision makers' willingness to pay for an additional unit of outcome [21].

Table 4. Costs and health utilities in the ROSSINI trial, base-case analysis.

Variable	WEPD (n = 369)	Standard care (n = 366)
Costs (£), mean(SE)		
Total cost	5420 (246)	5130 (234)
Intervention cost (WEPD)	15	n/a
Cost of inpatient care	5089 (247)	4812 (234)
General surgical ward	3638 (128)	3460 (122)
Intensive therapy unit	1123 (197)	1053 (186)
High dependency unit	329 (47)	299 (43)
Cost of primary care	316 (29)	318 (29)
GP visits	16 (2)	19 (2)
Practice nurse visits	2 (0.5)	4 (1)
District nurse visits	252 (27)	261 (28)
Outpatient clinic visits	44 (6)	33 (4)
Medication	1 (0.2)	1 (0.3)
Health-related quality of life, mean (SE)		
QALY	0.0213 (0.0014)	0.0213 (0.0014)
EQ-5D score at baseline	0.751 (0.016)	0.752 (0.016)
EQ-5D score at 30 days	0.683 (0.016)	0.684 (0.016)

Note: Standard errors (SE) were calculated assuming a Gamma distribution for costs and a normal distribution for EQ-5D scores and QALYs.

Sensitivity analyses were performed to check the robustness of cost-effectiveness findings, as follows: a complete case analysis based on trial subjects with complete primary outcome, cost and EQ-5D data (n = 532); and adjusted analyses for both base-case and complete case scenarios, where differences between the trial's arms were investigated using generalized linear models. Total costs and EQ-5D scores were regressed against the following pre-specified covariates: intervention group, baseline utility (only for adjusting incremental QALYs), plan to create a stoma, plan to create a viscus (defined as any internal organ), elective/emergency surgery, age, body mass index, diabetes, current smoking status and SSI. The total cost and QALY values were regressed against the variables above using generalised linear models with an identity link [22]. A gamma distribution was assumed for costs and a normal distribution was assumed for QALYs. The analyses were performed using SAS 9.2 [23] and R 2.15.3 software [24].

Results

ROSSINI randomised 760 patients undergoing open abdominal surgery between the use of WEPD during and standard care. 735 patients were included in the primary analysis, of which 369 patients received the intervention and 366 patients received standard care. There was no evidence of benefit for WEPDs in terms of SSI reduction (OR 0.97; 95% CI 0.69 to 1.36) or hospital length of stay [25]. In total 20 patients died within 30 days of surgery: 12 in the control group and eight in the intervention group. For those patients who died within 30 days of surgery we carried forward the last available wound assessment, unless no information was available in which case they were treated as lost to follow-up.

Table 1 presents the unit costs which informed the cost calculations. Health care utilisation data by ROSSINI patients are presented in Table 2. There is no apparent difference between the two treatment groups for neither secondary care nor primary care services. The only exception is the number of practice nurse visits: patients in the standard care arm reported twice as many practice nurse contacts than WEPD patients. When resource utilisation was aggregated as nurse visits, there were no significant differences between the two arms (Table S1).

Despite very low levels of missing data for the primary outcome, the amount of missing data for resource utilisation and health utility was somewhat higher (Table 3). EQ-5D scores at 30 days post-operatively were not available for 14% of patients, while hospital and primary care data were unavailable cumulatively for less than 10% of patients (6.66%). Overall, 20.4% of patients had incomplete observations in terms of resource use or EQ-5D data. However, there was no imbalance between the two arms with respect to the levels of missing data.

Cost-effectiveness

The base-case analysis used information from all patients with complete primary outcome data (n = 735). The results of the multiple imputation process are presented in Appendix S3. Patients in the WEPD arm accessed health care worth £5,420 on average, compared to £5,130 for patients in the standard care arm (Table 4). The use of the WEPD was associated with 0.02131 QALYs, compared to 0.02133 QALYs in the control group. Overall, the WEPD strategy was on average £290 more costly (95%CI -£372 to £948) and 0.00002 QALYs (95%CI-0.0018 to 0.0017) less beneficial than standard care, thus suggesting that WEPD was technically dominated by standard care.

The cost-effectiveness plane (Figure 1) shows that both incremental cost and incremental QALY estimates are associated with considerable uncertainty. The cost-effectiveness acceptability curves (CEACs) communicate the probability for an intervention to be cost-effective for a range of willingness-to-pay thresholds (£/

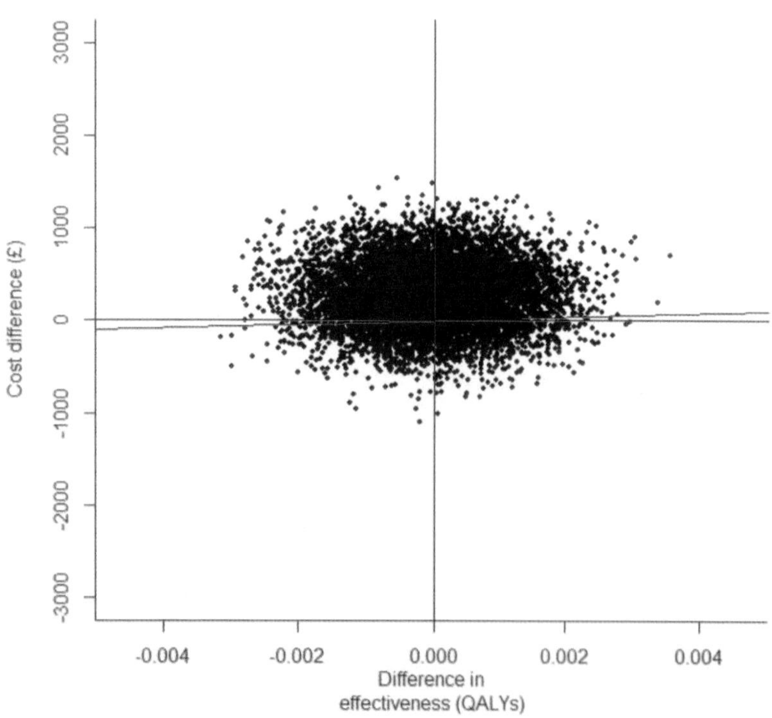

Figure 1. ROSSINI trial economic evaluation: cost-effectiveness plane for the base-case analysis.

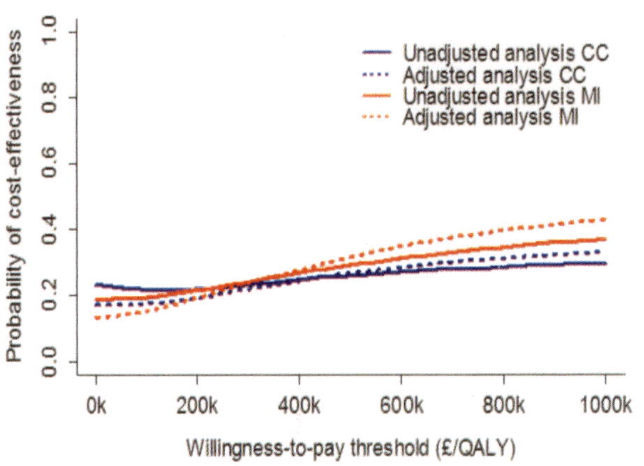

Figure 2. ROSSINI trial economic evaluation: comparison of cost-effectiveness acceptability curves across the analysed scenarios. Legend: MI - Base-case analysis; CC - complete case analysis.

QALY). CEACs suggest that the WEPD is less than 30% likely to be cost-effective in all analyses for the willingness-to-pay threshold range of £20,000 to £30,000 recommended by NICE (Figure 2).

Sensitivity Analysis

The results of the regression adjusted analyses were similar to the unadjusted results: in the base-case analysis, the incremental cost increased from £290 to £311, while the QALY gain increased from −0.00002 to 0.00018 (Table 5). The resulting ICER is in excess of £1.7 million/QALY and, thus, much higher than the threshold recommended by NICE. In the unadjusted complete case scenario the ICER was £740,000/QALY; after regression adjustment the WEPD became more costly and less effective than standard care (Table 5).

Discussion

Summary of Findings

The WEPD intervention was associated with higher costs and practically no QALY gains compared to standard care in the base-case analysis; the confidence intervals for both incremental costs and incremental QALYs show the extent of the uncertainty in the findings (Figure 1). Within the willingness-to-pay interval recommended by NICE [12], WEPDs were less than 30% likely to be cost-effective compared to standard care in all analyses (Figure 2). The result was robust to a range of sensitivity analyses. As such, WEPDs are unlikely to be cost-effective compared to standard care and their use cannot be recommended.

Although resource utilisation was comparable across the two trial arms, patients in the standard care arm appear to have received more practice nurse visits than intervention arm patients. We believe this difference may be due to mis-classification of patient reported visits on the trial case report forms (Appendix S2). A sensitivity analysis is presented in Table S1: when nurse and primary care contacts are aggregated, demonstrated that there is no significant difference between the two arms. This does not affect the cost-effectiveness findings.

Strengths and Limitations

To our knowledge, this study is the first economic evaluation of WEPDs against any comparator and in any setting. It was an integral part of the largest multi-centre RCT to date that investigated the benefits of WEPDs. A wide range of sensitivity analyses confirmed the robustness of base-case findings.

There are also several limitations. First, the choice of time horizon may be subject to debate. The 30-day time horizon was determined by the ROSSINI primary outcome i.e. the occurrence of SSI within 30 days post-operatively, in line with the international guidelines on SSI diagnosis [10,26]. A 30-day time horizon was also adopted in other decision models which evaluated interventions reducing SSI [27].

A further limitation refers to the complexity of SSI management, especially in primary care. NICE clinical guidelines on SSI care provide evidence that the weekly cost of wound dressings can be up to £100, depending on the type of wound and the type of dressing [28]. However, district nurses are the health care professional most likely to apply the wound dressings in a primary care setting and ROSSINI arms were more than comparable regarding the number of district nurse visits, which reduces the potential effect of not costing wound dressings (Table 2).

The uncertainty around the point estimates of incremental costs and QALYs, reflected in the width of the confidence intervals, is considerable. However, it is very unlikely that the ROSSINI trial was underpowered: the pre-specified sample size in the statistical analysis plan (n = 750), based on the best available evidence to date, assumed a 50% reduction in SSI and a 12% SSI rate in the study population. This suggests there may be a large amount of variability in the cost and QALY gains associated with the use of the WEPD. In support of this hypothesis, the primary outcome

Table 5. ROSSINI trial economic evaluation: summary of incremental costs and incremental QALYs across the analysed scenarios.

Scenario	Variable	Mean difference (WEPD – standard care)	95% BCa CI	ICER
Base-case unadjusted	Total cost (£)	290	−372 to 949	WEPD is dominated
	QALY	−0.00002	−0.0018 to 0.0017	
Base-case adjusted	Total cost (£)	311	−273 to 1012	1,712 k/QALY
	QALY	0.0002	−0.0015 to 0.0019	
Complete case unadjusted	Total cost (£)	237	−407 to 892	740 k/QALY
	QALY	0.0003	−0.0023 to 0.0016	
Complete case adjusted	Total cost (£)	369	−214 to 976	WEPD is dominated
	QALY	−0.0001	−0.0022 to 0.0019	

also exhibited considerable uncertainty (OR 0.97, 95% CI 0.69 to 1.36).

Relation to other Studies

We have no knowledge of economic evaluations of WEPDs, but there are published data on SSI costs. The most recent study on the costs SSI care in a primary setting in the UK collected data on 29 SSI patients following colorectal surgery and found that primary care costs amount to about 15% of total SSI costs (on average £1,563 out of £10,523 per SSI patient), thus suggesting that the largest part of the SSI cost burden comes from inpatient care [5]. This is compatible with ROSSINI findings: primary care cost accounted for less than 10% of total costs (Table 4). However, Tanner *et al.* reported total and average resource use and costs, respectively, without any mention of the variability around these quantities. Variability is an important aspect, as illustrated in the older study of Davey *et al.* [29]: out of seven patients with a SSI in primary care, one patient alone received 57 district nurse visits, another patient received two visits and the rest no visit at all.

Conclusion

The ROSSINI trial has shown WEPDs to be neither effective nor cost-effective in reducing SSI compared to standard care. This contradicts previous evidence, which suggested that WEPDs may be effective. ROSSINI is the largest and most robust trial investigating WEPDs to date and the first to have a pre-specified integral economic evaluation. WEPDs have been used to date at the surgeons' discretion in the NHS to reduce SSI but there are no official data on the WEPD utilisation and, as such, the current NHS spending on WEPDs cannot be estimated. Our analyses suggest that the use of WEPDs for SSI reduction cannot be justified and should be discontinued.

Supporting Information

Protocol S1 Trial Protocol.

Checklist S1 CONSORT Checklist.

Appendix S1 CHEERS Statement checklist for the ROSSINI within-trial economic evaluation.

Appendix S2 Case report forms used to capture resource use in the ROSSINI trial.

Appendix S3 Details of the multiple imputation exercise.

Appendix S4 ROSSINI trial: summary of resource use by treatment group, overview.

Acknowledgments

ROSSINI Trial steering group: T Pinkney (chair), D Bartlett, T Mak, H Youseff, G Harrison, W Hawkins, D Morton, S Wilson, M Calvert, G Dowswell, V Redman, R Ryan, L Magill, J Bradbury, M Gill, L Berkman, D Leaper.

Data monitoring committee: J Dunn (chair), J Hill, A Obichere.

Trial administration and site support: J Bradbury, G Dowswell, M Ghods-Ghorbani, R Haslop, V Redman.

Statistical expertise: M Calvert, A Gheorghe, T Roberts.

West Midlands research collaborative committee: D Bartlett, A Bhangu, K Futaba, G Harrison, E Hepburn, S Macleod, T Mak, P Marriott, P Mistry, T Pinkney, H Youssef.

Trials unit operations group: M Calvert (chair), G Dowswell, V Redman, R Haslop, S Warmington, A Gheorghe.

Local principle investigators: A Kingsnorth (Derriford Hospital, Plymouth); J Hardman (Good Hope Hospital, Sutton Coldfield); D Bowley (Heartlands Hospital, Birmingham); G Carlson (Hope Hospital, Manchester); S Selvaseter, A Khan (Leighton Hospital); A Hamouda (Maidstone Hospital); H Wegstapel (Medway Maritime Hospital); H Youssef (New Cross Hospital, Wolverhampton); S Clarke (Northwick Park, London); A Acheson (Queens Medical Centre, Nottingham); N Hurst (Royal Derby Hospital); P Boorman (Royal Devon and Exeter Hospital); R Patel (Russells Hall Hospital, Dudley); N Cruickshank (Sandwell Hospital); K Siddiqui (Tameside General Hospital, Manchester); R Pullan (Torbay Hospital); D Morton (University Hospital Birmingham); J Lengyel (University Hospital North Staffordshire); R Church (Walsall Manor Hospital); J Francombe (Warwick Hospital); M Paraoan (Wrightington, Wigan and Leigh).

Operating surgeons: S Aroori, M Bowles, S Brundell, A Kingsnorth, D Stell (Derriford Hospital, Plymouth); M Chapman, T Raju (Good Hope Hospital, Sutton Coldfield); D Bowley, C Hendrickse, S Karandikar, M Richardson, P Super (Heartlands Hospital, Birmingham); I Anderson, G Carlson, N Lees, D Speake, Jonathan Vickers, D Watson (Hope Hospital, Manchester); AU Khan, J Slavin (Leighton Hospital), S Bailey (Maidstone Hospital); S Andrews, W Garrett, P Gandhi, H Wegstapel (Medway Maritime Hospital); I Badger, F Curran, S Elgaddal, T Gardecki, B Isgar, M Manu, R Soulsby, GJ Williams, H Youssef (New Cross Hospital, Wolverhampton); S Clarke, I Jenkins, R Kennedy, R Phillips (Northwick Park, London); A Acheson, C Maxwell-Armstrong, J Simpson, J Willliams (Queens Medical Centre, Nottingham); N Hurst, S Y Iftikhar, M Larvin, J Lund, J Quarmby, J Reynolds, W Speake, G Tierney (Royal Derby Hospital); P Boorman, I Daniels, S Mansfield (Royal Devon and Exeter Hospital); A Jayatunga, A Kawesha, S Macleod, R Patel, R Pathak, A Rehman, A Savage, C Sellahewa, P Stonelake (Russells Hall Hospital, Dudley); N Cruickshank, K Gill, E Harper, H Joy, V Laloe, M Mirza, D Mobarak, M Sintler, V Thumbe, M Vairavan, K Wheatley (Sandwell Hospital); A Benhamida, K Siddiqui, M Solkar (Tameside General Hospital, Manchester); R Pullan (Torbay Hospital); O Adedeji, S Bach, D Gourevitch, T Ismail, C Keh, M Midwinter, D Morton, S Radley, N Suggett (University Hospital Birmingham), D Beardsmore, C Cheruvu, W Crisp, F Curran, R Dawson, M Deakin, D Durkin, M Farmer, R Kirby, J Lengyel (University Hospital North Staffordshire); R Church (Walsall Manor Hospital); K Busby, J Francombe, P Murphy, M Osborne (Warwick Hospital); A Azmi, A Blower, M Haque, R Harland, S Loganathan, N Mackenzie, M Paraoan (Wrightington, Wigan and Leigh).

Local investigators and wound reviewers: M Bowles, P Brockmann, F Coates, P Eardley, M Gavasingha, S Hornby, B Hyam, C Meachin, M Napier, A Page, S Price, S Read (Derriford Hospital, Plymouth); L Hanna, A Torrance, H Youssef (Good Hope Hospital, Sutton Coldfield); D Bowley, P Calderbank, W Hawkins, C Horrobin, A Munasinghe, S Nachrauthu, R Nandra (Heartlands Hospital, Birmingham); J Barker, E Barrow, C Downes, J Epstein, A Keen, V Shetty, D Speake, M Taylor (Hope Hospital, Manchester); V Adamson, C Hough, A Khan, C Mansfield, O Oshin (Leighton Hospital); J Bedo, R Einosas, A Hamouda, S Jones, L Tomlinson, A Wadoodi (Maidstone Hospital); T Akinola, R Casey, T Cumming, H Dent, R Evans (Medway Maritime Hospital); H Ali, S Ashraf, T AuYong, N Battersby, G Bonney, H Cheng, H Coop, H Cooper, S Dhanda, S Dhillon, S Elgaddal, C El-sayed Fi, M Green, J Long, G Markam, M Mascarentros, D McArthur, J Mohammed, S Pickering, T Pinkney, A Quigley, S Raichura, E Rahman, N Raza, C Richardson, S Roy, H Roberts, S Sahdev, T Sein, A Sharples, R Soulsby, M Treece, M Whitehouse, A Wong, H Youssef (New Cross Hospital, Wolverhampton); G Bashir, C Beaton, G Lee, G Rahbour, D Ramgoolam, S Rasheed, S Sakuma, S Sherman, C Thorn, S Wright (Northwick Park, London); E Barnes, D Humes, J Lynch, M Lythgoe, J Simpson, C Walter, K Ward (Queens Medical Centre, Nottingham); S Aggrawal, C Boereboom, E Collins, E Elsey, A Hall, S Hamandishe, L Kimber, O Peacock, S Pyke, D Reeves, J Smith, E Stobbs, N Watson (Royal Derby Hospital); S Harvey, R James, S Mansfield, Y Nijs, M Wiggins (Royal Devon andExeter Hospital); J Bate, A Bhangu, T Jennson, P Marriott, K McNamara, J Royle, P Singh, M Tan, J Walton, J Wheeler, L Wright, N Yassin (Russells Hall Hospital, Dudley); T Baldwin, M Ballentine, A

Bhangu, C Bell, A Beveridge, J Carter, J Chrickshank, J Colley, D Cox, N Cruickshank, N Cutmore, J Dasgin, K Davis, M Dixon, J Doyle, A Dudley, G Fisher, H Fletcher, F Fuerstenberg, B Gammon, C Garbutt, K Goonetilleke, D Harji, H Harper, J Harvey, L Henderson, I Jenkins, A John, P Kaur, P Marriott, S Poxon, C Parkes, D Pugh, L Rhodes, K Richardson, M Roper, V Rusius, B Sharip, J Smith, S Todd, B Turner, D Vijayan, M Wakewal, R Walker, K Wheatley, L Williams (Sandwell Hospital); S Cocks, E Curran, S Ridgway (Tameside General Hospital, Manchester); B George, A Hall, P Mercer, H Thatcher, J Watson (Torbay Hospital); D Bartlett, S Baijal, J Bradbury, M Coakes, L Crutch, H Edgar, K Futaba, P Guruswamy, A Leyland, N Mabena, T Mak, K Manan, N Manimaran, N Markarian, R Melhado, J Millington, N Mirza, D Mittapalli, A Munasinghe, M Naqvi, S Pandey, T Pinkney, S Ramcharan, R Ravikumar, L Ryder, G Sahota, M Singh, C Wearn, M White, K Wong (University Hospital Birmingham); S Bahia, D Beardsmore, C Bloom, N Briscoe, P Casey, S Dawson, M Deakin, M Denning, M Dennis, A Durber, M El-Shaeib, J Evans, L Fellows, S Hoswell, J Jackson, T Jones, M Lakhan, S Lord, W Hawkins, D Monnery, P Patel, F Rafati, M Reabin, E Rylands, O Sharifi, L Stevenson, F Tomlins (University Hospital North Staffordshire); R Church, A Kitchen, A Puligari, J Sidebotham, E Swan, A Tilley, L Wagstaff (Walsall Manor Hospital); J Barnes, L Clare, K Dasari, S Fallis, J Francombe, E Foster, K Futaba, E Leung, M McFarlane, S Rastall, N Silvey, G Waight, L Whisker (Warwick Hospital); M Antony, A Ahmed, S Baxendale, Y Chandler, M Corfield, Y Dunn, T Edwardson, N Fairclough, R Hodgkins, J Hughes, K Humayun, V Kaliyaperumal, S Lawton, J Leary, S Loganathan, N Mackenzie, M McDermott, M Paraoan, D Paterson, L Pender, P Prasad, J Smith, C Spence, L Roberts, A Robinson (Wrightington, Wigan and Leigh).

Author Contributions

Conceived and designed the experiments: TP MC DB DM. Performed the experiments: TP MC DB DM. Analyzed the data: AG MC TR TP DB. Contributed reagents/materials/analysis tools: AG MC TR TP DB. Wrote the paper: AG MC TR TP DB DM.

References

1. Smyth ETM, McIlvenny G, Enstone JE, Emmerson AM, Humphreys H, et al. (2008) Four country healthcare associated infection prevalence survey 2006: overview of the results. J Hosp Infect 69: 230–248.
2. Bruce J, Russell EM, Mollison J, Krukowski ZH (2001) The measurement and monitoring of surgical adverse events. Health Technology Assessment 5: 1–194.
3. Mangram AJ, Horan TC, Pearson ML (1999) Silver LC, Jarvis WR. Guideline for prevention of surgical site infection. American Journal of Infection Control 27: 97–132.
4. Coello R, Charlett A, Wilson J, Ward V, Pearson A, et al. (2005) Adverse impact of surgical site infections in English hospitals. J Hosp Infect 60: 93–103.
5. Tanner J, Khan D, Aplin C, Ball J, Thomas M, et al. (2009) Post-discharge surveillance to identify colorectal surgical site infection rates and related costs. J Hosp Infect 72: 243–250.
6. Gheorghe A, Calvert M, Pinkney TD, Fletcher BR, Bartlett DC, et al. (2012) Systematic review of the clinical effectiveness of wound-edge protection devices in reducing surgical site infection in patients undergoing open abdominal surgery. Annals of Surgery 255: 1017–1029.
7. Edwards JP, Adelyn HL, Tee MC, Dixon E, Ball CG (2012) Wound protectors reduce surgical site infection: a meta-analysis of randomized controlled trials. Annals of Surgery 256: 53–59.
8. Pinkney TD, Bartlett DC, Hawkins W, Mak T, Youssef H, et al. (2011) Reduction of surgical site infection using a novel intervention (ROSSINI): study protocol for a randomised controlled trial. Trials 12: 217.
9. Pinkney Thomas D, McCall J, Dumville Jo C, Edwards Francesca J, Gheorghe A, et al. (2013) Wound-edge protection devices for preventing surgical site infection in abdominal surgery. Cochrane Database Syst Rev. John Wiley & Sons, Ltd.
10. Health Protection Agency (2011) Protocol for the Surveillance of Surgical Site Infection London: Health Protection Agency.
11. The EuroQol Group (1990) EuroQol - a new facility for the measurement of health-related quality of life. Health Policy 16: 199–208.
12. National Institute for Health and Clinical Excellence (2013) Guide to the Methods of Technology Appraisal 2013. London: NICE.
13. 3M Healthcare (2011) 3M Steri-Drape Wound-edge protector. Available at http://solutions.3m.com/wps/portal/3M/en_US/infection-prevention-solutions/home/products/?PC_7_RJH9U52308DUB0IIL8TMGN3013_nid=PTDM8B1RG4bc4Q6TMNMMVPgl, accessed 14/11/2011.
14. Department of Health (2011) NHS Reference costs 2010–2011. Available at https://www.gov.uk/government/publications/2010-11-reference-costs-publication, accessed 04/09/2013.
15. Department of Health (2008) NHS Reference costs 2007–2008. Available at http://webarchive.nationalarchives.gov.uk/20130107105354/http://www.dh.gov.uk/en/Publicationsandstatistics/Publications/PublicationsPolicyAndGuidance/DH_098945, accessed 04/09/2013.
16. Curtis L (2011) Unit costs of health and social care 2011. Canterbury: Personal Social Services Unit, University of Kent.
17. Joint Formulary Committee (2011) British National Formulary. 61st edition. London: British Medical Association and Royal Pharmaceutical Society of Great Britain.
18. Manca A, Hawkins N, Sculpher MJ (2005) Estimating mean QALYs in trial-based cost-effectiveness analysis: the importance of controlling for baseline utility. Health Economics 14: 487–496.
19. Briggs AH, Mooney CZ, Wonderling DE (1999) Constructing confidence intervals for cost-effectiveness ratios: an evaluation of parametric and non-parametric techniques using Monte Carlo simulation. Statistics in Medicine 18: 3245–3262.
20. Black WC (1990) The CE plane: a graphic representation of cost-effectiveness. Medical Decision Making 10: 212–214.
21. Fenwick E, O'Brien BJ, Briggs A (2004) Cost-effectiveness acceptability curves - facts, fallacies and frequently asked questions. Health Economics 13: 405–415.
22. Dobson AJ, Barnett AG (2008) Introduction to Generalized Linear Models. Boca Raton, FL: Chapman and Hall/CRC.
23. Eborall H, Stewart M, Cunningham-Burley S, Price J, Fowkes FG (2011) Accrual and drop out in a primary prevention randomised controlled trial: qualitative study. Trials 12: 7.
24. R Development Core Team (2013) R: A language and environment for statistical computing. Vienna, Austria: R Foundation for Statistical Computing.
25. Pinkney TD, Calvert M, Bartlett DC, Gheorghe A, Redman V, et al. (2013) Impact of wound edge protection devices on surgical site infection after laparotomy: multicentre randomised controlled trial (ROSSINI Trial). BMJ 347.
26. Centers for Disease Control and Prevention (1999) Guideline for Prevention of Surgical Site Infection. Infection Control and Hospital Epidemiology 20: 247–278.
27. Cranny G, Elliott R, Weatherly H, Chambers D, Hawkins N, et al. (2008) A systematic review and economic model of switching from non-glycopeptide to glycopeptide antibiotic prophylaxis for surgery (Provisional abstract). Health Technology Assessment: 1–147.
28. National Institute for Health and Clinical Excellence (2008) Surgical site infection - prevention and treatment of surgical site infection. Clinical Guideline 78. London: RCOG Press.
29. Davey P, Lynch B, Malek M, Byrne D, Thomas P (1992) Cost-effectiveness of single dose cefotaxime plus metronidazole compared with three doses each of cefuroxime plus metronidazole for the prevention of wound infection after colorectal surgery. J Antimicrob Chemother 30: 855–864.

Duodenum Clamping Trauma Induces Significant Postoperative Intraperitoneal Adhesions on a Rat Model

Jingrui Bai[1]❡, Hongbin Liu[1,2]❡, Donghua Li[2], Lihua Cui[2], Xianzhong Wu[1,2]*

1 Graduate school of Tianjin Medical University, Tianjin, China, 2 Department of Pharmacology, Tianjin Nankai Hospital, Tianjin, China

Abstract

Objective: The purpose of this study was to investigate the histological and morphological changes in the first two postoperative weeks on a rat intraperitoneal adhesion model induced by duodenum clamping trauma.

Method: The rat model of postoperative intraperitoneal adhesions was established in 48 male Wistar rats by laparotomy, followed by the duodenum clamping trauma. Rats were sacrificed respectively on 1st, 3rd, 5th, 7th and 14th day after the operation. The control rats were sacrificed immediately after the operation (0 day). Then the intraperitoneal adhesions were assessed macroscopically. Histopathology and immunohistochemistry were performed to evaluate the fibrosis, inflammatory responses, neovascularization, and cells infiltration in adhesion tissues. In addition, the changes of the mesothelium covering the surgical sites were examined by scanning electron microscopy.

Results: Our study revealed that duodenum clamping trauma induced by mosquito hemostat can result in significant postoperative intraperitoneal adhesions formation. The extent and tenacity of intraperitoneal adhesions reached their peaks on 3rd and 5th days, respectively. Histopathological examination showed that all rats developed inflammatory responses at the clamped sites of duodenum, which was most prominent on 1st day; the scores of fibrosis and vascular proliferation increased slowly from 3rd to 5th day. Myofibroblasts proliferated significantly in the adhesion tissues from 3rd day, which were examined by immunohistochemical method. And the mesothelium covering the surgical sites and the adhesion tissues healed on 7th day.

Conclusion: This study suggests that clamping trauma to the duodenum can result in significant postoperative intraperitoneal adhesions formation, which represents an ideal rat model for intraperitoneal adhesions research and prevention. And myofibroblasts may play an important role in the forming process of intraperitoneal adhesions.

Editor: Shree Ram Singh, National Cancer Institute, United States of America

Funding: This investigation was financially supported by the Innovative Foundation of Tianjin Medical University (NO. 146#200022, Tianjin, China). The funders had no role in study design, data collection and analysis, decision to publish, or preparation of the manuscript.

Competing Interests: The authors have declared that no competing interests exist.

* E-mail: wuxianzhongdoctor@hotmail.com

❡ These authors contributed equally to the work.

Introduction

The intraperitoneal adhesions are pathological bonds usually be-tween the omentum, viscera and abdominal wall [1]. Etiological factors of intraperitoneal adhesions formation include peritonitis, endometriosis, radiotherapy, foreign body reaction, and so on, but the majority of intraperitoneal adhesions are caused by surgical procedures [2,3,4]. The incidence of intraperitoneal adhesions after operation was as high as 95% [5]. The formation of intraperitoneal adhesions is an almost inevitable complication following abdominal surgery, leading to severe clinical consequences, such as abdominal pain, adhesive small bowel obstruction and infertility [1,2].

The intraperitoneal adhesions always took shape within the first five to seven days after the injury to peritoneum [6]. It is the result of both insufficient fibrinolytic capacity and increased fibrin formation in response to an enhanced inflammatory status of the peritoneum [3]. In recent years, many managements and drugs for adhesions prevention were applied in experimental and clinical studies, but few were proved to be really effective and safe [7,8,9]. Better understanding of the forming process and pathologic mechanism of intraperitoneal adhesions will contribute to the promotion of prevention measures. However, results from animal studies investigating prevention or treatment of adhesions are limited, due to lack of consistency in existing animal models. In our present model, traumatizing the duodenum by clamping with a hemostat is the direct cause of intraperitoneal adhesions. The histological and morphological changes in the first two post-operative weeks were studied and the mechanisms were investigated.

Materials and Methods

Experimental Animal

The animal experiment was approved by Ethics Committee of Tianjin Nankai Hospital (Permit number: SCXK-Jin-2011-0011. Tianjin, China).

Male Wistar rats, twelve-weeks-old and weighed 250–270 g, were purchased from Academy of Military Medical Sciences (Tianjin, China). Rats were housed in accordance with current national guidelines regarding animal welfare. Before the experiment, rats were kept in special-pathogen-free conditions for one week, with standard laboratory chow and water available *ad libitum*. The environment was maintained at 18–26°C with a relative humidity of 30–70% and in a 12 hours light/12 hours dark cycle.

Surgical Procedure

The key surgical instrument for the model establishment is a mosquito hemostat with curved tips and full teeth (Jinzhong, Shanghai, China), which is 12.5 cm in length and has three ratchets. The teeth of the mosquito hemostat were shielded by a segment of a 12Fr rubber single Nelaton Catheter (Welllead, Guangzhou, Guangdong, China) (Figure 1). The mean value of clamping force by the second ratchet is 18.3±0.9 N, which was detected by electronic universal testing machine (HTE Model, Hounsfield Company, Surrey, England).

After fasting overnight before the operation, all animals were assigned randomly to six groups, 8 in each. All surgical procedures were performed by the initial under sterile conditions. Animals were anesthetized by intraperitoneal injection with 10% Chloral Hydrate solution (3 ml/kg bodyweight; Tianjin Chemical Reagent Company, Tianjin, China), after which the abdomen was shaved and swabbed with 75% alcohol. Then the prepared rat was fixed in the supine position and the abdomen was covered with a fenestrated sterile drape. Heat loss was prevented by placing the rat on a warming tray together with a hot incandescent light during the operation. An up midline incision was made to identify and expose the duodenum. Subsequently, from the pylorus down, grasp the duodenum in the clamp of the hemostat and squeeze the handle of hemostat to the second ratchet for 3 seconds. There were nine segmental clamping in total and at intervals of 0.5 cm.

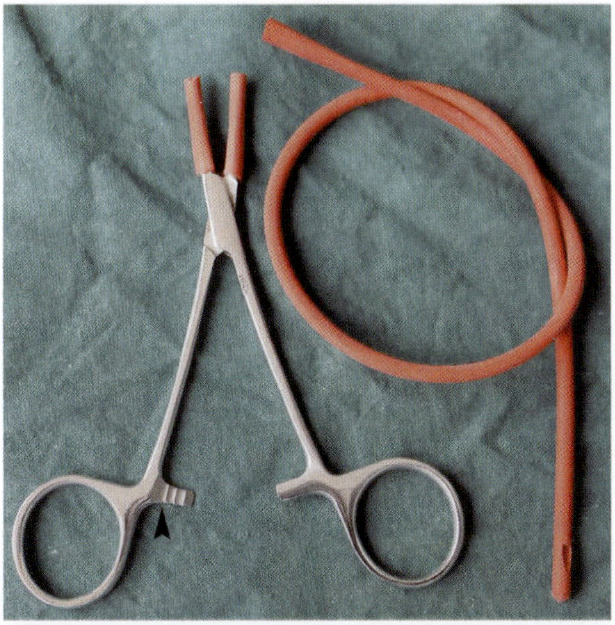

Figure 1. The special devise for the operation. A mosquito hemostat with curved tips and full teeth, which were shielded by a segment of rubber single Nelaton Catheter. (Black arrowhead: the second ratchet of the hemostat).

Then, the injured bowel was return into the abdominal cavity gently, and Bupivacaine (0.25%, 1.5 ml; Mintong, Zhuhai, China) was infiltrated into the abdominal wound for postoperative analgesia. Finally, close the peritoneum, fasciae and abdominal musculature applying simple running sutures, and close the skin applying simple interrupted sutures, using 4–0 silk nonabsorbable surgical suture (Cangsong, Shanghai, China) [10]. All procedures were finished with 10 minutes.

Postoperatively, the rats were transferred to individual cages, given O_2 by mask and infrared warming lamp irradiation until they were awake and moving. Rats were fasted for 24 hours, but free to water. No other analgesic and antibiotic drugs were given after the operation.

Macroscopical Evaluations

The animals were sacrificed by cervical dislocation after the surgery (0 day), and then on 1st, 3rd, 5th, 7th and 14th day. The abdominal cavity was opened in U-shaped incision and firstly examined for the incidence of intraperitoneal adhesions. The extent and tenacity of the adhesions were graded by two pathologists in a blinded fashion, using two different scoring systems that were respectively described by Nair [11] and Zuhlke [12] (Table 1).

Histological Evaluations

After macroscopical evaluations, specimens of injured duodenum containing adhesion tissues were excised, rinsed with 0.9% Normal Saline (Otsuka, Guangdong, China) and then carefully dissected into two parts. One was for light microscopy; the other was for scanning electron microscopy (SEM).

For light microscopy examination, the samples were immersed in 10% formalin solution (Tianjin Chemical Reagent Company, Tianjin, China) for 24 hours and dehydrated in a graded series of ethanol before embedded in paraffin. Serial sections were stained with Hematoxylin and Eosin (H&E). Each slide was selected five random visual fields (×200) and scored using the following scales (Table 2) [13,14,15], to evaluate the grade of fibrosis, inflammation and neovascularization of adhesion tissues. Immunohistochemistry staining of pan cytokeratin (PCK), vimentin (Vim) and α-smooth muscle actin (α-SMA) was carried out to evaluate the cellular infiltration in the forming process of adhesions (monoclonal mouse antibody, 1:200 dilution; labeled Streptavidin/Peroxidase biotin method, Boster, Wuhan, China), and the control sections were treated with phosphate buffered saline (PBS, PH = 7.0) rather than any of the first antibodies. The fibroblast was positive for PCK and Vim, but negative for α-SMA; nevertheless the myofibroblast stained positive for Vim and α-SMA, and negative for PCK.

All slides were evaluated by two pathologists in a blinded manner with light microscope (LEICA DM4000B, LAS Version 3.7.0, Germany). Image-Pro® Plus v 6.0 For Windows (Media Cybernetics, Silver Spring, Maryland, USA) was also used in the evaluations of Immunohistochemistry staining to account the value of integral optical density of the target areas.

For SEM, the specimens were fixed with 2.5% glutaraldehyde (Sigma-Aldrich, Saint Louis, USA) in PBS for 4 hours, dehydrated in increasing alcohol series, critical point dried (CPD-030, BAL-TEC, Switzerland), sputter coated with gold ion (SCD-005, BAL-TEC, Switzerland). Examination and photographs were obtained with scanning electron microscope (FEI Quanta 200, FEI, and Holland).

Table 1. Scales for macroscopical evaluations.

Score	Extent [11]	Tenacity [12]
0	No adhesions.	No adhesions.
1	Single band of adhesion between viscera or from one viscus to the abdominal wall.	Filmy adhesion, easy to separate by blunt dissection.
2	Two bands, either between viscera or from viscera to the abdominal wall.	Strong adhesion, blunt dissection possible, partly sharp dissection.
3	More than two bands between viscera or from viscera to the abdominal wall.	Stronger adhesion; sharp dissection necessary.
4	Multiple dense adhesions or viscera directly adherent to the abdominal wall, irrespective of number and extent of adhesive bands.	Very strong adhesion between organs; its division by sharp dissection damages organ serosa.

Statistics

Macroscopical and histological scores of intraperitoneal adhesions were expressed as mean±SD, and analysed by one-way ANOVA with post-hoc Bonferroni tests. A P-value<0.05 was considered statistically significant. Analysis was performed using IBM SPSS Statistics version 19 (IBM SPSS, Chicago, Illinois, USA).

Results

Macroscopically, no adhesion was found in all eight rats on 0 day. In other five groups, the incidence of adhesions was 87.5% (7/8) for 1st day, 100% (8/8) for 3rd day, 5th day, 7th day and 14th day. The surgical sites were oncotic and hemorrhagic in the first three days; fibrin appeared and deposited around the injured on 1st day, and filmy adhesions were detected on all rats on 3rd day. The intraperitoneal adhesions always formed among the duodenum, liver, omentum, even the stomach, diaphragma and abdominal wall. The extent of adhesions continuingly expanded till 3rd postoperative day, whereas the tenacity kept strengthening till 5th day (Figure 2).

Under light microscope, the mucosa, submucosa and even smooth muscle of the surgical intestine were damaged by the clamping of the hemostat (0 day). On 1st day, there was marked inflammatory cell infiltration in the injured tissues; and the number of these inflammatory cells decreased from 3rd day till 7th day. The fibrosis of the adhesion tissues developed over time, especially from 3rd day to 5th day after the operation. The neoformative vessels appeared in the adhesion tissues on 3rd day, and its number increased slightly in the following days (Figure 3).

The value of integral optical density of the target areas of Immunohistochemistry staining micrographs were quantified and analyzed by Image-Pro® Plus v6.0 For Windows (Figure 4). PCK was not detected in almost all the samples. Surprisingly, Vim and α-SMA were positive in the fibroblast-like cells with spindle nucleus in adhesion tissues; and their mean value of integral optical density kept increasing till 7th day (Figure 4).

The destruction and regeneration of peritoneal mesothelium covering the surgical sites were clearly demonstrated by SEM imagines (Figure 5). The normal visceral peritoneum covering the duodenum was composed of many flat mesothelial cells. These cells overlapped with each other tightly and with lots of microvilli on their surfaces. The mesothelium on the surgical sites was broken by the clamping trauma on 0 day; the mesothelial cells were swollen and deformed, the microvilli on which were disappeared; the cell junctions were lost and the basement membrane was exposed. Inflammatory cells including macrophages, and red blood cells (RBC) leaked out immediately after the operation. On 1st day, these transudatory cells were enwrapped by deposited fibrin; and blood clots were formed to stop bleeding. Then, on 3rd day, the injured sites adhered to the surrounding organs by fibroin net. The mesothelial cells, with sparse and short microvilli, began to proliferate from the edge of the injury; lots of inflammatory cells and few RBC could also be seen on the injured surface. On 5th day, most parts of the surgical sites were re-covered by mesothelial cells, which overlapped with each other loosely, and with very short microvilli. On 7th day, the mesothelial cells completely overlaid the surgical sites and the adhesion tissues; and on 14th day, the number and length of the microvilli improved significantly, which were rehabilitated to the normal condition.

In summary, the extent and tenacity of intro-peritoneal adhesions reached their peaks on 3rd and 5th days, respectively. The inflammation of the adhesion tissues was most serious on 1st day; the fibrosis and the neovascularization developed slowly from 3rd to 5th day. Myofibroblasts proliferated significantly in the adhesion tissues from 3rd day, which were examined by immunohistochemical method. And the mesothelium covering the surgical sites and the adhesion tissues healed on 7th day.

Discussion

The intraperitoneal adhesions following abdominal surgery remains an ongoing challenge, without ideal products or measures for adhesions reduction. A reliable animal model that allows for

Table 2. Scales for histological (H&E) evaluations [13,14,15].

Scale	Fibrosis	Inflammation	Microvessel density
0	None	None	None
1	Slight	Giant cell or foreign body-macrophages, lymphocytes and plasma cells.	1–3 capillaries
2	Moderate	As score 1 plus polymorphonuclear granulocytes and eosinophils.	4–10 capillaries
3	Severe	Abundant inflammatory cells and microabscesses.	More than 10 capillaries.

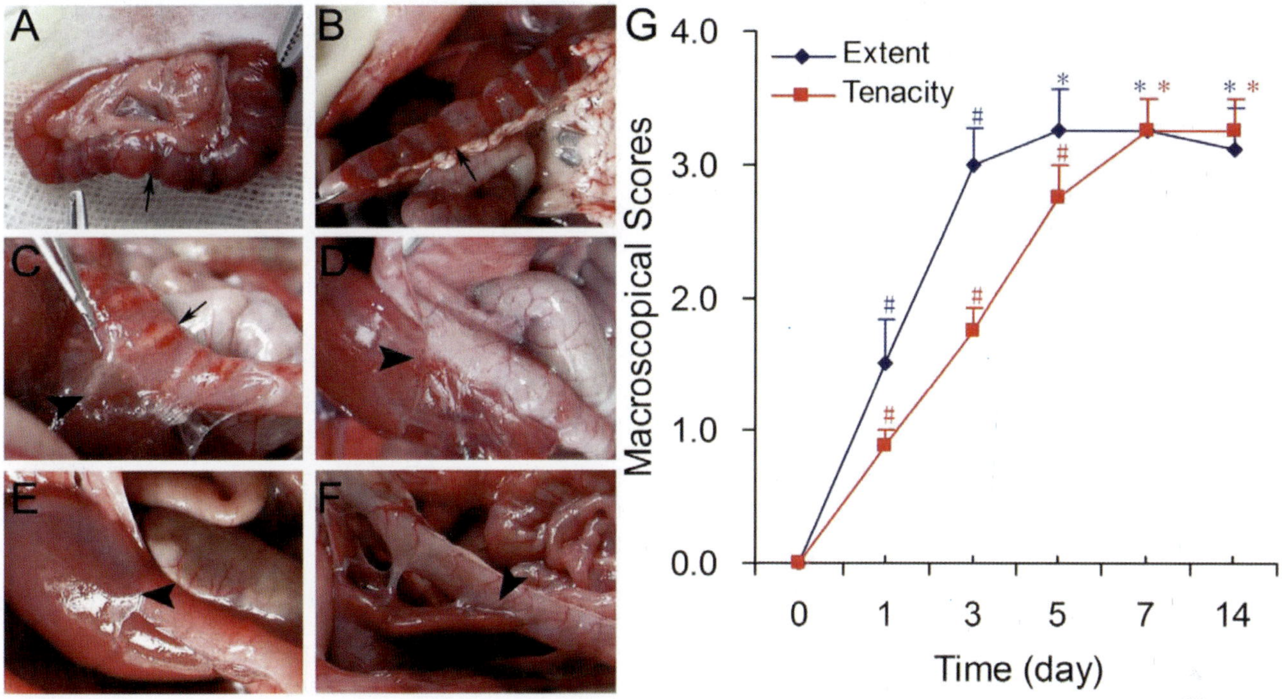

Figure 2. Representative macroscopical photos and adhesion scores. A–F) Macroscopical photos of 0 day, 1st, 3rd, 5th, 7th and 14th day. G) Mean of adhesion scores by macroscopical evaluations in all groups. n = 8, #: $P<0.05$, *: $P>0.05$. Vs. preceding group. (Surgical site: arrow; adhesion: arrowhead).

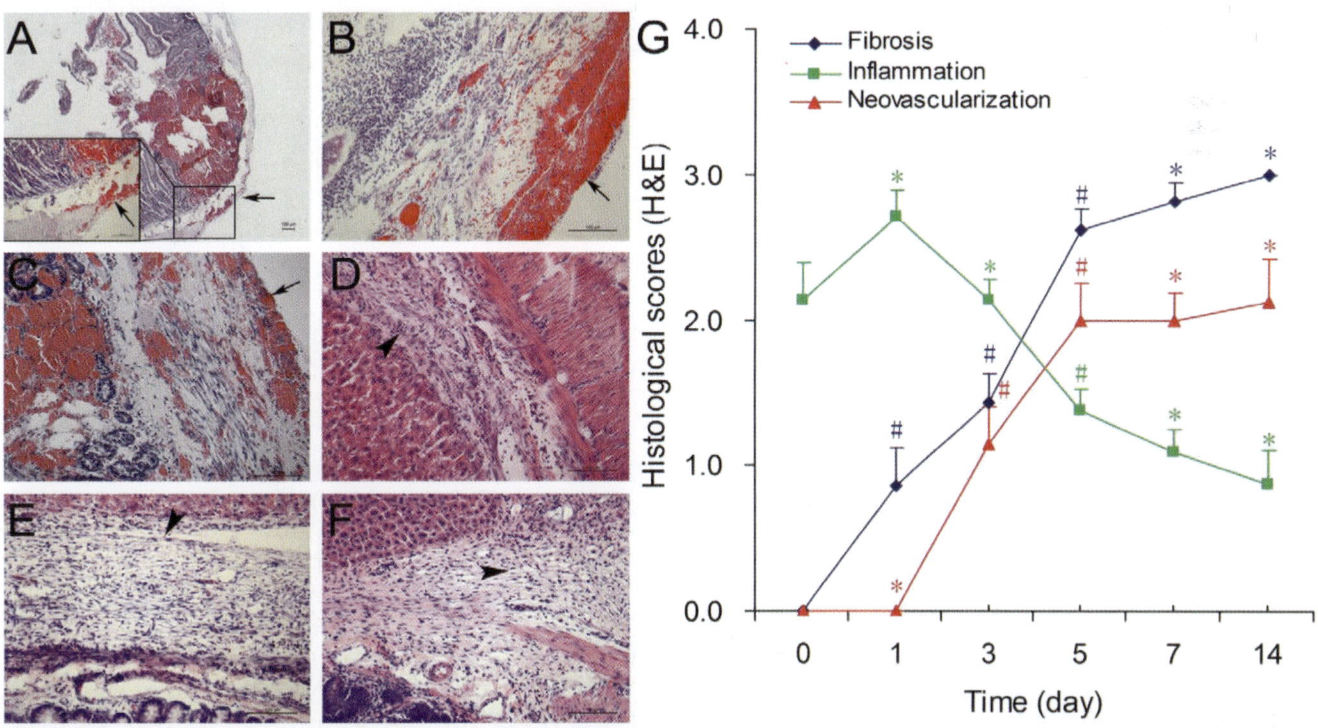

Figure 3. Histological micrographs and scores of fibrosis, inflammation and neovascularization (H&E). A) Micrograph of 0 day (×50, lower left corner; ×200, bar = 100 μm); B–F) Micrographs of 1st, 3rd, 5th, 7th and 14th day (×200, bar = 100 μm. Surgical site: arrow; adhesion: arrowhead). G) Mean of fibrosis, inflammation and neovascularization scores by histological evaluations in all groups. #: $P<0.05$, *: $P>0.05$. Vs. preceding group.

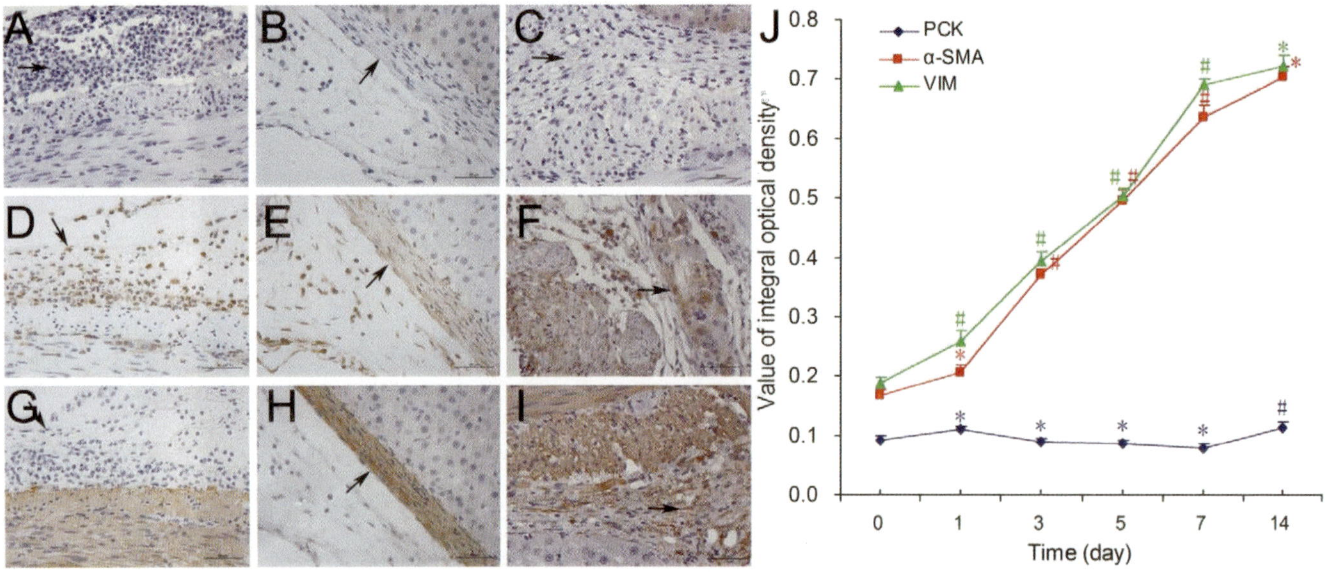

Figure 4. Micrographs of immunohistochemistry staining and the expression of PCK, Vim and α-SMA of 0, 7th and 14th day. Representative immunohistochemistry staining images stained with PCK (A–C), Vim (D–F) and α-SMA (G–I) antibody of 0 day (A, D, G), 7th day (B, E, H), 14th day (C, F, I) (×400, bar = 50 μm, target area: arrow). J) The values of integral optical density for PCK, Vim and α-SMA of 0 7th and 14th day. #: *P*<0.05, *: *P*>0.05. Vs. preceding group.

objective quantification of adhesions is a key component in elucidating the authenticity of various anti-adhesive strategies [16]. This study evaluated a novel animal model of intraperitoneal adhesions, and suggested this rat model induced by duodenum clamping trauma to be consistent, reliable and reproducible.

Methods of intraperitoneal adhesion model include abdominal sidewall defect, cecal abrasion, peritoneal excision or abrasion, uterine horn injuries, and so on [15], but the results are inconsistent. Many proposed adhesion models were criticized because of observer bias and the subjective nature of recording the adhesions characteristics. For example, Gaertner *et al.* evaluated the conventional sidewall models involving cecal abrasion and peritoneal excision or abrasion, and found the classical sidewall models showed inconsistent patterns of adhesions formation and were difficult to evaluate [17]. In addition, although Whang *et al.* suggested the peritoneal button technique to be a most consistent and reproducible technique for intraperitoneal adhesion model [16]; some researchers criticized this approach, claiming that the peritoneal button technique leads to exaggerated results when evaluating anti-adhesive measures [18]. Therefore, it is imprecise to deduce definitive conclusions from anti-adhesive proposals if no credible adhesion model is available. A readily reproducible adhesion model will ensure better evaluation of the anti-adhesive measures, because confounding results from the model will be minimized.

In this study, we developed an intraperitoneal adhesion model induced by duodenum clamping trauma. We shielded the hemostat teeth with rubber single lumen Nelaton Catheter to avoid the injury caused by direct collision between the metal teeth, which can lead the injured duodenum to necrosis. Therefore, with this new devise, on the one hand, clamping the duodenum can lead to adequate injury both to duodenal serosa and inner-lumen mucosa, which will result in intraperitoneal adhesions; on the other hand, this clamping trauma is moderate and the model animal can survive with the formation of adhesions. Although the classical sidewall models involving cecal abrasion and peritoneal excision or abrasion popularly used by many investigators [19], it was impossible to accurately control the damage given to each animal, because the area and degree excised or abrased are difficult to keep consistent in all animals, and the adhesions can not be scored exactly [17]. However, on the duodenum clamping trauma rat model, the adhesions always formed among the duodenum, liver and omentum, which were more stable and easily to score because of the standardized and controllable surgical procedures.

In addition, adhesions secondary to operations in upper abdominal region occurred more frequently in recent years, due to the increase of surgical treatments on diseases of liver, gall and pancreas [20]. But most of the previous adhesion models focus on adhesions in lower abdominal region and pelvic cavity, such as the classical sidewall defect model and the uterine horn injuries model. The rat model we recommended is accurately located on the duodenum, which imitates the adhesions in the upper abdominal region.

The peritoneal mesothelium is a highly specialized monolayer of polarized flat epithelial cells that covering the entire surface of the abdominal cavity. It serves as a protective anatomical barrier, as a non-adhesive frictionless interface for the movement of abdominal organs and is involved in the formation and turnover of abdominal fluid [21,22]. Injury to the peritoneum is often associated with structural and functional alterations of the mesothelium, which may result in peritoneal healing and adhesions formation [23]. Histopathogenesis of inflammation and repair of the mesothelium are involved in the process of adhesions formation. Moreover, postoperative peritoneal adhesions are considered as a consequence of redundant fibrin formation and insufficient fibrinolytic activity in response to enhanced inflammatory status revoked by peritoneal impairment [24]. Under normal conditions, the generation and degradation of fibrin could be a dynamic balance, which was broken under pathological conditions [25].

In our present model, the damage to the duodenum was accurately located and carried out by hemostat-clamping, leading to the injured sites congestive and swollen when the operation was

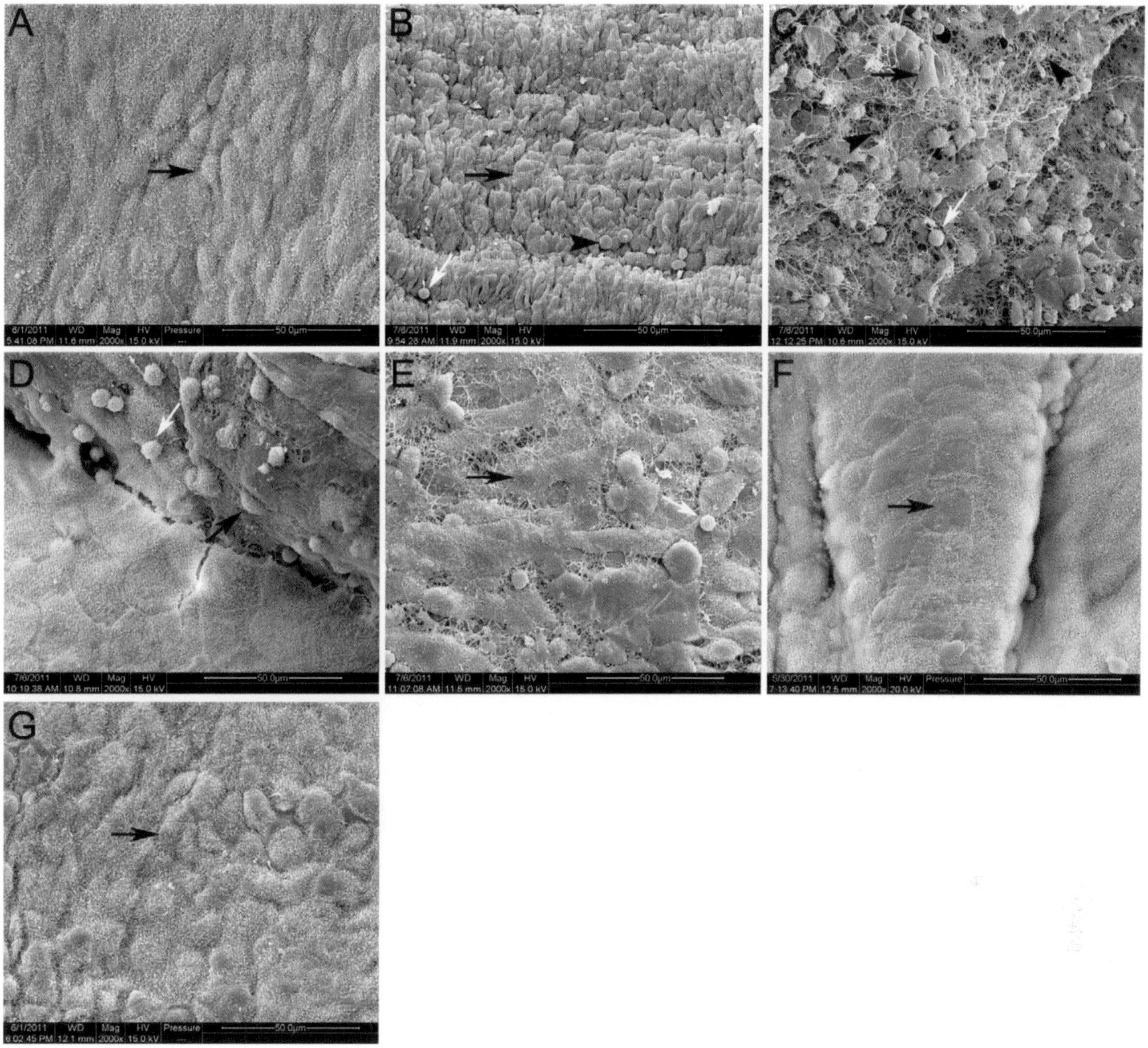

Figure 5. SEM images of mesothelium covering the duodenum and adhesion tissues. A) Normal control from additional rats. B–G) Micrographs showed the destruction and regeneration of the mesothelium on 0 day, 1st, 3rd, 5th, 7th and 14th day (×2000, bar = 50 μm. Mesothelial cell: black arrow; RBC: black arrowhead; inflammatory cell: white arrow).

finished. Local inflammatory response was triggered in the clamping sites, resulting in fibrin-rich exudates formed nearby [26]. Simultaneously, the mesothelial monolayer covering the duodenum was damaged seriously. The mesothelial cells lost their original form and cell junctions, and infiltrated by inflammatory cells on 1st postoperative day, which was confirmed by diZerega [27]. The fibrin deposited on the damaged areas contributing to hemostasis and tissue repair of the injury. Nevertheless, if not degradated by 3rd day, the deposited fibrin became filmy adhesion tissues connecting the injured duodenum and the adjacent organs or tissues, such as the liver, the omentum and the abdominal wall. Some people believed that adhesions formation occurred when two injured peritoneal surfaces were apposed [27,28]. However, in this new adhesion model, adhesions formed between the injured duodenum and the surrounding tissues, which were protected in the operation. There were two possibilities about this phenomenon: the first one is the surfaces of the adjacent tissues are destroyed by the local inflammation; the second one is that the adhesions form once one of the apposed surfaces is injured.

From 1st postoperative day, lots of fibroblast-like cells with spindle nucleus intruded into the deposited fibrin and proliferated, bringing about more extracellular matrix (ECM) including collagen [27]. New blood vessels appeared in adhesion tissues from 3rd postoperative day [29]. At the same time, the range of adhesions enlarged very slowly; in contrast, the strength needed to separate the adhesions increased greatly. On the SEM photomicrograph of 1st day, various inflammation cells appeared on the injured surface, simultaneously with a lot of elongated, flattened, irregularly shaped cells [30,31]. These mesothelial cells, which connected with each other loosely, covered most part of the injured surface on 5th day; but their microvilli were still very sparse and short.

On 7th day, the adhesions were too strong to be separated by blunt dissection. The adhesion tissues were full of fibroblast-like cells [27]. New vessels of different diameters presented. The number of mesothelial cells increased significantly compared with 5th day; they completely overlaid the injured surface, regularly and tightly, although the microvilli on which were still very short. On 14th day, the macroscopical and histological evaluations changed little compared to 7th day, except that the microvilli of the mesothelial cells were more and longer, similar to the normal [31,32].

Here we got a question: what were the fibroblast-like cells in the adhesion tissues? For a long time, fibroblasts were considered to be the main cells that secrete fibrin and transform deposited fibrin into fibrous, permanent adhesions [27,32,33,34]. In our experiment, immunohistochemistry staining of PCK, Vim and α-SMA was employed to validate this hypothesis. However, the results showed that it's myofibroblasts who proliferated prominently in the adhesion tissues.

In fact, the myofibroblast is a special form of fibroblast, characteristically expressing α-SMA$^+$and acquisition of contractile features. It can be differentiated form multiple sources, such as local primary producers, epithelial cells, mesenchymal cells and endothelial cells, when stimulated by cytokines and mechanical tension in wound healing [35,36,37]. During the acute inflammation period after operation, a variety of cytokines and chemotactic factors were secreted into the ECM. Myofibroblast progenitors proliferated and migrated within provisional matrix of the wound clot containing the platelet-derived growth factor, and transformed into myofibroblasts by transforming growth factor beta, which could induce myofibroblasts decreasing by apoptosis in normal wound healing [38,39,40]. However, under many pathological situations, myofibroblasts persisted and continued to remodel the ECM by synthesizing ECM components such as collagen types I and III, resulted in adhesions formation or even fibrosis of organs [41]. And in patients after surgery, postoperative complications such as abdominal pain, vomiting, and adhesive illus may relate to the contractile feature of myofibroblast.

In conclusion, clamping trauma to the duodenum can induce significant postoperative intraperitoneal adhesions formation, which represents an ideal animal model for intraperitoneal adhesions research and prevention. And myofibroblasts may play an important role in the forming process.

Author Contributions

Conceived and designed the experiments: XW HL JB. Performed the experiments: DL JB LC. Analyzed the data: JB. Contributed reagents/materials/analysis tools: DL HL. Wrote the paper: JB HL.

References

1. Arung W, Meurisse M, Detry O (2011) Pathophysiology and prevention of postoperative peritoneal adhesions. World J Gastroenterol 17: 4545–4553.
2. Liakakos T, Thomakos N, Fine PM, Dervenis C, Young RL (2001) Peritoneal adhesions: Etiology, pathophysiology, and clinical significance - Recent advances in prevention and management. Digestive Surgery 18: 260–273.
3. Hellebrekers BW, Kooistra T (2011) Pathogenesis of postoperative adhesion formation. Br J Surg 98: 1503–1516.
4. Ellis H, Moran BJ, Thompson JN, Parker MC, Wilson MS, et al. (1999) Adhesion-related hospital readmissions after abdominal and pelvic surgery: a retrospective cohort study. Lancet 353: 1476–1480.
5. Lauder CI, Garcea G, Strickland A, Maddern GJ (2010) Abdominal adhesion prevention: still a sticky subject? Dig Surg 27: 347–358.
6. Harris ES, Morgan RF, Rodeheaver GT (1995) Analysis of the kinetics of peritoneal adhesion formation in the rat and evaluation of potential antiadhesive agents. Surgery 117: 663–669.
7. Johns A (2001) Evidence-based prevention of post-operative adhesions. Hum Reprod Update 7: 577–579.
8. Duron JJ (2007) Postoperative intraperitoneal adhesion pathophysiology. Colorectal Dis 9 Suppl 2: 14–24.
9. Brochhausen C, Schmitt VH, Planck CN, Rajab TK, Hollemann D, et al. (2012) Current strategies and future perspectives for intraperitoneal adhesion prevention. J Gastrointest Surg 16: 1256–1274.
10. Mingsan M, Feipeng Z (2007) Animal model commonly used in medicine research. Beijing: People's medical publishing house. 604 p.
11. Nair SK, Bhat IK, Aurora AL (1974) Role of proteolytic enzyme in the prevention of postoperative intraperitoneal adhesions. Archives of surgery (Chicago, Ill. : 1960) 108: 849–853.
12. Zuhlke HV, Lorenz EM, Straub EM, Savvas V (1990) Pathophysiology and classification of adhesions. Langenbecks Arch Chir Suppl II Verh Dtsch Ges Chir: 1009–1016.
13. Lalountas M, Ballas KD, Michalakis A, Psarras K, Asteriou C, et al. (2012) Postoperative adhesion prevention using a statin-containing cellulose film in an experimental model. British Journal of Surgery: 423–429.
14. Irkorucu O, Ferahkose Z, Memis L, Ekinci O, Akin M (2009) Reduction of postsurgical adhesions in a rat model: a comparative study. Clinics (Sao Paulo) 64: 143–148.
15. Durmus AS, Yildiz H, Yaman M, Simsek H (2011) The effects of heparin and pentoxifylline on prevention of intra-abdominal adhesions in rat uterine horn models : histopathological. Revue: 198–203.
16. Whang SH, Astudillo JA, Sporn E, Bachman SL, Miedema BW, et al. (2011) In search of the best peritoneal adhesion model: comparison of different techniques in a rat model. J Surg Res 167: 245–250.
17. Gaertner WB, Hagerman GF, Felemovicius I, Bonsack ME, Delaney JP (2008) Two experimental models for generating abdominal adhesions. J Surg Res 146: 241–245.
18. Ozel H, Avsar FM, Topaloglu S, Sahin M (2005) Induction and assessment methods used in experimental adhesion studies. Wound Repair Regen 13: 358–364.
19. Diamond MP, Linsky CB, Cunningham T, Constantine B, DiZerega GS, et al. (1987) A model for sidewall adhesions in the rabbit: reduction by an absorbable barrier. Microsurgery 8: 197–200.
20. Beckingham IJ, Krige JE (2001) ABC of diseases of liver, pancreas, and biliary system: Liver and pancreatic trauma. BMJ 322: 783–785.
21. Chegini N (2002) Peritoneal molecular environment, adhesion formation and clinical implication. Front Biosci 7: e91-e115.
22. Elkins TE, Stovall TG, Warren J, Ling FW, Meyer NL (1987) A histologic evaluation of peritoneal injury and repair: implications for adhesion formation. Obstet Gynecol 70: 225–228.
23. Stadlmann S, Raffeiner R, Amberger A, Margreiter R, Zeimet AG, et al. (2003) Disruption of the integrity of human peritoneal mesothelium by interleukin-1beta and tumor necrosis factor-alpha. Virchows Arch 443: 678–685.
24. Herington JL, Crispens MA, Carvalho-Macedo AC, Camargos AF, Lebovic DI, et al. (2011) Development and prevention of postsurgical adhesions in a chimeric mouse model of experimental endometriosis. Fertil Steril 95: 1295–1301.
25. Ellis H (1971) The cause and prevention of postoperative intraperitoneal adhesions. Surgery, gynecology & obstetrics 133: 497–511.
26. DiZerega GS (1997) Biochemical events in peritoneal tissue repair. Eur J Surg Suppl: 10–16.
27. DiZerega GS, Campeau JD (2001) Peritoneal repair and post-surgical adhesion formation. Hum Reprod Update 7: 547–555.
28. Haney AF, Doty E (1994) The formation of coalescing peritoneal adhesions requires injury to both contacting peritoneal surfaces. Fertil Steril 61: 767–775.
29. Bigatti G, Boeckx W, Gruft L, Segers N, Brosens I (1995) Experimental model for neoangiogenesis in adhesion formation. Hum Reprod 10: 2290–2294.
30. Baptista ML, Bonsack ME, Felemovicius I, Delaney JP (2000) Abdominal adhesions to prosthetic mesh evaluated by laparoscopy and electron microscopy. J Am Coll Surg 190: 271–280.
31. Maciver AH, McCall MD, Edgar RL, Thiesen AL, Bigam DL, et al. (2011) Sirolimus drug-eluting, hydrogel-impregnated polypropylene mesh reduces intra-abdominal adhesion formation in a mouse model. Surgery 150: 907–915.
32. Yang B, Gong C, Zhao X, Zhou S, Li Z (2012) Preventing postoperative abdominal adhesions in a rat model with PEG-PCL-PEG hydrogel. International Journal: 547–557.
33. Lucas PA, Warejcka DJ, Young HE, Lee BY (1996) Formation of abdominal adhesions is inhibited by antibodies to transforming growth factor-beta1. J Surg Res 65: 135–138.
34. Zhou J, Elson C, Lee TD (2004) Reduction in postoperative adhesion formation and re-formation after an abdominal operation with the use of N, O - carboxymethyl chitosan. Surgery 135: 307–312.
35. Quan TE, Cowper SE, Bucala R (2006) The role of circulating fibrocytes in fibrosis. Current rheumatology reports 8: 145–150.
36. Kalluri R, Neilson EG (2003) Epithelial-mesenchymal transition and its implications for fibrosis. J Clin Invest 112: 1776–1784.
37. Wight TN, Potter-Perigo S (2011) The extracellular matrix: an active or passive player in fibrosis? Am J Physiol Gastrointest Liver Physiol 301: G950–G955.
38. Serini G, Gabbiani G (1999) Mechanisms of myofibroblast activity and phenotypic modulation. EXPERIMENTAL CELL RESEARCH 250: 273–283.

Incidence of Incisional Hernia after Cesarean Delivery

Anna J. M. Aabakke[1]*, Lone Krebs[1], Steen Ladelund[2], Niels J. Secher[3,4]

1 Department of Obstetrics and Gynecology, University of Copenhagen, Holbæk Hospital, Holbæk, Denmark, 2 Clinical Research Center, University of Copenhagen, Hvidovre Hospital, Hvidovre, Denmark, 3 The Research Unit Women's and Children's Health, The Juliane Marie Center, Copenhagen University Hospital, Copenhagen, Denmark, 4 Department of Obstetrics and Gynecology, Aarhus University Hospital, Aarhus, Denmark

Abstract

Objective: To estimate the incidence of incisional hernias requiring surgical repair after cesarean delivery over a 10-year period.

Methods: This population- and register-based cohort study identified all women in Denmark with no history of previous abdominal surgery who had a cesarean delivery between 1991 and 2000. The cohort was followed from their first until 10 years after their last cesarean delivery within the inclusion period or until the first of the following events: hernia repair, death, emigration, abdominal surgery, or cesarean delivery after the inclusion period. For women who had a hernia repair, hospital records regarding the surgery and previous cesarean deliveries were tracked and manually analyzed to validate the relationship between hernia repair and cesarean delivery. Data were analyzed with a competing risk analysis that included each cesarean delivery.

Results: We identified 57,564 women who had had 68,271 cesarean deliveries during the inclusion period. During follow-up, 134 of these women had a hernia requiring repair. Of these 68 (51% [95% CI 42–60%]) were in a midline incision although the transverse incision was the primary approach at cesarean delivery during the inclusion period. The cumulated incidence of a hernia repair within 10 years after a cesarean delivery was 0.197% (95% CI 0.164–0.234%). The risk of a hernia repair was higher during the first 3 years after a cesarean delivery, with an incidence after 3 years of 0.157% (95% CI 0.127–0.187%).

Conclusions: The overall risk of an incisional hernia requiring surgical repair within 10 years after a cesarean delivery was 2 per 1000 deliveries in a population in which the transverse incision was the primary approach at cesarean delivery.

Editor: Katariina Laine, Oslo University Hospital, Ullevål, Norway

Funding: This work was supported by grants from the Faculty of Health, University of Copenhagen (www.sund.ku.dk), The Region Zealand Health Sciences Research Foundation (http://www.regionsjaelland.dk/sundhed/forskning/praktisk%20om%20forskning/sider/den-regionale-forskningsfond.aspx), and Department of Obstetrics and Gynecology, University of Copenhagen, Holbæk Hospital. The funders had no role in study design, data collection and analysis, decision to publish, or preparation of the manuscript.

Competing Interests: The authors have declared that no competing interests exist.

* Email: aabakke@gmail.com

Introduction

Cesarean delivery is the most common surgical procedure in the United States, and the rates are increasing worldwide [1,2]. In the United States, Latin America, Australia, and several European countries cesarean delivery rates are presently above 30% [3–6]. Several studies have found both short- and long-term complications related to cesarean delivery [7–11]. Incisional hernia is a well-known long-term complication of abdominal surgery, with a reported incidence of 3.0–20.6% in association with midline incisions and 0–2.1% with lower transverse incisions [12–19]. Two meta-analyses have confirmed that the risk of developing an incisional hernia after abdominal surgery is higher after a midline than a transverse incision [20,21]. However, only one study, with 6 to 12 months follow-up, has focused on incisional hernia after cesarean delivery [12]. The authors found no incisional hernias after 280 cesarean deliveries performed through a transverse incision. Studies have found that more than 50% of incisional hernias occur more than 1 year after surgery, indicating that the incidence of incisional hernia after cesarean delivery might be underreported [16,22].

The objective of this study was to estimate the incidence of incisional hernias requiring surgical repair after cesarean delivery in a large cohort during a 10-year period.

Materials and Methods

This was a population-based cohort study with data obtained from the Danish National Patient Register and the Danish Medical Birth Register.

In Denmark all in- and out-patient hospital contacts are registered in the Danish National Patient Register established in 1977 and all births in the Danish Medical Birth Register established in 1968 [23,24]. Both registers were administered by the Danish National Board of Health at the time of data extraction. All Danish citizens have a unique personal identification number, and information in the registers is linked to this number. The registers contain information on age, gender, surgical procedure, diagnosis, readmission, and reoperation, but no surgical details (e.g. type of incision and suture material). Surgical procedures have since 1996 been recorded based on codes according to the NOMESCO classification of surgical procedures (a common Nordic classification) [25]. Before 1996, surgical registrations were based on a national classification of treatments and surgical procedures. The completeness of the registration in the Danish National Patient Register is 98–100%, and the validity of the system in terms of the type of surgical procedure has been proven to be high [26–28].

This study was based on a search in the two registries. The main inclusion criterion was a cesarean delivery between January 1, 1991 and December 31, 2000 in women with no history of previous abdominal surgery. Women who had had a cesarean delivery during the inclusion period were identified through the codes for cesarean delivery (sectio_u and, sectio_f [1991–95], and KMCA 10, 11, 12a, 12b [1996–2000]). The cohort was followed from their first cesarean delivery until 10 years after their last cesarean delivery in the inclusion period for an event of hernia repair. Hernia repairs performed during 1991–95 were identified by the codes herniotomia incisionalis (40680), herniotomia ventralis (42400), herniotomia parietis abdominis (40600), hernioplastica cum implantation (40800), hernioplastica cum implantatione laparascopica (40801), and herniotomia (40740, 42900, and no previous diagnosis of inguinal hernia). Hernia repairs during 1996–2000 were identified by the code for surgeries of incisional hernia (KJAD). We registered only the primary hernia repair, and any recurrences were not included. We also registered events of death, emigration, abdominal surgery, and cesarean deliveries during the follow-up period. The surgical codes for hernia repair do not contain information about the anatomical location of the hernia. Therefore, for women with a hernia repair, hospital records of the primary examination, description of surgery, and discharge letter were retrieved as were the descriptions of the previous cesarean deliveries. The records were manually analyzed by two investigators (AA and LK) to validate the relationship between hernia repair and cesarean delivery and to determine the type of incision. When in doubt, consensus was obtained through discussion. Before study initiation, the following exclusion criteria for the hernia repairs were defined: Diastasis recti without hernia, hernia not in the cesarean incision, and no hernia. Cases in which no validation information was accessible were maintained in the cohort as confirmed cases so that the incidence of hernia repair was not falsely underestimated.

Ethics Statement

The results of the study were reported following the STROBE recommendations for strengthening the reporting of observational studies in epidemiology [29].

The study was approved by the Danish Data Protection Agency (reg. no. 2013-41-2155). Ethical approval was not required. Written informed consent was not required and therefore not obtained for the clinical records to be used in the study. However, patient records and the data-set were anonymized before analysis.

Statistics

The cumulative risk of a hernia repair after cesarean delivery was estimated by a competing risk analysis [30]. Each cesarean delivery during the inclusion period was analyzed individually. The competing endpoints that mutually excluded each other were hernia repair, death, abdominal surgery, and a consecutive cesarean delivery. Emigration during the follow-up period caused censoring. Right censoring also occurred after 10 years if the woman did not meet any of the endpoints mentioned above.

Continuous data were analyzed by unpaired t test when normally distributed and by Mann Whitney test when not. Nominal data were analyzed by chi^2 test or, when relevant, Fischer's exact test. P values <0.05 were regarded as statistically significant.

The analyses were performed using R 3.0.2 (R Foundation for Statistical Computing, Vienna, Austria) with the add-on library cmprsk [30], and IBM SPSS Statistics 21 (SPSS Inc., Chicago, IL, USA).

Results

Between January 1991 and December 2000, 57,564 unique women, with no history of previous abdominal surgery, had a total of 68,271 cesarean deliveries. Of these, 158 were identified as having a subsequent hernia repair performed within 10 years after their cesarean delivery within the inclusion period. Analysis of the hospital records excluded 24 cases. Of these, 4 women had a history of previous abdominal surgery, 4 had abdominal surgery after the cesarean delivery but before the hernia repair, one had the hernia repair done coincidently with the including cesarean delivery, 9 hernias were not in the cesarean incision, 5 had diastasis recti without hernia, and 1 had no hernia. A total of 134 cases of hernia repair were included in the analysis. In 20 patients, hospital records from the hernia repair surgery were not available, primarily due to destruction of medical records after 10 years of inactivity. In 68 cases (51% [95% CI 42–59%]) the hernias treated were in a midline incision, in 50 cases (37% [95% CI 29–46%]) in a transverse incision, and in 16 cases (12% [95% CI 7–19%]) in an incision of unknown type due to missing cesarean delivery records. Study design and flow including information on competing events are illustrated in Figure 1. The basic characteristics of the hernia repairs based on type of incision did not differ and are shown in Table 1. There was no change over time in either the frequency of cesarean deliveries resulting in hernia repairs or the distribution of transverse and midline incisions among the hernias requiring hernia repair (data not shown).

The cumulated incidence of a hernia repair within 10 years after a cesarean delivery was 0.197% (95% CI 0.164–0.234%) (Figure 2). The risk of a hernia repair was higher within the first 3 years after a cesarean delivery, with a cumulated incidence at 3 years of 0.157% (95% CI 0.127–0.187%) (Figure 2 and Table 2). Among women who developed an incisional hernia requiring surgical repair the median time from cesarean delivery to repair was 1.36 years (IQR 0.79–2.27 years).

Discussion

This prospective cohort study found a cumulated risk of 0.197% of developing an incisional hernia requiring surgical repair within 10 years after a cesarean delivery. The risk of a hernia repair was higher during the first 3 years after a cesarean delivery.

Less than half of the hernia repairs were performed within the first year after the cesarean delivery (Table 2). Our study thereby confirms previous studies showing that less than half of incisional hernias develop within the first year after surgery [22]. However, it cannot be ruled out that women who developed an incisional hernia within the first year after a cesarean delivery postponed repair of various reasons.

Through validation, we found that the repairs identified in this study were of hernias in both midline and transverse incisions and that more than half of them were of hernias in midline incisions. During the study period, the majority of cesarean deliveries in

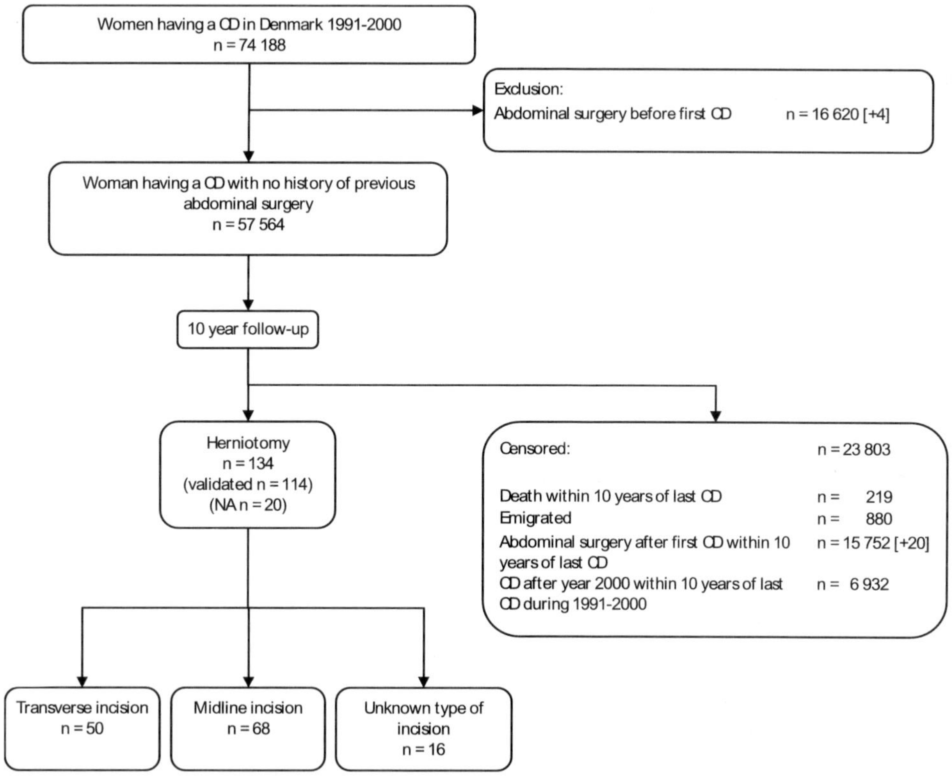

Figure 1. Flow through the study. Number in brackets is number of excluded and censored cases found through validation. CD: cesarean delivery. NA: Not available.

Denmark were performed through a transverse incision, but, unfortunately, the distribution of the two types of incisions during the study period is unknown. We therefore can only try to make an estimate of the risk of surgical repair of a hernia in transverse incisions based on previously published data: In order not to underestimate the risk, unknown incision types are assumed to be transverse and the following assumptions regarding midline incisions are made. The lowest found incidence of incisional hernia in midline incisions is reported to be 3.0% in gynecological surgeries [13]. Additionally, one study found that 16% of incisional hernias occurring within 10 years of laparotomy are surgically repaired [16]. Based on these findings, surgical hernia repair was performed on 0.48% of all midline incisions in the study population. Under these assumptions surgical repair of transverse incision hernias was performed after 66 of 54.104 cesarean deliveries during a 10 year period corresponding to an overall crude incidence of 0.12%. The risk of a hernia in a transverse incision requiring repair is therefore probably lower than the risk found in this study. Previous studies have found that the risk of developing a hernia in a midline compared with a transverse incision is increased, with odds ratios of 1.68 to 3.33 [20,21]. This difference most likely explains why more than half the hernia repairs in our study were performed on hernias in midline incisions, although the percentage of midline incisions in the cesarean delivery cohort was low. We found no statistically significant differences between the hernia repairs performed in a midline compared with transverse incision regarding time from cesarean delivery to repair, number of previous cesarean deliveries, age at the cesarean delivery, or percentage performed as an emergency procedure.

Factors other than the type of incision have been suggested to influence the development of incisional hernias. The suture material and suture technique used to close the fascia have been shown to affect the risk of incisional hernia in midline incisions. A

Table 1. Basic characteristics of surgical repairs performed on hernias in midline and transverse incisions.

	Transverse incision (n = 50)	Midline incision (n = 68)	*P*
Age at last cesarean delivery before hernia repair (years) [Mean (SD)]	32 (5)	32 (5)	0.836*
Number of cesarean deliveries before hernia repair [Median (IQR)]	1.5 (1.0–2.0)	2.0 (1.0–2.8)	0.139†
Time from cesarean delivery to hernia repair (months) [Median (IQR)]	18.5 (9.6–26.0)	21.7 (11.4–60.8)	0.078†
Acute hernia repair [n (%)]	2 (4.5%)	2 (3.1%)	1.000‡

Data analyzed with *unpaired *t*-test, †Mann Whitney test, and ‡ Fischer's exact test.

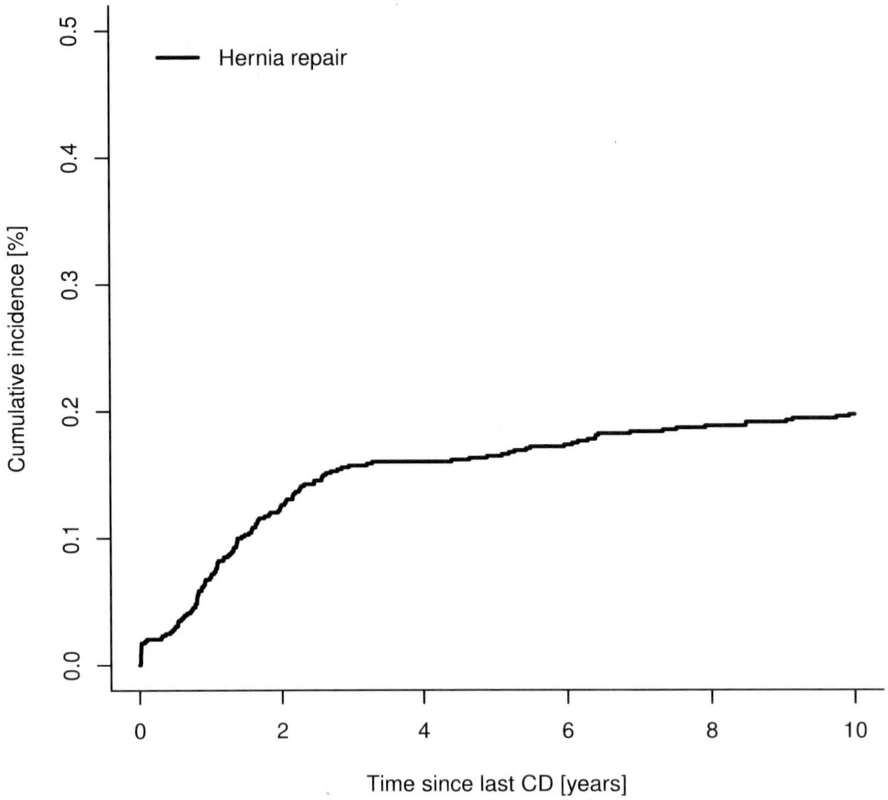

Figure 2. Cumulative incidence of incisional hernias requiring repair after cesarean delivery. CD: cesarean delivery.

suture technique with continuous sutures placed 1 cm apart and 1 cm from the incision using a suture 4 times the length of the incision has been shown to prevent hernias [31]. Additionally, a meta-analysis found that slowly absorbable suture material caused fewer hernias [32]. Unfortunately, there are no studies on closure techniques of the fascia in transverse incisions for cesarean delivery. The risk of incisional hernia after cesarean delivery seems to be so low that randomized trials with incisional hernia as the primary outcome would need a very large number of participants and at least 3 years of follow-up. And unfortunately, two current multifactorial randomized trials with long-term follow-up after cesarean delivery are not exploring methods to close the fascia [33,34]. The development of incisional hernias may also be influenced by factors such as BMI and post-cesarean complications including infection. Unfortunately these variables were not available in the Danish registers during the study period and were not uniformly registered in the available medical records, and could therefore not be included in this analysis. A case-control study could theoretically evaluate differences in various risk factors between cases with a hernia repair and a control group. However, since data about BMI, post-operative infection, and surgical technique for fascial closure were not consistently registered in the records in the 1990s, the study would only be able to add information about risk differences due to incision type and confirm previously estimated odds ratios.

This is the largest study to date that gives an estimate of the risk of developing an incisional hernia requiring repair after cesarean delivery and the first study with a follow-up time of more than 1 year. However, the study has some limitations that need to be considered. Register studies are dependent on the rate, completeness, and accuracy of the registration. Both the registration rate and the validity of type of surgical procedures in the Danish National Patient Register have been shown to be high, and we assume that our data are representative [26–28]. The surgical codes for hernia repair do not contain information about anatomical location of the hernia explaining the relatively high rate of hernia repairs that were found to be unrelated to a previous cesarean delivery through validation. We excluded women with previous abdominal surgery from our cohort, and there may have been some cases of hernia repairs after a cesarean delivery in this group. However, it is unlikely that the incidence is different in the excluded group compared with our cohort, and thus exclusion of these women should not have affected our results.

Table 2. Cumulative incidence of incisional hernias requiring surgical repair 1, 3, and 10 years after a cesarean delivery.

	1 year	3 years	10 years
Hernia repair	0.072 (0.052–0.092)	0.157 (0.127–0.187)	0.197 (0.164–0.231)

Data are expressed as % (95% confidence interval).

The Danish National Patient Register was established in 1977, and patients with abdominal surgeries performed before 1977 could not be identified and excluded from our cohort. Additionally, we excluded some cases of hernia repair in the process of validation due to the identification of previous abdominal surgeries. This may have caused us to underestimate the actual incidence of hernia repair after cesarean delivery. But there are also some factors that may have led to an overestimation of the actual incidence of hernia repair after cesarean delivery. During the process of validation, a number of hospital records were not retrievable. We maintained these unconfirmed cases in the cohort in order to avoid underestimation. Additionally, more than half the repairs were of hernias in midline rather than transverse incisions, the latter being the preferred incision for cesarean delivery in the Western world [35]. Unfortunately, the distribution of the two types of incisions in Denmark in the 1990s is unknown, although the transverse incision was the incision of choice. We were therefore not able to separately estimate the risk of a hernia repair in the two types of incisions.

The risk of developing an incisional hernia after a cesarean delivery that does not require repair was not investigated in this study. The validity of diagnostic codes in the Danish registries have been shown to be poor [36,37] and we therefore selected the surgical code of hernia repair. Medical treatment is free in Denmark and we therefore assume that clinically important incisional hernias were treated surgically due to the risk of serious adverse events (e.g. incarceration). But small hernias may be left un-treated, and thus the risk of an incisional hernia might be higher than the risk of surgical hernia repair found in this study.

In conclusion, this study found that the overall risk of having an incisional hernia requiring repair within 10 years of a cesarean delivery was 2 per 1000 cesarean deliveries. Most hernias were in midline incisions in a population in which the transverse incision was the primary approach at cesarean delivery. Consequently the risk of developing a hernia in a transverse cesarean incision following current surgical recommendations is very low and should not restrict the use of cesarean delivery.

Acknowledgments

We thank Steen Rasmussen, University of Copenhagen, Hvidovre Hospital for his assistance with data management. He was paid for the service through project funds.

Edwin Stanton Spencer edited the language in the article and was paid for the service through project funds.

Author Contributions

Conceived and designed the experiments: AA LK SL NJS. Performed the experiments: AA LK SL. Analyzed the data: AA SL. Contributed reagents/materials/analysis tools: SL AA. Contributed to the writing of the manuscript: AA.

References

1. Berghella V, Baxter JK, Chauhan SP (2005) Evidence-based surgery for cesarean delivery. Am J Obstet Gynecol 193: 1607–1617.
2. (2006) National Institutes of Health state-of-the-science conference statement: Cesarean delivery on maternal request March 27–29, 2006. Obstet Gynecol 107: 1386–1397.
3. EURO-PERISTAT (2012) European Perinatal Health Report. Health and Care of Pregnant Women and Babies in Europe in 2010. Available: http://www europeristat com/images/doc/Peristat%202013%20V2 pdf. Accessed 10 March 2014.
4. Villar J, Valladares E, Wojdyla D, Zavaleta N, Carroli G, et al. (2006) Caesarean delivery rates and pregnancy outcomes: the 2005 WHO global survey on maternal and perinatal health in Latin America. Lancet 367: 1819–1829.
5. Martin JA, Hamilton BE, Ventura SJ, Osterman MJK, Mathew T J (2013) Births: Final data for 2011. Hyattsville, MD: National Center for Health Statistics. Available: http://www.cdc.gov/nchs/data/nvsr/nvsr62/nvsr62_01. pdf. Accessed 20 February 2014.
6. Li Z, Zeki R, Hilder L, Sullivan E A (2013) Australia's mothers and babies 2011. Perinatal Statistics series no. 28. Cat.no. PER 59. Canberra: Australian Institute of Health and Welfare, National Perinatal Epidemiology and Statistics Unit. Available: http://www.aihw.gov.au/WorkArea/DownloadAsset. aspx?id=60129545698. Accessed 20 February 2014.
7. Silver RM (2012) Implications of the First Cesarean: Perinatal and Future Reproductive Health and Subsequent Cesareans, Placentation Issues, Uterine Rupture Risk, Morbidity, and Mortality. Seminars in Perinatology 36: 315–323.
8. Liu S, Liston RM, Joseph KS, Heaman M, Sauve R, et al. (2007) Maternal mortality and severe morbidity associated with low-risk planned cesarean delivery versus planned vaginal delivery at term. CMAJ 176: 455–460.
9. Schneider KT (2002) [Cesarean section on demand–must risk of morbidity be considered?]. Gynakol Geburtshilfliche Rundsch 42: 12–14.
10. Souza JP, Gulmezoglu A, Lumbiganon P, Laopaiboon M, Carroli G, et al. (2010) Caesarean section without medical indications is associated with an increased risk of adverse short-term maternal outcomes: the 2004–2008 WHO Global Survey on Maternal and Perinatal Health. BMC Med 8: 71.
11. Villar J, Carroli G, Zavaleta N, Donner A, Wojdyla D, et al. (2007) Maternal and neonatal individual risks and benefits associated with caesarean delivery: multicentre prospective study. BMJ 335: 1025.
12. Adesunkanmi AR, Faleyimu B (2003) Incidence and aetiological factors of incisional hernia in post-caesarean operations in a Nigerian hospital. J Obstet Gynaecol 23: 258–260.
13. Biswas KK (1973) Why not Pfannenstiel's incision? Obstet Gynecol 41: 303–307.
14. Israelsson LA, Jonsson T (1996) Incisional hernia after midline laparotomy: a prospective study. Eur J Surg 162: 125–129.
15. Luijendijk RW, Jeekel J, Storm RK, Schutte PJ, Hop WC, et al. (1997) The low transverse Pfannenstiel incision and the prevalence of incisional hernia and nerve entrapment. Ann Surg 225: 365–369.
16. Mudge M, Hughes LE (1985) Incisional hernia: a 10 year prospective study of incidence and attitudes. Br J Surg 72: 70–71.
17. Seiler CM, Bruckner T, Diener MK, Papyan A, Golcher H, et al. (2009) Interrupted or continuous slowly absorbable sutures for closure of primary elective midline abdominal incisions: a multicenter randomized trial (INSECT: ISRCTN24023541). Ann Surg 249: 576–582.
18. Veljkovic R, Protic M, Gluhovic A, Potic Z, Milosevic Z, et al. (2010) Prospective clinical trial of factors predicting the early development of incisional hernia after midline laparotomy. J Am Coll Surg 210: 210–219.
19. Wissing J, van Vroonhoven TJ, Schattenkerk ME, Veen HF, Ponsen RJ, et al. (1987) Fascia closure after midline laparotomy: results of a randomized trial. Br J Surg 74: 738–741.
20. Brown SR, Goodfellow PB (2005) Transverse verses midline incisions for abdominal surgery. Cochrane Database Syst Rev 4: CD005199.
21. Grantcharov TP, Rosenberg J (2001) Vertical compared with transverse incisions in abdominal surgery. Eur J Surg 167: 260–267.
22. Hoer J, Lawong G, Klinge U, Schumpelick V (2002) [Factors influencing the development of incisional hernia. A retrospective study of 2,983 laparotomy patients over a period of 10 years]. Chirurg 73: 474–480.
23. Lynge E, Sandegaard JL, Rebolj M (2011) The Danish National Patient Register. Scand J Public Health 39: 30–33.
24. Knudsen LB, Borlum KF (1986) Monitoring perinatal mortality and perinatal care with a national register: content and usage of the Danish Medical Birth Register. Community Med 8: 29–36.
25. Nordic Medico-Statistical Committee (2010) NOMESCO Classification of Surgical Procedures (NCSP). Available: http://nomesco-eng.nom-nos.dk/filer/ publikationer/NCSP%201_15.pdf. Accessed 13 December 2013.
26. Helgstrand F, Rosenberg J, Kehlet H, Bisgaard T (2011) Low risk of trocar site hernia repair 12 years after primary laparoscopic surgery. Surg Endosc 25: 3678–82.
27. Ottesen M (2009) [Validity of the registration and reporting of vaginal prolapse surgery]. Ugeskr Laeger 171: 404–408.
28. Bay-Nielsen M, Kehlet H, Strand L, Malmstrom J, Andersen FH, et al. (2001) Quality assessment of 26,304 herniorrhaphies in Denmark: a prospective nationwide study. Lancet 358: 1124–1128.
29. Vandenbroucke JP, Elm Ev, Altman DG, Gotzsche PC, Mulrow CD, et al. (2007) Strengthening the Reporting of Observational Studies in Epidemiology (STROBE): explanation and elaboration. Epidemiology 18: 805–835.
30. Gray RJ (1988) A class of k-samle tests for comparing the cumulative incidence of a competing risk. The Annals of Statistics 16: 1141–1154.
31. Jargon D, Friebe V, Hopt UT, Obermaier R (2008) Risk Factors and Prevention of Incisional Hernia - What is Evidence-Based? Zentralbl Chir 133: 453–457.
32. Diener MK, Voss S, Jensen K, Buchler MW, Seiler CM (2010) Elective midline laparotomy closure: the INLINE systematic review and meta-analysis. Ann Surg 251: 843–856.

33. The CORONIS Collaborative Group (2013) CORONIS - International study of caesarean section surgical techniques: the follow-up study. BMC Pregnancy Childbirth 13: 215.
34. The CAESAR study Collaborative Group (2010) Caesarean section surgical techniques: a randomised factorial trial (CAESAR). BJOG 117: 1366–1376.
35. Maaløe N, Aabakke AJM, Secher NJ (2014) Midline versus transverse incision for cesarean delivery in low-income countries. Int J Gynecol Obstet 125: 1–2.
36. Thisted DL, Mortensen LH, Hvidman L, Rasmussen SC, Larsen T, et al. (2014) Use of ICD-10 codes to monitor uterine rupture: validation of a national birth registry. Eur J Obstet Gynecol Reprod Biol 173: 23–28.
37. Lykke JA, Bare LA, Olsen J, Lagier R, Tong C, et al. (2012) Vascular associated gene variants in patients with preeclampsia: results from the Danish National Birth Cohort. Acta Obstet Gynecol Scand 91: 1053–1060.

Predicting Perioperative Venous Thromboembolism in Japanese Gynecological Patients

Masae Ikeda[1]*, Hidetoshi Kan-no[1], Masaru Hayashi[1], Hitomi Tsukada[1], Masako Shida[1], Takeshi Hirasawa[1], Toshinari Muramatsu[1], Yoichi Ogushi[2], Mikio Mikami[1]

1 Department of Obstetrics and Gynecology, Division of Specialized Clinical Science, Tokai University School of Medicine, Isehara, Kanagawa, Japan, **2** Department of Medical Informatics, Division of Basic Medical Science and Molecular Medicine, Tokai University School of Medicine, Isehara, Kanagawa, Japan

Abstract

Objective: To develop a convenient screening method that can predict perioperative venous thromboembolism (VTE) and identify patients at risk of fatal perioperative pulmonary embolism (PE).

Methods: Patients hospitalized for gynecological abdominal surgery (n = 183) underwent hematology tests and multidetector computed tomography (MDCT) to detect VTE. All statistical analyses were carried out using the SPSS software program (PASWV19.0J)

Results: The following risk factors for VTE were identified by univariate analysis: plasmin-alpha2-plasmin inhibitor complex (PIC), thrombin-antithrombin III complex (TAT), and prolonged immobility (all $p<0.001$); age, neoadjuvant chemotherapy (NAC), malignancy, hypertension, past history of VTE, and hormone therapy (all $p<0.01$); and hemoglobin, transverse tumor diameter, ovarian disease, and menopause (all $p<0.05$). Multivariate analysis using these factors revealed that PIC, age, and transverse tumor diameter were significant independent determinants of the risk of VTE. We then calculated the incidence rate of perioperative VTE using PIC and transverse tumor diameter in patient groups stratified by age. In patients aged $\leqq 40$ years, PIC ≥ 1.3 µg/mL and a transverse tumor diameter ≥ 10 cm identified the high-risk group for VTE with an accuracy of 93.6%. For patients in their 50 s, PIC ≥ 1.3 µg/mL identified a high risk of VTE with an accuracy of 78.2%. In patients aged ≥ 60 years, a transverse tumor diameter ≥ 15 cm (irrespective of PIC) or PIC ≥ 1.3 µg/mL identified the high-risk group with an accuracy of 82.4%.

Conclusions: We propose new screening criteria for VTE risk that are based on PIC, transverse tumor diameter, and age. Our findings suggest the usefulness of these criteria for predicting the risk of perioperative VTE and for identifying patients with a high risk of fatal perioperative PE.

Editor: Shannon M. Hawkins, Baylor College of Medicine, United States of America

Funding: These authors have no support or funding to report.

Competing Interests: The authors have declared that no competing interests exist.

* E-mail: ikedam@tokai-u.jp

Introduction

Venous thromboembolism (VTE) is a serious preventable complication of gynecological surgery and it has been known for decades that acute pulmonary embolism (PE) is relatively frequent in postoperative gynecological patients. VTE, comprising deep venous thrombosis (DVT) and PE, does not generally present with specific symptoms or findings and there are no simple definitive diagnostic procedures for these conditions. A recent study demonstrated the globally inadequate provision of VTE prophylaxis for acute inpatients [1]. Thus, there is a high incidence of VTE during hospitalization and it is still among the major postoperative complications and causes of death, even in the present era of supposedly advanced prophylaxis, diagnosis, and treatment.

Measurement of D-dimer is widely used at present. This test is highly sensitive and can accurately exclude VTE, but it has a low specificity and low positive predictive value, so patients with high D-dimer levels do not always have VTE [2]. Therefore, while measurement of D-dimer can be used to exclude VTE, it is necessary to find a new marker to reliably detect perioperative VTE.

Accordingly, the purpose of this study was to develop a convenient screening method that could predict perioperative VTE and identify patients with a high risk of fatal perioperative PE based on preoperative laboratory parameters, imaging findings, and patient background characteristics.

Materials and Methods

The subjects were 183 ethnic Japanese patients who were admitted to Tokai University Hospital for planned gynecological abdominal surgery between October 2002 and March 2006. The patients underwent laboratory tests and multidetector computed tomography (MDCT) to detect VTE within two weeks before laparotomy, and MDCT was repeated prior to walking on the first

Table 1. Characteristics of the 183 patients.

Characteristic	Mean ± SD
Age (years)	48.06±13.34
Body mass index (kg/m^2)	23.21±3.87
Thrombin-antithrombin III complex (ng/mL)	6.53±8.73
Plasmin-alpha2-plasmin inhibitor complex (μg/mL)	1.22±1.56
Hemoglobin (g/dL)	12.15±1.77
Hematocrit (%)	37.43±5.05
Platelet count (×10^4/μL)	27.11±8.67
Mean platelet volume (fl)	10.01±0.78
International normalized ratio	0.99±0.10
Longitudinal tumor diameter (cm)	11.35±5.80
Anteroposterior tumor diameter (cm)	9.23±4.41
Transverse tumor diameter (cm)	10.69±5.31
Operating time (minutes)	189.43±96.79
Blood loss (ml)	1000.79±1281.79

Abbreviation: SD, Standard Deviation.

day after surgery (Tables 1 and 2). We then followed the prognosis of these patients up to April 2012. Only patients having elective abdominal surgery were enrolled in this study, with those undergoing emergency surgery, laparoscopic procedures, and transvaginal operations being excluded.

The Institutional Review Board for Clinical Research of Tokai University School of Medicine approved this study. Written informed consent was obtained at the time of enrollment and this study was performed in conformity with the Declaration of Helsinki.

To identify risk factors for VTE, the following variables were evaluated by univariate analysis (Mann-Whitney U test) to assess the relation with the risk of VTE occurring: plasmin-alpha2-plasmin inhibitor complex (PIC) (μg/mL), thrombin-antithrombin III complex (TAT) (ng/mL), age (years), body mass index (BMI) (kg/m^2), hemoglobin (g/dL), hematocrit (%), platelet count (×10^4/μL), mean platelet volume (MPV) (fl), international normalized ratio (INR), longitudinal/transverse/anteroposterior tumor diameters (cm), operating time (min), blood loss (g), malignancy (present/absent), site of lesion (uterus/ovary/others), blood transfusion (yes/no), neoadjuvant chemotherapy (NAC) (yes/no), smoking (yes/no), hypertension (present/absent), diabetes mellitus (present/absent), hyperlipidemia (present/absent), history of VTE (present/absent), varicose veins (present/absent), menopause (yes/no), hormone therapy (yes/no), prolonged immobility (yes/no), and history of malignant disease (present/absent). For measurement of lesion dimensions, endometrial cancer was measured as the uterine body, while the actual dimensions of cervical cancer, ovarian tumors, and solitary uterine myoma were measured. In patients with multiple uterine myomata, the largest transvers diameter of the entire uterus was measured.

Table 2. Characteristics of the 183 patients (continued).

Characteristic	yes	no	
Malignancy	78	105	
Transfusion	74	109	
Neoadjuvant chemotherapy	13	170	
Smoking	20	163	
Hypertension	26	157	
Diabetes	6	177	
Hyperlipidemia	12	171	
History of venous thromboembolism	1	182	
Varicose veins	1	182	
Menopause	67	116	
Hormone replacement therapy	1	182	
Prolonged immobility	2	181	
History of malignancy	4	179	
Lesion	**uterus**	**ovary**	**others**
	106	72	5

Risk factors that were found to be significant by univariate analysis were subsequently assessed by multiple logistic regression analysis with forward selection of variables to identify significant independent determinants of the risk of VTE. Then a screening method for high-risk patients was devised by combining factors that were found to be independently related to the risk of VTE, and its sensitivity and specificity were evaluated by performing receiver operating characteristic (ROC) analysis.

All statistical analyses were carried out using SPSS software (PASWV19.0J).

Results

Of the 183 patients enrolled, 23 patients (12.6%) were found to have VTE by preoperative and/or postoperative MDCT. Eighteen patients (9.8%) had preoperative VTE. DVT was located distal to the popliteal fossa (e.g., in the popliteal, tibial, fibular, or soleal veins) in 7 patients, proximal to the popliteal fossa (e.g., in the femoral or iliac veins, inferior vena cava, or pulmonary artery) in 5 patients, and affected both regions in 6 patients. Five other patients (2.7%) were found to have VTE on postoperative MDCT. None of these 5 patients had any evidence of VTE on preoperatively, but it was found when MDCT was performed prior to walking on the first day after the operation.

Of the 18 patients with preoperative VTE, 13 patients (72.2%) underwent surgery for malignancy, including ovarian cancer in 10 patients (55.6%), endometrial cancer in 2 patients (11.1%), and cervical cancer in 1 patient (5.6%). The other five patients (27.8%) underwent surgery for benign diseases, including uterine myoma in 4 patients (22.2%) and ovarian cyst (5.6%) in 1 patient. Among the 5 patients with postoperative VTE, 3 patients (60%) received surgery for malignancy (all 3 had ovarian cancer) and 2 patients (40%) had surgery for benign disease (both had uterine myoma).

Follow up of the 183 patients was performed between October 2002 and March 2012. Among the18 patients with preoperative VTE, there was one PE-related death (5.6%) while the patient was receiving chemotherapy. Seven patients (38.9%) died of cancer, one of whom developed VTE at three years and ten months postoperatively. The survivors were 5 patients (27.8%) with cancer and 5 patients (27.8%) with benign disease. The five patients who developed postoperative VTE all survived irrespective of whether they had cancer or benign disease. Among all 183 patients, there was one PE-related death (0.55%), while 30 patients (16.4%) died of cancer, one patient (0.55%) died of unknown causes, 51 patients (27.9%) survived with cancer, and 100 patients (54.6%) survived with benign diseases.

Univariate analysis (Mann-Whitney U test) revealed the following significant independent risk factors for VTE: PIC, TAT, and prolonged immobility (all $p<0.001$); age, malignancy, NAC, hypertension, history of VTE, and hormone therapy (all $p<0.01$); and hemoglobin, transverse tumor diameter, ovarian disease, and menopause (all $p<0.05$) (Table 3).

Three factors were judged to be inappropriate for multivariate analysis because of the small sample size (history of VTE, hormone therapy, and prolonged immobility) and one factor was deleted due to unclear criteria (hypertension). Accordingly, multiple logistic regression analysis was performed by the forward selection method using PIC, TAT, hemoglobin, age, transverse tumor diameter, ovarian disease, malignancy, NAC, and menopause as independent variables, while VTE (yes/no) was the dependent variable. This analysis identified PIC ($p<0.001$), transverse tumor diameter ($p<0.01$), and age ($p<0.05$) as significant independent risk factors for VTE (Table 4).

We then calculated the incidence rate of perioperative VTE in our gynecological patients using PIC and transverse tumor diameter stratified by age (Table 5). To devise a convenient algorithm for bedside assessment of VTE risk, we categorized the patients into 4 age groups, which were ≦39 years old, 40–49 years old, 50–59 years old, and ≧60 years old. We also divided PIC into 2 categories (≦1.2 μg/ml and ≧1.3 μg/ml) and transverse tumor diameter into 3 categories (≦9 cm, 10–14 cm, and ≧15 cm).

Because a standard PIC value for diagnosis of VTE has not been established, we used ROC analysis to determine the optimal cut-off value. ROC analysis of the data showed that the optimum sensitivity and specificity were obtained at a PIC value of 1.25 μg/mL, with a sensitivity of 78.3%, specificity of 78.7%, positive predictive value of 78.3%, and area under the ROC curve (ROC-AUC) of 0.816. ROC analysis of the transverse tumor diameter

Table 3. Risk factors for venous thromboembolism.

Factor	p value
Age	0.006
Body mass index	n.s.
Thrombin-antithrombin III complex	0.000
Plasmin-alpha2-plasmin inhibitor complex	0.000
Hemoglobin	0.042
Hematocrit	n.s.
Platelet count	n.s.
Mean platelet volume	n.s.
International normalized ratio	n.s.
Longitudinal tumor diameter	n.s.
Anteroposterior tumor diameter	n.s.
Transverse tumor diameter	0.021
Lesion (uterus/ovary/others)	0.041
Malignancy	0.005
Operating time	n.s.
Blood loss	n.s.
Transfusion	n.s.
Neoadjuvant chemotherapy	0.004
Smoking	n.s.
Hypertension	0.003
Diabetes	n.s.
Hyperlipidemia	n.s.
History of venous thromboembolism	0.008
Varicose veins	n.s.
Menopause	0.010
Hormone replacement therapy	0.008
Prolonged immobility	0.000
History of malignancy	n.s.

Table 4. Results of multiple logistic regression analysis.

Factor	SEM	Probability	Odds Ratio	95% Confidence Interval	
				Lower limit	Upper limit
PIC	0.240	0.000	2.485	1.552	3.977
age	0.020	0.011	1.053	1.012	1.096
Transverse	0.044	0.005	1.130	1.037	1.232

Abbreviation: PIC, Plasmin-alpha2-plasmin inhibitor complex. Transverse, Transverse tumor diameter. SEM, Standard error of the mean (n = 183).

Table 5. Incidence rate of perioperative venous thromboembolism in patients groups stratified by age.

≦39 years old			
		PIC: ≦1.2 μg/mL	PIC : ≧1.3 μg/mL
Transverse: ≦9 cm		1.5%	12.3%
Transverse:10–14 cm		2.6%	19.7%
Transverse: ≧15 cm		8.2%	41.8%
Accuracy	93.6%		
40–49 years old			
		PIC: ≦1.2 μg/mL	PIC : ≧1.3 μg/mL
Transverse: ≦9 cm		1.7%	14.0%
Transverse:10–14 cm		3.0%	22.2%
Transverse: ≧15 cm		8.2%	45.4%
Accuracy	93.6%		
50–59 years old			
		PIC: ≦1.2 μg/mL	PIC : ≧1.3 μg/mL
Transverse: ≦9 cm		2.7%	20.3%
Transverse:10–14 cm		4.6%	30.9%
Transverse: ≧15 cm		12.3%	56.6%
Accuracy	78.2%		
≧60 years old			
		PIC: ≦1.2 μg/mL	PIC : ≧1.3 μg/mL
Transverse: ≦9 cm		4.6%	30.9%
Transverse:10–14 cm		7.8%	44.0%
Transverse: ≧15 cm		19.7%	69.7%
Accuracy	82.4%		

Abbreviation: PIC, Plasmin-alpha2-plasmin inhibitor complex. Transverse, Transverse tumor diameter.

revealed the optimum sensitivity and specificity at a diameter of 10.5 cm, with a sensitivity of 69.6%, specificity of 61.2%, and positive predictive value of 69.6%.

For patients ≦39 years old or aged 40–49 years who had a PIC level ≥1.3 μg/ml and a transverse tumor diameter ≥10 cm, the predicted incidence of perioperative VTE exceeded 20%, and the accuracy of this new screening method was 93.6%. For patients aged 50–59 years with a PIC ≥1.3 μg/ml, the predicted incidence of perioperative VTE was also >20% and the accuracy was 78.2%. For patients ≥60 years old with a transverse tumor diameter ≥15 cm (irrespective of PIC) or those with a PIC ≥1.3 μg/ml, the predicted incidence of perioperative VTE was >20% as well and the accuracy was 82.4%.

Discussion

We devised a new screening method based on PIC, transverse tumor diameter, and age for predicting the risk of perioperative VTE in patients undergoing elective gynecological surgery.

PIC is a marker of the activation of fibrinolysis [3]. Its half-life is about 6 hours and it is a satisfactory indicator of an enhanced fibrinolytic state in vivo, particularly because it is almost undetectable in normal persons. Fibrinolytic activity refers to the so-called secondary fibrinolysis that occurs after a fibrin clot forms in vivo, so elevation of PIC provides evidence of thrombosis [4].

D-dimer is a degradation product of cross-linked fibrin from blood clots and is commonly employed as a highly sensitive (>95%) test for acute VTE that is very accurate for excluding this condition (its negative predictive value is 97%) [5,6]. Measurement of D-dimer is particularly useful to exclude VTE in outpatients [2]. However, this test has a low specificity (30%) and low positive predictive value, which means that patients with high D-dimer levels do not necessarily have VTE [7–9], and there have been reports about no appreciable elevation of D-dimer during the stage of distal thrombus formation in patients with extensive thromboembolism [10–12]. Thus, measurement of D-dimer should only be used for excluding VTE.

Measurement of PIC enables assessment of fibrinolytic activity, and thus is expected to be more useful for the clinical evaluation of perioperative VTE, especially in patients who have a high risk of fatal postoperative PE and no evidence of preoperative VTE. The disadvantage of PIC is that one to two days is required to obtain the result, so this test is not suitable for emergency assessment.

The risk of VTE is strongly associated with age, and its incidence rises sharply with aging. Patients ≦39 years old generally have a low risk of VTE, while patients ≥40 old have a higher risk and the risk increases dramatically in patients ≥60 years old [13,14]. Compared with the general population, the incidence of VTE is five-fold higher in patients aged ≥75 years (10 per 1000). With aging, decreased myodynamia and muscle tone in the lower limbs can lead to failure of venous pump function, resulting in a high rate of VTE in elderly patients [15,16].

Unlike younger patients, elderly patients often do not have typical symptoms and imaging findings of VTE, suggesting that perioperative management needs to be modified according to age [17,18].The majority of preventable deaths for VTE are ascribed to missed or late diagnosis rather than to failure of therapy [19].

Because an intrapelvic mass compresses the pelvic veins, a large ovarian tumor or uterine myoma can cause stasis of blood in the lower extremities, leading to the development of DVT in the venous sinuses of the soleus muscle or in the tibial and peroneal veins. Subsequent damage to the venous valves results in cephalad progression of the thrombus and the formation of free thrombi in the popliteal and femoral vein, which can be followed by the occurrence of PE.

Compared with the longitudinal and anteroposterior directions, compression of the pelvic veins by a mass lesion is more likely to occur in the transverse direction because of the relation to the pelvic bones. Vascular compression increases as a pelvic mass (especially an ovarian tumor) becomes larger, resulting in a high frequency of VTE. The size of a pelvic mass can be easily determined by imaging modalities clinically available to gynecologists.

The mortality of PE in untreated patients is reported to be as high as 30%, but this can be reduced to 2–8% by starting appropriate treatment, such as anticoagulant therapy, at an early stage [20].

Our follow up investigation of 23 patients with perioperative VTE revealed PE-related death during chemotherapy in only one patient, while the other 22 patients died of cancer or survived with malignant or benign diseases, so the cause of death was the primary disease and not VTE. This result emphasizes the importance of accurately diagnosing perioperative VTE at an early stage. If perioperative VTE is accurately diagnosed and treated early, it will generally be possible to prevent fatal PE. To achieve this objective, a convenient method of testing for perioperative VTE and assessing the risk factors for individual patients is essential because a delayed or missed diagnosis can result in death or long-term complications.

In the present study, we calculated the predicted incidence rate of perioperative VTE using the PIC level and the transverse tumor diameter stratified by age. Based on our findings, we propose the following algorithm for preoperative assessment of the risk of VTE.

After measurement of PIC and the transverse tumor diameter for screening, the incidence of VTE is predicted with adjustment for age. When the predicted risk of VTE is 20% or higher, MDCT should be performed within two weeks before surgery and prior to walking on the first postoperative day to detect proximal DVT and/or PE.

The main limitation of our study is that it was not designed to predict the actual incidence rate of perioperative VTE. Our screening method only extracts a high-risk group for perioperative VTE among patients having elective gynecological surgery. In order to actually identify VTE, it is necessary to perform further examinations such as MDCT in the high-risk group. Another limitation of our approach includes lack of data on important clinical symptoms for making a diagnosis of VTE such as pain, swelling, tenderness, and redness of the legs

In conclusion, PIC, transverse tumor diameter, and age are useful factors for predicting the risk of perioperative VTE. The new screening method that we developed is based on these three factors and can identify patients with a high risk of perioperative VTE/fatal PE. It is an easy method for gynecologists to adopt in daily clinical practice.

Acknowledgments

The authors wish to extend their heartfelt gratitude to Mr. Shinichi Yamamoto, M.T. (Tokai University) for his expertise and cooperation with this investigation.

Author Contributions

Conceived and designed the experiments: MI. Performed the experiments: MI HK MH HT MS TH TM MM. Analyzed the data: MI YO. Contributed reagents/materials/analysis tools: MI YO. Wrote the paper: MI.

References

1. Cohen AT, Tapson VF, Bergmann JF, Goldhaber SZ, Kakkar AK, et al. (2008) Venous thromboembolism risk and prophylaxis in the acute hospital care setting (ENDORSE study): a multinational cross-sectional study. Lancet 371: 387–394.
2. Righini M, Perrier A, De Moerloose P, Bounameaux (2008) D-Dimer for venous thromboembolism diagnosis: 20 years later. J Thromb Haemost 6: 1059–1071.
3. Asakura H (2011) Interpretation of hemostatic and fibrinolytic markers. Rinsho Byori 59: 970–977. (in Japanese)
4. Jinnin M, Ihn H, Yamane K, Asano Y, Yazawa N, et al. (2003) Plasmin-α2-plasmin inhibitor complex levels are increased in systemic sclerosis patients with pulmonary hypertension. Rheumatology 42: 240–243.
5. Vermeer HJ, Ypma P, Van Strijen MJ, Muradin AA, Hudig F, et al. (2005) Exclusion of venous thromboembolism: evaluation of D-Dimer PLUS for the quantitative determination of D-dimer. Thromb Res 115: 381–386.
6. Di Nisio M, Squizzato A, Rutjes AW, Büller HR, Zwinderman AH, et al. (2007) Diagnostic accuracy of D-dimer test for exclusion of venous thromboembolism: a systematic review. J Thromb Haemost 5: 296–304.
7. Wells PS (2006) Advances in the diagnosis of venous thromboembolism. J Thromb Thrombolysis 21: 31–40.
8. Caprini JA, Glase CJ, Anderson CB, Hathaway K (2004) Laboratory markers in the diagnosis of venous thromboembolism. Circulation 109: 14–18.
9. Merli GJ (2004) Pulmonary embolism in medical patients: improved diagnosis and the role of low-molecular-weight heparin in prevention and treatment. J Thromb Thrombolysis 18:117–125.
10. Merli G (2005) Diagnostic assessment of deep vein thrombosis and pulmonary embolism. Am J Med (Suppl 8A): 3S–12S.
11. Mansencal N, Joseph T, Vieillard-Baron A, El Hajjam M, Bendaoud M, et al. (2003) Negative D-dimers and peripheral pulmonary embolism. Arch Mal Coeur Vaiss 96: 1143–1148. (in French)
12. Engelberger RP, Aujesky D, Calanca L, Staeger P, Hugli O, et al. (2011) Comparison of the diagnostic performance of the original and modified Wells score in inpatients and outpatients with suspected deep vein thrombosis. Thromb Res 127: 535–539.
13. Geerts WH, Heit JA, Clagett GP, Pineo GF, Colwell CW, et al. (2001) Prevention of venous thromboembolism. Chest 119: 132S–175S.
14. Stein PD, Hull RD, Kayali F, Ghali WA, Alshab AK, et al. (2004) Venous thromboembolism according to age. Arch Intern Med 164: 2260–2265.
15. White RH (2003) The epidemiology of venous thromboembolism. Circulation 107: I-4–I-8.
16. Di Nisio M, Di Iorio A, Porreca E, Abate M, Ferrante N, et al. (2011) Obesity, poor muscle strength, and venous thromboembolism in older persons: the InCHIANTI study. J Gerontol A Biol Sci Med Sci 66A(3): 320–325.
17. Le Gal G, Righini M, Roy PM, Meyer G, Aujesky D, et al. (2005) Differential value of risk factors and clinical signs for diagnosing pulmonary embolism according to age. J Thromb Haemost 3(11): 2457–2464.
18. Siccama RN, Janssen KJ, Verheijden NA, Oudega R, Bax L, et al. (2011) Systematic review: Diagnostic accuracy of clinical decision rules for venous thromboembolism in elderly. Ageing Res Rev. 10(2): 304–313.
19. Fedullo PF, Tapson VF (2003) The evaluation of suspected pulmonary embolism. N Engl J MED 349: 1247–1256
20. Carson JL, Kelley MA, Duff A, Weg JG, Fulkerson WJ, et al. (1992) The clinical course of pulmonary embolism. N. Engl. J. Med. 326: 1240–1245.

Systematic Review of the Literature and Evidence-Based Recommendations for Antibiotic Prophylaxis in Trauma: Results from an Italian Consensus of Experts

Daniele Poole[1]*, Arturo Chieregato[2], Martin Langer[3], Bruno Viaggi[2], Emiliano Cingolani[4], Paolo Malacarne[5], Francesca Mengoli[6], Giuseppe Nardi[4], Ennio Nascimben[7], Luigi Riccioni[4], Ilaria Turriziani[6], Annalisa Volpi[8], Carlo Coniglio[6], Giovanni Gordini[6], on behalf of the Trauma Update Working Group

1 U.O. Anestesia e Rianimazione, Ospedale S. Martino, Belluno, Italy, **2** SOD Anestesia e Area Intensiva CTO, AOU Careggi, Firenze, Italy, **3** Dipartimento di Anestesia e Rianimazione, Fondazione IRCCS Istituto Nazionale dei Tumori e Università degli Studi di Milano, Milano, Italy, **4** UOC Shock e Trauma, AO San Camillo-Forlanini, Roma, Italy, **5** U.O. Anestesia e Rianimazione - P.S., Azienda Ospedaliera Universitaria Pisana, Pisa, Italy, **6** U.O. Rianimazione 118, Ospedale Maggiore, Bologna, Italy, **7** Neurorianimazione Ospedale S. Maria di Ca' Foncello, Treviso, Italy, **8** Anestesia e Rianimazione 1, Azienda Ospedaliero-Universitaria di Parma, Parma, Italy

Abstract

Background: Antibiotic prophylaxis is frequently administered in severe trauma. However, the risk of selecting resistant bacteria, a major issue especially in critical care environments, has not been sufficiently investigated. The aim of the present study was to provide guidelines for antibiotic prophylaxis for four different trauma-related clinical conditions, taking into account the risks of antibiotic-resistant bacteria selection, thus innovating previous guidelines in the field.

Methods: The MEDLINE database was searched for studies comparing antibiotic prophylaxis to controls (placebo or no antibiotic administration) in four clinical traumatic conditions that were selected on the basis of the traumatic event frequency and/or infection severity. The selected studies focused on the prevention of early ventilator associated pneumonia (VAP) in comatose patients with traumatic brain injury, of meningitis in severe basilar skull fractures, of wound infections in long-bone open fractures. Since no placebo-controlled study was available for deep surgical site-infections prevention in abdominal trauma with enteric contamination, we compared 24-hour and 5-day antibiotic prophylaxis policies. A separate specific research focused on the question of antibiotic-resistant bacteria selection caused by antibiotic prophylaxis, an issue not adequately investigated by the selected studies. Randomised trials, reviews, meta-analyses, observational studies were included. Data extraction was carried out by one author according to a predefined protocol, using an electronic form. The strength of evidence was stratified and recommendations were given according to the Grading of Recommendations Assessment, Development and Evaluation (GRADE) criteria.

Results: Uncertain evidence deserving further studies was found for two-dose antibiotic prophylaxis for early VAP prevention in comatose patients. In the other cases the risk of resistant-bacteria selection caused by antibiotic administration for 48 hours or more, outweighed potential benefits.

Conclusions: When accounting for antibiotic-resistant bacteria selection we found no evidence in favour of antibiotic prophylaxis lasting two or more days in the studied clinical conditions.

Editor: Zhi Zhou, Purdue University, United States of America

Funding: The authors have no support or funding to report.

Competing Interests: The authors have declared that no competing interests exist.

* Email: daniele.poole@alice.it

Introduction

In the attempt to investigate antibiotic prophylaxis in several trauma-related clinical conditions, taking into account the potential ecological risk, innovating previous approaches, in February 2013 a meeting of experts was held in Bologna in the context of the 8th edition of the *Trauma Update and Organization* conference.

Infection is the consequence of contamination due to the contact between normally sterile tissues and microorganisms from the external environment or from internal sites. The inoculation occurs when the trauma breaks natural barriers against infections.

All attempts to reduce the bacterial charge in the tissues should be made. Cleaning, irrigation, disinfection of wounds, followed by the appropriate early surgical treatment when indicated, are crucial for infection prevention. Antimicrobial prophylaxis is only one element integrating these interventions and should be limited to the period immediately after the trauma.

One major drawback of exposure to antibiotics is the emergence of drug-resistant bacteria strains, as the result of selection pressure on resistant colonizing strains or on bacteria with newly acquired mutations. Unfortunately, most studies dealing with antibiotic prophylaxis have not adequately investigated this issue, which is particularly relevant in critical care settings where bacterial resistance to antibiotics has become a major problem. Here, we focused on studies comparing antibiotic prophylaxis and placebo in reducing infections in several trauma-related conditions taking into account the risk of antibiotic-resistant bacteria selection to produce a fair risk/benefit ratio assessment, in contrast with other guidelines addressing similar issues [1,2].

In the present paper, we report the contents of the review, the analysis and discussion of the literature, and the conclusions of the conference.

Methods

The works was organized in three sequential steps:

Step 1: The Coordinating Committee formed by five intensivists selected an initial list of topics. Head, thorax, abdomen, and limbs trauma were considered. Because of time constraints (there were only two days to discuss the issues during the convention) only four clinical conditions were selected based on traumatic event frequency and/or infection severity. The scenarios included antibiotic prophylaxis for 1) early VAP in comatose patients, 2) meningitis in severe skull fractures, 3) wound infection in long-bone open fractures (we initially focused on osteomyelitis but found no study specifically investigating this issue), 4) deep surgical-site infections in abdominal trauma with hollow viscus perforation. We also considered but discarded pneumonia in thoracic contusion, empyema after chest tube insertion, surgical-site infection for long-bone closed fractures, infection after soft tissues open injuries, abdominal trauma without bowel perforation, and inhalation pneumonia in pre-hospital intubation.

The Coordinating Committee then generated the queries for the literature search and selected the articles fulfilling the criteria established for each subject. The fundamental criterion, shared by all the investigated issues, was the comparison between adult patients subjected to antibiotic prophylaxis and controls. When such studies were not available comparison between groups receiving different pharmacological protocols were considered.

The MEDLINE database was searched using the free PubMed provider. Randomised trials, reviews, meta-analyses, or observational studies were selected. Pediatric and animal studies, and articles not written in English, were excluded. The MEDLINE search covered a period between January 1970 and January 2014. This search was integrated with the consultation of reference lists of retrieved articles.

The Coordinating Committee members unanimously selected the articles after reviewing the abstracts, with the help of one of the authors with specific expertise in statistics and research methodology. Full-texts were then retrieved and a further selection was carried out.

The statistical and methodological expert also performed data extraction according to a predefined plan (the protocol was not pre-registered), using a dedicated electronic form that automatically performed all planed computations and plot generation. The electronic form was developed *ad hoc* for this revision, and tested and refined using the studies on early VAP prevention with antibiotic prophylaxis.

Data collected included study inclusion criteria, antibiotic class and dose, duration of prophylaxis, antibiotic-resistant bacteria selection when investigated, infection rates, and mortality rates when available, along with information needed for the GRADE evidence quality assessment.

Data were presented as event rates in treatment arms and controls, absolute risks, absolute risk reductions, and relative risks. Adjusted odds ratios were reported when dealing with multivariate analysis results in observational studies. Numbers needed to treat were also calculated. Confidence intervals were computed for all the above measures. Relative risks were graphically represented in Forest plots.

Design heterogeneity among selected studies advised against their combination in meta-analyses. For the same reason statistical approaches to investigate presence of asymmetry and potential publication bias were not carried out [3].

The queries and the results of the summarised results were submitted to the External Scientific Advisory Panel, formed by four intensivists with expertise in the field of infections and trauma in critical care settings, who discussed them together with Coordinating Committee members.

Evidence provided by randomised controlled trials (RCTs) and observational studies was ranked on the basis of the Grading of Recommendations Assessment, Development and Evaluation (GRADE) criteria. [4–6] The GRADE provides a framework to guide reviewers for the assessment of the strength of evidence, taking into account that different reviewers or reviewing groups can evaluate the same evidence differently. [7] Moreover, it eliminates automatic links between the strength of the recommendation and the strength of the evidence, leaving to the reviewers the possibility of grading recommendations based on other variables relevant to clinical decisions, besides evidence.

The GRADE stratifies quality of evidence on a four-level scale, ranging from high to very low, [7], in favour or against intervention. In the middle of this scale an absence of evidence level was added. This event occurs frequently in studies with small sample size, where the alternative hypothesis and statistical power have not been adequately taken into account. In our opinion, negative results from such studies should thus not be considered indicative of no effect, but rather of an unresolved issue [8].

The reporting of RCTs was evaluated on the basis of currently shared standards. [9] We considered quasi-randomised studies, in which treatment allocation is based on non-random methods such as alternation, leading to severe bias in regards to sequence generation and allocation concealment.

Our evaluation of meta-analyses was restrictive, according to the principle that heterogeneity among studies in terms of inclusion criteria, study design, study treatment, type of outcome, which are not accounted for by statistical methods focused on heterogeneity of outcome rates, [10] should contraindicate the merging of their results. [11] When dealing with observational studies we discarded al investigations that reported only crude-data comparisons without performing adjustment for potential confounders.

Step 2: The results were presented to the physicians invited to the symposium - intensivists, infectious disease specialists, surgeons, emergency physicians, radiologists, and physiatrists – and the issues were collectively discussed. The discussion was audio-recorded and at a later stage revised by members of the Coordinating Committee to identify and highlight the main opinions that emerged from the discussion.

Step 3: the scientific advisors and the Coordinating Committee members formed the jury that provided recommendations that were presented as preliminary results on the final day of the conference, but discussed and refined in the following months by e-mail. A final meeting was held one year after the conference, to discuss diverging opinions until unanimity was reached. To develop the recommendations the panel followed the GRADE framework. This is based on four points: quality of evidence, balance between desirable and undesirable effects, values and preferences, uncertainty about whether the intervention represents a wise use of resources [12].

The GRADE initially attributes a high default level of evidence to RCTs and a low level to observational studies. [7] RCTs can then be up- or downgraded according to the following criteria: study limitations due to insufficient internal validity, indirectness of evidence, imprecision of results, inconsistency between studies, and selective publication of studies. [13–17] While the first three are related to single studies, the last two points take into account the relation with other studies in terms of inconsistent results and publication bias, respectively. We added an *other* criterion which included other weak features of the study, such as the unbalance in important variables between study arms in RCTs that may occur when the sample size is small.

For RCTs the first criterion, i.e. bias, takes into account allocation concealment and blinding, completeness of follow-up and adherence to the intention-to-treat principle, premature study interruptions for benefit, and selective reporting of outcomes. [17] The last criterion takes into account the existence and availability of a study protocol or on the clear omission to report important outcomes. [17] We were not able to comply with this criterion because, for most RCTs, protocols were not available. For each of these items, concerns can be serious or very serious, down-scoring the evidence by one and two points respectively. For example, a RCT with an initial high-evidence grading can be downgraded to moderate or low, or even very low, if there are other weak points.

Limits in observational studies can include lack of controls, as in case series, or, when controls are present, lack of adjustment for important covariates, which may be unevenly distributed between study groups [17].

Initially, evidence is rated only one point up when the relative risk is between 0.5 and 0.2 or between 2 and 5, and two points up when lower than 0.2 or higher than 5, obviously when dealing with statistically significant results. However, even in the presence of large effects, when imprecision is strong (i.e. wide 95% confidence intervals) and negligible effects cannot be ruled out, upgrading is not performed. The rating can also be increased when a dose-response is evident or plausible potential confounders would only increase the confidence in the results [7,18].

The strength of recommendations can be strong or weak, in favour or against interventions. [19] Only when an intervention with a strong likelihood of effectiveness had not been sufficiently investigated (i.e. absence of evidence as defined above) we considered the possibility of not giving any recommendation, although we usually gave a weak negative recommendation in most cases of absence of evidence, in the light of the limited resources available.

The conference dealt with four different issues of broad clinical interest but focusing especially on relevance for critically ill patients and from the point of view of intensive care unit (ICU) and emergency department physicians.

To investigate the main undesirable effects of prophylaxis, we preliminarily performed a systematic research on the effect of short antibiotic administration on bacterial antibiotic-resistance selection, to provide a fair assessment of the balance between benefits and risks. The results of this investigation integrated, when appropriate, the evidence concerning antibiotic prophylaxis in the clinical conditions we explored.

A transparent report of the reviewing process and of evidence grading is provided for each query in the supporting information.

The review was conducted complying with the Preferred Reporting Items for Systematic Reviews and Meta-Analyses (PRISMA) statement recommendations (Table S6 in File S6) [20].

Results

We tried to find an answer to the following question: *Does short antibiotic prophylaxis cause resistant bacteria selection?* To do this we explored the influence of short antibiotic course on resistant bacteria selection at two levels: at the patient's level, investigated before and after exposure, and at the centre level, comparing restrictive and liberal antibiotic prescription strategies between centres or within a single centre before and after the policy change.

We also assumed that there is strong evidence that prolonged antibiotic exposure (say, 7–10 days) increases the risk of colonization with resistant bacterial strains, [21] and without formally investigating this issue with the GRADE approach, we attributed to it a default high level of evidence.

Selection of antibiotic-resistant bacteria in patients exposed to prophylaxis

The contemporaneous combination of the mutant bacteria and antibiotic exposure determines the spread of antibiotic-resistant bacteria. [22] Although patients admitted to the hospital after trauma are usually young and healthy, given the presence of resistant bacteria also within the community, the possibility that they may be already colonized by such strains cannot be ruled out. [23,24] Moreover, colonization in non-colonized patients can occur because of newly acquired bacterial mutations, selection of bacterial resistant strains among heterogeneous populations, [25] and horizontal transfer, [26] the latter being particularly relevant in ICU environments. [27] We made an extensive literature revision focusing on antibiotic-resistant colonization in patients undergoing short antibiotic treatment, but RCTs in this field were unavailable. Thus, we had to rely on the few observational studies found (Table S5 in File S5).

In a study carried out on a cohort of 2,641 patients receiving antibiotic prophylaxis for cardiac surgery, of 1,094 undergoing cultures 426 were shown to harbour bacteria resistant to the antibiotic they were exposed to. Logistic regression, adjusting for many possible confounders, indicated an increased risk of resistance selection in case of antibiotic prophylaxis lasting more than 48 hours. [28] Overall the description of the statistical procedures was scanty, hindering quality assessment. One major limitation was that only part of the patients were submitted to cultures and that physicians in the centre were "encouraged" to keep antibiotic prophylaxis duration within 48 hours, potentially introducing selection biases that logistic regression may have not accounted for. Moreover, colonization status was not assessed before prophylaxis was administered, so it is not known whether the patients had previous colonization or acquired the resistant pattern during therapy or during the postoperative stay in a high-risk environment as the ICU.

In a before/after study involving 5 wards, the rate of acquisition within 30 days from initial antibiotic exposure, was 3% for MRSA (22/724), 2% for vancomycin-resistant enterococci (VRE) (10/430), and 1% (11/840) for ciprofloxacin-resistant *Pseudomonas Aeruginosa* (CRPA). [29] Forty per cent of newly acquired colonization with resistant bacteria was detected 48 hours from the first antibiotic dose. The initial colonization rate was 16% of 864 patients for MRSA, 50% for VRE, and 3% for ciprofloxacin-resistant *Pseudomonas Aeruginosa*. Cephalosporins, quinolones, and macrolides were the antibiotics more frequently administered (31, 29, 19% of cases, respectively). Absence of control (i.e. patient not exposed to antibiotics) although not irrelevant was not a major issue, in our opinion, because we do not expect factors other than antibiotic pressure to affect the colonization rate within a 48-hour period. A low colonization rate, as in this study, is still clinically relevant if we account for the duration and possibility of horizontal spread of resistant bacterial colonization, especially in environments such as the ICU [27,30].

Another study investigated 29 patients undergoing cardiac surgery and 10 coronary angioplasty, receiving prophylaxis for three days with a first or a second-generation cephalosporin. [31] Cultures were collected at time 0 and on the third day. The investigators detected colonization by methicillin-resistant coagulase-negative staphylococci in 36 of 43 cultured sites (84%) previously not colonized and a quantitative colonization increase in 17 of 28 sites (61%) harbouring low-level colonization before antibiotic administration. The main limitation of the study was that multiple samples were collected from each patient that may have borne the same resistant bacteria, inflating the final count of true events. A reliable quantitative estimation of resistant bacteria selection was hence impossible. This study was also limited by its small sample size.

Finally, in a study investigating the effect of a five-day course with clarithromycin, 5 patients colonised by susceptible enterococcus strains few days after the end of treatment developed resistant types, which in 3 cases persisted for one year or more. [32] Although, almost a case report, this study is indicative of how antibiotic pressure can select resistant strains and how long the effects can last over time.

Effect of liberal vs. aggressive antibiotic prescriptive strategies

The limitation of antibiotics use is widely recognized as an effective strategy for the reduction in bacterial resistance. [33,34] However, the role of antibiotic prophylaxis policies, corresponding to strong limitations in antibiotic use, have never been investigated in relation to antibiotic-resistance acquisition. Indeed a recent review concerning the influence of antibiotic exposure on MRSA diffusion, the shortest period of antibiotic administration considered was 7 days. [21] In a before/after study dealing with late-generation cephalosporin administration policy, surgical prophylaxis was among the exceptions to restriction, indicating that the authors did not feel it was significant for the purposes of their policy [35].

Conclusions: there is low evidence indicating that antibiotic prophylaxis lasting 48 hours or more is capable of determining the colonization with resistant bacterial strains, that is the *undesirable effect* reported in the text and tables for each of the interventions under scrutiny.

Question 1: is antibiotic prophylaxis for the prevention of ventilator-associated lower respiratory tract infections effective in intubated patients with traumatic head injury (TBI) and coma, i.e. Glasgow Coma Scale (GCS) ≤8?

Results: the MEDLINE search provided only three studies, two RCTs and one observational study, [36–38] all complying with our inclusion criteria. Although, the studies did not deal exclusively with TBI patients, the results can be reasonably extended to this category of patients. The two RCTs are described in Table 1, Table S1 in File S1, and Figure S1 and tested respectively a 3-day and a single-day antibiotic prophylaxis. Both RCTs reported a statistically significant reduction of early-VAP, but no reduction of late-onset pneumonia and ICU mortality. Besides other flaws, major limitations of both RCTs were the absence of blinding, the small sample size and the lack of power to detect increases in antibiotic-resistant infections in the treatment group (outcome investigated only in the first RCT). [36] Moreover, the second RCT was not specifically focused on comatose patients. [37] The premature interruption of the first RCT after the first interim analysis when only 38 patients were randomised, on the basis of the reduction of early-onset pneumonia incidence in the treatment arm, while no difference in mortality was detected, is a questionable choice. Finally, the beneficial effect of the postponement of pneumonia in a phase of minor vulnerability of the brain in severe brain injury is only theoretical and was not demonstrated with a robust outcome, such as the long-term mortality/severe disability rate. The main undesirable effect, i.e. antibiotic-resistant bacteria selection, according to the evidence we collected, was likely to occur after three days of antibiotic administration, while probably irrelevant when only two doses are given.

The results of a recent observational study, including 129 patients suggested that a single dose of ceftriaxone was an independent predictor of reduced incidence of early-onset pneumonia. [38] The regression analysis was performed including a propensity score and the variable "antibiotic prophylaxis" in a regression model, but the number of outcomes (overall 15 cases of early-onset VAP) did not justify the inclusion of the two above variables according established rules. [39,40] Moreover, the sample size and the number of events were small, and the model was underpowered to include potential important covariates capable of influencing the significance of ceftriaxone administration in the predictive model. The observational study appeared to be, hence, unreliable and was not taken into account in our final evaluation.

Conclusions: The two RCTs had substantial different interventions and outcomes, thus we provided recommendations for two different queries (Table 2).

Intervention 1. Three-day course with a beta-lactamase-protected penicillin for the prevention of ventilator-associated early-VAP in intubated patients with TBI and coma:

Level of evidence in favour: Very low evidence.

Level of evidence against: Low evidence.

Recommendation: Weak against intervention.

Intervention 2. 2-dose wide spectrum antibiotic administration for the prevention of early-VAP in intubated patients with TBI and coma.

Level of evidence in favour: Very low evidence.

Level of evidence against: No evidence.

Recommendation: Weak against intervention.

Table 1. Antibiotic prophylaxis for early-VAP prevention in comatose patients: patients, interventions, and outcomes.

			Desirable effect		Undesirable effect		Desirable effect			
Sample	**Treatment**	**Control**	**Outcome**	**Outcome quality**	**Outcome**	**Outcome quality**	**Treatment arm % (95%-CI)**	**Controls % (95%-CI)**	**Difference % (95%-CI)**	**RR (95%-CI)**
Ventilated patients, cerebral haemorrhage, GCS ≤8	Ampicillin-sulbactam 3-day course - 19 patients	No placebo -19 patients	Early VAP	Weak, surrogate of death/severe disability	Antibiotic- resistant bacteria selection not Adequately investigated	Robust, Clinically relevant for the patient/crucial for the health-care organization	21.1 (8.5 to 43.3)	57.9 (36.3 to 76.9)	-36.8 (-59.6 to -5.8)	0.36 (0.14 to 0.94)
Ventilated patients, cerebral haemorrhage, GCS ≤12	2-dose cefuroxime - 50patients	No placebo - 50 patients	Early VAP	Weak, surrogate of death/severe disability	Antibiotic- resistant bacteria selection not investigated	Robust, Clinically relevant for the patient/crucial for the health-care organization	16 (8.3 to 28.5)	36 (24.1 to 49.9)	-20 (-35.8 to -2.8)	0.44 (0.21 to 0.93)

Question 2: is antibiotic prophylaxis effective in patients with basilar skull fractures from non-penetrating head trauma to decrease the occurrence of meningitis?

Results: of 146 studies found only four were RCTs. One was discarded because only 10 patients were randomised while 129 were the object of a retrospective evaluation and therefore included among observational studies. [41] The remaining were single-centre trials, including 109, 37, and 52 patients respectively, all providing negative results, but the three studies were underpowered to demonstrate clinically relevant differences (Table 3, Table S2 in File S2, Figure S2). [42–44] The 37 patients enrolled in the second study with basilar fractures were a subset of 196 with either basilar or skull open fractures. Thus the findings of interest for our review were the result of a subgroup analysis, and as such biased. [45] The other two trials also suffered from methodological bias. Most important long-lasting antibiotic prophylaxis was administered (5-day ceftriaxone, 3-day ceftriaxone or ampicillin-sulbactam, and 8-day average penicillin course, respectively) and no monitoring of antibiotic-resistant bacteria selection was investigated. This was a major undesirable effect of such prolonged antibiotic prophylaxis, as supported by the literature revision we carried out.

The negative evidence regarding this issue are summarised in a recent Cochrane review and meta-analysis [46] that also includes the study of the randomised ten patients mentioned above and a RCT published as correspondence. [47] Although the studies were not heterogeneous in terms of meningitis odds ratios, they were heterogeneous in terms of meningitis absolute rates, inclusion criteria, duration of antibiotic treatment, ceftriaxone dose in the two studies that used this antibiotic, [43,44] and number of patients lost to follow-up, advising against their inclusion in a meta-analysis. Two other non-recent meta-analyses were biased by the merging of RCTs and observational studies [48,49].

We found four observational studies matching the inclusion criteria, none of which performed adjusted comparisons, thus not providing any acceptable evidence in favour of or against antibiotic prophylaxis [41,50–52].

Conclusions: The three studies under scrutiny all investigated prolonged antibiotic administration, that was thus the object of our query (Table 4).

Intervention. Three or more days of antibiotic prophylaxis for the prevention of meningitis in patients with basal-skull fractures:

Level of evidence in favour: No evidence.

Level of evidence against: Low evidence.

Recommendation: Strong against intervention.

Question 3: is antibiotic prophylaxis beneficial for the reduction of wound infection rate in patients with long-bone open fractures?

Results: of 174 studies fulfilling the search criteria, only three trials, [53–55] one observational study, [56] and one meta-analysis [57] matched the inclusion criteria. The studies were carried out in between the 1970s and the 1980s. In the first RCT, patients with open-fractures were only a subset of the randomised sample, [53] the findings thus being the result of a subgroup analysis and as such inadequate to provide conclusive answers. [45] The second study [54] was of higher level, but still the reporting was insufficient to allow a thorough assessment of its quality according to current standards. [9] In these two studies, the diagnosis required positive cultures. The third study was very low quality,

Table 2. Antibiotic prophylaxis for early-VAP prevention in comatose patients - Level of evidence and recommendations.

Patients and intervention	Desirable effect	Undesirable effect*	Benefit/risk profile	Values and preferences	Resource use	Recommendation	Rationale
Ventilated patients, cerebral haemorrhage, GCS≤8 – Ampicillin-sulbactam 3-day course	Very low evidence in favour of intervention +□□□	Low evidence against intervention ++□□	Unfavourable	Not available	Unwise	Weak against intervention	The benefit/risk ratio was unfavourable. Resistant bacteria selection was considered a likely event for a three-day antibiotic course, a more robust and thus prevalent outcome compared to early-VAP reduction, a surrogate of middle term death and severe disability.
Ventilated patients, cerebral haemorrhage, GCS≤8-2-dose cefuroxime	Very low evidence in favour of intervention +□□□	No evidence against intervention □□□□	Uncertain	Not available	Not assessable	Weak against intervention	The intervention requires further investigation focused on hard outcomes such as death and severe disability. The selection of resistant bacteria appears to be unlikely with two doses of antibiotic although it cannot be ruled out. Notwithstanding the large effect size (RR 0.44), given the high degree of imprecision a limited reduction of early VAP (lower 95%-CI = 0.93) is possible, corresponding to a 2.8 absolute risk reduction and a NNTB of 36, a small effect at the price of an excessively high number of patients to expose to antibiotics, especially in the context of the ICU.

*Not investigated in the studies, evidence could be found from external sources. NNTB = number needed to treat for benefit.

Table 3. Antibiotic prophylaxis for the prevention of meningitis in basilar skull fractures: patients, interventions, and outcomes. NC = not computable.

			Desirable effect		Undesirable effect		Desirable effect			
Sample	**Treatment**	**Control**	**Outcome**	**Outcome quality**	**Outcome**	**Outcome quality**	**Treatment arm % (95%-CI)**	**controls % (95%-CI)**	**Difference % (95%-CI)**	**RR (95%-CI)**
Open skull fractures or basilar skull fractures	3-day course ceftriaxone or ampicillin-sulphadiazine - 25 patients	No placebo - 12 patients	Meningitis reduction	Robust, Prognostically relevant outcome	Antibiotic- resistant bacteria selection not investigated	Robust, Clinically relevant for the patient/crucial for the health-care organization	0 (0 to 13.3)	8.3 (1.5 to 35.4)	-8.3 (-35.4 to 6.6)	NC
Acute traumatic pneumo-cephalus verified by CT scan	5-day course ceftriaxone - 53 patients	No placebo - 56 patients	Meningitis reduction	Robust, Prognostically relevant outcome	Antibiotic- resistant bacteria selection not investigated	Robust, Clinically relevant for the patient/crucial for the health-care organization	18.9 (10.6 to 31.4)	21.4 (12.7 to 33.8)	-2.6 (-17.5 to 12.7)	0.88 (0.42 to 1.86)
Traumatic rhinorrhoea or otorrhoea	Average 7.7 days course penicillin - 26 patients	Placebo - 26 patients	Meningitis reduction	Robust, Prognostically relevant outcome	Antibiotic-resistant bacteria selection not investigated	Robust, Clinically relevant for the patient/crucial for the health-care organization	0 (0 to 12.9)	3.8 (0.7 to 18.9)	-3.8 (-18.9 to 9.4)	NC

with no blinding and no placebo, and a partial report of the results. It was carried out on open fractures due to gunshot, with infections diagnosis not based on cultures. [55] This study was negative, since 2 cases out of 32 were reported in the single-day cefazolin group and 2 out of 35 in the group not receiving antibiotic. We considered this study methodologically too weak to be considered a reliable source of evidence.

The antibiotic tested in the first two RCTs (Table 5, Table S3 in File S3, Figure S3) were instead dicloxacillin or benzyl penicillin, [53] and cloxacillin, [54] respectively. In the first study treatment was continued for 48 hours and, in the second, for ten days. The influence of prophylaxis on bacterial resistance to antibiotics was not investigated in any of these studies. We assumed that a 10-day antibiotic administration would certainly greatly increase the risk of antibiotic-resistant bacteria selection. We attributed, instead, a lower level of evidence to a 48-hour treatment (Table 6).

A 13.3 and 22.6% wound-infection rate decrease was found in the antibiotic-prophylaxis arms in the two studies, corresponding respectively to an almost statistically significant result and a fully statistically significant result. Interestingly, in the second study, infections occurring within six weeks were considered early infections, including infections that, reasonably, should have not been influenced by early antibiotic prophylaxis. In the first study, instead, the duration of the "window" period was not specified.

The observational study that matched the inclusion criteria suggested a protective effect of antibiotic prophylaxis, but since it was based only on the crude infection rate, it was not included in the analysis [56].

The meta-analysis included, besides the three RCT mentioned above, two other studies that we excluded because one was written in German [58] and the other including hand, foot, and fingers fracture, pediatric patients and gunshot injuries, without performing any subgroup analysis on long-bone fractures. [59] The meta-analysis concluded that antibiotic prophylaxis is effective in reducing wound infections. However, study designs, inclusion criteria, treatment protocols, and quality of the trials, were so heterogeneous to question the reliability of their merging in a single sample. We hence considered this study a potential source of misleading information.

We did not find any study comparing no antibiotic prophylaxis with 24-hours antibiotic prophylaxis, an option recommended by other guidelines presumably on the basis of indirect evidence [1,2,60,61].

Conclusions: Two different antibiotic strategies were adopted in the two studies that were included in the final evaluation, leading to two answers to two different queries (Table 6).

Intervention 1. 2-day antibiotic administration for the prophylaxis of wound infections (not specifically osteomyelitis).

Level of evidence in favour: No evidence.

Level of evidence against: Low evidence.

Recommendation: Weak against intervention.

Intervention 2. Prolonged (ten-day) antibiotic prophylaxis for the prevention of wound infections (not specifically osteomyelitis).

Level of evidence in favour: Low evidence.

Level of evidence against: High evidence.

Recommendation: Strong against intervention.

Table 4. Antibiotic prophylaxis for the prevention of meningitis in basilar skull fractures - Level of evidence and recommendations.

Patients and intervention	Desirable effect	Undesirable effect*	Benefit/risk profile	Values and preferences	Resource use	Recommendation	Rationale
Open skull fractures or basilar skull fractures - 3-day course ceftriaxone or ampicillin/sulphadiazine	No evidence in favour of intervention □□□□	Low evidence against intervention ‡‡□□	Unfavourable	Not available	Unwise	Strong against intervention	
Acute traumatic pneumocephalus verified by CT scan - 5-day course ceftriaxone	No evidence in favour of intervention □□□□	Low evidence against intervention ‡‡□□	Unfavourable	Not available	Unwise	Strong against intervention	Results of the RCTs were negative. The studies were seriously biased The risk of resistant bacteria selection is a likely and relevant undesirable effect when prolonged antibiotic prophylaxis is administered.
Traumatic rhinorrhoea or otorrhoea - Average 7.7 days course penicillin	No evidence in favour of intervention □□□□	Low evidence against intervention ‡‡□□	Unfavourable	Not available	Unwise	Strong against intervention	

*Not investigated in the studies, evidence could be found from external sources.

Question 4: is antibiotic prophylaxis indicated to reduce the risk of deep surgical site infections in patients with abdominal trauma and enteric abdominal contamination submitted to emergent surgery?

Results: out of 504 articles resulting from the literature search, none compared treatment and no-treatment arms. Our results were consistent with those of two recent Cochrane meta-analyses that did not find any RCTs investigating the effectiveness of antibiotic prophylaxis compared to placebo in reducing infections following penetrating abdominal trauma [62,63].

Since no direct evidence exists with regard to the effectiveness of antibiotic prophylaxis in abdominal trauma compared to placebo, under the assumption that antibiotic prophylaxis is effective in preventing surgical site infections, [64] we oriented the query towards the duration of antibiotic prophylaxis as it was studied by three RCTs focused on penetrating abdominal trauma and deep surgical infections occurrence, [65–67] and excluded a fourth one because it did not report the rate of deep surgical site infections. [68] The main limitation of the studies was that only a minority of the patients had associated hollow viscus injury. Moreover, the infection rate for those who bore intestinal perforations was not reported, making it impossible to analyse subgroup performance. Thus, it was only possible to study the number of events in relation to the overall sample, including those without perforation. Another weakness was that no evidence concerning blunt trauma, a common event in abdominal trauma, was available.

The first two studies dealt almost exclusively with deep surgical site infections, i.e. intra-abdominal abscess, peritonitis, and necrotizing fasciitis, while the third one reported disaggregated data concerning deep and superficial surgical site infections. Thus, we were able to analyse data concerning deep surgical infections. The studies recruited 317, 515, and 300 patients respectively, and infections rates were 10 vs. 8% in the 5-day and 24-hour treatment arms in the first two studies, and 6% in both arms in the third one (Table 7). Although the studies were underpowered to detect clinically meaningful differences in the outcome rate (the power to detect a 5% difference ranged between 40 and 60% in the three RCTs), looking at the range of the absolute-difference 95%-confidence intervals, there is little chance that a clinically relevant superiority of 5-day prophylaxis is present (Table 7, Table S4 in File S4, Figure S4). Moreover, on the basis of our specific evidence assessment, five days of antibiotic administration have a high probability of determining resistant-bacterial selection unlike a 24-hour therapy.

In the studies, surgical management was carried out within few hours from the injury, and early surgery appears to be a reasonable condition for short (i.e. $\leq$24 hours) antibiotic prophylaxis. We adopted the Infective Disease Society of America (IDSA) definition of early surgery (i.e. carried out within 12 hours from trauma). [69] There is currently no clear proof in favour of this cut-off but it, nevertheless, seems reasonable.

Conclusions: The review was focused on different antibiotic strategies under the assumption that antibiotic prophylaxis is effective in reducing infections compared to placebo (Table 8).

Intervention. Administration of 24-hour is equivalent to 5-day antibiotic prophylaxis for surgical abdominal trauma with hollow viscus injury and surgical repair within 12 hours of trauma:

Level of evidence in favour: Very low evidence.

Level of evidence against: No evidence.

Recommendation: Weak in favour intervention.

Table 5. Antibiotic prophylaxis for the prevention of wound infections in long-bone open fractures: patients, interventions, and outcomes.

			Desirable effect		Undesirable effect		Desirable effect			
Sample	**Treatment**	**Control**	**Outcome**	**Outcome quality**	**Outcome**	**Outcome quality**	**Treatment arm % (95%-CI)**	**Controls % (95%-CI)**	**Difference %(95%-CI)**	**RR (95%-CI)**
Long-bone open fractures	48-hour course, dicoxacillin or penicillin - 60 patients	Placebo - 30 patients	Wound infection (not specifically osteomyelitis)	Weak, Minor prognostic relevance	Antibiotic- resistant bacteria selection, not investigated by the study	Robust, Clinically relevant for the patient/crucial for the health-care organization	6.7 (2.6 to 15.9)	20 (9.5 to 37.3)	−13.3 (−31.1 to 0.7)	0.33 (0.1 to 1.09)
Long-bone open fractures	cloxacillin 10-day course - 43 patients	Placebo - 44 patients	Wound infection (not specifically osteomyelitis)	Weak, Minor prognostic relevance	Antibiotic- resistant bacteria selection, not investigated by the study	Robust, Clinically relevant for the patient/crucial for the health-care organization	4.7 (1.3 to 15.5)	27.3 (16.3 to 41.8)	−22.6 (−37.6 to −7.3)	0.17 (0.04 to 0.72)

Table 6. Antibiotic prophylaxis for the prevention of wound infections in long-bone open fractures - Level of evidence and recommendations.

Patients and intervention	Desirable effect	Undesirable effect*	Benefit/risk profile	Values and preferences	Resource use	Recommendation	Rationale
Long-bone open fractures - 48-hour course dicoxacillin or penicillin	No evidence in favour of intervention □□□□	Low evidence against intervention ++□□	Unfavourable	Not available	Unwise	Weak against intervention	The study was slightly negative but the power was insufficient to detect clinically significant differences. Being the result of a subgroup analysis the effectiveness of the intervention is only hypothetical. There is evidence of risk for resistant bacteria selection even with a two-day antibiotic course. Wound infections (excluding osteomyelitis) are not as relevant an outcome as resistant bacteria selection, given the potentially high number needed to treat (Table S3 in File S3).
Long-bone open fractures - 10-day course cloxacillin	Low evidence in favour of intervention ++□□	High evidence against intervention ++++	Unfavourable	Not available	Unwise	Strong against intervention	It is common knowledge that 10-day antibiotic prophylaxis has a very high chance of determining resistant bacteria selection, which outweighs wound. infections prevention, generating an unfavourable benefit/risk profile.

*Not investigated in the studies, evidence could be found from external sources.

Table 7. Antibiotic prophylaxis for the prevention of deep surgical-site infections in abdominal trauma with enteric contamination: patients, interventions, and outcomes.

			Desirable effect		Undesirable effect		Desirable effect			
Sample	Treatment	Control	Outcome	Outcome quality	Outcome	Outcome quality	Treatment arm % (95%-CI)	Controls % (95%-CI)	Difference % (95%-CI)	RR (95%-CI)
Penetrating abdominal trauma	24-hour cefoxitin or cefotetan - 265 patients	5-day cefoxitin or cefotetan - 250 patients	Deep surgical site infections	Robust, Prognostically relevant outcome	Antibiotic-resistant bacteria selection, not investigated in the study	Robust, Clinically relevant for the patient/ crucial for the health-care organization	7.9 (5.2 to 11.8)	10 (6.9 to 14.3)	-2.1 (-7.2 to 2.9)	0.79 (0.46 to 1.38)
Penetrating abdominal trauma	24-hour ampicillin-sulbactam - 158 patients	5-day ampicillin-sulbactam - 159 patients	Deep surgical site infections	Robust, Prognostically relevant outcome	Antibiotic-resistant bacteria selection, not investigated in the study	Robust, Clinically relevant for the patient/crucial for the health-care organization	8.2 (4.9 to 13.6)	10.1 (6.3 to 15.7)	-1.8 (-8.4 to 4.7)	0.82 (0.41 to 1.64)
Penetrating abdominal trauma	24-hour cefoxitin - 148 patients	5-day cefoxitin - 152 patients	Deep surgical site infections	Robust, Prognostically relevant outcome	Antibiotic-resistant bacteria selection, not investigated in the study	Robust, Clinically relevant for the patient/crucial for the health-care organization	6.1 (3.2 to 11.2)	5.9 (3.1 to 10.9)	0.2 (-5.5 to 5.9)	1.03 (0.42 to 2.52)

Discussion

The main limitation of our study is that the literature search was limited to the MEDLINE database and only to publications in English, because of financial constraints. However, the issues we have dealt with have been largely investigated in previous reviews, and the guidelines included in the literature we have scrutinized wee used as an alternative source of references. We are therefore confident that we did not miss important publications in this field.

It is our firm belief that our recommendations, and guidelines in general, should not be clinical rules that impose specific clinical behaviours on doctors, but only indications applicable to an average patient, and should never replace the complex and individualised decisional process that physicians follow for individual patients [70].

In studying the role of antibiotic prophylaxis in trauma we found that in many cases the studies did not provide sufficient information for GRADE categories to be fully applied. Specifically, the assessment of the overall benefit/risk profile requires the comparison between desirable and undesirable effects. In the case of prolonged antibiotic prophylaxis (in several scrutinized studies antibiotic were administered for three days or more), the undesirable effect is the selection of antibiotic-resistant bacteria, an outcome not investigated in most of the studies. [71] Thus we had to integrate studies investigating exclusively infection prevention with evidence from other sources dealing with selection of resistant bacteria, a novel approach compared to other experiences that have proposed a different interpretation of evidence in this field [1,2].

The risk of resistant mutant selection due to short antibiotic pressure has not been investigated with RCTs. We had therefore to rely on before-after studies investigating either the colonization of single patients after treatment or the effect of antibiotic policies changes in single centres.

We were able to find observational studies suggesting that a 2/3-day antibiotic course could already result in the selection of antibiotic-resistant bacteria. We graded this evidence as low or very low, due to several limitations of the studies. However, in the face of similar strength of evidence in favour and against the intervention, as in the case of the 3-day antibiotic prophylaxis for wound infections in open-fractures or early-VAP prevention in comatose patients, we considered the antibiotic-resistant resistant selection the main concern in terms of clinical impact and social relevance of the outcome., Antibiotic-resistant bacteria spread constitutes an emergency for the global health-care system, given its high burden of mortality and resource consume. [72–74] Since resistant mutations are widespread in hospitals and extending within the community, the solution to this problem appears to be the restoration of susceptible bacteria by strongly limiting antibiotic use. [22] Our concern is that the common use of antibiotics in prophylaxis, even for short periods, might significantly worsen this problem. Our recommendations go in this direction.

In conclusion, we would like to mention a striking report from a neurosurgical centre that in the late 1960s had to face an outbreak of resistant *Klebsiella Aerogenes*, which at its peak caused urinary infections in 1 of 4 patients, respiratory infections in 1 of 8, and 9 cases of meningitis 8 of which were fatal. [75–77] Though antibiotic treatment was targeted on sensitivity tests and despite the major increase in antibiotic consumption in the ward between 1966 ad 1969 the outbreak was out of control. As the authors state, "in desperation", antibiotic use whether for treatment or prophylaxis was abandoned. This resulted in an immediate reduction of infections and the elimination of the Klebsiella from the ward without any serious adverse event being reported as the consequence of this strategy. This report although deviating from the paradigm of

Table 8. Antibiotic prophylaxis for the prevention of deep surgical-site infections in abdominal trauma with enteric contamination - Level of evidence and recommendations.

Query	Desirable effect	Undesirable effect*	Benefit/risk profile	Values and preferences	Resource use	Recommendation	Rationale
Penetrating abdominal trauma - 24-hour cefoxitin or cefotetan vs. 5-day cefoxitin or cefotetan	Very low evidence in favour of intervention ✚□□□	No evidence against intervention □□□□	Favourable	Not available	Wise	Weak in favour of intervention	Only part of the patients had intestinal perforation, but no specific data is available for this subset; this hampers conclusive answers regarding patients with perforation, the focus of the review. However, the risk of resistant bacteria selection is itself a sufficient
Penetrating abdominal trauma - 24-hour ampicillin-sulbactam vs. 5-day ampicillin-sulbactam	Very low evidence in favour of intervention ✚□□□	No evidence against intervention □□□□	Favourable	Not available	Wise	Weak in favour of intervention	condition to contraindicate the 5-day antibiotic course. We assume that single-day prophylaxis is effective on the basis of indirect evidence from elective abdominal-surgery antibiotic prophylaxis studies and less dangerous in terms of antibiotic-resistant bacteria selection than a 5-day treatment. This issue however deserves further investigations.
Penetrating abdominal trauma - 24-hour cefoxitin vs. 5-day cefoxitin	Very low evidence in favour of intervention ✚□□□	No evidence against intervention □□□□	Favourable	Not available	Wise	Weak in favour of intervention	

*Not investigated in the studies, no evidence could be found from external sources.

evidence base medicine (we are dealing with a single-centre epidemiological descriptive report with no statistical analysis performed and no precise design) nevertheless provides a demonstration of the effectiveness of a drastic antibiotic containment strategy, a potential choice when "the going gets tough".

Supporting Information

Figure S1 Absolute proportions differences and relative risks for the studies concerning the first query.

Figure S2 Absolute proportions differences and relative risks for the studies concerning the second query.

Figure S3 Absolute proportions differences and relative risks for the studies concerning the third query.

Figure S4 Absolute proportions differences and relative risks for the studies concerning the fourth query.

File S1 MEDLINE database search, flow diagram illustrating the literature selection process, and Table S1 illustrating evidence assessment for the first query.

File S2 MEDLINE database search, flow diagram illustrating the literature selection process, and Table S2 illustrating evidence assessment for the second query.

File S3 MEDLINE database search, flow diagram illustrating the literature selection process, and Table S3 illustrating evidence assessment for the third query.

File S4 MEDLINE database search, flow diagram illustrating the literature selection process, and Table S4 illustrating evidence assessment for the fourth query.

File S5 MEDLINE database search, flow diagram illustrating the literature selection process, and Table S5 illustrating evidence assessment for antibiotic-resistant bacteria (undesirable effect).

File S6 Preferred Reporting Items for Systematic Reviews and Meta-Analyses (PRISMA) statement recommendations checklist (Table S6).

Acknowledgments

The authors would like to thank Fulvia Zerri for her help in the organization of the meetings and for her extraordinary support to the works of the panel.

Author Contributions

Conceived and designed the experiments: DP AC ML BV. Analyzed the data: DP. Contributed to the writing of the manuscript: DP AC ML BV. Interpretation of data: DP AC ML BV EC PM FM GN EN LR IT AV CC GG. Drafting the work and revising it critically for important intellectual content: DP AC ML BV EC PM FM GN EN LR IT AV CC GG.

References

1. Hauser CJ, Adams CA Jr, Eachempati SR, Council of the Surgical Infection S (2006) Surgical Infection Society guideline: prophylactic antibiotic use in open fractures: an evidence-based guideline. Surg Infect (Larchmt) 7: 379–405.
2. Luchette FA, Bone LB, Born CT, DeLong WG, Hoff WS, et al. (2000) EAST Practice Management Guidelines Workgroup: Practice management guidelines for prophylactic antibiotic use in open fractures. Eastern Association for the Surgery of Trauma.
3. Ioannidis JP, Trikalinos TA (2007) The appropriateness of asymmetry tests for publication bias in meta-analyses: a large survey. CMAJ 176: 1091–1096.
4. Atkins D, Eccles M, Flottorp S, Guyatt GH, Henry D, et al. (2004) Systems for grading the quality of evidence and the strength of recommendations I: critical appraisal of existing approaches The GRADE Working Group. BMC Health Serv Res 4: 38.
5. Guyatt G, Oxman AD, Akl EA, Kunz R, Vist G, et al. (2011) GRADE guidelines: 1. Introduction-GRADE evidence profiles and summary of findings tables. J Clin Epidemiol 64: 383–394.
6. Guyatt GH, Oxman AD, Vist GE, Kunz R, Falck-Ytter Y, et al. (2008) GRADE: an emerging consensus on rating quality of evidence and strength of recommendations. BMJ 336: 924–926.
7. Balshem H, Helfand M, Schunemann HJ, Oxman AD, Kunz R, et al. (2011) GRADE guidelines: 3. Rating the quality of evidence. J Clin Epidemiol 64: 401–406.
8. Altman DG, Bland JM (1995) Absence of evidence is not evidence of absence. BMJ 311: 485.
9. Moher D, Schulz KF, Altman DG, Consort G (2001) The CONSORT statement: revised recommendations for improving the quality of reports of parallel-group randomized trials. Ann Intern Med 134: 657–662.
10. Higgins JP, Thompson SG, Deeks JJ, Altman DG (2003) Measuring inconsistency in meta-analyses. BMJ 327: 557–560.
11. Feinstein AR (1995) Meta-analysis: statistical alchemy for the 21st century. J Clin Epidemiol 48: 71–79.
12. Andrews JC, Schunemann HJ, Oxman AD, Pottie K, Meerpohl JJ, et al. (2013) GRADE guidelines: 15. Going from evidence to recommendation-determinants of a recommendation's direction and strength. J Clin Epidemiol 66: 726–735.
13. Guyatt GH, Oxman AD, Kunz R, Brozek J, Alonso-Coello P, et al. (2011) GRADE guidelines 6. Rating the quality of evidence–imprecision. J Clin Epidemiol 64: 1283–1293.
14. Guyatt GH, Oxman AD, Kunz R, Woodcock J, Brozek J, et al. (2011) GRADE guidelines: 8. Rating the quality of evidence–indirectness. J Clin Epidemiol 64: 1303–1310.
15. Guyatt GH, Oxman AD, Kunz R, Woodcock J, Brozek J, et al. (2011) GRADE guidelines: 7. Rating the quality of evidence–inconsistency. J Clin Epidemiol 64: 1294–1302.
16. Guyatt GH, Oxman AD, Montori V, Vist G, Kunz R, et al. (2011) GRADE guidelines: 5. Rating the quality of evidence–publication bias. J Clin Epidemiol 64: 1277–1282.
17. Guyatt GH, Oxman AD, Vist G, Kunz R, Brozek J, et al. (2011) GRADE guidelines: 4. Rating the quality of evidence–study limitations (risk of bias). J Clin Epidemiol 64: 407–415.
18. Guyatt GH, Oxman AD, Sultan S, Glasziou P, Akl EA, et al. (2011) GRADE guidelines: 9. Rating up the quality of evidence. J Clin Epidemiol 64: 1311–1316.
19. Andrews J, Guyatt G, Oxman AD, Alderson P, Dahm P, et al. (2013) GRADE guidelines: 14. Going from evidence to recommendations: the significance and presentation of recommendations. J Clin Epidemiol 66: 719–725.
20. Liberati A, Altman DG, Tetzlaff J, Mulrow C, Gotzsche PC, et al. (2009) The PRISMA statement for reporting systematic reviews and meta-analyses of studies that evaluate health care interventions: explanation and elaboration. PLoS Med 6: e1000100.
21. Tacconelli E, De Angelis G, Cataldo MA, Pozzi E, Cauda R (2008) Does antibiotic exposure increase the risk of methicillin-resistant Staphylococcus aureus (MRSA) isolation? A systematic review and meta-analysis. J Antimicrob Chemother 61: 26–38.
22. Levy SB (2002) The 2000 Garrod lecture. Factors impacting on the problem of antibiotic resistance. J Antimicrob Chemother 49: 25–30.
23. Naimi TS, LeDell KH, Como-Sabetti K, Borchardt SM, Boxrud DJ, et al. (2003) Comparison of community- and health care-associated methicillin-resistant Staphylococcus aureus infection. JAMA 290: 2976–2984.
24. Valverde A, Grill F, Coque TM, Pintado V, Baquero F, et al. (2008) High rate of intestinal colonization with extended-spectrum-beta-lactamase-producing organisms in household contacts of infected community patients. J Clin Microbiol 46: 2796–2799.
25. Schentag JJ, Hyatt JM, Carr JR, Paladino JA, Birmingham MC, et al. (1998) Genesis of methicillin-resistant Staphylococcus aureus (MRSA), how treatment of MRSA infections has selected for vancomycin-resistant Enterococcus faecium,

and the importance of antibiotic management and infection control. Clin Infect Dis 26: 1204–1214.
26. Lipsitch M, Samore MH (2002) Antimicrobial use and antimicrobial resistance: a population perspective. Emerg Infect Dis 8: 347–354.
27. Bonten MJ, Slaughter S, Ambergen AW, Hayden MK, van Voorhis J, et al. (1998) The role of "colonization pressure" in the spread of vancomycin-resistant enterococci: an important infection control variable. Arch Intern Med 158: 1127–1132.
28. Harbarth S, Samore MH, Lichtenberg D, Carmeli Y (2000) Prolonged antibiotic prophylaxis after cardiovascular surgery and its effect on surgical site infections and antimicrobial resistance. Circulation 101: 2916–2921.
29. Tacconelli E, De Angelis G, Cataldo MA, Mantengoli E, Spanu T, et al. (2009) Antibiotic usage and risk of colonization and infection with antibiotic-resistant bacteria: a hospital population-based study. Antimicrob Agents Chemother 53: 4264–4269.
30. Filius PM, Gyssens IC, Kershof IM, Roovers PJ, Ott A, et al. (2005) Colonization and resistance dynamics of gram-negative bacteria in patients during and after hospitalization. Antimicrob Agents Chemother 49: 2879–2886.
31. Kernodle DS, Barg NL, Kaiser AB (1988) Low-level colonization of hospitalized patients with methicillin-resistant coagulase-negative staphylococci and emergence of the organisms during surgical antimicrobial prophylaxis. Antimicrob Agents Chemother 32: 202–208.
32. Sjolund M, Wreiber K, Andersson DI, Blaser MJ, Engstrand L (2003) Long-term persistence of resistant Enterococcus species after antibiotics to eradicate Helicobacter pylori. Ann Intern Med 139: 483–487.
33. Gould IM (1999) A review of the role of antibiotic policies in the control of antibiotic resistance. J Antimicrob Chemother 43: 459–465.
34. Tacconelli E (2009) Antimicrobial use: risk driver of multidrug resistant microorganisms in healthcare settings. Curr Opin Infect Dis 22: 352–358.
35. Rahal JJ, Urban C, Horn D, Freeman K, Segal-Maurer S, et al. (1998) Class restriction of cephalosporin use to control total cephalosporin resistance in nosocomial Klebsiella. JAMA 280: 1233–1237.
36. Acquarolo A, Urli T, Perone G, Giannotti C, Candiani A, et al. (2005) Antibiotic prophylaxis of early onset pneumonia in critically ill comatose patients. A randomized study. Intensive Care Med 31: 510–516.
37. Sirvent JM, Torres A, El-Ebiary M, Castro P, de Batlle J, et al. (1997) Protective effect of intravenously administered cefuroxime against nosocomial pneumonia in patients with structural coma. Am J Respir Crit Care Med 155: 1729–1734.
38. Valles J, Peredo R, Burgueno MJ, Rodrigues de Freitas AP, Millan S, et al. (2013) Efficacy of single-dose antibiotic against early-onset pneumonia in comatose patients who are ventilated. Chest 143: 1219–1225.
39. Babyak MA (2004) What you see may not be what you get: a brief, nontechnical introduction to overfitting in regression-type models. Psychosom Med 66: 411–421.
40. Peduzzi P, Concato J, Kemper E, Holford TR, Feinstein AR (1996) A simulation study of the number of events per variable in logistic regression analysis. J Clin Epidemiol 49: 1373–1379.
41. Ignelzi RJ, VanderArk GD (1975) Analysis of the treatment of basilar skull fractures with and without antibiotics. J Neurosurg 43: 721–726.
42. Klastersky J, Sadeghi M, Brihaye J (1976) Antimicrobial prophylaxis in patients with rhinorrhea or otorrhea: a double-blind study. Surg Neurol 6: 111–114.
43. Demetriades D, Charalambides D, Lakhoo M, Pantanowitz D (1992) Role of prophylactic antibiotics in open and basilar fractures of the skull: a randomized study. Injury 23: 377–380.
44. Eftekhar B, Ghodsi M, Nejat F, Ketabchi E, Esmaeeli B (2004) Prophylactic administration of ceftriaxone for the prevention of meningitis after traumatic pneumocephalus: results of a clinical trial. J Neurosurg 101: 757–761.
45. Assmann SF, Pocock SJ, Enos LE, Kasten LE (2000) Subgroup analysis and other (mis)uses of baseline data in clinical trials. Lancet 355: 1064–1069.
46. Ratilal BO, Costa J, Sampaio C, Pappamikail L (2011) Antibiotic prophylaxis for preventing meningitis in patients with basilar skull fractures. Cochrane Database Syst Rev: CD004884.
47. Hoff JT, Brewin A, U HS (1976) Letter: Antibiotics for basilar skull fracture. J Neurosurg 44: 649.
48. Brodie HA (1997) Prophylactic antibiotics for posttraumatic cerebrospinal fluid fistulae. A meta-analysis. Arch Otolaryngol Head Neck Surg 123: 749–752.
49. Villalobos T, Arango C, Kubilis P, Rathore M (1998) Antibiotic prophylaxis after basilar skull fractures: a meta-analysis. Clin Infect Dis 27: 364–369.
50. Dagi TF, Meyer FB, Poletti CA (1983) The incidence and prevention of meningitis after basilar skull fracture. Am J Emerg Med 1: 295–298.
51. Zrebeet HA, Huang PS (1986) Prophylactic antibiotics in the treatment of fractures at the base of the skull. Del Med J 58: 741–748.
52. Frazee RC, Mucha P Jr, Farnell MB, Ebersold MJ (1988) Meningitis after basilar skull fracture. Does antibiotic prophylaxis help? Postgrad Med 83: 267–268, 273–264.
53. Bergman BR (1982) Antibiotic prophylaxis in open and closed fractures: a controlled clinical trial. Acta Orthop Scand 53: 57–62.
54. Braun R, Enzler MA, Rittmann WW (1987) A double-blind clinical trial of prophylactic cloxacillin in open fractures. J Orthop Trauma 1: 12–17.
55. Dickey RL, Barnes BC, Kearns RJ, Tullos HS (1989) Efficacy of antibiotics in low-velocity gunshot fractures. J Orthop Trauma 3: 6–10.
56. Patzakis MJ, Wilkins J, Moore TM (1983) Use of antibiotics in open tibial fractures. Clin Orthop Relat Res: 31–35.
57. Gosselin RA, Roberts I, Gillespie WJ (2004) Antibiotics for preventing infection in open limb fractures. Cochrane Database Syst Rev: CD003764.
58. Rojczyk M (1983) Treatment results in open fractures, aspects of antibiotic therapy. Hefte Unfallheilkd 162: 33–38.
59. Patzakis MJ, Harvey JP Jr, Ivler D (1974) The role of antibiotics in the management of open fractures. J Bone Joint Surg Am 56: 532–541.
60. Hoff WS, Bonadies JA, Cachecho R, Dorlac WC (2011) East Practice Management Guidelines Work Group: update to practice management guidelines for prophylactic antibiotic use in open fractures. J Trauma 70: 751–754.
61. Hospenthal DR, Murray CK, Andersen RC, Bell RB, Calhoun JH, et al. (2011) Guidelines for the prevention of infections associated with combat-related injuries: 2011 update: endorsed by the Infectious Diseases Society of America and the Surgical Infection Society. J Trauma 71: S210–234.
62. Brand M, Goosen J, Grieve A (2009) Prophylactic antibiotics for penetrating abdominal trauma. Cochrane Database Syst Rev: CD007370.
63. Brand M, Grieve A (2013) Prophylactic antibiotics for penetrating abdominal trauma. Cochrane Database Syst Rev 11: CD007370.
64. Bratzler DW, Houck PM, Surgical Infection Prevention Guidelines Writers W, American Academy of Orthopaedic S, American Association of Critical Care N, et al. (2004) Antimicrobial prophylaxis for surgery: an advisory statement from the National Surgical Infection Prevention Project. Clin Infect Dis 38: 1706–1715.
65. Fabian TC, Croce MA, Payne LW, Minard G, Pritchard FE, et al. (1992) Duration of antibiotic therapy for penetrating abdominal trauma: a prospective trial. Surgery 112: 788–794; discussion 794–785.
66. Kirton OC, O'Neill PA, Kestner M, Tortella BJ (2000) Perioperative antibiotic use in high-risk penetrating hollow viscus injury: a prospective randomized, double-blind, placebo-control trial of 24 hours versus 5 days. J Trauma 49: 822–832.
67. Bozorgzadeh A, Pizzi WF, Barie PS, Khaneja SC, LaMaute HR, et al. (1999) The duration of antibiotic administration in penetrating abdominal trauma. Am J Surg 177: 125–131.
68. Cornwell EE III, Dougherty WR, Berne TV, Velmahos G, Murray JA, et al. (1999) Duration of antibiotic prophylaxis in high-risk patients with penetrating abdominal trauma: a prospective randomized trial. J Gastrointest Surg 3: 648–653.
69. Solomkin JS, Mazuski JE, Bradley JS, Rodvold KA, Goldstein EJ, et al. (2010) Diagnosis and management of complicated intra-abdominal infection in adults and children: guidelines by the Surgical Infection Society and the Infectious Diseases Society of America. Clin Infect Dis 50: 133–164.
70. Hurwitz B (1999) Legal and political considerations of clinical practice guidelines. BMJ 318: 661–664.
71. Guyatt GH, Oxman AD, Kunz R, Atkins D, Brozek J, et al. (2011) GRADE guidelines: 2. Framing the question and deciding on important outcomes. J Clin Epidemiol 64: 395–400.
72. de Kraker ME, Davey PG, Grundmann H, group Bs (2011) Mortality and hospital stay associated with resistant Staphylococcus aureus and Escherichia coli bacteremia: estimating the burden of antibiotic resistance in Europe. PLoS Med 8: e1001104.
73. de Kraker ME, Wolkewitz M, Davey PG, Koller W, Berger J, et al. (2011) Burden of antimicrobial resistance in European hospitals: excess mortality and length of hospital stay associated with bloodstream infections due to Escherichia coli resistant to third-generation cephalosporins. J Antimicrob Chemother 66: 398–407.
74. de Kraker ME, Wolkewitz M, Davey PG, Koller W, Berger J, et al. (2011) Clinical impact of antimicrobial resistance in European hospitals: excess mortality and length of hospital stay related to methicillin-resistant Staphylococcus aureus bloodstream infections. Antimicrob Agents Chemother 55: 1598–1605.
75. Price DJ, Sleigh JD (1970) Control of infection due to Klebsiella aerogenes in a neurosurgical unit by withdrawal of all antibiotics. Lancet 2: 1213–1215.
76. Price D, Sleigh JD (1970) Infection due to Klebsiella aerogenes in a neurosurgical unit. J Clin Pathol 23: 378.
77. Price DJ, Sleigh JD (1972) Klebsiella meningitis report of nine cases. J Neurol Neurosurg Psychiatry 35: 903–908.

Permissions

All chapters in this book were first published in PLOS ONE, by The Public Library of Science; hereby published with permission under the Creative Commons Attribution License or equivalent. Every chapter published in this book has been scrutinized by our experts. Their significance has been extensively debated. The topics covered herein carry significant findings which will fuel the growth of the discipline. They may even be implemented as practical applications or may be referred to as a beginning point for another development.

The contributors of this book come from diverse backgrounds, making this book a truly international effort. This book will bring forth new frontiers with its revolutionizing research information and detailed analysis of the nascent developments around the world.

We would like to thank all the contributing authors for lending their expertise to make the book truly unique. They have played a crucial role in the development of this book. Without their invaluable contributions this book wouldn't have been possible. They have made vital efforts to compile up to date information on the varied aspects of this subject to make this book a valuable addition to the collection of many professionals and students.

This book was conceptualized with the vision of imparting up-to-date information and advanced data in this field. To ensure the same, a matchless editorial board was set up. Every individual on the board went through rigorous rounds of assessment to prove their worth. After which they invested a large part of their time researching and compiling the most relevant data for our readers.

The editorial board has been involved in producing this book since its inception. They have spent rigorous hours researching and exploring the diverse topics which have resulted in the successful publishing of this book. They have passed on their knowledge of decades through this book. To expedite this challenging task, the publisher supported the team at every step. A small team of assistant editors was also appointed to further simplify the editing procedure and attain best results for the readers.

Apart from the editorial board, the designing team has also invested a significant amount of their time in understanding the subject and creating the most relevant covers. They scrutinized every image to scout for the most suitable representation of the subject and create an appropriate cover for the book.

The publishing team has been an ardent support to the editorial, designing and production team. Their endless efforts to recruit the best for this project, has resulted in the accomplishment of this book. They are a veteran in the field of academics and their pool of knowledge is as vast as their experience in printing. Their expertise and guidance has proved useful at every step. Their uncompromising quality standards have made this book an exceptional effort. Their encouragement from time to time has been an inspiration for everyone.

The publisher and the editorial board hope that this book will prove to be a valuable piece of knowledge for researchers, students, practitioners and scholars across the globe.

List of Contributors

Li Shao, Feng-Ju Jia, Hui-Qin Wang, Li Liu, Meng-Ying An and Xiu-Hua Zhang
Department of Operation Room, The First Teaching Hospital of Xinjiang Medical University, Urumqi, Xinjiang Uygur Autonomous Region, China

Hao Wen
Department of Surgery, The First Teaching Hospital of Xinjiang Medical University, Urumqi, Xinjiang Uygur Autonomous Region, China

Hong Zheng
Department of Anesthesiology, The First Teaching Hospital of Xinjiang Medical University, Urumqi, Xinjiang Uygur Autonomous Region, China

Qi Sun
Department of Statistic Counseling, The First Teaching Hospital of Xinjiang Medical University, Urumqi, Xinjiang Uygur Autonomous Region, China

Hao Lai, Xianwei Mo, Yang Yang, Jun Xiao, Jiansi Chen and Yuan Lin
Department of Gastrointestinal Surgery, Affiliated Cancer Hospital of Guangxi Medical University, Nanning, Guangxi Autonomous Region, China

Ke He
Department of Neck and Head Surgery, Affiliated Cancer Hospital of Guangxi Medical University, Nanning, Guangxi Autonomous Region, China

Shu Li, You-zhong An and Feng-xue Zhu
Department of Critical Care Medicine, Peking University People's Hospital, Beijing, China

Jing-yi Ren and Hong Chen
Department of Cardiology, Peking University People's Hospital, Beijing, China

Chuan Qin, Lin Chen and Ying-bin Xiao
The Department of Cardiovascular Surgery, Xinqiao Hospital, the Third Military Medical University, Chongqing, PR China

Shijiang Liu
Department of Anesthesiology, The First Affiliated Hospital of Nanjing Medical University, Nanjing, China

Jie Sun
Department of Anesthesiology, The First Affiliated Hospital of Nanjing Medical University, Nanjing, China

Xing Chen
Department of Project Management, Jiangsu New Energy Development Company, Jiangsu Guoxin Investment Group, Nanjing, China

Yingying Yu
Department of Anesthesiology, The First Affiliated Hospital of Nanjing Medical University, Nanjing, China

Xuan Liu
Department of Anesthesiology, General Hospital of TISCO, TaiYuan, China

Cunming Liu
Department of Anesthesiology, The First Affiliated Hospital of Nanjing Medical University, Nanjing, China

Robert B. Dorman, Daniel B. Leslie, Federico J. Serrot, Bridget Slusarek, Henry Buchwald and Sayeed Ikramuddin
Department of Surgery, University of Minnesota, Minneapolis, Minnesota, United States of America

Christopher J. Miller and John E. Connett
Division of Biostatistics, University of Minnesota, Minneapolis, Minnesota, United States of America

Sanghoon Lee, Hyojun Park, Jong Man Kim, Jae Berm Park, Choon Hyuck David Kwon and Jae-Won Joh
Department of Surgery, Samsung Medical Center, Sungkyunkwan University School of Medicine, Seoul, Korea

Sung Joo Kim
Department of Surgery, Samsung Medical Center, Sungkyunkwan University School of Medicine, Seoul, Korea
SHIST, Samsung Medical Center, Sungkyunkwan University School of Medicine, Seoul, Korea

Sang Yun Ha and Seung Eun Lee
Department of Pathology, Samsung Medical Center, Sungkyunkwan University School of Medicine, Seoul, Korea

Yoon-La Choi
Department of Pathology, Samsung Medical Center, Sungkyunkwan University School of Medicine, Seoul, Korea

SHIST, Samsung Medical Center, Sungkyunkwan University School of Medicine, Seoul, Korea

Kwang Yeol Paik
Department of Surgery, The Catholic University of Korea, Yeouido St. Mary's Hospital, Seoul, Korea

Masaki Sano, Hiroki Tanaka, Kazunori Inuzuka, Naoto Yamamoto and Naoki Unno
Division of Vascular Surgery, Applied Medical Photonics Laboratory, Medical Photonics Research Center, Hamamatsu City, Shizuoka, Japan
Second Department of Surgery, Hamamatsu University School of Medicine, Hamamatsu, Shizuoka, Japan

Takeshi Sasaki and Kohji Sato
Department of Anatomy and Neuroscience, Applied Medical Photonics Laboratory, Medical Photonics Research Center, Hamamatsu City, Shizuoka, Japan

Satoshi Hirakawa and Junichi Sakabe
Department of Dermatology, Applied Medical Photonics Laboratory, Medical Photonics Research Center, Hamamatsu City, Shizuoka, Japan,

Mikako Ogawa
Department of Molecular Imaging, Applied Medical Photonics Laboratory, Medical Photonics Research Center, Hamamatsu City, Shizuoka, Japan

Satoshi Baba
Department of Diagnostic Pathology, Hamamatsu University School of Medicine, Hamamatsu, Shizuoka, Japan

Mitsutoshi Setou
Department of Cell Biology and Anatomy, Hamamatsu University School of Medicine, Hamamatsu, Shizuoka, Japan,

Nobuhiro Zaima
Department of Cell Biology and Anatomy, Hamamatsu University School of Medicine, Hamamatsu, Shizuoka, Japan
Department of Applied Biological Chemistry, Kinki University, Osaka, Japan

Hiroyuki Konno
Second Department of Surgery, Hamamatsu University School of Medicine, Hamamatsu, Shizuoka, Japan

Xiaohong Tian, Jun Fan, Miao Yu, Shuling Bai, Weijian Hou and Hao Tong
Department of Tissue Engineering, College of Basic Medical Sciences, China Medical University, Shenyang, Liaoning, P. R. China

Yu Zhao
Department of Plastic Surgery, Shengjing Hospital of China Medical University, Shenyang, Liaoning, P. R. China

Yan Fang
Department of Anatomy, Liaoning Medical University, Jinzhou, Liaoning, P. R. China

Maria Antonella Burza, Per-Arne Svensson, Kajsa Sjöholm, Lars Sjöström and Lena M. S. Carlsson
Department of Molecular and Clinical Medicine and Center for Cardiovascular and Metabolic Research, Sahlgrenska Academy, University of Gothenburg, Gothenburg, Sweden

Stefano Romeo
Department of Molecular and Clinical Medicine and Center for Cardiovascular and Metabolic Research, Sahlgrenska Academy, University of Gothenburg, Gothenburg, Sweden
Clinical Nutrition Unit, Department of Medical and Surgical Sciences, University Magna Graecia, Catanzaro, Italy

Markku Peltonen and Anna Kotronen
Department of Chronic Disease Prevention, National Institute for Health and Welfare, Helsinki, Finland

Jarl S. Torgerson
Department of Health Care, Regional Secretariat, Västra Götaland Region, Gothenburg, Sweden

Anna-Karin Lindroos
Nutrition Department, National Food Administration, Uppsala, Sweden

Sanderland J. T. Gurgel
Department of Anesthesiology, Faculdade de Medicina de Botucatu, UNESP, Univ Estadual Paulista, Brazil; and UNINGÁ University, Maringá, Paraná, Brazil

Regina El Dib
Department of Anesthesiology, Faculdade de Medicina de Botucatu, UNESP, Univ Estadual Paulista, Brazil; and McMaster Institute of Urology, McMaster University, Canada

Paulo do Nascimento, Jr.
Department of Anesthesiology, Faculdade de Medicina de Botucatu, UNESP, Univ Estadual Paulista, Brazil

Hope T. Jackson and Katherine P. Davenport
Sheikh Zayed Institute for Pediatric Surgical Innovation Children's National Medical Center, Washington DC, United States of America

Emmanuel F. Mongodin and Claire M. Fraser
Institute for Genome Sciences, University of Maryland School of Medicine, Baltimore, Maryland, United States of America

Anthony D. Sandler
Department of Pediatric Surgery, and the Sheikh Zayed Institute for Pediatric Surgical Innovation Children's National Medical Center, Washington DC, United States of America

Steven L. Zeichner
Center for Cancer and Immunology Research, Children's Research Institute, Children's National Medical Center, Washington DC, United States of America
Departments of Pediatrics and Microbiology, Immunology, and Tropical Medicine George Washington University, Washington DC, United States of America

James Fung, Wai-Kay Seto, Ching-Lung Lai and Man-Fung Yuen
Department of Medicine, The University of Hong Kong, Hong Kong, China

Ronnie T. P. Poon, Wan-Ching Yu, See-Ching Chan, Albert C. Y. Chan, Kenneth S. H. Chok, Tan-To Cheung and Chung-Mau Lo
Department of Surgery, The University of Hong Kong, Hong Kong, China

Tommy Supit and Camden Lo
Monash Institute of Medical Research, Clayton, Victoria, Australia

Daniela Ulrich
Monash Institute of Medical Research, Clayton, Victoria, Australia
Medical University Graz, Graz, Austria
Department of Obstetrics and Gynaecology and Monash Micro Imaging, Monash Medical Centre, Monash University, Clayton, Victoria, Australia

Caroline E. Gargett
Monash Institute of Medical Research, Clayton, Victoria, Australia
Department of Obstetrics and Gynaecology and Monash Micro Imaging, Monash Medical Centre, Monash University, Clayton, Victoria, Australia

Sharon L. Edwards, Jacinta F. White, Jerome A. Werkmeister and John A. M. Ramshaw
CSIRO Materials Science and Engineering, Clayton, Victoria, Australia

Anna Rosamilia
Department of Obstetrics and Gynaecology and Monash Micro Imaging, Monash Medical Centre, Monash University, Clayton, Victoria, Australia

Bianca K. Itariu, Maximilian Zeyda and Thomas M. Stulnig
Division of Endocrinology and Metabolism, Department of Medicine III, Medical University Vienna, Vienna, Austria
Christian Doppler Laboratory for Cardio-Metabolic Immunotherapy, Medical University Vienna, Vienna, Austria

Gerhard Prager
Department of Surgery, Medical University of Vienna, Vienna, Austria

Po-Li Wei
Division of General Surgery, Department of Surgery, Taipei Medical University Hospital, Taipei, Taiwan
Department of Surgery, School of Medicine, College of Medicine, Taipei Medical University, Taipei, Taiwan

Shih-Ping Liu
Department of Urology, National Taiwan University Hospital and College of Medicine, Taipei, Taiwan

Joseph J. Keller
School of Public Health, Taipei Medical University, Taipei, Taiwan

Herng-Ching Lin
School of Health Care Administration, Taipei Medical University, Taipei, Taiwan

Hong Gil Jeon, Hyeong Uk Ju and Jae-Bum Jun
Department of Internal Medicine, Ulsan University Hospital, University of Ulsan College of Medicine, Ulsan, Republic of Korea

Gyu Yeol Kim
Department of Surgery, Ulsan University Hospital, University of Ulsan College of Medicine, Ulsan, Republic of Korea

Joseph Jeong
Department of Laboratory Medicine, Ulsan University Hospital, University of Ulsan College of Medicine, Ulsan, Republic of Korea

Min-Ho Kim
Biomedical Research Center, Ulsan University Hospital, University of Ulsan College of Medicine, Ulsan, Republic of Korea

Zhipeng Xu, Yuanlin Dong, Yiying Zhang and Zhongcong Xie
Geriatric Anesthesia Research Unit, Department of Anesthesia, Critical Care and Pain Medicine, Massachusetts General Hospital and Harvard Medical School, Charlestown, Massachusetts,

Hui Wang
Geriatric Anesthesia Research Unit, Department of Anesthesia, Critical Care and Pain Medicine, Massachusetts General Hospital and Harvard Medical School, Charlestown, Massachusetts
Department of Anesthesia, Beijing Chaoyang Hospital, Capital Medical University, Beijing, P. R. China

Deborah J. Culley and Gregory Crosby
Department of Anesthesia, Brigham and Women's Hospital and Harvard Medical School, Boston, Massachusetts

Edward R. Marcantonio
Divisions of General Medicine and Primary Care and Gerontology, Department of Medicine, Beth Israel Deaconess Medical Center and Harvard Medical School, Boston, Massachusetts

Rudolph E. Tanzi
Genetics and Aging Research Unit, Mass General Institute for Neurodegenerative Disease, Department of Neurology, Massachusetts General Hospital and Harvard Medical School, Charlestown, Massachusetts

Yen Chu, Yi-Cheng Wu, Ming-Ju Hsieh, Tzu-Ping Chen, Ying-Kai Chao, Ching-Yang Wu, Po-Jen Ko, Yun-Hen Liu and Hui-Ping Liu
Department of Thoracic Surgery, Chang Gung Memorial Hospital, Chang Gung University, Taoyuan, Taiwan

Chien-Ying Liu
Department of Thoracic Medicine, Chang Gung Memorial Hospital, Chang Gung University, Taoyuan, Taiwan

Hsu-Chia Yuan
Laboratory Animal Center, Chang Gung Memorial Hospital, Chang Gung University, Taoyuan, Taiwan

Hon-Yi Shi and Wen-Hsien Ho
Department of Healthcare Administration and Medical Informatics, Kaohsiung Medical University, Kaohsiung, Taiwan

King-Teh Lee
Department of Healthcare Administration and Medical Informatics, Kaohsiung Medical University, Kaohsiung, Taiwan
Division of Hepatobiliary Surgery, Department of Surgery, Kaohsiung Medical University Hospital, Kaohsiung, Taiwan

Hao-Hsien Lee
Department of Surgery, Chi Mei Medical Center, Liouying, Taiwan

Chong-Chi Chiu
Department of Surgery, Chi Mei Medical Center, Liouying, Taiwan
Department of General Surgery, Chi Mei Medical Center, Tainan, Taiwan
Taipei Medical University, Taipei, Taiwan
Chia Nan University of Pharmacy and Science, Tainan, Taiwan

Jinn-Tsong Tsai
Department of Computer Science, National Pingtung University of Education, Pingtung, Taiwan

Chieh-Fan Chen
Emergency Department, Kaohsiung Municipal United Hospital, Kaohsiung, Taiwan
Department of Health Business Administration, Meiho University, Pigntung, Taiwan

Adrian Gheorghe
Primary Care Clinical Sciences, University of Birmingham, Birmingham, United Kingdom

Melanie Calvert
Primary Care Clinical Sciences, University of Birmingham, Birmingham, United Kingdom
West Midlands Research Collaborative, Birmingham, United Kingdom

Tracy E. Roberts
Health Economics Unit, University of Birmingham, Birmingham, United Kingdom

Thomas D. Pinkney and Dion Morton
Academic Department of Surgery, University of Birmingham, Birmingham, United Kingdom
West Midlands Research Collaborative, Birmingham, United Kingdom

David C. Bartlett
West Midlands Research Collaborative, Birmingham, United Kingdom

Jingrui Bai
Graduate school of Tianjin Medical University, Tianjin, China

Hongbin Liu and Xianzhong Wu
Graduate school of Tianjin Medical University, Tianjin, China

Department of Pharmacology, Tianjin Nankai Hospital, Tianjin, China

Donghua Li and Lihua Cui
Department of Pharmacology, Tianjin Nankai Hospital, Tianjin, China

Anna J. M. Aabakke and Lone Krebs
Department of Obstetrics and Gynecology, University of Copenhagen, Holbæk Hospital, Holbæk, Denmark

Steen Ladelund
Clinical Research Center, University of Copenhagen, Hvidovre Hospital, Hvidovre, Denmark

Niels J. Secher
The Research Unit Women's and Children's Health, The Juliane Marie Center, Copenhagen University Hospital, Copenhagen, Denmark
Department of Obstetrics and Gynecology, Aarhus University Hospital, Aarhus, Denmar

Masae Ikeda, Hidetoshi Kan-no, Masaru Hayashi, Hitomi Tsukada, Masako Shida, Takeshi Hirasawa, Toshinari Muramatsu and Mikio Mikami
Department of Obstetrics and Gynecology, Division of Specialized Clinical Science, Tokai University School of Medicine, Isehara, Kanagawa, Japan

Yoichi Ogushi
Department of Medical Informatics, Division of Basic Medical Science and Molecular Medicine, Tokai University School of Medicine, Isehara, Kanagawa, Japan

Daniele Poole
U.O. Anestesia e Rianimazione, Ospedale S. Martino, Belluno, Italy

Arturo Chieregato and Bruno Viaggi
SOD Anestesia e Area Intensiva CTO, AOU Careggi, Firenze, Italy

Martin Langer
Dipartimento di Anestesia e Rianimazione, Fondazione IRCCS Istituto Nazionale dei Tumori e Universita` degli Studi di Milano, Milano, Italy

Emiliano Cingolani, Giuseppe Nardi and Luigi Riccioni
UOC Shock e Trauma, AO San Camillo-Forlanini, Roma, Italy

Paolo Malacarne
U.O. Anestesia e Rianimazione - P.S., Azienda Ospedaliera Universitaria Pisana, Pisa, Italy

Francesca Mengoli, Ilaria Turriziani, Carlo Coniglio and Giovanni Gordini
U.O. Rianimazione 118, Ospedale Maggiore, Bologna, Italy

Ennio Nascimben
Neurorianimazione Ospedale S. Maria di Ca' Foncello, Treviso, Italy

Annalisa Volpi
Anestesia e Rianimazione 1, Azienda Ospedaliero-Universitaria di Parma, Parma, Italy

Index